Human Placenta: Recent Progress and Research

Human Placenta: Recent Progress and Research

Edited by **Betty Hong**

FOSTER
ACADEMICS

New Jersey

Published by Foster Academics,
61 Van Reypen Street,
Jersey City, NJ 07306, USA
www.fosteracademics.com

Human Placenta: Recent Progress and Research
Edited by Betty Hong

International Standard Book Number: 978-1-63242-237-8 (Hardback)

Printed in China.

Contents

Preface

It is often said that books are a boon to mankind. They document every progress and pass on the knowledge from one generation to the other. They play a crucial role in our lives. Thus I was both excited and nervous while editing this book. I was pleased by the thought of being able to make a mark but I was also nervous to do it right because the future of students depends upon it. Hence, I took a few months to research further into the discipline, revise my knowledge and also explore some more aspects. Post this process, I begun with the editing of this book.

The recent progress as well as research in the field of human placenta has been illustrated in this book. It includes contributions from eminent scholars and experts related to the human placenta. It aims at providing a broad overview on human placenta, providing insights into recent advances and future prospects in the early detection, recognition and management of placental abnormalities along with common placental structure and functions, infections, toxicology and pathologies. It also discusses the extremely debatable topic of therapeutic applications of the human placenta. The book provides recent findings and up-to-date developments in the field of placental research for biomedical researchers, medical students and practicing clinicians in the domains of genetics, obstetrics, and pediatrics.

I thank my publisher with all my heart for considering me worthy of this unparalleled opportunity and for showing unwavering faith in my skills. I would also like to thank the editorial team who worked closely with me at every step and contributed immensely towards the successful completion of this book. Last but not the least, I wish to thank my friends and colleagues for their support.

Editor

Part 1

Screening Tests and Application of Placentas

1

Human Placenta as a Biomarker of Environmental Toxins Exposure – Long-Term Morphochemical Monitoring

Monika Zadrożna, Barbara Nowak, Maria Żołnierek,
Lucyna Zamorska and Józef Niweliński
Department of Pharmacobiology, Medical College, Jagiellonian University, Poland

1. Introduction

A healthy lifestyle, concerning the choice of diet and physical activity, has become increasingly important to human choice. However, even with the best of intentions and the best individual lifestyle choices, unfortunately we are not able to control all of the factors affecting our body, even in the simplest terms of chemical and physical pollutants of the ambient environment. Biomonitoring is the sphere of human interest regarding how a variety of environmental factors affect living organisms. In practice this means most frequently the elucidation of the adverse effects of environmental pollution, and looking for meaningful markers of such effects, which demonstrate not only the causal relationship with the agent but also a dose-proportionality of the causative agent. The efforts related to the monitoring make sense here, and can ultimately lead to the elimination of negative acting stimuli. In a large number of cases this is possible. Choice of human placenta for monitoring pollutants proven to be detrimental to human health has enabled us to lead real-time monitoring and long-term monitoring. With the exception of hair and placenta, ie transient organ which serves the needs of developing embryo and fetus, the other specimens used for real time monitoring require invasive procedures, or are obtained post-mortem.

The placenta binds two genetically distinct individuals, the mother and the fetus, and serves as an intermediary between maternal and fetal circulations. It is not merely a passive barrier between the maternal and fetal circulations, but has many physiological functions, including the exchange of respiratory gasses, metabolites, nutrients and waste products as well as the production of hormones and the metabolism of xenobiotics. The understanding of the mechanisms and rates of the maternal-fetal transport of chemicals at the placental level and the contribution of placental binding, storage and the metabolism of compounds is still being intensively studied, but offers many of scientific and practical benefits for vulnerable human populations.

The placenta is a unique sample requiring no invasive procedure, offers possibilities for real time monitoring, and serves for evaluating the pollutant burden exerted on the mother as well as on the embryo and fetus can provide powerful dosimeters for investigating reproductive effect.

1.1 Brief outline of placental biomonitoring

The possibility of using the placenta as an indicator of the chemical pollution and, accordingly, of the ecological value of human environments arose in the 1960s from the need to procure insight into the effect of fluorine compounds emitted by the Skawina Aluminium Smelter near Cracow on its employees and their families. At the same time the whole surroundings of Cracow used to be covered with a heavy metal dust fall and also oxides of carbon, sulphur, nitrogen and extremely many compounds of fluorine (Zamorska 1979, 1982/1983; Zamorska & Niweliński 1982/1083). The data elaborated in those years by Prof. Niweliński and Dr. Zamorska, pioneers of placental biomonitoring in Poland, have been handed over to the corresponding institution and finally contributed to the closure of the smelter in the 1980s. This was the first case of immobilization of the smelter as a result of social and scientific world protests in Poland. Many striking enzymatic and structural differences that were observed between the placentas of the Skawina women and those collected in mountainous, non-polluted regions of southern Poland, encouraging the use of the human placenta in the further monitoring of environmental pollution. This data supported by simultaneous analytical detection of trace elements and xenobiotics helped to control the excessive emission of industrial pollutants. Using the results of these first effective placento-ecological researches and their practical worth as a basis, the Department of Cytobiology and Histochemistry of Jagiellonian University opened in 1986 a new stage of researches for the monitoring of the environment pollution of a number of vulnerable South Poland regions, Upper Silesia and the Copper Basin, and as the comparative material placentas from the Carpathian Mountains - Bieszczady were taken. The choice of this Polish region was dictated not only by the distance from the industrial centers but also by the transport accessibility as well. Generally, Bieszczady is estimated as the least polluted region in South Poland and that is why Bieszczady placentas could be applied as the comparative material. During our 18 years of studies on the effect of environmental factors on the enzymatic and structural characteristics of the human placenta nearly 500 full term placentas from uncomplicated pregnancies of mostly non-smoking women, were collected in different regions of southern Poland and studied using histochemical, immunohistochemical and histological methods. In selected cases, a trace elements examination was applied. Prolonged studies of the effect of environmental chemical pollution on the biochemical and microanatomical organization of the human placenta show that this organ, when influenced by toxic factors, undergoes changes that are approximately proportional to the intensity of the pollution. The primary change consists of a histochemically detectable deterioration of cytochrome c oxidase in the villous syncytiotrophoblast when compared with the activity shown by placentas from sites of low pollution. This consequently results in a lack of energy supply and imminent placental insufficiency.

The researches of full-term human placentas as the substrate of monitoring lead to wide information both in the action for protection of the natural environment and in medical prophylaxis; especially in gynaecology and paediatrics.

1.2 Placental biomonitoring – examples of other challenges

Several other national scientific centers have developed programmes with a focus on ambient air pollution and the outcome of pregnancies and many these studies are of practical importance.

In the 1990s, an investigation "Teplice Program"was performed in the Czech Republic to evaluate the impact of air pollution on genetic material and reproductive outcomes (Binkova et al, 1999; Sram et al., 1996). Then the possible impact of air pollution on human reproductive quality was studied in the Pregnancy Outcome Project in the period 1994 - 1999. The effects of all monitored pollutants were studied in the background of a wide spectrum of potential confounding factors (parental biological, social and lifestyle parameters, ethnicity, seasonal factors, etc.) using logistic regression models. The most important findings of the Teplice Program were that air pollution may have an impact on adverse reproductive outcomes, DNA adducts and some genotypes are sensitive biomarkers of exposure and PAHs are an important source of the genotoxic and embryotoxic activities of organic mixtures associated with urban air particles. The Czech studies of the effect of air-pollution have demonstrated also a pronounced effect on intrauterine growth retardation (Dejmek et al., 2000), which is even more pronounced than the effect of active and passive smoking.

Bobak and Leon (Bobak & Leon, 1999) conducted an ecological study of low birth weight and the level of nitrous and sulfur oxides in many districts of the Czech Republic in 1986-1988. They concluded that only SO2 was related to these adversary outcomes of gestation. Then, in the subsequent study (Bobak et al., 2001), they tested the hypothesis that air pollution is related to low birth weight on the data from a British cohort in 1946, and after researching and controlling a number of potential confounding variables ultimately found a strong association between birth weight and the air pollution index based on coal consumption (Sram et al., 2005). Ukrainian study was designed to analyze the effect of environmental oxidative stress on human placental monooxygenases, glutathione S-transferase (GST) activity and polycyclic aromatic hydrocarbon (PAH)-DNA adducts in human term placentas from radioactivity-contaminated and chemically-polluted areas of the Ukraine and Belarus, and to compare these biomarkers to the newborn's general health status. Environmental oxidative stress was related to an increase in anemia, threatened abortions, toxemia, fetal hypoxia, spontaneous abortions and fetal hypotrophy (Obolenskaya et.al., 2010). Further Polish data of study on children (Kubiak et al., 1993) confirms the cytogenic damages from environmental exposures. Although a detailed review of the studies on the effects of pollution on reproductive outcome is beyond the volume of this scope, this gives a view of interest concerning the problem of children's vulnerability in the first period of their development and generally reproductive effect to the state of the environment.

2. Morphoenzymatic monitoring

2.1 Area of interest – Ecological background

The ecological hazard area is the territory where, as a result of intense human activity, the degradation of the components of the natural environment lead to the infringement of the ecological balance. Degradation is the result of repeated and prolonged doses of water and air pollution exceeding the considered safe limit.

2.1.1 Upper Silesia

The Polish Ministry Cabinet decided in 1983r that the Upper Silesia region was recognized as an ecologically impendent/hazard one. The extremely dramatic state of the environment in this region was the consequence of a greater emission of gases and dust pollutions coming from the developing industry in the main coal basin in Poland. The mining of not only coal but also other raw materials (zinc and lead ores, etc) and their processing caused irreversible changes on the natural environment. The industrial refuses of Upper Silesia amounted to one third of the refuses in the entire country and, additionally, 1/6 of the total municipal waste amount produced in the country. A significant percentage of untreated toxic wastewater used to enter into rivers. Improvement of the ecological environment both in the air's sanitary state and in the quality of surface flowing waters could be observed after two decades of continuous monitoring (for details see fig. 10), although the state of health of the Upper Silesia population left much to be desired. Very importantly, it was revealed that a high number of mortality and morbidity among children was simultaneous with the high coefficient of prematurity and supermortality of newborn children (Burton et al., 1989).

2.1.2 Polish Copper Basin

The Polish Copper Basin is the one of main industry centers in Poland and the one of the biggest centers of copper in the world. The copper industry development, not always well organized considering the ecological responsibilities, generated a huge amount of gas impurities as well as metallurgical dust. The emission of pollution was so high in this region that the Copper Basin was claimed to be the most ecologically hazardous region in the 1980s. It was not until in the '90s that a significant decreasing of the emission dimension (both gases and dust) to the atmosphere was observed. Analysis of data from 1980-1995 (Hławiczka, 1998) proved that the main components of emitted compounds were the following metals: copper, lead, arsenic and zinc. In spite of the diminishing emission level of the heavy metals, the purity of the atmosphere, plants and soil were still disappointing. The effect of pollution immediately was transposed into human health, especially children. According to the researches of the Foundation for Children from the Copper Basin, it turned out that the number of children with a higher level of Pb concentration in their blood, which is more than 10 μg/dl, was in 1996 yet 13.6% (Strugała-Stawik & Stawik, 1999). Moreover, amongst the Copper Basin population, diseases of the respiratory system, blood system, stomach-intestinal troubles, liver dysfunctions evidenced human intoxication in SO_2 and Cu were more commonly observed.

2.2 Samples collection and methods

The examined material consisted of 493 full term human placentas from non-complicated pregnancies. Among them, 197 placentas were collected during the years 1985-2002 in Upper Silesia, 69 - during the years 1995-1998 in the Copper Basin and 227 during the period of 1985-2002 in the low polluted South-Eastern Carpathian Mountains. The latter placentas served as control material. All the mothers (placenta donors) were healthy and free from alcoholic and smoking habits and throughout their gestation time they did not change their dwelling places. All the neonates were healthy. A detailed inquiry was made with each of the women who supplied the placentas. The inquiry pertained to the woman`s age, her general health state, genetic constitution and diseases she had in the past. Similarly, the corresponding data and sex of each neonate was noted.

2.2.1 Tissue preparation

Immediately after parturition the cord was clamped. The umbilical cord, the blood coagula and membranes were then carefully trimmed and each placenta weighed and the volume measured by fluid displacement. Approximately 12 full thickness cores of placental tissue (fetal subchorial to maternal parabasal surface) were generated, at an equal rate, from the area close to the umbilical cord insertion, from the peripheral region and from the interspaces between them in a random manner. A part of the tissue cores was processed to paraffin using routine laboratory techniques. For histochemical purposes the blocks were instantly frozen using dry ice and cut to meet the requirement for vertical full depth slices, yet haphazardly of the x,y - cutting plane to ensure isotropy to the estimation surface cross-section and numerical density of placental structures. For investigation into the concentration of trace elements, full-thickness tissue samples were uniformly excised from the central and pericentral areas of each placentas and from fetal membranes using sterile conditions and materials. All specimens were kept frozen until further use.

2.2.2 Histochemistry

The frozen placental portions were sectioned at 6 μm in a cryostat and processed for the detection of the following oxidative enzymes: cytochrome c oxidase (CCO - EC 1.9.3.1) by the modified Burstone method (Stoward & Pearse, 1991), NADH dehydrogenase (NADD – EC 1.6.99.3) by the method of Pearse (Pearse, 1972) and glucose-6-phosphate dehydrogenase (G6PD – EC 1.1.1.49) according to Van Noorden and Vogels (Stoward & Pearse, 1991). We detected also lactate dehydrogenase (LDH - EC 1.1.1.27) and LDH-1 and LDH-5 isoenzymes by the standard method of Mac Millan (Mac Millan, 1967). The histochemical reaction applied for NADH made it possible to simultaneously study the morphological character of the structures of interest.

2.2.3 Trace element study

The concentration of trace elements in the placental and fetal membrane samples were studied using the total reflection X-ray fluorescence (TRXRF) method. This research was conducted in the Institute of Physics, Świętokrzyska Academy of Kielce, Poland. The TXRF method is known to be well suited to study trace elements in biomedical samples. For details of this method see ref. (Majewska et al., 1999). Moreover, the semiquantitative evaluation of the contents of mineral deposits in placental tissue, using an arbitrary scale of five degrees (from 0 to 4 in ascending gradation order), was performed.

2.2.4 Morphometric analysis

Morphological analysis was undertaken at a light microscopy level aided by the computer software Multiscann 6.08 and using histochemical placental tissue sections processed for the demonstration of the NADD activity. This was because the histochemical procedure did not produce the shrinking effect in the internal structures which generally, otherwise, appear in tissues treated with histological fixatives. All tissue sections were coded and subsequently examined blindly with the environmental information. An average of 6 randomly selected serial sections from central and pericentral placental areas were analyzed. Test point counting was used to estimate the placental intervillous space density. Diameters of the villi were estimated by direct measurement. The total counting number of villi and this number then divided into classes with increasing dimensional was referred to as the 1mm^2 placental cross-section area yielding numerical density value. A villi classification scheme describes Tab. 2 and its relation to this as described by Mayhew (Mayhew, TM. 2002, Benirschke, K. 2006), classes 1 and 2 both refer to terminal villi, class 3 refers to the largest terminal villi and to intermediate mature villi, class 4 embraces large immature intermediate villi and class 5 - stem villi. To ensure the uniformity of measurement approximately 60 systematic random microscopic fields of view were analyzed per placenta.

2.2.5 Statistical analysis

Statistical analysis was accomplished using the t-Student test and its most sensitive nonparametric analogue the Mann-Whitney U test to show the differences between the two groups. To compare with each other more than two groups, the Kruskal-Wallis test and Dunn`s post-hoc test were applied. The median test was used to assess the significance of the differences between the data found in the rank order. To assess correlation values between the selected parameters, the Pearson or Spearman correlation were used. The p values below 0.05 were considered as significant.

2.3 Some aspects of the development and morphology of the placenta in the context of monitoring

Prior to entering into details of the complicated effect of the xenobiotic factor on the morphological and histoenzymatic characters of the human placenta it seems reasonable to have a general view of the structure and function of this materno-fetal organ, at least in respect of its use in biomonitoring. A well-developed placenta consists of a chorionic plate, which is of embryonic descent and of a basal plate whose essential layer is the decidua, a derivative of the endometrium. Between these two plates there is a voluminous intervillous space.

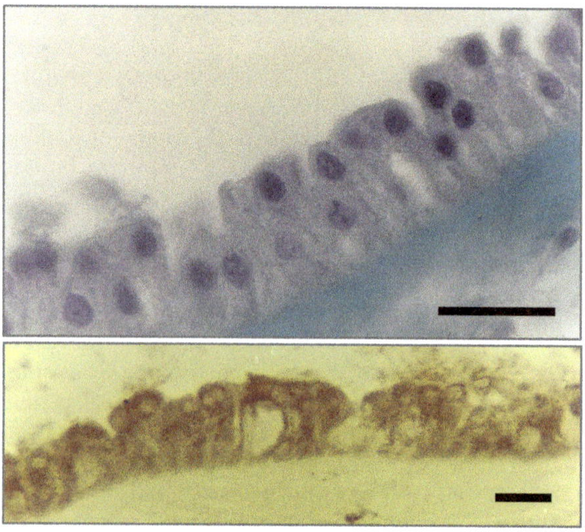

Fig. 1. Cryostat cross-section through fetal membranes from the control material. Histological trichrome Masson stain (upper panel) and histochemical reaction for cytochrome c oxidase. Bar: 20 μm.

The upper surface of the chorionic plate is covered by the rather uniform amniotic epithelium (Bilic et al., 2004), which is in contact with amniotic fluid directly, whereas the lower surface of that plate presents an abundance of villous tress which are ramified and richly vascularized outgrowths of the plate. Each villous tree consists of a stem villus (over 300 um in diameter) whose cells by gradual proliferation progressively arborize and form branches in descending order of length and thickness. The thinnest and shortest branches of every villous tree are the placental terminal villi, which are structures of the uppermost functional importance for placental efficiency.

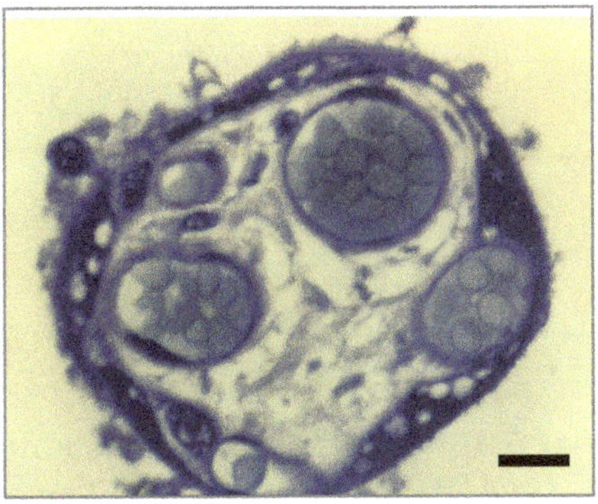

Fig. 2. Paraffin cross-section through crucial for transplacental exchange terminal villous (methyl blue stain). It comprises of outher trophoblastic epithelium which surrounds mesodermal stroma containing fetoplacental capillaries. The cpithelium is composed of proliferative cytotrophoblast cells and a superficial terminally-differentiating syncytiotrophoblast. Bar: 15 μm.

It is through the walls of these villi that the great majority of the exchange of materials between the fetal blood in the villous blood vessels and the maternal blood flowing through the intervillous space occurs. The surface of the villous trees is coated by a double layer of trophoblast, under which there is a well vascularized mesenchymal core. The superficial layer of the trophoblast is a syncytium; i.e. the syncytiotrophoblast that abuts on the underlying layer of the cytotrophoblast. The cytotrophoblast is capable of mitotic divisions that do not occur in the syncytiotrophoblast. Throughout the gestation period, the cytotrophoblast replenishes and restores the syncytiotrophoblastic layer which with the progress of time gradually becomes used up and destroyed by forming the syncytial knots. The whole trophoblast coat also gradually expands and finally completely covers the entire wall of the intervillous space. The cytotrophoblastic cells enter and dilate the spiral maternal arteries in the basal plate and thus augment the maternal blood supply to the feto-placental unit. This blood is rich in indispensable oxygen and nutrients obtained from the mother.

The previously emphasized great role of the terminal villi is made possible by the many activities of the syncytiotrophoblast which, above all, is responsible for the adequate oxygen supply to the fetus. Amino acids, polypeptides and proteins including maternal antibodies protecting the fetus against dangerous antigens and infections, plus many vitamins, pass from the maternal to the fetal blood by active transport accomplished by the syncytiotrophoblast.

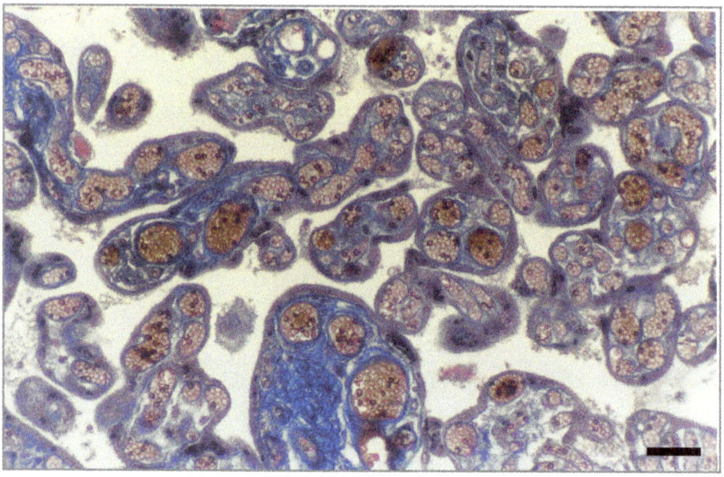

Fig. 3. Paraffin cross-section of a full term control placenta. Histological trichrome Masson stain. Bar: 30 μm.

Active transport as the process occurring against chemical gradients requires expenditure of placental energy accumulated in ATP, which is produced by the trophoblastic mitochondria only in the presence of oxygen. Other important functions of the syncytiotrophoblast are synthesis, metabolism and secretion of hormones including human chorionic gonadotropin, human chorionic somatotropin, steroid hormones progesterone and oestrogens hypothalamic hormones, e.g. the corticotropin releasing hormone (factor) CRH. Removal of fetal waste products also requires cooperation of the syncytiotrophoblast. All these facts demonstrate the absolutely essential role of the villous trophoblast in the placental and fetal physiology (Benirshke et al., 2006).

2.4 Maternal and neonatal findings

By contrast to the maternal characteristic, e.g. mothers age and gestational age, the neonatal findings (tab. 1), were significantly different between groups. A newborn child's birth weight and length from the polluted environment show significantly lower values. More detailed studies revealed that differences in the weight of the neonatal of different sexes were much more pronounced in the polluted area (3189 g for female newborn and 3369 g for male newborn; $p < 0,05$) than in the control (respectively 3443 g and 3490 g). Also, the placental weight, although not its volume, was significantly lower in the contaminated environment. Measurements of weight and length of newborns from Upper Silesia showed a strong Pearson correlation in respect of one another; i.e. newborns weight terms of placental weight ($r = 0.6738$, $p < 0.001$), newborn weight terms of its length ($r = 0.7479$, $p < 0.001$) and placental weight terms of the length of the newborn ($r = 0.6738$, $p < 0.001$).

These findings strongly suggest that ambient air pollution, industrial emissions accurately and/or other factors associated with residence near a exposed region during the pregnancy, affect fetal growth. A great number of other studies of air pollution and birth outcomes also clearly evidenced that pregnancies are susceptible to the adverse effects of air pollution and the evidences are sufficient to infer causal relationship between air pollution and birth

	Upper Silesia (n = 197)	Control (n = 227)	p value
Mothers age (years)	26.2 ± 1.1 (median - 25)	27.1 ± 1.1 (median - 26)	NS
Gestational age (weeks)	39.6 ± 0.1 (38-42)	39.5 ± 0.1 (38-42)	NS
Newborn`s birth weight (g)	3262 ± 35 (2100-4420)	3571 ± 33 (2950-4700)	p = 0,003
Newborn`s length (cm)	54.1 ± 0.2 (48-62)	55.3 ± 0.2 (48-64)	p < 0.001
Placental weight (g)	461 ± 8.3 (220-650)	497.6 ± 7.9 (260-780)	p = 0.015
Placental volume (cm^3)	465 ± 15.4 (230-680)	486 ± 9.6 (300-800)	NS

Table 1. The clinical characteristics of studied groups. Data are presented as mean ± SEM.; (range or median); t-Student test for comparison of two studied groups was used. NS, not significant.

weight (Bobak & Leon 1999b; Bobak et al.; 2001; Rich et. al 2009) in addition to other adverse reproductive outcomes, including premature births, intrauterine growth retardation and ultimately infant deaths, whose range does not overlap with our study.

2.5 Morphological changes in placentas from polluted areas

The data presented above evidenced that in conditions of severe ambient exposure decrease not only infant's weight but also impair the development of the placenta. Therefore it was necessary to try to explain how it changes the internal placental structure which is closely affiliated with their functions. It was therefore necessary to examine how this changed their internal morphology, which after all is closely affiliated with their functions. Our presented data provides clear evidence of rebuilding the structure of villous trees. The numerical density of the villi measured in placentas' cross-sections strongly increases (tab. 2). This increase was primarily generated by the small dimensional terminal villi. Our working distinction of terminal villi to two separate classes enabled us to realize that there was an increase in the density of small dimensional terminal villi (class 1), while the terminal villi of typical dimensions (class 2) remained at the same level of density than in the control placentas. It should be underlined here that only fully histological qualified terminal villi were included to class 1, avoiding syncytial knots and trophoblast sprouts, and even neck regions with unclear characteristics. Also, other types of placental villi, i.e. intermediate mature villi and immature ones, and mesenchymal villi, included in other classes, did not show the revised density. Therefore we claim that because of the overproduction of small dimensional terminal villi, the differences in the percentage of individual villous class terms of the other ones became statistically significant. Furthermore, we consider the phenomenon of overproduction of terminal villi with small dimensions to be an important indicator of the impact of a polluted ambient environment on human placental developmental processes. It can be assumed that this change is caused by adaptive processes in the direction of increasing the surface area of the gas transfer and transport of nutrients.

The structure of the villous tree develops on the basis of proliferative and angiogenic processes, and the functions of angiogenic factors (Mayhew, TM. 2002). Intraplacental oxygen status has effect on the control of the angiogenic growth factor production, and in consequence villous differentiation. A lot of the phenomena regarding changes in the placental morphology and the adaptive processes are explained on the ground of materno-placento-fetal hypoxia (Mayhew et al., 2004). Hypoxia has been sub-classified into pre-placental, uteroplacental and post-placental in source (Bush et al., 2000). Preplacental hypoxia means that maternal blood is hypoxaemic when it enters the intervillous space. In uteroplacental hypoxia, normoxic maternal blood flows into intervillous space, but disturbances appear locally in the blood flow and the placenta suffers from a heterogenous oxygen supply. In postplacental hypoxia, fetal oxygen extraction from the placenta is diminished (Kingdom & Kaufmann, 1997). Oxygen-dependent growth factors are essential in regulating angiogenesis and switch this process into a branching or non-branching path and promote or inhibit terminal villous development (Egbor et al., 2006; Kaufmann et al., 2004). There is now a reasonable body of evidences that the placental villous trees with adverse stimuli can adapt to the attendance in order to maintain an effective level of transport for the gasses and nutrients. In pregnancies under the impact of fetal hypoxic stress (high altitude or anemia), changes in transport efficiency are variable and may reflect the differences in sources of hypoxia (Mayhew et al., 2004). The comparisons show that the pattern of changes in pregnancies exposed to all industrial pollution is not fully consistent with any other patterns but are close to that of uteropplacental hypoxia with reduced intraplacental oxygenation. The main point of a coherent with a uteroplacental pattern of hypoxia is that it causes predominantly branching angiogenesis following by terminal villous overproduction. Formation of new villi is not the only consequence, as branching angiogenesis leads to reduced vascular impedance in the fetal blood vessel. Simultaneously, a denser villous arrangement takes up intervillous space (tab. 2, fig. 2) which restricts, on the other hand, the maternal blood supply and the physical abilities to diffusion and nutrient transport. In other words the incorrect switching towards the hypermature differentiation results that despite its highly differentiated villi, placenta may not provide enough exchange level.

	Diameter (in relation to classes of villi)	Upper Silesia (n = 197)	Control (n - 227)	p value
Density of all villi classes (per 1 mm²)		142.92 ± 3.4	125.27 ± 3.1	p < 0.001
Class 1 of villi (per 1 mm²)	below 40.50 μm	32.81 ± 2.6	13.77 ± 2.5	p < 0.001
Class 1 of villi (%)		21.81 ± 1.6	10.71 ± 1.3	p < 0.001
Class 2 of villi (per 1 mm²)	40.51 μm - 59.50 μm	69.45 ± 2.9	68.76 ± 2.4	NS
Class 2 of villi (%)		48.74 ± 1.6	54.01 ± 1.6	p = 0.003
Class 3 of villi (per 1 mm²)	59.51 μm - 89.50 μm	30.62 ± 1.1	31.64 ± 1.3	NS
Class 3 of villi (%)		22.07 ± 08	25.39 ± 0.7	p < 0.001
Class 4 of villi (per 1 mm²)	89.51 μm - 119.50 μm	6.57 ± 0.5	7.62 ± 0.4	NS
Class 4 of villi (%)		4.81 ± 0.4	6.28 ± 0.3	p = 0.002
Class 5 of villi (per 1 mm²)	119.51 μm - 159.50 μm	2.18 ± 0.2	2.63 ± 0.2	NS
Class 5 of villi (%)		1.67 ± 0.1	2.18 ± 0.1	p = 0.015
Intervillous space (%)		20.46 ± 0.5	25.19 ± 0.5	p < 0.001

Table 2. The numerical density of all villi classes and percentage of intervillous space. Data are presented as mean ± SEM.; t-Student test for comparison of two studied groups was used. NS, not significant.

In the proper developmental processes through the third trimester, the mesenchymal villi become preferentially transformed into mature intermediate villi. The surface of the latter, as we said, is protruded by elongating and looping fetal capillaries resulting in protrusion of highly specialized of materno-fetal exchange terminal villi. There is no longer transformation of mesenchymal villi into mature intermediate villi - the remaining population of immature intermediate villi differentiate into stem villi. Thus their number steeply decreases toward the term and, together with this the base for the formation of new mesenchymal villi sprouts, and the growth capacity of the villous trees gradually slows (Benirshke et al., 2006, Castellucci et al., 2000). Meanwhile, immature intermediate villi are constantly strongly represented in the exposed placentas (tab. 2).

2.6 Histoenzymatic changes in placentas from polluted areas

The morphological adaptations previously described are affiliated by variations in the normal metabolic paths in the placenta. We investigated the following oxidative enzymes: cytochrome c oxidase, NADH dehydrogenase and glucose-6-phosphate dehydrogenase. We detected also lactate dehydrogenase LDH-1 and LDH-5 isoenzymes in villous trophoblast and fetal membranes.

Cytochrome c oxidase is the ultimate enzyme of the mitochondrial electron transport chain located in the mitochondrial membrane and its activity is required for the cell energy supply. In placental trophoblast nutrient transport, protein synthesis and other processes need a continuous supply of energy and in this perspective cytochrome c oxidase is the key enzyme in the regulation of placental functions. Placental insufficiency to energy delivery restricts fetal growth. We observed a significant decrease in the histochemically detectable activity of mitochondrial cytochrome c oxidase in the trophoblast of exposed placentas. A detailed discussion of the origin of mitochondrial insufficiency or causal link between exposure and hypoxia is beyond our present scope. Decreased cytochrome c oxidase activity or the decrease of cytochrome c oxidase positive mitochondria may be a result from placental ischemia which is an inherent occurance in pre-eclampsia. While the mechanism of the reduced cytochrome c oxidase activity observed here is unknown, such a reduction may impair the production of placental energy, resulting in placental insufficiency in patients and the deterioration of the newborn. Damage to the cytochrome c oxidase activity, which is responsible for the intensity of aerobic oxidation and thus for the intensity of metabolism, is causally related to compensatory efforts that the feto-placental unit undertakes to save its function and homeostasis (tab. 3, fot. 4, 5).

		The mean activity of enzymes (optical degrees)		
Enzymes		Upper Silesia (n = 197)	Control (n = 227)	p value
Cytochrome c oxidase	trophoblast of villi	79.9 ±2.7	123.8 ± 1.9	$p < 0.001$
	amniotic epithelium	66.2 ± 4.7	120.2 ± 3.7	$p < 0.001$
NADH dehydrogenase	trophoblast of villi	155.3 ± 2.2	167.2 ± 1.1	$p < 0.001$
	amniotic epithelium	171.8 ± 4.6	184.4 ± 3.6	$p = 0.009$
Glucose-6-phosphate dehydrogenase	trophoblast of villi	106.1 ± 3.9	127.6 ± 1.8	$p < 0.001$
	amniotic epithelium	112.8 ± 7.5	149.6 ± 5.4	$p < 0.001$
Lactate dehydrogenase LDH-1	trophoblast of villi	56.3 ± 4.6	80.5 ± 2.9	$p < 0.001$
	amniotic epithelium	35.2 ± 5.5	70.8 ± 4.3	$p < 0.001$
Lactate dehydrogenase LDH-5	trophoblast of villi	35.4 ± 3.5	26.2 ± 1.7	$p = 0.031$
	amniotic epithelium	133.8 ± 8.7	106.5 ± 6.7	$p = 0.002$

Table 3. The mean activity of intracellular enzymes in optical degrees. Data are presented as mean ± SEM. t-Student test for comparison of two studied groups was used.

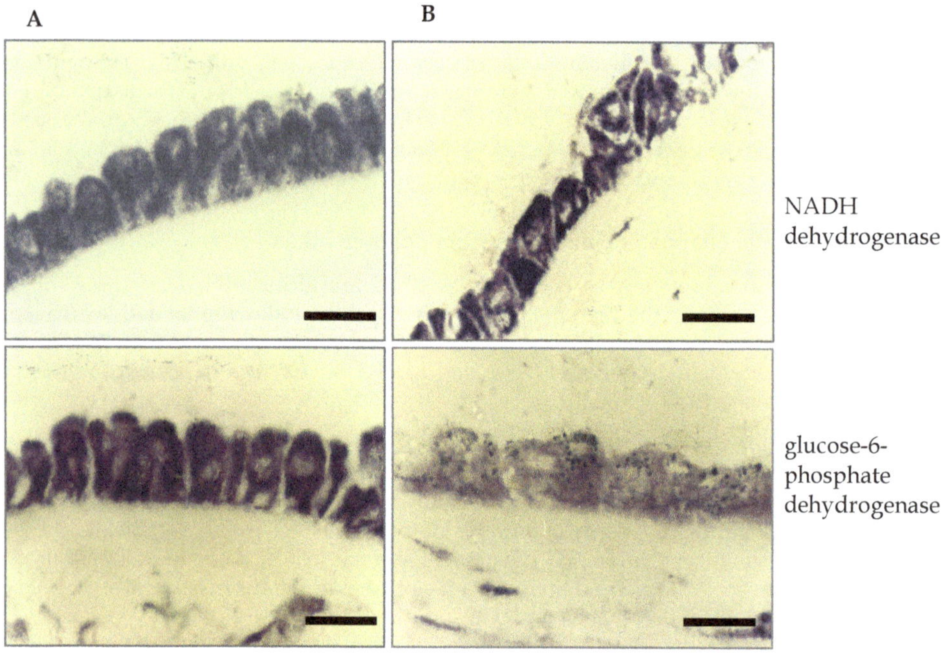

Fig. 4. Cryostat cross-section through amniotic membranes from control (column A) and polluted (column B) environments. Histochemical reactions for intracellular enzymes. Bar: 20 μm.

Similar changes, although with not as dramatic a reduction in activity, were observed in the case of NADD, which is an enzyme located in the inner mitochondrial membrane and catalyzes the transfer of electrons from the NADH to coenzyme Q, and is claimed to be the "entry enzyme" of oxidative phosphorylation in the mitochondria (tab. 3, fot. 4, 5).

Glucose-6-phosphate dehydrogenase also showed a decreased activity in the villous trophoblast of exposed placentas (tab. 3, fot. 4, 5). G6PDH catalyses the first step of the pentose phosphate pathway and then generates the reducing form of NADPH and produces pentose phosphates necessary for nucleotide biosynthesis and ultimately serves as the path of entry for pentoses to the glycolytic pathway. In the placenta, which is the transport gate for substances to the fetal bloodstream, and at the same time a barrier for many other ones, the reducing power of NADPH cannot be overestimated, due to its relationship with glutathione disulfide reductase. Glutathione and its disulfide protect the cell against the undesirable effect of noxious chemicals, which might be transferred from maternal blood (Myllynen et al., 2005). Next to the generation of reducing equivalents, the pentose phosphate pathway contributes to the production of ribose-5-phosphate used in the synthesis of nucleotides and nucleic acids, and erythrose-4-phosphate, used in the synthesis of aromatic amino acids. In valid metabolism, the increased utilization of NADPH would trigger G6PDH activity. Meanwhile, in the case of exposed placentas we observed a diminishing G6PDH activity in villous trophoblast and fetal membranes, which in turn, in accordance with prescribed metabolic directions impacts on fetal growth.

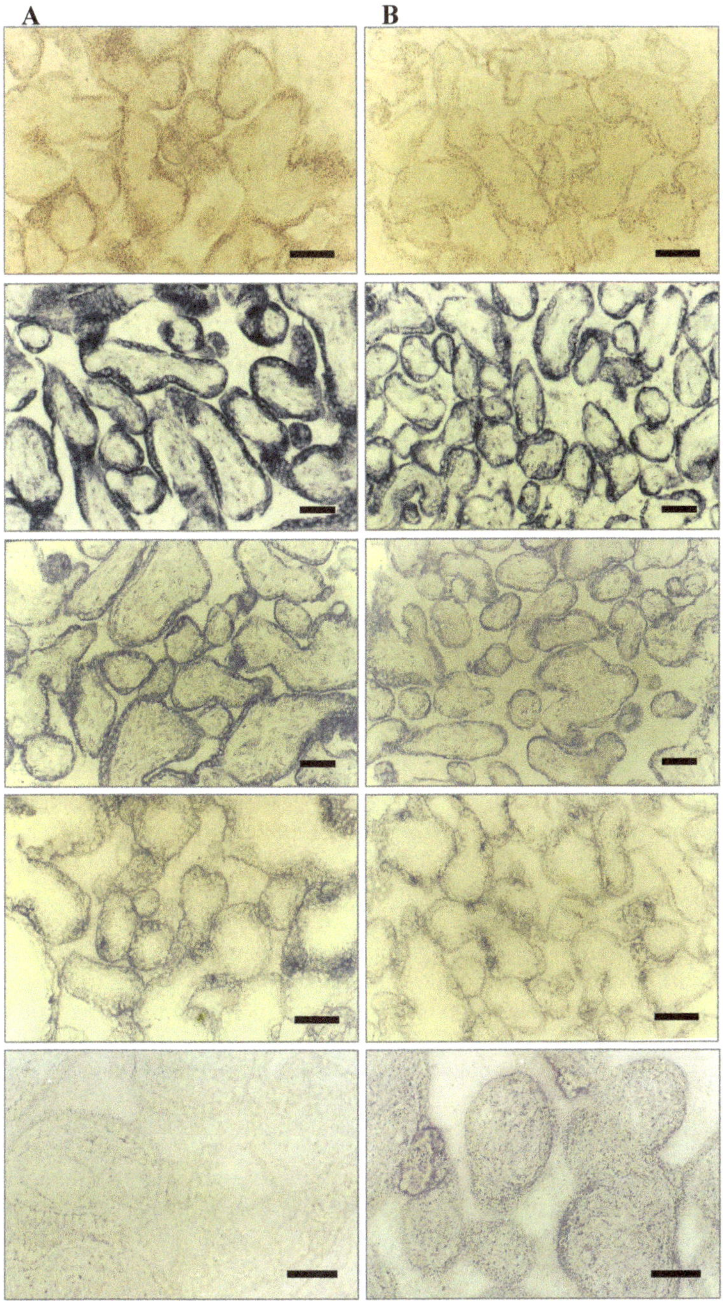

Fig. 5. Cryostat cross-section through full term placentas from control (column A) and polluted (column B) environments. Histochemical reactions for intracellular aerobic and anaerobic enzymes. Bar: 25 μm.

A very expressively presented the distribution of isoenzymes of lactate dehydrogenase. LDH is responsible for pyruvate conversion to lactate through the glycolysis and is an important enzyme in the placenta because glucose is its main metabolic substrate and glycolysis is the major metabolic pathway. LDH-5 isoenzyme efficiently catalyzes pyruvate to lactate regenerating co-factor NAD+ under anaerobic conditions (Tsoi et al., 2000). This study is the first, to our knowledge, to demonstrate there is a differential expression of LDH isozymes in placental tissue when exposed to noxious ambient air. We found that exposed to ambient pollution placenta predominantly express the LDH-5 isoenzyme in villous trophoblast. Selective expression of LDH isoenzymes in syncytiotrophoblasts and villous matrix cells in the villi may reflect functional differences in LDH isoenzyme activity related to energy. As the LDH-5 isoenzyme has a higher affinity binding to pyruvate and NADH than the LDH-1 isoenzyme, it is more directly responsible for the production of lactate and NAD+. The high level of LDH-5 expression in a polluted environment, proves that villous trophoblast may be more capable of utilizing pyruvate as an energy source through anaerobic glycolysis under a hypoxic environment. The LDH-5 gene is a well-characterized hypoxia-inducible gene among many other glycolytic enzyme genes (Semenza et al., 1994). Given the upregulation of the LDH-5 gene expression shown in this study, the evidence supports the role for hypoxia within the metabolic/morphological changes in the placenta. In contrast to LDH-5, the LDH-1 isoenzyme is expressed constitutively and is the predominant enzyme in the cytotrophoblasts throughout the normal development of the placenta, as also evident in our study (fot. 4, tab. 3). On the other hand, the ascending lactate production has an effect on the VEGF level increase (Kay et al., 2007), which contributes in turn to the branching angiogenesis associated with hypoxia and the consequently observed generation of a new population of terminal villi (discussed above).

2.7 Placental indicators based on the long-time monitoring

The placentas of donors dwelling in polluted regions showed an advanced degradation of the activity of cytochrome c oxidase (fig. 6) and other oxidative enzymes of utter importance to the sustaining of life processes, particularly for the generation of energy indispensable for the active transport of substances exchanged between the mother and her fetus to occur. The substantial changes included an increase in the number of the terminal placental villi and thus an enlargement production of the inner exchange surface of the pollution affected placentas at the cost of the dimension of the placental intervillous space (fig. 9) and lessened supply of nutrients to the fetus. The children born with placentas showing histochemical changes were remarkable for their poor birth weight. Both the placentas and children in the low polluted region presented a full contrast with their counterparts from Upper Silesia (fig. 7).

The considerable amount of reciprocal correlations in turn of various features identified in exposed placentas give the strong confirmation of hypothesis on morphological and metabolic modifications in follow of intraplacental hypoxia (tab.4, fig. 6-9). The particular attention is paid to placental markers based on the strong correlations found in exposed placentas between the oxygen-dependent and this operated in lack of proper oxygenation metabolic and morphologic features: inverse correlations between the CCO activity vs the mineral deposit occupancy ($r = -0.2468$, $p = 0.012$), the numerical density of small dimensional terminal villi (tab. 4, fig. 9), and the LDH-5 activity (tab. 4, fig. 9), and in turn positive correlation between the LDH-5 activity vs the numerical density of small

List of Pearson correlations for Upper Silesia samples		
CCO vs LDH-1	r = 0.5550	$p < 0.001$
CCO vs NADD	r = 0.3703	$p < 0.001$
CCO vs G6PD	r = 0.2752	p = 0.038
CCO vs LDH-5	r = - 0.2715	p = 0.034
NADD vs LDH-1	r = 0.4666	$p < 0.001$
NADD vs G6PD	r = 0.3353	p = 0.011
CCO vs total number of villi (per mm^2)	r = - 0.2633	p = 0.013
CCO vs class 1 (per mm^2)	r = - 0.5248	$p < 0.001$
CCO vs class 1 (%)	r = - 0.5378	$p < 0.001$
CCO vs class 2 (%)	r = 0.4033	$p < 0.001$
CCO vs IVS	r = 0.3669	$p < 0.001$
LDH-1 vs total number of villi (per mm^2)	r = - 0.3106	p = 0.028
LDH-1 vs class 1 (per mm^2)	r = - 0.4955	$p < 0.001$
LDH-1 vs class 1 (%)	r = - 0.5284	$p < 0.001$
LDH-1 vs class 2 (%)	r = 0.4379	p = 0.002
NADD vs class 1 (%)	r = - 0.2269	p = 0.037
NADD vs class 2 (%)	r = 0.2733	p = 0.012
G6PD vs class 1 (per mm^2)	r = - 0.3267	p = 0.027
G6PD vs class 1 (%)	r = - 0.4122	p = 0.004
LDH-5 vs class 1 (%)	r = 0.2950	p = 0.048

Table 4. List of Pearson correlations for findings from Upper Silesia samples.

dimensional terminal villi (tab. 4, fig. 9). On the other hand, in the control placentas the LDH-5 activity correlated negatively with small dimensional terminal villi. It is worth noting that the introduction of improved industrial technology and of unleaded fuel over the last 20 years (fig. 10) has led to an increase in the levels of cytochrome c oxidase and LDH-1 activity in placentas from Upper Silesia regions .

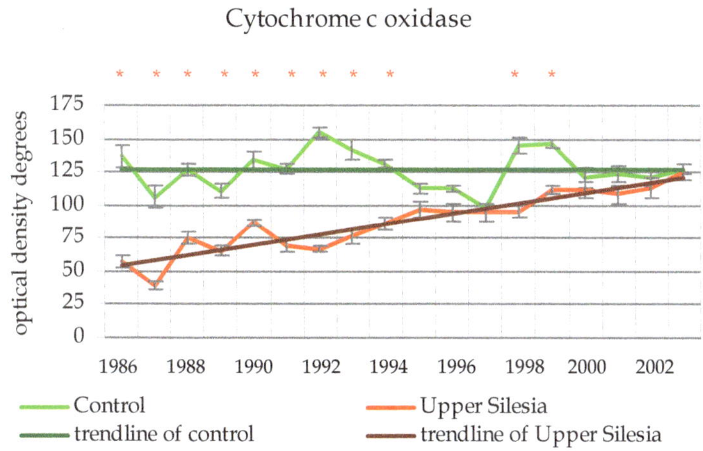

Fig. 6. The mean annual cytochrome c oxidase activity of Upper Silesia and control placentas in period 1986 - 2003.

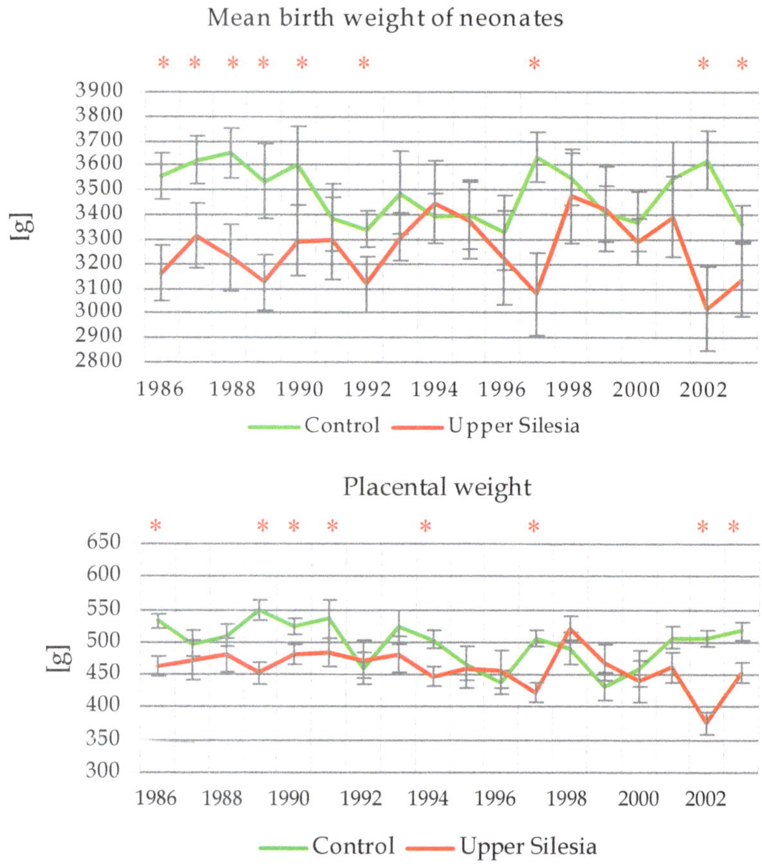

Fig. 7. The mean annual birth weight of neonates and placental weight in period 1986 - 2003. Comparison between control and Upper Silesia regions.

3. Essential and toxic elements in placentas and fetal membranes from Polish Copper Basin and their relationship to neonates birth weight and sex

The results of numerous studies conducted in recent years confirm the negative effect of the environmental contamination with heavy metals on the health and general biological condition of the population living in the areas threatened ecologically. The harmful effects of the environmental exposures depends on the type of contaminants, their concentrations and duration of exposure, as well as from the so-called ontogenic susceptibility.

Pregnant women, especially from industrial areas, are exposed to a wide variety of environmental toxins. During pregnancy, all of them are transferred from mother to fetus across the placenta. The placenta functions as a selective barrier and often bioaccumulates specific environmental toxic substances, including metals (Kantola et al., 2000). They may interfere with placental functions, causing placental damage and a change in the transport of essential trace metals to the fetus.

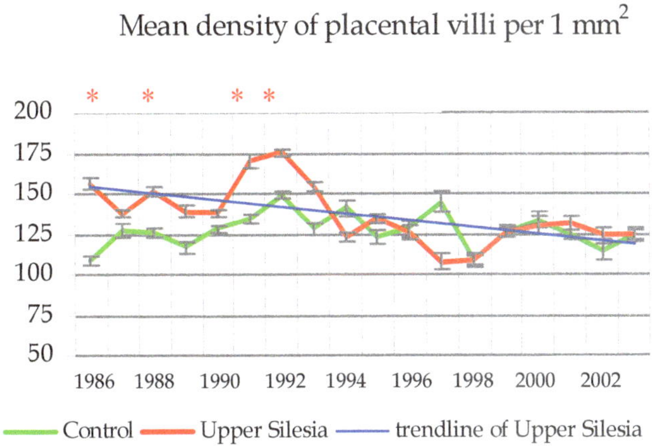

Fig. 8. The mean density of placental villi per 1 mm² of cross-section of Upper Silesia and control placentas in period 1986 - 2003.

Environmental exposure to heavy metals such as mercury, cadmium and lead is a serious growing problem throughout the world. These metals serve no biological function and their presence in tissues reflects contact of the organism with its environment. Their toxicity is frequently the result of long term, low level exposure to pollutants. Metal toxins have the ability to impair not just a single cell or tissue, but many of the body's systems that are responsible for our behavior, mental health, and proper physiological functioning. Essential minerals, such as zinc, copper, iron, selenium, chromium, manganese and calcium, may play an important role in decreasing the risk of the toxicity of heavy metals. On the other hand, a deficiency of these essential elements increases the toxicity of heavy metals (Sorell & Graziano, 1990; Kantola et al., 2000). Knowledge of the mineral interactions is essential in order to counteract the harmful effects of environmental exposure.

In the present study, we investigated some of the essential elements such as zinc, copper, chromium, manganese, calcium and toxic metals such as lead and mercury concentrations as well as mineral deposit contents in the placentas and fetal membranes of male and female neonates from the Polish Copper Basin.

3.1 The clinical characteristics of the studied groups

The examined material consisted of 88 placentas and 68 fetal membranes collected in the years 1995-1988. Of these, 50 placentas and 32 fetal membranes were collected in the Copper Basin and 38 placentas and 36 fetal membranes in the Carpathian Mountains – the control region. To avoid the seasonal variations in metal content, all of the samples were obtained during the autumn. The clinical characteristics of the studied groups are detailed in table 5.

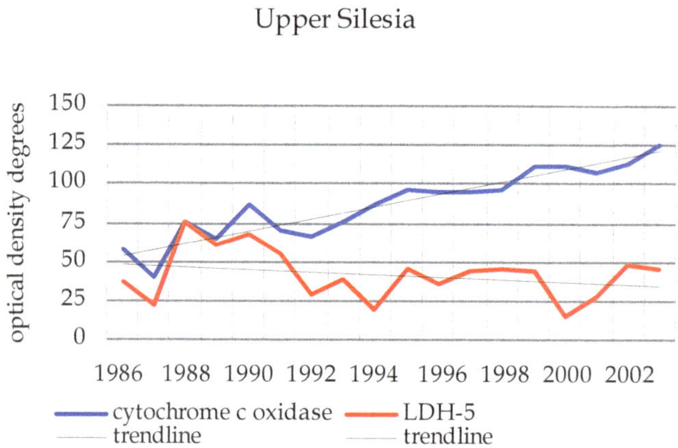

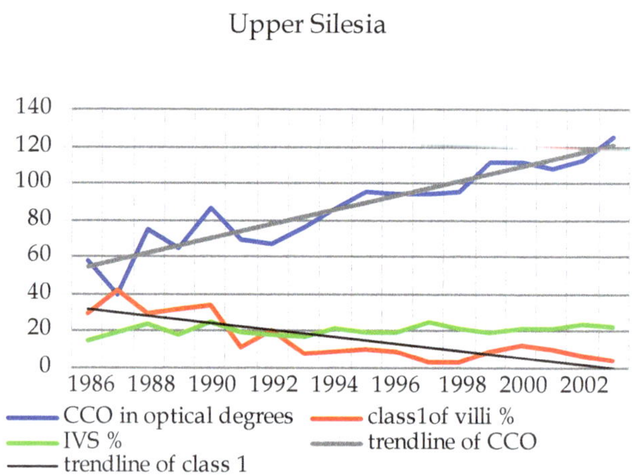

Fig. 9. The relationship of some placental characteristics for Upper Silesia region. The upper figure in clear manner shows inverse correlation between the activities of oxygen dependent cytochrome c oxidase in term of hypoxia-inducible LDH-5 isoenzyme. The lower one serves to clarify reverse dependencies of the cytochrome c oxidase activity and small dimensional terminal villi generation affiliated by decrease (in term of control material) intervillous space volume. Incredibly suggestive is elucidation of the cytochrome c oxidase activity increase during the research period on the background of improvement parameters of environmental conditions in Upper Silesia region (compare with fig. 10).

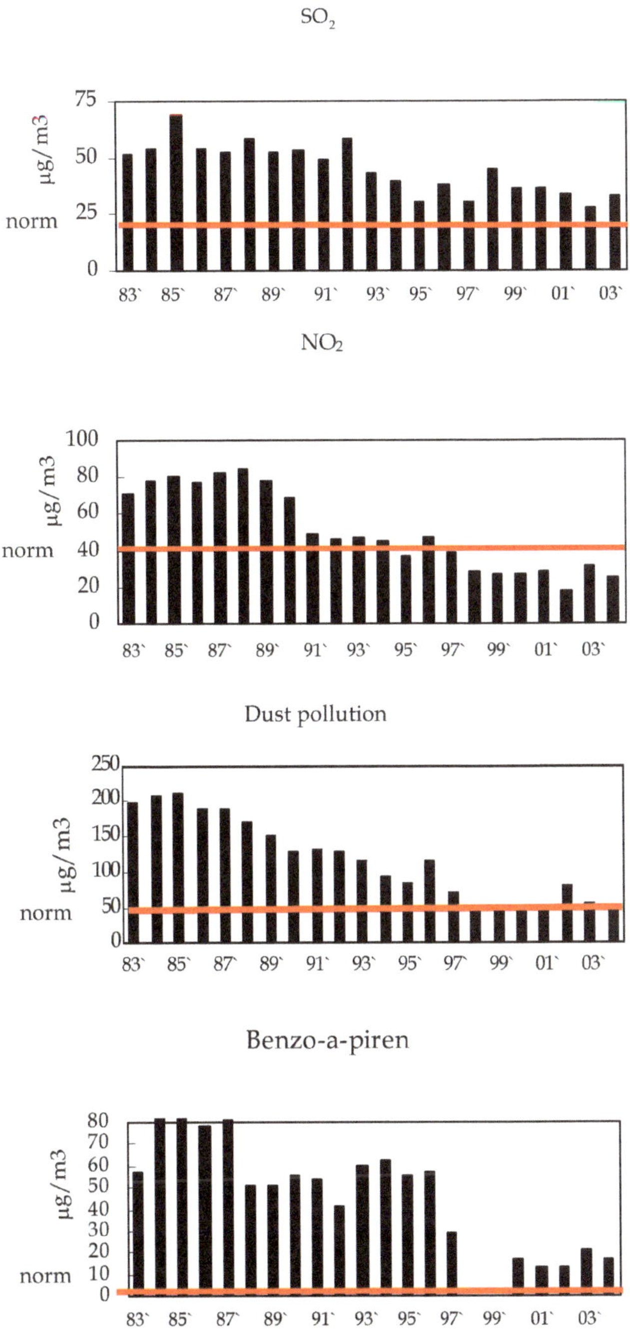

Fig. 10. The average annual emissions of SO_2, NO_2, dust and benzo-a-piren pollutants for Upper Silesia region in period 1983 - 2003.

	Copper Basin		Control		
	Male (n = 26)	Female (n = 24)	Male (n = 18)	Female (n = 20)	p value
Mothers age (years)	24.9 ± 1.0 (17-37)	23.2 ± 1.1 (19-35)	27.5 ± 1.1 (19-38)	26.7 ± 1.5 (17-38)	NS
Gestational age (weeks)	39.9 ± 0.2 (38-42)	40.2 ± 0.3 (38-42)	39.4 ± 0.2 (38-42)	39.6 ± 0.3 (38-42)	NS
Newborn`s birth weight (g)	3551 ± 90 *a* (2600-4150)	3360 ± 123 *b* (2400-3290)	3571 ± 122 (2900-4050)	3511 ± 92 *c* (2900-3970)	*a,b* p <0,05 *b,c* p <0,05
Newborn`s length (cm)	55.1 ± 0.5 (49-61)	54.3 ± 0.8 (48-60)	56.0 ± 0.6 (50-63)	54.9 ± 0.6 (48-59)	NS
Placental weight (g)	518 ± 16 *a* (350-720)	466 ± 29 *b* (330-690)	508 ± 22 (330-710)	446 ± 16 (350-570)	*a,b* p <0,05

Table 5. The clinical characteristics of the studied groups. Data are presented as mean ± SEM.; (range); NS, not significant; Kruskal-Wallis and post-hoc Dunn test.

The mother's age and gestational age showed no differences between the studied groups. Birth weight was significantly lower for girls than boys but only from the Copper Basin region. Girls of the copper basin also had a significantly lower birth weight than girls from the control region. Similarly, neonatal length and placental weight were lower for girls than boys, but only the differences between the placental weight of girls and boys from the Copper Basin region were statistically significant.

According to many reports (Bleker et al., 1979; Kato, 2004), the average birth weight of boys is usually slightly higher than the birth weight of girls in a healthy population. Studies of the Carpathian newborns (low polluted control material) for over 18 years, showed no statistically significant differences between the birth weight of boys and girls (3490 ± 58.2; n = 108 vs 3443 ± 64.4; n = 119 respectively). However, in healthy newborns from high polluted areas, these differences were visible (Upper Silesia: boys 3369 ± 53.1, n = 102 vs girls 3189 ± 61.8, n = 95, $p < 0.05$; Copper Basin: see table 5). This may indicate a greater susceptibility of female fetuses to harmful environmental factors.

3.2 The concentrations of heavy metals and essential minerals in placentas and fetal membranes

The concentrations of copper, manganese and chrome in the placentas of the studied regions were found to be statistically different. An increase in the concentration of copper (34%) and a decrease of manganese (38%) and chromium (30%) in placentas from the Copper Basin, when compared to the control samples, was observed. For fetal membranes, the statistically significant increase of concentration of copper (84%), manganese (230%), chromium (58%) and mercury (60%) in samples from the Copper Basin, when compared to the control group, was found. The mean concentrations of trace elements in the placentas and fetal membranes of neonates of both sexes from studied regions are summarized in table 6.

Element	Placenta		Fetal membranes	
	Control (38)	Copper Basin (50)	Control (36)	Copper Basin (32)
Cu	*2.15 ± 0.19* * (0.75-5.58)	*2.89 ± 0.23* (1.02-7.84)	*2.56 ± 0.17* *** (0.31-4.95)	*4.71 ± 0.29* (0.98-10.71)
Zn	16.97 ± 1.31 (7.72-36.44)	16.24 ± 1.42 (7.81-38.01)	7.54 ± 0.34 (4.75-14.99)	8.81 ± 0.43 (3.67-18.50)
Mn	*1.55 ± 0.34* * (0.18-7.86)	*0.96 ± 0.21* (0.00-6.67)	*0.27 ± 0.06* * (0.00-1.37)	*0.89 ± 0.24* (0.16-3.82)
Cr	*1.99 ± 0.28* * (0.59-5.55)	*1.38 ± 0.36* (0.51-5.08)	*0.92 ± 0.41* * (0.14-4.52)	*1.45 ± 0.58* (0.41-7.09)
Pb	0.78 ± 0.10 (0.35-1.75)	0.80 ± 0.28 (0.17-3.85)	0.61 ± 0.19 (0.00-1.28)	0.64 ± 0.17 (0.11-1.90)
Hg	1.07 ± 0.25 (0.00-1.95)	1.11 ± 0.19 (0.41-1.99)	*0.51 ± 0.29* * (0.00-2.13)	*0.83 ± 0.19* (0.00-1.75)
Ca	1546 ± 420 * (416-6598)	3161 ± 928 (740-24100)	210 ± 10.2 (122-369)	313 ± 32.1 (106-922)

Table 6. The mean concentrations (in µg/g) of trace elements in the placentas and fetal membranes of neonates of both sexes from the Copper Basin and control regions. Data are presented as mean ± SEM.; (range). *$p<0.05$, ***$p<0.001$, Mann-Whitney U test.

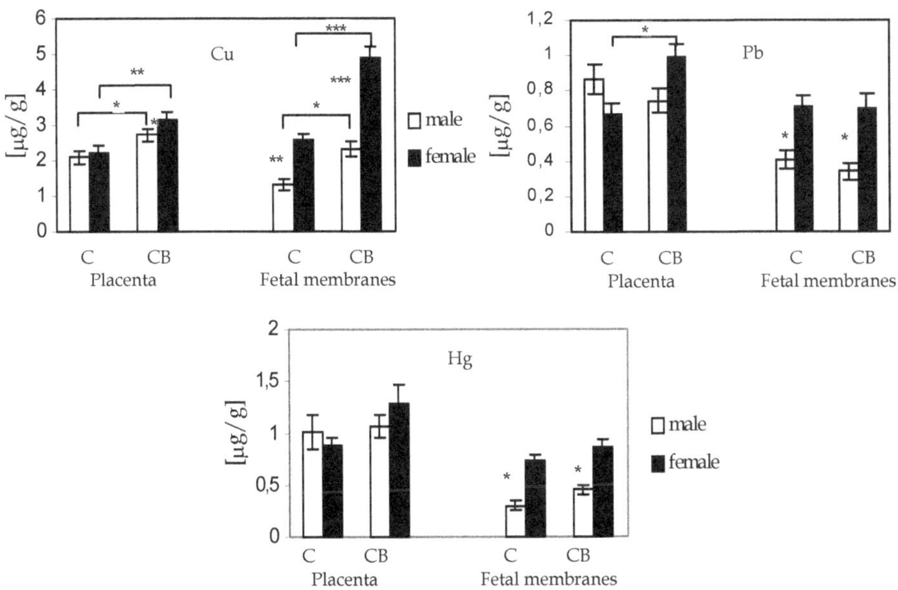

Fig. 11. Mean concentration ± SEM of copper, lead and mercury in male and female placentas and fetal membranes of Copper Basin (CB) and control (C) regions. *$p<0.05$, **$p<0.01$, ***$p<0.001$, Kruskal-Wallis and post-hoc Dunn test.

The levels of elements such as zinc, manganese, chrome, mercury and calcium were higher in the placenta than in fetal membranes mainly in the control group. Conversely, the level of copper was twice as high in the fetal membranes than in the placenta, but only in the Copper Basin group. Lead levels did not differ between the placenta and fetal membranes.

A comparison between the afterbirths of male and female neonates from the Copper Basin and control regions showed interesting differences in the concentrations of copper, lead and mercury. Generally, the higher contents of these metals was found in the female versus male placentas from the Copper Basin. The concentration of copper was higher by 14% ($p<0.05$), lead by 25% ($p<0.05$) and mercury by 16%, as illustrated in figure 11. The controls` female placentas had significantly lower concentrations of the studied metals than female placentas from the Copper Basin. For fetal membranes, the statistically significant increase in the concentration of the studied metals in female samples when compared to the male ones, was found both in the Copper Basin and control materials, figure 11 .

3.2.1 Copper

It is known that copper toxicity is an acute episode usually resulting from copper contamination of drinking water or other beverages. However, relatively little information is available about the effect of long-term exposure to copper on the human body. Copper is essential for the human body. As a basic bioelement, it is a component of numerous enzymes including cytochrome c oxidase (Yewey & Caughey, 1988). However, due to the high rate of copper bioaccumulation and the big extent of its anthropogenic activation, it causes a risk to the local environment via contamination. On the Copper Basin, this risk arises from the long-term operation and processing of copper ore. An excessive copper drop, when accompanied by other metals and contaminating compounds, leads to the degradation of all the ecosystems when it exceeds the level of its acceptable environmental concentration. In cells, copper accumulates mainly in the mitochondria and binds to DNA, RNA, and the nucleus. With its ability to bind with nucleic acids, copper can cause permanent changes in their structure and thus alter their biological properties (Kabata-Pendias & Pendias 1993). Copper and its ions have a very high affinity for sulfhydryl groups of various enzymes and a significant share in the creation of the reactive oxygen species that initiate the peroxidation of lipids in cell membranes, thus leading to the inactivation of enzymes associated with these membranes (Chan et al., 1982). Sokol et al. (Sokol et al., 1993), especially in the mitochondrial lipid peroxidation induced by copper toxical action, which is considered the reason of the cytochrome c oxidase activity decrease. The activity of this enzyme and glucose-6-phosphate dehydrogenase was significantly lower in the investigated placentas from the Copper Basin in relation to control materials, both in the placental villi and in the amniotic epithelium (Zadrożna, 2003). Moreover, the activity of these enzymes significantly negatively correlated with a high copper concentration in the placentas and fetal membranes from the Copper Basin. We observed negative correlations between: the cytochrome c oxidase activity of placental villi and placental copper concentration ($r = -0.2952$, $p < 0.05$), cytochrome c oxidase activity of amniotic epithelium and copper concentration in fetal membranes ($r = -0.3055$, $p < 0.05$) and glucose-6-phosphatase dehydrogenase activity of amniotic epithelium and copper concentration in the fetal membranes ($r = -0.3471$, $p < 0.05$). Additionally, the relationship between sex and the copper content in the placentas and fetal membranes was demonstrated. A significantly higher concentration of copper in female versus male afterbirths was observed.

It is reported that, during pregnancy, maternal serum has twice the level of copper found in it than normal healthy adults, which suggests an important role of this mineral during gestation (Krachler et al., 1999). The placenta can accumulate copper either from ceruloplasmin or from low molecular complexes (McArdle & van den Berg, 1992). The level of copper in the placenta is largely dependent on interactions with other minerals. Especially, zinc interacts directly with copper. The researchers propose that zinc may interfere with copper absorption by competing for binding sites on metallothionein, which regulate the transportation such a metals as zinc, copper and cadmium (Itoh, 1996; Milnerowicz, 1993). Animal studies report that zinc deficiency increases plasma copper levels (O`Dell, 1976, as cited in Massaro, 1997). Conversely, the high levels of zinc induce symptoms of a copper deficiency in laboratory animals (Klevy, et al., 1994; Oestreicher & Cousin, 1985). However, in our study, the levels of zinc in the placentas and fetal membranes did not differ between two studied regions. In addition to zinc, copper also interacts with calcium. The level in the placentas from the Copper Basin was two times higher than in the control. The studies of laboratory animals indicate that copper increases the loss of calcium from the bone (Wang & Bhattacharyya, 1993). Yet, on the other hand, high intakes of calcium and phosphorus lead to reportedly lower copper retention in the human body (Spencer et al., 1984, as cited in Massaro, 1997). Also, iron deficiency increases copper levels in the placenta (McArdle et al., 2008), but this metal has not been tested in our study.

3.2.2 Manganese and chromium

The next comparison of the Copper Basin and control materials allowed us to note the different concentration of manganese in placentas and fetal membranes. The placentas from the Copper Basin contained 38% less manganese than the control placentas while the fetal membranes from the Copper Basin were richer in manganese by 70% than the control ones. These similar proportions were observed relative to chrome in the studied materials. Overall, in the control material, the concentrations of manganese and chromium in placentas were relatively high, while they were low in the fetal membranes. In turn, in the material from the Copper Basin, the average concentrations of these metals in placentas and fetal membranes were similar. The above results from our observation are apparently an effect of the interactions between chromium, manganese and calcium. The limited research that exists indicates that calcium inhibits manganese absorption in laboratory animals (Van Barveveld & Van den Hamer, 1984).

Manganese is an essential element for growth and bone development. This confirms the positive correlation ($r = 0.6011$, $p = 0.02$) between the birth weight of girls and placental concentrations of manganese found in the material from the Copper Basin. The lower concentration of manganese and chromium in the placentas from the Copper Basin in relation to the control, and higher concentrations of these metals in the fetal membranes, may indicate on increase in the placental barrier permeability for chromium and manganese under conditions of prolonged exposure to environmental toxins.

3.2.3 Lead

It is universally accepted that lead represents a potentially toxic agent in humans. On the basis of numerous reports (Korpela et al. 1986; Lagerkvist et al. 1996), it is known that lead can cross the placenta and have consequences upon the developing fetus. Many older papers have proved that high doses of lead can cause miscarriage (Ernhart, 1992), and epidemiological data indicated the negative effect of lead contamination during pregnancy on newborn children and during early childhood (Shukla et al. 1989). However, more recent reports (Rudkowski, 1999) pay attention to the fact that the already observed destructive results of lead in children were not considered as dangerous till now. Dietrich (Dietrich, 1987) and Needleman (Needleman, 1990) proved that the so-called low levels of lead found in the blood of pregnant women exposed to environmental lead could cause not only abnormal fetal development but also impaired postnatal mental development. It is very important to note that, during pregnancy, there can occur the mobilization of lead (together with calcium) from the bone, which has collected there as a result of prior accumulation, especially since the half-life of lead in bones takes approximately 20-30 years (O'Flaherty, 1995; Gulson, 1997). Currently, on the basis of numerous epidemiological studies concerning the concentration of lead in children's blood, that may cause harmful effects, is calculated at 100 μg/l (Dutkiewicz, 1993). According to data by the Foundation for Children from the Copper Basin (Strugała-Stawik, 1999), the percentage of children tested in this area, in which the concentration of lead in blood was higher than 100 μg/l, was respectively 16.0%, 13.6% and 11.6% in the years 1995-1997. This data also showed a higher concentration of lead in the blood of boys than girls. It is well documented (Iyengar & Rapp, 2001; Lagerkvist et al., 1996; Loiacono et al., 1992), based on studies of the lead levels in maternal blood, umbilical cord blood and placenta that, that lead does not accumulate in the placenta and that the placenta does not impede, to any significant extent, the transfer of lead from the mother to the fetus. It is therefore concluded that the placenta is not suitable material for use in the monitoring of environmental lead exposure. This is in line with our research findings. In our study, the concentrations of lead in the placentas and fetal membranes from the Copper Basin did not demonstrate differences in comparison to the control, although the previously cited data showed that lead mikrointoxication was a serious problem in this territory. No differences in lead content between placenta and fetal membrane samples in both groups were also observed. A lack of expected differences in the lead concentration in the investigated materials may also be the result of lead interactions with other metals. In the human body lead is accompanied usually by calcium. Lead and calcium interact in a negative manner. Calcium deficiency raises lead toxicity, and an adequate calcium intake decreases lead toxicity. In human infants, lead absorption decreases as dietary calcium increases (Ziegler et al., 1978 as cited in Massaro, 1997). Also, higher calcium intakes decrease lead absorption in human adults (Blake & Mann, 1983).

However, analyzing separately male and female afterbirths from the Copper Basin, a higher lead concentration ($p < 0.05$) in placentas as well as in fetal membranes of female neonates was visible than in the male ones. This would suggest the higher ability of the lead accumulation by a female afterbirth in dangerous environment circumstances.

3.2.4 Mercury

Mercury is a ubiquitous environmental toxicant. There are three main forms of mercury: elemental, inorganic, and organic compounds (methyl and ethyl mercury). Humans are exposed to all of its forms and even relatively low doses of mercury containing compounds can have serious adverse neurodevelopmental impacts (Choi et al., 1978). Mercury exposure has a potentially negative effect on fetal development (Ask at al., 2002), because it can interfere with the developing nervous system. Mercury exposure for the fetus and nursing infants comes both from mercury stored in the woman's body prior to pregnancy, and from mercury to which the woman is exposed during pregnancy and breast feeding. The organic mercury can easily pass through the placental barrier and accumulates in the fetus. Some recent researches (Rudge at al., 2009; Stern & Smith, 2003) indicate that the cord's blood mercury concentration was almost twice as higher than the maternal. The results obtained through examining maternal blood, placental tissue and umbilical cord blood from an urban region showed a higher total mercury content in the placenta than in maternal and cord blood (Tsuchyia et al., 1984). The opposite results were obtained earlier by Hubermont et al. (Hubermont et al., 1978), who showed the highest levels of mercury was in blood samples from newborns when compared to the maternal blood and placenta from rural areas of Belgium. Based on these results, Iyengar and Rapp (Iyengar & Rapp, 2001) conclude that higher mercury content in the umbilical cord blood and placental tissue than in maternal blood indicated the presence of the transplacental pathway of mercury. The placentas from urban areas have slightly more ability to retain mercury in their tissues.

The results of our research showed no differences in the placental total mercury concentrations, but not in fetal membranes, between a polluted and rural region. The concentration of mercury in the fetal membranes from the Copper Basin were higher ($p < 0.05$) than in the control. Also, only female fetal membranes had a significantly higher mercury content than the male membranes, both in the material of the Copper Basin and in the control group. Methylmercury toxicity studies conducted on laboratory animals have shown variation among sexes. Female mice revealed a higher resistance to methylmercury acute toxicity than the males (Yasutake et al., 1990), and upon life-long exposure to methylmercury, male mice and rats manifested neurotoxic symptoms earlier than the females (Mitsumori et al., 1990).

4. Mineral deposits and calcium levels in high polluted placentas

The placentas from Upper Silesia and the Copper Basin of both sexes were richer in mineral deposits than the control, figure 12. In female placentas from the Copper Basin, the big amounts of mineral deposits were found more often than in male placentas, although the differences were statistically non-significant.

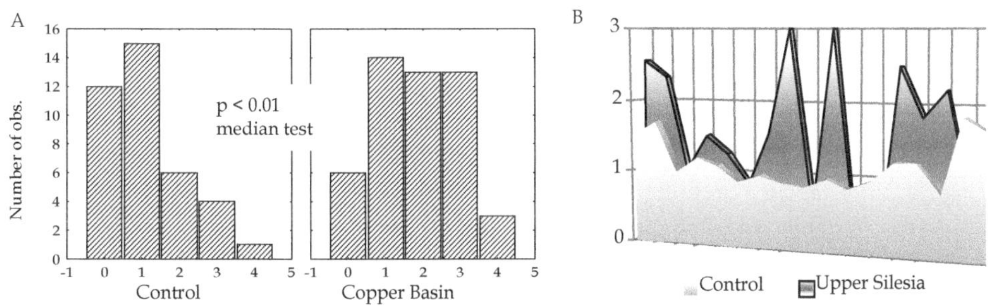

Fig. 12. A. The frequency distribution of mineral deposits occurrence in the Copper Basin and control placentas. B. The mean abundance of mineral deposits in placentas from Upper Silesia and control regions during the years 1986-2003; $p < 0.01$, median test. Scale: from 0 to 4 in ascending gradation order.

Mineral deposits usually occur in anomalous fibrous and hyaline connective tissue structures in stem and terminal villi as well as in blood vessel walls and cytotrophoblastic islets. Mineral deposits appear yellow or brown and stippled, and occur in irregular quantities. In the tissue sections they are visible in the form of transparent crystals, figures 13, 14.

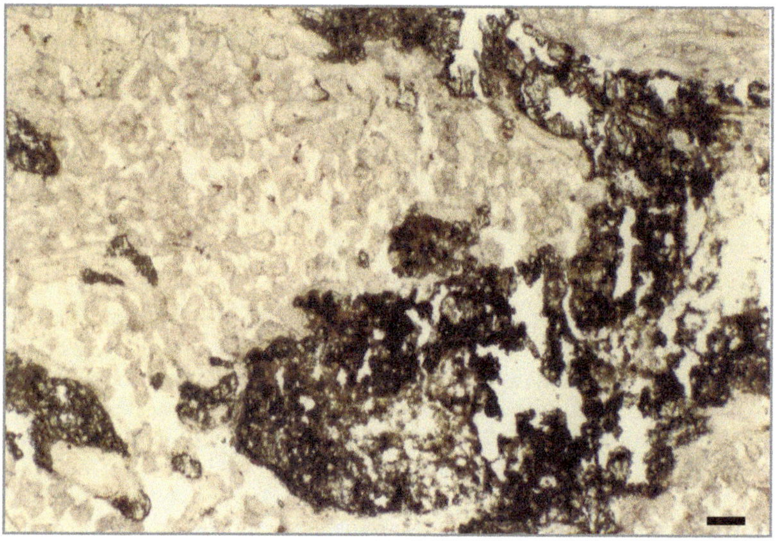

Fig. 13. Cryostat cross-section through a full term placenta from Upper Silesia. The giant mineral deposit; and in the background histochemical reactions for cytochrome c oxidase. Bar: 50 μm.

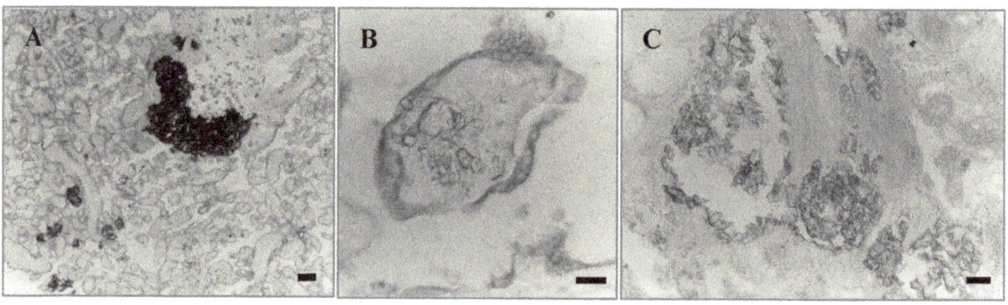

Fig. 14. Cryostat cross-section through a full-term placentas collected in the Copper Basin territory. A. Numerous of mineral deposits deposited within the cytotrophoblastic island and the intervillous space. Bar: 100 μm. B. Mineral deposits within the placental villous. Bar: 20 μm. C. Mineral deposits in the chorionic plate. Bar: 50 μm.

Necrosis of placental tissues and excess of calcium ions are believed to be one of the reasons for mineral deposits originating. The researches of the placentas collected from the aluminum smelter territory (Zamorska, 1982/1983)) have revealed adverse effects of fluorine compounds on the condition of placentas and newborns, and also a significant increase in the content of mineral deposits and richness of fluoride in these deposits. The placenta, as it is known, limits the passage of fluoride ions from the maternal blood to fetal blood, binding them mainly with calcium or magnesium ions and forming insoluble salts (Shen & Taves, 1974). In this way the placenta protects the fetus from an excess of fluoride when the maternal fluoride intake is high. These observations confirm the results of studies on the fluoride and calcium distribution in the placenta (Chlubek et al., 1998). The high positive correlation between fluoride and calcium concentrations in the marginal part of placentas of women residing in an area with a relatively low water and air fluoride content was found.

In our studied materials, the chemical analysis proved that there was twice as much concentration of calcium in the placentas from the Copper Basin than in the control ($p < 0.05$). Moreover, we found a strong positive correlation ($r = 0.4877$; $p < 0.000$) between the calcium concentration and the mineral deposits, and a negative correlation between calcium and a newborn`s length ($r = - 0.543$; $p < 0.05$).

It is known that the calcium excess can cause the alteration of cell metabolism as a consequence of interaction with a series of cellular trace elements (Miller & Groziak, 1997), and in extremal cases it causes cell death by necrosis or apoptosis (Leist & Nicotera, 1998). In cytotoxicity induced by the calcium ions there is a substantial participation of mitochondria (Kang, 1997). They are able to cumulate the calcium ions and in this way reduce their concentration in cytoplasm, and consequently prevent their toxic activity (Rutter et al., 1993). On the other hand, the calcium ion excess in mitochondria leads to their dysfunction and thereby to the decrease of ATP production (Bernardi, 1996). The statistically significant negative correlation ($r = - 0.3224$; $p = 0.011$) between cytochrome c oxidase activity of placental villi and placental calcium concentration in the Copper Basin samples was found. Moreover, the strong negative correlation between activity of cytochrome c oxidase of the placental villi and mineral deposits was observed both in the Copper Basin ($r = - 0.2416$; $p < 0.001$) and Upper Silesia materials ($r = - 0.2468$; $p = 0.012$).

In examining the placentas from low polluted regions, we observed that cigarette smoking by pregnant women is also associated with the occurrence of large amounts of mineral deposits in the placenta.

5. Conclusion

The hypothesis that the morphology of the feto-placental unit is sensitive to the impact of all environmental pollutants is fully confirmed here, and the presented changes are of a dose-dependent effect type. We found that enzyme histochemistry is a very useful tool for studying placental physiology and for metabolic and morphological connections. Our presented placental studies are the only ones, as far as we are aware, which covers the longest monitoring period and because of it we seriously rely on the strength of our arguments.

Our prolonged studies of the effect of environmental chemical pollution on the biochemical and microanatomical organization of the human placenta showed that this organ, when influenced by toxic factors, undergoes changes. The primary change consists in histochemically detectable deterioration of the oxidative enzymes activity in the villous syncytiotrophoblast as compared with the activity shown by placentas from sites of low pollution. Especially the measurement of cytochrome c oxidase activity is a good indicator of oxygen availability in utero-placental environment and thus a good marker of energy supply for the fetus. This consequently results in placental hypoxia and in compensatory increase in numerical density of the small dimensional villi.

The presented morphological measurements do not meet the requirements of today's stereology (Mayhew, TM., 2008, 2009). It is worth noting, however, that in the 1980s, the reciprocal presuppositions of contemporary placental stereology were shaped. The data collected for so many years using the same assumptions provides a strong basis for the outcome of comparisons between environments.

Our study also showed an interesting variation among sexes. In the highly polluted environment, female afterbirths accumulated more copper, lead and mercury. Simultaneously the female newborns had a significantly lower average birth weight than male infants, but there was no direct correlation with a higher content of studied metals in the placenta. One interesting observation is a positive correlation between the mean weight of newborns and manganese content, which in the placentas from the Copper Basin was significantly less.

The human placenta is not a sensitive indicator of environmental contamination of toxic trace elements because, as it is clear from many studies, it is not a barrier for metals such as lead or mercury. If, however, despite this, the concentration of toxic trace elements in placentas increases, this information could be used to diminish postnatal exposure of the fetus or maternal exposure during subsequent pregnancies, as suggested Iyengar (Iyengar & Rapp, 2001).

The systematic collection of reliable information on concentrations of lead, cadmium, copper, themselves recognized as major contributors to environmental pollution, in the human body is the most effective method for evaluating the effectiveness of activities aimed at protecting the environment and the health of residents.

6. Acknowledgment

We would like to thank to staff members of Department of Cytobiology and Histochemistry of Jagiellonian University in Krakow for assistance in the collection of placental samples.

We are grateful to the staff of the gynecological and obstetric hospitals in Brzozów, Lesko, Ustrzyki Dolne, Bytom, Chorzów, Zabrze, Legnica, Zlotoryja, and Głogów.

This work we would like to dedicate memory of Prof. Józef Niweliński and Dr. Lucyna Zamorska who pioneered the ecological study of human placentas in Poland.

7. References

Aksoy, Y.; Ögüs, LH. & Özer, N. (2001). Purification and Some Properties of Human Placental glucose-6-Phosphate Dehydrogenase. *Protein Expression And Purification*, Vol.21, No.2, (March 2001), pp. 286-292, ISSN 1046 - 5928

Ask, K.; Akesson, A.; Berglund, M. & Vahter, M. (2002). Inorganic mercury and methylmercury in placentas of Swedish women. *Environmental Health Perspectives*, Vol.110, No.5, (April 2002), pp. 523-526, ISSN 02110523

Benirschke, K.; Kaufmann, P. & Baergen, R. (2006). *Pathology of the human placenta.* (5th edn), Springer, ISBN 0-387-26738-7, New York

Bernardi, P. (1996). The permeability transition pore: Control points of a cyclosporin A-sensitive mitochondrial channel involvet in cell death. *Biochimica et Biophysica Acta,* Vol.1275, No.1-2, pp. 5-9, ISSN 0304-4165

Bilic, G.; Ochsenbein-KÖlble, N.; Hall, H.; Huch, R. & Zimmermann R. (2004). In vitro lesion repair by human amnion epithelial and mesenchymal cells. *American Journal of Obsterics and Gynecology,* Vol.190, No.2, (February2004), pp. 87-92, ISSN 0002 - 9378

Binkova, B.; Veselý, D.; Vesela, D.; Jelinek, R. & Sram, RJ. (1999). Genotoxicity and embryotoxicity of urban air particulate matter collected during winter and summer period in two different districts of the Czech Republic. *Mutation Research,* Vol.440, No.1 (January 1999), pp. 45-58, ISSN 0027-5107

Bleker, OP.; Breur, W. & Huidekoper, BL. (1979). A study of birth weight, placental weight and mortality of twins as compared to singletons. *British Journal of Obstetrics and Gynecology,* Vol.86, No.2, (February 1979), pp. 111-118, ISSN 1471-0528

Bobak, M.; Leon, DA. (1999b). Pregnancy outcomes and outdoor air pollution: an ecological study in district of the Czech Republic. *Journal of Occupational and Environmental Medicine,* Vol.56, No. 8, (September 1999), pp. 539-543, ISSN 1076-2752

Bobak, M.; Richards, M. & Wadsworth, M. (2001). Air pollution and birth weight in Britain in 1946. *Epidemiology,* Vol.12, No.3, (May 2001), pp. 358-359, ISSN 1044-3983

Burton, GJ.; Mayhew, TM. & Robertson, LA. (1989). Stereological re-examination of the effects of varying oxygen tensions on human placental villi maintained in organ culture for up to 12 h. *Placenta,* Vol.10, No.3, pp. 263-273, ISSN 0143-4004

Bush, PG.; Mayhew, TM.; Abramovich, DR.; Aggent, PJ.; Burke, MD.; & Page, RK. (2000) A Quantitative Study on the Effects of Maternal Smoking on Placental Morphology and Cadmium Concentration. *Placenta,* Vol.21, No.2-3, (March 2000), pp. 247-256, ISSN 0143-4004

Castelluci, M.; Kosanke, G.; Verdenelli, F.; Huppertz, B. & Kaufmann P. (2000). Villous sprouting: fumdamental mechanisms of human placenta development. *Human Reproduction Update,* Vol. 6, No. 2, (February 2000), pp. 185-194, ISSN 1355-4786

Chan, PC.; Peller, OG. & Kesner, I. (1982). Copper (II) - catalyzed lipid peroxidation in liposomes and erythrocyte membranes. *Lipids,* Vol.17, No.2, (February 1982), pp. 331-337, ISSN 2090-3030

Chlubek, D.; Poreba, R. & Machalinski, B. (1998). Fluoride and calcium distribution in human placenta. *Fluoride,* Vol.31, No.3, pp. 131-136, ISSN 0015-4725

Choi, BH.; Lapham, LWW.; Amin-Zaki, L. & Asleem, T. (1978). Abnormal neuronal migration, deranged cerebral cortical organization and diffuse white matter astrocytosis of human fetal brain: a major effect of methylmercury poisoning in utero. *Journal of Neuropathology and Experimental Neurology,* Vol.37, No.6, (June 1978), pp. 719-733, ISSN 0022-3069

Dejmek, J.; Solansky, I.; Benes. I.; Lenicek, J. & Sram, RJ. (2000). The Impact of Polycyclic Aromatic Hydrocarbons and Fine Particles on Pregnancy Outcome. *Environmental Health Perspectives,* Vol.108, No.12 (December 2000), pp. 1159-1164, ISSN 0091-6765

Dietrich, KN. (1987). Low level foetal lead exposure effect on neurobehavioral development in early infancy. *Pediatrics,* Vol.80, No.5, (November 1987), pp.721-730, ISSN 0031-4005

Dutkiewicz, T. & Kulka, E. (1993). Reference levels of lead in children with clean Polish regions. *Medycyna Pracy*, Vol.44, No.2, (April 1993), pp.77-84, ISSN 0465-5893 (in Polish)

Egbor, M.; Ansari, T.; Morris, N.; Green, CJ. & Sibbons, PD. (2006). Pre-eclampsia and fetal growth restriction: How Morphometrically Different is the Placenta?, *Placenta*, Vol.27, No.6-7 (June -July 2006), pp. 727-734, ISSN 0143-4004

Ernhart, CB. (1992). A critical review of low-level prenatal lead exposure in the human: 1. Effects on the fetus and newborn. *Reproductive Toxicology*, Vol.6, No.1, (January 1992), pp. 9-19, ISSN 0890-6238

Gulson, B. (1997). Pregnancy increases mobilization of lead from maternal skeleton. *Journal of Laboratory and Clinical Medicine*, Vol.130, No.1, (January 1997), pp. 51-62, ISSN 0022-2143

Hławiczka, S.(1998). Assessment of heavy metal emissions to air from Polish territory. Part. II. Emissions in 1980 - 1995. *Archiwum Ochrony Środowiska*, Vol.24, No.4, pp. 91-108, ISSN 0324-8461

Hubermont, G.; Buchet, JP.; Roels, H. & Lauwerys, R. (1978). Placental transfer of lead, mercury and cadmium in women in a rural area. *International Archives of Occupational and Environmental Health*, Vol.41, pp. 117-124, ISSN 0340-0131

Itoh, N.; Nakanishi, H.; Kawai, Y.; Mayumi, T.; Hwang, GS.; Min, K.; Onosaka, S.; Muto, N. & Tanaka, K. (1996). Binding of Cd to metallothionein in the placenta of Cd-treated mouse. *The Journal of Toxicological Sciences*, Vol.21, No.1, pp. 19-27, ISSN 1880-3989

Iyengar, GV. & Rapp, A. (2001). Human placenta as a dual biomarker for monitoring fetal and maternal environment with special reference to potentially toxic trace elements. Part 3: Toxic trace elements in placenta and placenta as a biomarker for these elements. *The Science of the Total Environment*, Vol.280, pp. 221-238, ISSN 0048-9697

Kang, J. (1997). Mechanisms of cell death induced by metals. In: *Handbook of Human Toxicology*, Massaro, pp. 256-275, CRC Press, ISBN 0-8493-4493-X, Boca Raton, New York

Kabata-Pendias, A.& Pendias, H. (1993). *Biogeochemistry of trace elements*. Polish Sci. Publ., ISBN 83-01-11257-3, Warsaw, (in Polish)

Kaufmann, P.; Mayhew, TM. & Charnock-Jones, DS. (2004). Aspects of human fetoplacental vasculogenesis and angiogenesis. II. Changes during normal pregnancy. *Placenta*, , Vol.25, No.2-3, (February-March 2004), pp. 114-26, ISSN 0143-4004

Kato, N. (2004). Reference birth weight range for multiple birth neonates in Japan. *BMC Pregnancy and Childbirth*, Vol.4, No.2, (February 2004), pp. 1-9, ISSN 1471-2393

Kay, HH.; Zhu, S. & Tsoi, S. (2007). Hypoxia and lactate production in trophoblast cells. *Placenta*, Vol.28, No.8-9, (August-September 2007), pp. 854-860, ISSN 0143-4004

Kingdom, JCP. & Kaufmann, P. (1997). Oxygen and placental villous development: origins of fetal hypoxia. *Placenta*, Vol.18, pp. 613-626, ISSN 0143-4004

Klevy, L.; Pond, W. & Medeiros, D. (1994). Decreased high density lipoprotein cholesterol and apoprotein A-1 in plasma and ultra structural pathology in cardiac muscle of young pigs fed a diet high in zinc. *Nutrition Research*, Vol.14, No.8, pp. 1227-1239, ISSN 0271-5317

Korpela, H.; Loueniva, R.; Yrjänheikki, E. & Kauppila, A. (1986). Lead and cadmium concentrations in maternal and umbilical cord blood, amniotic fluid, placenta and amniotic membranes. *American Journal of Obstetrics and Gynecology*, Vol.155, No.5, (May 1986), pp. 1086-1089, ISSN 0002-9378

Krachler, M.; Rossipal, E. & Micetic-Turk, D. (1999). Trace element transfer from the mother to the newborn investigations on triplets of colostrums, maternal and umbilical cord sera. *European Journal of Clinical Nutrition*, Vol.53, No.6, pp. 486-494, ISSN 0954-3007

Kubiak, R.; Rudek, Z.; Cieszkowski, J. & Garlicki, S. (1993). Cytogenetic studies in biomonitoring of inhabitants of the surrounding of "Sendzimir" steel work in Krakow", Folia Medica Cracoviensia: 188-197 (in Polish). ISSN 0015-5616

Lagerkvist, BJ.; Sandberg, S.; Frech, W. & Jin, T. (1996). Is placenta a good indicator of cadmium and lead exposure? *Archives of Environmental Health*, Vol.51, No.5. (May 1996), pp. 389-394, ISSN 0003-9896

Leist, M. & Nicotera, P. (1998). Calcium and neuronal death. *Reviews of Physiology, Biochemistry and Pharmacology*, Vol.132, pp. 79-125, ISSN 0303-4240

Loiacono, NJ.; Graciano, JH.; Kline, JK.; Popovac, D.; Ahmedi, X.; Gashi, E.; Mehmeti, A. & Rajovic, B. (1992). Placental cadmium and birth weight in women living near a lead smelter. *Archives of Environmental Health*, Vol.47, No.4, pp. 250-255, ISSN 0003-9896

Majewska, U.; Braziewicz, J.; Banaś, D.; Kubala-Kukuś, A.; Góźdź, S.; Pajek, M.; Zadrożna, M.; Jaskóla, M. & Czyżewski, T. (1999). Some aspects of statistical distribution of trace element concentrations in biomedical samples. *Nuclear Instruments and Methods in Physics Research B: Beam Interactions with Materials and Atoms*, Vol. 150, No. 1-4, (April 1999), pp. 254-259, ISSN 0168-583X

Massaro, EJ. (Ed(s).). (1997). *Handbook of human toxicology*. CRC Press, ISBN 0-8493-4493-X, Boca Raton, New York

Mayhew, TM. (2002). Angiogenesis and villous development in human placenta. Journal of Anatomy. Vol.200, No.5, (May 2002), pp. 523–534, ISSN 0021 8782

Mayhew, TM. (2008). Taking Tissue Samples from the Placenta: An Illustration Of Principles and Strategies. *Placenta*, Vol. 29, No.1, (January 2008), pp. 1-14, ISSN 0143-4004

Mayhew, TM. (2009). A stereological perpective on placental morphology in normal and complicated pregnancies. *Journal of Anatomy*, Vol.215, pp. 77-90, ISNN 1469-7580

Mayhew, TM.; Wijesekara, J.; Baker, PN.; & Ong SS. (2004). Morphometric Evidence that Villous Development and Fetoplacental Angiogenesis are Compromised by Intrauterine Growth Restriction but not by pre-eclampsia. *Placenta*, Vol.25, pp. 829-833, ISSN 0143-4004

McArdle, HJ. & van den Berg, GJ. (1992). The accumulation of copper by microvillar vesicles isolated from human placenta. *The Journal of Nutrition*, Vol.122, No.6, pp. 1260-1265, ISSN 0022-3166

McArdle, HJ.; Andersen, HS.; Jones, H. & Gambling, L. (2008). Copper and Iron Transport Across the Placenta: Regulation and Interactions. *Journal of Neuroendocrinology*, Vol.20, No.4, (April 2008), pp.427-431, ISSN 1365-2826

McMillan, PJ.(1967). Differential demonstration of muscle and heart type lactic dehydrogenase of rat muscle and kidney. *Journal of Histochemistry & Cytochemistry*, Vol.15, No.1, pp. 21-31, ISSN 0022-1554

Miller, GD. & Groziak, SM. (1997). Essential and nonessential mineral interactions. In: *Handbook of Human Toxicology*, Massaro, pp. 369-407, CRC Press, ISBN 0-8493-4493-X, Boca Raton, New York

Milnerowicz, H. (1993). Metalloproteins in human placenta and fetal membranes in non-smoking and smoking women. *Acta Biochimica Polonica*, Vol.40, No.1, pp. 179-181, ISSN 1734-154X

Mitsumori, K.; Hirano, M.; Ueda, H.; Maita, K. & Shirasu, Y. (1990). Chronic toxicity and carcinogenicity of methylmercury chloride in B6C3F1 mice. *Fundamental and Applied Toxicology*, Vol.14, No.1, ISSN 0272-0590

Needleman, H. (1990). The long term effects of exposure to low doses of lead in childhood - an 11 years follow - up report. *The New England Journal of Medicine*, Vol.322, No.2, pp. 83-88, ISSN 0028-4793

Obolenskaya, MY., Teplyuk, NM., Divi, RL., Poirier, MC., Filimonova, NB., Zadrozna, M. & Pasanen, MJ. (2010). Human placental glutathione S-transferase activity and polycyclic aromatic hydrocarbon DNA adducts as biomarkers for environmental oxidative stress in placentas from pregnant women living in radioactivity- and chemically-polluted regions. *Toxicology Letters*, Vol.196, No.2. (July 2010), pp. 80-86, ISSN 0378-4274

Oestreicher, P. & Cousin, R. (1985). Copper and zinc absorption in the rat: mechanism of mutual antagonism. *The Journal of Nutrition*, Vol.115, No.2, pp. 159-166, ISSN 0022-3166

O'Flaherty, E. (1995). Physiologically based models for bone - seeking elements. V. Lead absorption and deposition in childhood. *Toxicology and Applied Pharmacology*, Vol.131, No.2, pp. 297-308, ISSN 0041-008X

Pearse, AGE. (1972). *Histochemistry, Theoretical and Applied*, (3th edn.), Churchill Livingstone, ISBN 0-443-00865-5, Edinburgh & London

Rich, DQ.; Demissie, K.; Lu, SE..; Kamat1, L.; Wartenberg, D. & Rhoads, GG. (2009). Ambient air pollutant concentrations during pregnancy and the risk of fetal growth restriction. *Journal of Epidemiology and Community Health*, Vol.63, No.6, ISSN 0143-005X

Rudge, CV.; Röllin, HB.; Nogueira, CM.; Thomassen, Y.; Rudge, MC. & Odland, J. (2009). The placenta as a barrier for toxic and essential elements in paired maternal and cord blood samples of South African delivering women. *Journal of Environmental Monitoring*, Vol.11, No.7, (July 2009), pp. 1322-1330, ISSN B903805A

Rudkowski, Z. (1999). The impact of xenobiotic and physiological metals in immunological reactions. *Pediatria Polska*, Supplement, pp. 39-44, ISSN 0031-3939, (in Polish)

Rutter, GA.; Theler, JM.; Murgia, M.; Wollheim, CB.; Pozzan, T. & Rizzuto, R. (1993). Stimulated Ca^{++} influx raises mitochondrial free Ca^{++} to supramicromolar levels in a pancreatic □□cell line. Possible role in glucose and agonist-induced insulin secretion. *The Journal of Biological Chemistry*, Vol.268, No.30, (October 1993), pp. 22385-22390, ISSN 0021-9258

Semenza, GL.; Roth, PH.; Fang, HM. & Wang, GL. (1994). Transcriptional regulation of genes encoding glycolytic enzymes by hypoxia-inducible factor. *The Journal of Biological Chemistry*, Vol.269, pp. 23757–23763, ISSN 0021-9258

Shen, YW. & Taves, D. (1974). Fluoride concentrations in the human placenta in maternal and cord blood. *American Journal of Obstetrics and Gynecology*, Vol.119, No.1, (January 1974), pp. 205-207, ISSN 0002-9378

Shukla, R.; Bornschein, RL.; Dietrich, KN.; Buncher, CR.; Berger, O.; Hammond, PB. & Succop, PA. (1989). Effects of fetal and infant lead exposure on growth and stature. *Pediatrics*, Vol.84, No.4, pp. 604-612, ISSN 1098-4275

Sokol, RJ.; Devereaux, MA.; O'Brien, K.; Khandwala, RA. & Loehr, JP. (1993). Abnormal hepatic mitochondrial respiration and cytochrome c oxidase activity in rats with long-term copper overload. *Gastroenterology*, Vol.105, pp. 178-187, ISSN 1007-9327

Sorell, TL. & Graziano, JH. (1990). Effect of oral cadmium exposure during pregnancy on maternal and fetal zinc metabolism in the rat. Toxicol Appl Pharmacol Vol.102, No.3, pp. 537-545, ISSN 0041-008X

Sram, RJ.; Binkova, B.; Rössner, P.; Rubes, R.; Topinka, J. & Dejmek, J. (1999). Adverse reproductive outcomes from exposure to environmental mutagens. *Mutation Research*, 428: 203-215. ISSN 0027-5107

Sram, RJ.; Binkova, B.; Dejmek, J. & Bobak, M. (2005). Ambient Air Pollution and pregnancy Outcomes: A review o the Literature. *Environmental Health Perspectives*, Vol.113, No.4, (april 2005), pp. 375-382, ISSN 0091-6765

Stern, AH. & Smith, AE. (2003). An assessment of the cord blood: maternal blood methylmercury ratio: implications for risk assessment. *Environmental Health Perspective*, Vol.111, No.5, (May 2003), pp. 1465–1470, ISSN 0091-6765

Stoward, PJ. & Pearse, AGE. (1991). *Histochemistry, Theoretical and Applied,* (4th edn.), Churchill Livingstone, ISBN 0-443-02996-2, Edinburgh, London, Melbourne, New York and Tokyo

Strugała-Stawik, H. & Stawik, K. (1999). Monitoring of the lead concentration in blond in children from Legnica Copper Basin in years 1996-1999. *Pediatria Polska,* Supplement, pp. 59-64, ISSN 0031-3939, (in Polish)

Tsoi, SCM.; Zheng, J.; Xu, K. & Kay HH. (2000). Differential Expression of Lactate Dehydrogenase isozymes (LDH) in human placenta with high expression of LDH-A4 isozyme in the endothelial cells of pre-eclampsia villi. *Placenta,* Vol.22, No.4, pp. 317–322, ISSN 0143-4004

Tsuchiya, H.; Mitani, K.; Kodama, K. & Nakata, T. (1984). Placental transfer of heavy metals in normal pregnant Japanese women. *Archives of Environmental Health,* Vol.39, No.1, (January 1984), 11-17, ISSN 0003-9896

Wang, C. & Bhattacharyya, MH. (1993). Effect of cadmium on bone calcium and 45 Ca in nonpregnant mice on a calcium-deficient diet: evidence of direct effect of cadmium on bone. *Toxicology and Applied Pharmacology*, Vol.120, No.2, pp. 228-239, ISSN 0041-008X

Van Barveveld, A. & Van den Hamer, C. (1984). The influence of calcium and magnesium on manganese transport and utilization in mice. *Biological Trace Element Research,* Vol.6, pp. 489-493, ISSN 0163-4984

Yasutake, A.; Hirayama, K. & Inouye, M. (1990). Sex difference in acute renal dysfunction induced by methylmercury in mice. Renal Failure, Vol.12, pp. 233-240, ISSN 0886-022X

Yewey, GL. & Caughey, WS. (1988). Metals of bovine heart cytochrome c oxidase. In: *Cytochrome oxidase : structure, function and physiopathology*. Brunori & Chance, Vol.550, Annals of the New York Academy of Science, ISBN 0-89766-484-1, New York

Zadrożna, M. (2003). Recent environmental toxic effect in the Polish Copper Mining Territory on human reproduction. Part I. Response of the placenta to the chemical stress. *Folia Biologica*, Vol.51, No.3-4, (September 2003), pp. 201-205, ISSN 0015-5497

Zamorska, L.(1979). Lactate dehydrogenase isozymes as genetic characters in human placentae from selected regions of Poland. *Folia Biologica*, Vol.27, pp. 343-353, ISSN 0015-5497

Zamorska, L. (1982/1983). The activity of oxidative enzymes and morphology of the full-term human placentas collected in the area surrounding the smelter aluminum in Skawina. *Folia Medica Cracoviensia*, Vol.24, pp. 67-88, ISSN 0015-5616 (in Polish)

Zamorska, L. & Niweliński, J. (1982/1983). Some aspects of reproduction in humans in the current ecological situation of Cracow. *Folia Medica Cracoviensia*, Vol.24, pp.203-209, ISSN 0015-5616 (in Polish)

2

Early Pregnancy Screening for Complications of Pregnancy: Proteomic Profiling Approaches

Murray D. Mitchell and Gregory E. Rice
University of Queensland Centre for Clinical Research, Herston, Queensland, Australia

1. Introduction

The keystone to improving health outcomes remains the timely and accurate diagnosis of the predisposition to, or early detection of, disease. Early detection of disease risk and onset is the first step in implementing efficacious treatment and improving patient outcome. (Figure 1). In the context of antenatal screening, the objective of proteomic approaches is to identify proteins and peptides that are informative of the risk of asymptomatic early pregnant women subsequently developing complications of pregnancy. That is, how the antecedents of complications of pregnancy alter the expression of the genome and how this is manifested as altered protein and peptide expression. Informative proteins and peptides identified may be used to develop classification models (*e.g.* multiple biomarker diagnostic

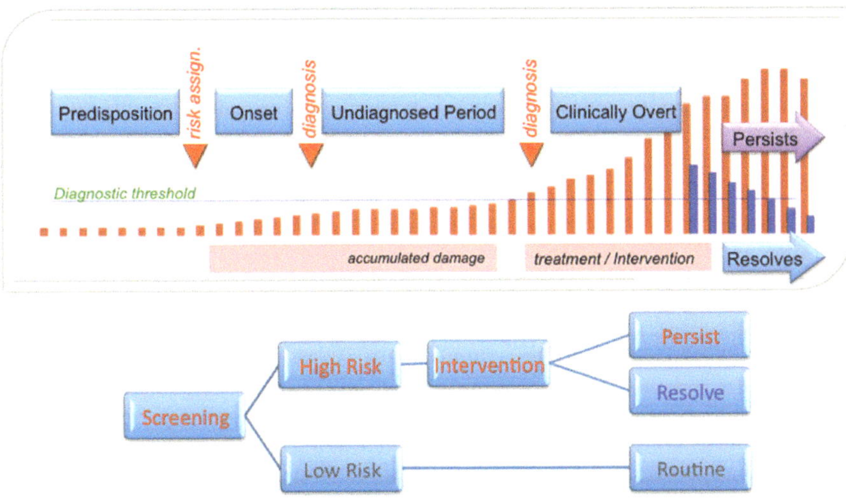

Fig. 1. The putative benefit of early pregnancy screening. A theoretical profile of disease progression in which disease onset is determined by diagnostic threshold. Once diagnosed, the condition can be treated and either persists or resolves. The rationale for both early screening and assessment of disease risk is early diagnosis of disease. Early diagnosis of disease affords the opportunity for early treatment and reduced adverse effects.

or prognostic tests) that assign the likelihood that an individual test sample came from a normal or "at risk" group. Such tests (as with all in vitro diagnostics, IVDs) inform clinical decision-making and provide an opportunity for timely and appropriate intervention. The performance of the test determines the quality of the information provided and ultimately the course of patient management. The bailiwick of proteomics, thus, extends beyond simply establishing the protein complement of a given sample and includes its contribution to the healthcare system.

Proteomic profiling technologies have undergone rapid development and diversification over the past decade, however, issues relating to the analysis of complex biological samples (such as plasma), achieving biomolecular bandwidth (*i.e.* the coverage of a given proteome that any one technique can attain) and translating outcomes into clinical practice remain (Rice *et al*, 2006). The objective of this brief commentary is to provide a conceptual and applications-based overview of how proteomic technologies may contribute to the development of IVDs for assigning risk of disease in both symptomatic and asymptomatic patients. At this time, there have been few Phase 2 (Pepe *et al*, 2001) (retrospective case control cohorts) and Phase 3 biomarker trials (longitudinal, cohort studies) completed that target the early pregnancy period (*i.e.* 6-12 weeks of gestation) and even fewer that consider complications other than chromosomal abnormalities or pre-eclampsia (PE).

2. Complications of pregnancy

Of the 130 million babies born each year, 8 million die before their first birthday. Four million babies die in the first 4 weeks of life (during the neonatal period). Three million of neonatal deaths occur in the first week, with the highest risk of death on the first day of life. More than 7 newborn babies die every second from what are ostensibly preventable causes (Zupan *et al*, 2005),(Lawn *et al*, 2005). A significant contributing factor in many of these deaths is poor pregnancy outcome as a result of a complication of pregnancy. Pre-eclampsia, intrauterine growth restriction (IUGR), gestational diabetes (GDM) and preterm birth (PTB) are the most important complications of pregnancy that have no effective antenatal treatment other than steroid administration and timely delivery. Each occurs with an incidence of 5-10% and are responsible for the majority of obstetric and paediatric morbidity and mortality and can permanently impact on life-long health. For example, PTB alone accounts for up to 2.7 million deaths per annum and ~50% of long-term neurological impairment. While, pre-eclampsia accounts for 10-15% of the 500,000 maternal deaths each year (Khan *et al*, 2006).

These complications of pregnancy are not usually clinically manifested until third trimester (*i.e.* > 24 weeks of pregnancy) thus limiting the window of opportunity to ameliorate adverse effects. Currently, there are no proven means of identifying asymptomatic women during the first trimester who subsequently develop complications of pregnancy (other than past obstetric history). Early detection of women at risk of complications of pregnancy would afford opportunity to develop and evaluate timely and appropriate intervention strategies to limit acute adverse sequelae (Figure 2).

The clinical imperative for the development of biomarkers for screening and monitoring pregnancy derives from the significant impact that undiagnosed, untreated and/or late-treated complications of pregnancy have on both the wellbeing of the mother and the newborn (including perinatal, neonatal and childhood development and adult susceptibility

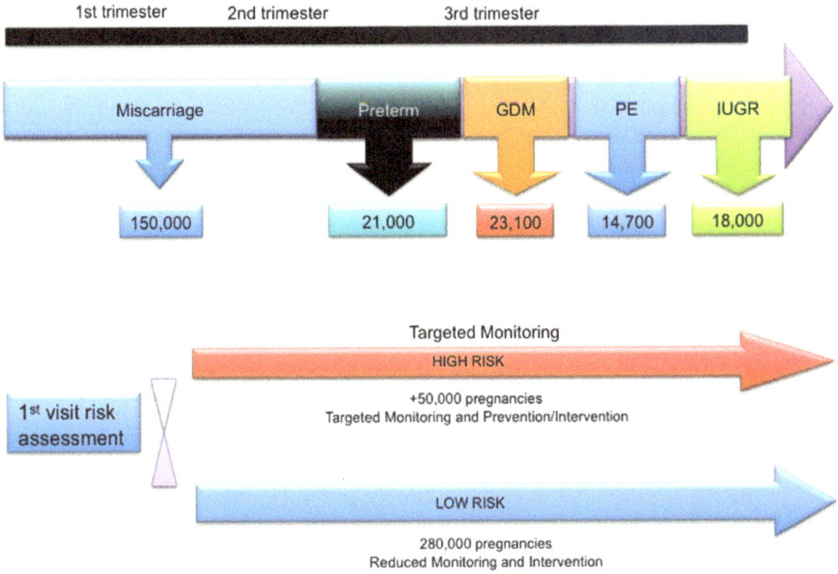

Fig. 2. In Australia in 2008, there were 294,700 live births (Laws *et al*, 2010). More than 60,000 women gave birth associated with a complication of pregnancy. 21,000 babies were born preterm (*i.e.* < 37 completed weeks of gestation). 18,000 babies were of low birthweight (<2500g). 23,100 pregnancies were complicated by GDM and 14,700 developed PE. Assessment of risk of developing a complication of pregnancy at first antenatal visit would provide opportunity to triage women to high- and low-risk management.

to disease). The development of predictive and diagnostic utilities for use at the first antenatal visit would provide, at least, an opportunity for more intensive monitoring of high-risk women and, at best, implementation of appropriate interventions.

Complications of pregnancy may represent symptom-defined manifestations of a single lesion. The available evidence supports the hypothesis that the etiology of complications of pregnancy (including for example PE, IUGR) may begin during 1st trimester (Brosens *et al*, 2002); (Meekins *et al*, 1994); (Jauniaux *et al*, 2006); (Norwitz, 2006). Such complications may originate from aberrant or suboptimal implantation and/or sequestration of the maternal uterine blood vessels. If pregnancy complications share a common etiology or elicit a common maternal response then changes in the profile (or specific patterns) of plasma proteins measured during early and /or mid-pregnancy may be informative in identifying women at risk. Identification of such proteins would provide opportunity to develop clinically useful early pregnancy screening tests to identify women at risk of developing complications during pregnancy. If this can be achieved it would provide an opportunity for early identification of risk and the implementation of an alternative clinical management to improve outcome for both mother and baby.

In addition to the acute effects on maternal and newborn morbidity and mortality, complications of pregnancy may adversely affect life-long disease susceptibility of the newborn and intergenerational health via epigenetic modification of the fetal genome (Weaver *et al*, 2004; WHO, 2006). Epigenetic modification is defined as alteration of the regulation of genomic information by means that do not result in a change in DNA sequence, but have a significant impact on the development and phenotype of an organism (Santos & Dean, 2004). The epigenome is responsive to external environmental factors including, but not limited to, nutrition and endocrine disruptors. Epimutations in the germline that become permanently programmed may be transmitted as epigenetic transgenerational phenotypes. The "external" environment for the placenta (and fetus) is maternal blood. The placenta and fetal membranes play a critical role in filtering or buffering environmental influences (Myatt, 2006). Changes in the external *milieu* (*e.g.* blood pressure, hyperglycemia (Brasacchio *et al*, 2009); (El-Osta *et al*, 2008); ischemia (Kumral *et al*, 2009; Parker *et al*, 2008)) and/or diet (e.g. butyrate (Vidali *et al*, 1978), organosulfur (Tissenbaum & Guarente, 2001), dietary polyphenols (Howitz *et al*, 2003), folate, and choline (Fang & Xiao, 2003)) may induce adaptive or compensatory epigenetic modifications within the placental and/or fetal genomes. Thus, periconceptional and early pregnancy events may affect the placental and/or fetal epigenome. This may be particularly relevant for women who experience complications of pregnancy that impact on placental structure and function. Early detection of women at risk of complications of pregnancy would afford opportunity to develop and evaluate timely and appropriate intervention strategies to limit long-term and intergenerational adverse sequelae.

The rationale for developing antenatal screening tests, thus, is not only for the management of the contemporaneous pregnancy but also to optimise life-long and intergenerational health. The diagnostic performance of antenatal screening tests may not need to be high to be effective. Unlike diseases such as cancer where IVDs need to be exquisitely specific (Edgell *et al*, 2010a; Edgell *et al*, 2010b; Rice *et al*, 2010), a useful antenatal screening test would ideally be highly sensitive, but not necessarily highly specific. The consequence of a false positive would be no worse than an erroneous triage to high-risk care.

3. Early pregnancy screening

Previous approaches to develop an early pregnancy-screening test for women at risk of developing complications of pregnancy have not been of great success. For example, with respect to pre-eclampsia, while it has been possible to identify blood-borne biomarkers that have pre-symptomatic predictive potential (including: activin-A (Diesch *et al*, 2006), C-reactive protein (Mihu *et al*, 2008), placenta growth factor and its receptor FLT (Shokry *et al*), leptin (Sucak *et al*), transforming growth factor-β1 and plasminogen activator inhibitor (Belo *et al*, 2002)), such markers have proven of limited clinical utility, lacking suitable sensitivity and specificity. No single marker has been described permitting early prediction of pre-eclampsia in the individual.

It is now widely acknowledged that single biomarkers are unlikely to deliver significant incremental gain in sensitivity and specificity that will be required for the development of effective screening and classification tests requisite for the implementation of personalized medicine. New approaches based upon the measurement of multiple biomarkers of disease risk afford opportunity to increase diagnostic test sensitivity and specificity. Even the use of two biomarkers can deliver improved performance. For example, cardiovascular risk classification is significantly improved by simply combining LDL-cholesterol and C-reactive protein data (Rifai & Ridker, 2003). The use of modelling algorithms to combine multiple known biomarkers (*e.g.* candidate-based approaches) similarly may increase diagnostic efficiency and deliver classification models of clinical utility (Fushiki *et al*, 2006; Kikuchi & Carbone, 2007; Kikuchi *et al*, 1989; Listgarten & Emili, 2005). Both candidate-based applications (*i.e.* in which the identity of the analytes being measured are well-established) and signature profiling applications (*i.e.* in which characteristic patterns or motifs within a signal profile are identified) may be utilized in the development of multivariate modelling strategies for the delivery of more informative diagnostic tests (Anderson, 2005).

Recent advances in the acquisition of proteomic and peptidomic data, methods of analysis and multivariate modelling approaches afford opportunities to deliver IVDs with increased diagnostic efficiencies. In the case of higher prevalence diseases, such as complications of pregnancy, these new approaches may contribute to the development of "first-visit" antenatal screening programs.

Using a similar rationale, (Horgan *et al*) recently reported that metabolomic profiles identified using ultra performance liquid chromatography-mass spectrometry were able to characterize a phenotypic signature for small for gestational age (SGA) babies. The authors concluded that the finding of a consistent discriminatory metabolite signature in early pregnancy plasma preceding the onset of SGA offers insight into disease pathogenesis and offers the promise of a robust pre-symptomatic screening test.

4. Defining the proteome

The proteome is the manifestation of the conditional expression of the genome. Proteomics, thus, defines the regional and temporal expression of proteins (and peptides) that characterize a given phenotype and how changes in expression impact the structure and function of the organism. It is the systematic, reproducible, differential and/or quantitative characterization of the peptide or protein complement under a defined biological state(s). In particular, its *raison d'être* is to elucidate networks and pathways that ensure coordinated and appropriate development of biologic organisms and to maintain homeostasis in response to physiological or pathological challenges. In its simplest form, proteomics is a reductive approach that reduces system complexity to more basic components, thus, enabling classical hypothesis testing. It affords the opportunity to characterize physiology and pathophysiology in terms of defined and specific changes in proteins and peptides that comprise the human proteome.

In recent years, it has been recognized that the complexity of the mammalian transcriptome and its functional expression as proteins far exceeds previous expectations. It is now estimated that only ~1.2% of the human genome contains protein-coding information. The expression of these ~21,000 genes, the elaboration of ~10^5 transcripts (*via* alternative splicing, alternate promoters and RNA editing) and the post-translational modification account for more than 10^6 proteins comprising the human proteome. It has been estimated, in some cases, that up to 100 different proteins may be derived from the expression of a single gene. An informed understanding of the ontogeny and complications of pregnancy, therefore, will include not only genomic and transcriptomic analysis but also information as to how global protein expression changes. This is the bailiwick of proteomics - defining the conditional expression of the genome.

As alluded to above, proteomic methodologies, however, now extend beyond the mapping of the protein complement of defined proteomes to proteome-wide profiling approaches

(Patterson & Aebersold, 2003). New approaches offer opportunities to: define protein expression profiles that reflect phenotypic change; and contribute to the development of prognostic and diagnostic applications. Such approaches apply preceptive filters to the proteome (*e.g.* knowledge-data bases, in the case of targeted proteomics or multivariate mathematical modelling in the case of protein/peptide profiling strategies) to extract data of contextual relevance. Proteomics affords opportunity to identify changes in specific subsets of proteins that are associated with variance from normal and to interrogate their role in the etiology of pregnancy complications.

There are three common approaches to the application of proteomics: cartographic or expression proteomics - the definition of normal expression profiles of proteins and peptides, how they are modified and processed (Di Quinzio *et al*, 2007); comparative profiling - in which protein expression profiles from different physiologic and/or pathologic states are compared for the purpose of identifying condition- or treatment-associated changes (Di Quinzio *et al*, 2008) and targeted profiling - in which specific known subsets of proteins are monitored (Heng *et al*, 2009) (Georgiou *et al*, 2008).

Common to the successful application of all approaches is the capacity to reduce sample complexity and to target a subfraction of the proteome for analysis, as no currently available platform provides proteome-wide display (Ahmed & Rice, 2005). With respect to sample complexity, a major challenge has been the identification of low abundance proteins that may reflect biological and/or clinical circumstance in the presence of overwhelming concentrations of high abundance protein species. Both depletion and enrichment sub-fractionation approaches have been employed with varying degrees of success, including affinity depletion of albumin (Ahmed *et al*, 2003), other high abundance proteins (Georgiou *et al*, 2001)) and affinity-capture enrichment of low abundance species (Callesen *et al*, 2009). It is becoming increasingly evident that combinations of multiple approaches and targeting of specific display bandwidths will be required to achieve the display resolution required to identify putative low abundance biomarkers.

5. Proteomic approaches for profiling early pregnancy

The identification of protein and peptide signatures or motifs contained within biological samples for the purpose of donor classification is a burgeoning area within the domain of diagnostic and predictive medicine. The premise upon which such initiatives are based is that: the expression of specific proteins or peptides and/or their metabolites is altered by and reflective or informative of the attendant pathophysiology; and the measurement and combination of multiple biomarkers of disease, may increase diagnostic sensitivity and specificity. Once established, reference profiles measured from healthy sample cohorts may be used as a template to detect variance and thus deliver a diagnostic or predictive capacity. Several proteomic-based approaches have been applied to identify informative biomarkers of complications of pregnancy, including protein solution array, 1 and 2 dimensional gel electrophoresis and mass spectrometry-based peptide profiling.

5.1 Solution array

Multiplex protein solution array has a number of advantages over current analyte quantification technologies, including: measurement of many biomarkers (theoretically, up to 100 different analytes) in a single sample; wider operational dynamic range; and increased sensitivity and specificity derived from multivariate modelling of combinations of biomarker analytes. This system utilizes a sandwich ELISA-like protocol, in which capture antibodies are coupled to spectrally distinct beads. Biotinylated sandwich antibody and streptavidin- phycoerytherin fluorophore are used as a reporter complex. Bead identity and analyte-specific fluorescence are assessed using a flow cytometer.

Georgiou *et al*, 2008 utilized protein solution array to measure multiple plasma biomarkers at 11 weeks of gestation in women who subsequently experienced normal pregnancy outcomes and women who subsequently developed gestational diabetes. Of the biomarkers considered, three biomarkers (adiponectin, insulin and blood glucose) displayed informative diagnostic characteristics (*i.e.* area under the receiver operator characteristic curve, AUC, adiponectin =0.867; insulin =0.872 and glucose =0.827). When these markers were combined in a multivariate classification and predicted posterior probability values generated, the classification model generated significantly outperformed individual biomarkers (model AUC = 0.94). This simple example demonstrates the putative benefit of a multimarker approach for improving diagnostic efficiency. While this Phase 1 biomarker trial delivered promising data, a much larger trial is required to establish diagnostic performance in an obstetric population.

5.2 Gel-based profiling

The gel-based platforms such as 1-dimensional and 2-dimensional polyacrylamide gel electrophoresis (2D PAGE) and fluorescence 2D difference gel electrophoresis (DIGE) have been used in both expression and comparative studies to define plasma protein abundance and disease-associated or treatment-induced changes. The advantage of these approaches resides in their ability to identify post-translational modified protein isoforms. The limitation of gel-based systems is their relatively low throughput, the necessity for sample processing and fractionation prior to display and limited mass range (~10-200 kDa). In addition, procedural protein losses and the overall experimental variation in estimating endpoints by 2D PAGE may be considerable. Procedural losses of proteins during 2DE PAGE display have been reported to be as high as 80% but this can vary depending on the initial protein load. As with any other technique, variation is apportioned between technical replication, both within assay and between assay, and biologic variation (*i.e.* sample-to-sample). Estimates of the variation attributable to technical replication average 25-40%. Biological variation has been estimated to be between 24 and 70% (Molloy *et al*, 2003).

We have utilized a 2D-PAGE approach to identify putative plasma biomarkers of GDM. Using a traditional 2D PAGE approach, maternal plasma proteome from women with a normal pregnancy were compared with women who subsequently developed GDM. Using this approach more than 600 protein spots were visualized. Of these more than 20 proteins were differentially-expressed in pre-symptomatic women. Some of these protein spots are unique to pre-GDM while others are also differentially-expressed during overt disease. In some cases only specific isomers of a particular protein were differentially-expressed (Figure 3).

Using this approach, gestation-associated changes in plasma protein expression changes can be established for individual patients (Figure 4). This latter application may be of utility in the development of personalized medicine approaches to risk assessment and disease monitoring during pregnancy.

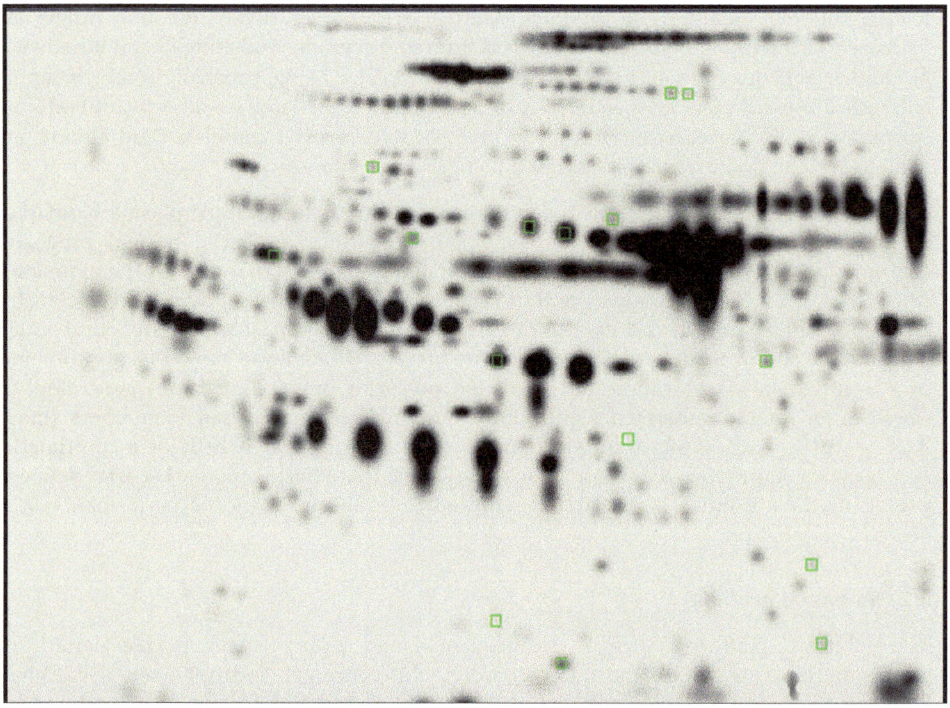

Fig. 3. 2D-PAGE Gaussian image of human plasma obtained at approximately 12 weeks' gestation. Boxes indicate protein spots that were significantly differentially-expressed in women who subsequently developed GDM compared to gestation-matched women who had a normal pregnancy.

The limitations of this methodology include (i) tedious and sometimes unreliable matching of hundreds of spots in multiple gels, (ii) problems associated with spot normalization, (iii) limited in-built statistical capacity to compare protein abundance, (iv) difficulty with excision of spots especially in small gel formats, and (v) the failure to reliably characterize proteins by MALDI-ToF mass spectrometry due to low protein abundance. This necessitates the need to up-scale methods for protein characterization (orthogonal identification).

Some of the limitations of gel-based approaches have been overcome with the development of difference gel electrophoresis. This minimal labeling approach using fluorescent cyanine dyes increases throughput by reducing sample processing and both gel-to-gel and analytical variation by combining case and control samples into a single processing step, and by the use of an internal standard for normalization of data across gels (as described above). DIGE also delivers useful relative quantification of protein expression profiles where the dyes are purported to have sub-nanogram sensitivity and a linear response to protein concentrations of over five orders of magnitude. The dyes are also compatible with mass spectrometric analysis. With respect to analyzing the plasma proteome, DIGE is still limited by the compositional complexity of plasma and similarly benefits from sample fractionation and the removal of high-abundance proteins.

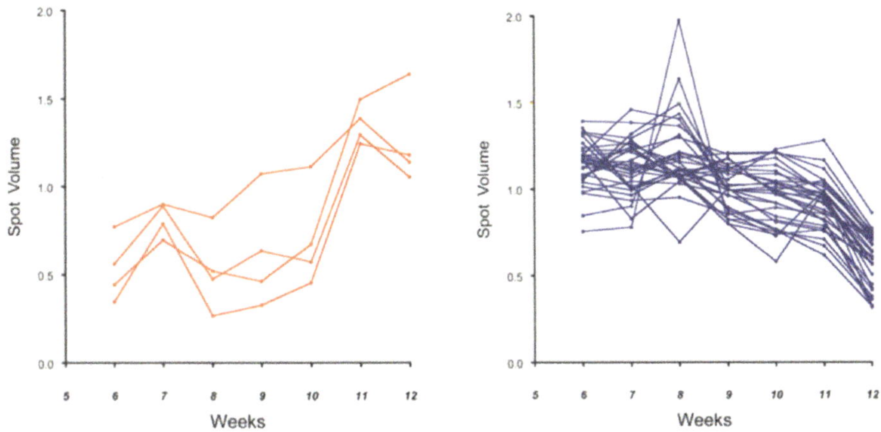

Fig. 4. Variation in plasma proteins displayed during early pregnancy (6-12 weeks of gestation). Serial peripheral blood samples were collected from women and displayed using 2D-DIGE. The data presented represent normalized spot volumes for protein spots identified that either increased or decreased during early gestation.

5.3 Mass spectrometry-based profiling

Mass spectrometry-based approaches for identifying and establishing relative changes in biomarker abundance included: stable isotope labeling techniques and label-free strategies. Stable isotope labeling has the advantage of being more sensitive and reproducible than gel-based methods. These approaches utilize either a mass tag coding strategy (*e.g.* ICPL - Isotope Coded Protein Labeling, ICAT - Isotope Coded Affinity Tag) or iTRAQ - isobaric Tag for Relative and Absolute Quantitation) that allow pooling of samples to reduce technical variation. Label-free quantitation is an approach that holds the promise of true MudPIT-type 'shotgun' quantitation and has some advantages in sample preparation, cost and the challenge of normalizing the data so that accurate quantitation can be done across multiple samples and multiple analyses.

In addition to its analytical applications, mass spectrometry affords opportunities to identify signature profiles contained within biological samples for the purpose of classification. The application of mass spectrometry is a burgeoning area within the domain of diagnostic and predictive medicine. This approach now affords the opportunity to develop disease-specific patterns or profiles based upon the presence of specific peptides in a patient sample. MS-based protein profiling relies on the presence and spatial relationships between peptide peaks to facilitate the classification of biological samples into different categories (*e.g.* normal and disease). Based upon the analysis of a training sample set (*e.g.* disease-free patients), pattern recognition software and multivariate modelling are employed to build peptide profiles or motifs that characterize a disease-free condition. Once established, such reference profiles may be used as a template to detect variance and thus deliver a diagnosis or predictive capacity.

Over the past 5 years, our research groups have utilized two mass spectrometry-based profiling approaches to identify peptides that may be informative of disease risk: affinity-capture MALDI-ToF and iTRAQ. In an initial prospective study of plasma samples collected from women (at 6-12 weeks' and 26-30 weeks' gestation), samples were analyzed after removal of high abundance proteins and following a single fractionation process. Immobilized Metal Affinity Chromatography (IMAC, ClinProt™), Bruker Daltonics) was used to capture a subpopulation of peptides for subsequent MALDI-ToF mass spectrometry profiling. Complication-specific, differentially-expressed peptide ion peaks were identified (*e.g.* Figure 5) that provided classification models of promising utility.

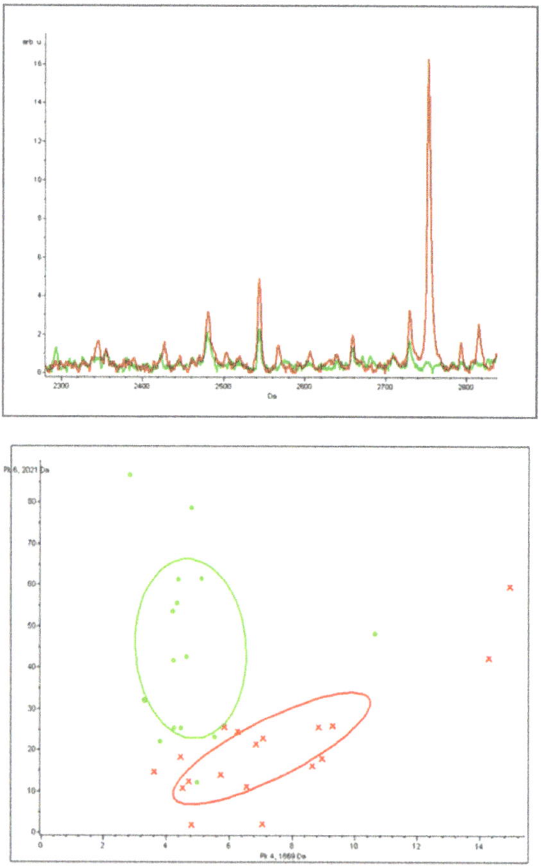

Fig. 5. An example of MALDI-ToF peptide profiling and bivariate cluster analysis. **Top.** Example of the average peptide profiles over a limited spectral range (2300-2800 m/z) is presented to illustrate identified differences in peptide profiles between women with a normal pregnancy (red, n=19, 12 weeks) and women who subsequently developed GDM (green, n=16, 12 weeks). **Bottom.** A peptide peak cluster plot highlighting the potential for using differentially-expressed peptides to classify women into low- and high-risk groups for subsequent development of GDM. The plot presents the data (integrated area) of two peptide peaks (1669 vs 2021 m/z) observed in plasma obtained from women (12 weeks' gestation) who subsequently experienced a normal (red) or GDM pregnancy (green). Standard deviation envelopes are presented.

Both bivariate cluster plots and multivariate modelling discriminated between women who subsequently experienced normal or complicated pregnancies. Disease-specific differentially-detected peptide ion peaks were identified and used to develop multivariate classification models (Support Vector Machine and Genetic Mutation Models) that discriminated between women who subsequently experienced a normal or GDM pregnancy. For example, using a genetic mutation classification model, 5 peptides were selected that had the ability to correctly classify 100% of women to a low-risk group (i.e. those women who subsequently experienced a normal pregnancy). Furthermore, the model correctly classified greater than 93% of those women who subsequently experienced a GDM pregnancy. While this Phase 1 biomarker trial has delivered promising data a further larger trial is required to validate these findings.

Of considerable note, was the observation that when data were combined into a normal and complicated group (*i.e.* all complications), both cluster analysis (Figure 6) and modelling algorithms of diagnostic utility were generated. This approach may be of use in the development of personalized medicine approaches to assess disease risk during pregnancy.

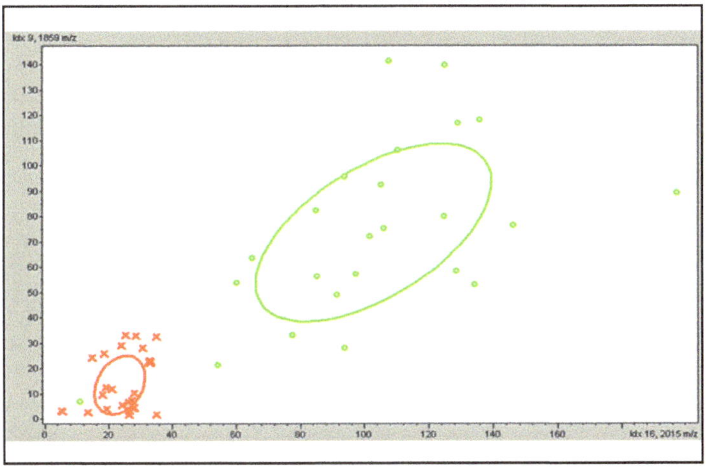

Fig. 6. A peptide peak cluster plot highlighting the potential for using differentially-expressed peptides to classify women into low- and high-risk groups for subsequent complication of pregnancy (PE, IUGR, GDM and PTB) . The plot presents the data (integrated area) of two peptide peaks (1859 vs 2015 m/z) observed in plasma. The plot depicts data obtained from women who subsequently experienced a normal (red) or experienced a complicated pregnancy (green). Standard deviation envelopes are presented.

Additionally, an iTRAQ mass spectrometry-based approach has been used to identify and quantify (relative to control) disease-specific peptide ion abundance in maternal plasma samples. This isotopic labeling method is arguably the benchmark for relative protein quantification. One significant benefit is that it allows sample multiplexing. High-abundance protein depleted plasma pools were generated from asymptomatic pregnant women at 12-18 weeks' gestation. Samples were digested with trypsin and each digested sample was labeled with one of four different iTRAQ reagents (normal 114, IUGR 116, GDM 118 and Macrosomia 121) and analyzed by LC-MS/MS for simultaneous protein identification and peptide quantification. Relative abundance of proteins in depleted plasma was determined by comparing the peak heights of reporter ions. Using this approach, 22 proteins that were differentially-expressed in maternal plasma in association with complications of pregnancy were unambiguously identified. Further studies are currently assessing the performance of these biomarkers in IVD panels.

6. Signature profiling and IVD development

A recent trend in the development of more efficient diagnostic tests has been the use of algorithm-based multivariate index assays (IVDMIAs). With the development of this new class of IVD, the discipline has sought new biostatistical approaches for assessing and quantifying incremental gains in diagnostic efficiency. Traditionally, the area under the receiver operator characteristic curve (AUC) has been used as a measure and comparator of diagnostic efficiency. Several investigators have argued that this measure alone may be imperfect and inefficient for comparing the true clinical usefulness of alternative marker panels (Pencina *et al*; Pencina *et al*, 2008). These authors reviewed several biomarker studies and observed that when evaluating improvement in risk assignment of biomarkers, very large odds ratios were often associated with very small increases in the AUC. This feature of the receiver operator characteristic curve analysis limits its utility in identifying putative beneficial contributions of new biomarkers to algorithm-based models. Pencina *et al*, therefore, proposed the use of two new methods for evaluating the diagnostic efficiency of biomarkers. These two methods are: (i) Net Reclassification Improvement (NRI); and (ii) Integrated Discrimination Improvement (IDI). The NRI is based on counts of the number of true positives showing an increase in probability of an event and the number of true negatives showing a decrease in probability of an event. The IDI is based on the integral of sensitivity and specificity of all possible thresholds. These new methods provide alternative statistical approaches for validating biomarkers and IVDMIAs.

7. Concluding comments

Complications of pregnancy remain a major health issue of the 21st century. They result in preventable mortality and morbidity to both mother and baby. Too few studies have focused on the development of early pregnancy risk assessment modalities. As a consequence, it has not been possible to robustly evaluate any putative early pregnancy intervention strategies that may improve pregnancy and life-long outcomes. Indeed, driven by health economic imperatives, it is becoming increasingly more difficult to establish longitudinal early pregnancy study cohorts (*i.e.* from 6 weeks of pregnancy) in our tertiary care hospitals. With recent advances in proteomic and peptidomic technologies and the development of formalized approaches for establishing and validating multivariate index assays, it is not unrealistic to suggest that more informative antenatal screening tests will be implemented within the next 5-10 years. Such IVDs would allow, at least, the triage of women at 6-12 weeks of pregnancy into high- and low-risk clinical management pathways.

Furthermore, we recognize the imperative to establish not only early pregnancy clinics but also preconception clinics to ensure an optimal start to life and lower risk of adult disease.

8. Acknowledgements

Aspects of the experimental data presented herein were funded by NHMRC Grants 509127, 526686 and 586651. GER was in receipt of an NHMRC Principal Research Fellowship.

9. References

Ahmed N, Barker G, Oliva K, Garfin D, Talmadge K, Georgiou H, Quinn M, Rice G (2003) An approach to remove albumin for the proteomic analysis of low abundance biomarkers in human serum. *Proteomics* 3: 1980-7

Ahmed N, Rice GE (2005) Strategies for revealing lower abundance proteins in two-dimensional protein maps. *Journal of Chromatography B: Analytical Technologies in the Biomedical & Life Sciences* 815: 39-50

Anderson L (2005) Candidate-based proteomics in the search for biomarkers of cardiovascular disease. *J Physiol (Lond)* 563: 23-60

Belo L, Santos-Silva A, Rumley A, Lowe G, Pereira-Leite L, Quintanilha A, Rebelo I (2002) Elevated tissue plasminogen activator as a potential marker of endothelial dysfunction in pre-eclampsia: correlation with proteinuria. *Bjog-an International Journal of Obstetrics and Gynaecology* 109: 1250-1255

Brasacchio D, Okabe J, Tikellis C, Balcerczyk A, George P, Baker EK, Calkin AC, Brownlee M, Cooper ME, El-Osta A (2009) Hyperglycemia Induces a Dynamic Cooperativity of Histone Methylase and Demethylase Enzymes Associated With Gene-Activating Epigenetic Marks That Coexist on the Lysine Tail. *Diabetes* 58: 1229-1236

Brosens JJ, Pijnenborg R, Brosens IA (2002) The myometrial junctional zone spiral arteries in normal and abnormal pregnancies: a review of the literature. *Am J Obstet Gynecol* 187: 1416-23

Callesen AK, Madsen JS, Vach W, Kruse TA, Mogensen O, Jensen ON (2009) Serum protein profiling by solid phase extraction and mass spectrometry: A future diagnostics tool? *Proteomics* 9: 1428-1441

Di Quinzio MKW, Georgiou HM, Holdsworth-Carson SJ, Ayhan M, Heng YJ, Walker SP, Rice GE, Permezel M (2008) Proteomic analysis of human cervico-vaginal fluid displays differential protein expression in association with labor onset at term. *J Proteome Res* 7: 1916-1921

Di Quinzio MKW, Oliva K, Holdsworth SJ, Ayhan M, Walker SP, Rice GE, Georgiou HM, Permezel M (2007) Proteomic analysis and characterisation of human cervico-vaginal fluid proteins. *Aust N Z J Obstet Gynaecol* 47: 9-15

Diesch CH, Holzgreve W, Hahn S, Zhong XY (2006) Comparison of activin A and cell-free fetal DNA levels in maternal plasma from patients at high risk for preeclampsia. *Prenat Diagn* 26: 1267-1270

Edgell T, Martin-Roussety G, Barker G, Autelitano DJ, Allen D, Grant P, Rice GE (2010a) Phase II biomarker trial of a multimarker diagnostic for ovarian cancer. *J Cancer Res Clin Oncology* 3: 1079-89.

Edgell TA, Barraclough DL, Rajic A, Dhulia J, Lewis KJ, Armes JE, Barraclough R, Rudland PS, Rice GE, Autelitano DJ (2010b) Increased plasma concentrations of anterior gradent 2 protein are positively associated with ovarian cancer. *Clin Sci (Lond)* 118: 717-725

El-Osta A, Brasacchio D, Yao DC, Pocai A, Jones PL, Roeder RG, Cooper ME, Brownlee M (2008) Transient high glucose causes persistent epigenetic changes and altered gene expression during subsequent normoglycemia. *J Exp Med* 205: 2409-2417

Fang JY, Xiao SD (2003) Folic acid, polymorphism of methyl-group metabolism genes, and DNA methylation in relation to GI carcinogenesis. *J Gastroenterol* 38: 821-9

Fushiki T, Fujisawa H, Eguchi S (2006) Identification of biomarkers from mass spectrometry data using a "common" peak approach. *BMC Bioinformatics* 7: 358

Georgiou HM, Lappas M, Georgiou GM, Marita A, Bryant VJ, Hiscock R, Permezel M, Khalil Z, Rice GE (2008) Screening for biomarkers predictive of gestational diabetes mellitus. *Acta Diabetologica* 45: 157-165

Georgiou HM, Rice GE, Baker MS (2001) Proteomic analysis of human plasma: failure of centrifugal ultrafiltration to remove albumin and other high molecular weight proteins. *Proteomics* 1: 1503-6

Heng YJJ, Di Quinzio MKW, Permezel M, Rice GE, Georgiou HM (2009) Multiple Novel Predictors of Human Labor. *Reproductive Sciences* 16: 160

Horgan RP, Broadhurst DI, Walsh SK, Dunn WB, Brown M, Roberts CT, North RA, McCowan LM, Kell DB, Baker PN, Kenny LC Metabolic Profiling Uncovers a Phenotypic Signature of Small for Gestational Age in Early Pregnancy. *J Proteome Res* 10: 3660-3673

Howitz KT, Bitterman KJ, Cohen HY, Lamming DW, Lavu S, Wood JG, Zipkin RE, Chung P, Kisielewski A, Zhang LL, Scherer B, Sinclair DA (2003) Small molecule activators of sirtuins extend Saccharomyces cerevisiae lifespan. *Nature* 425: 191-6

Jauniaux E, Poston L, Burton GJ (2006) Placental-related diseases of pregnancy: Involvement of oxidative stress and implications in human evolution. *Hum Reprod Update* 12: 747-55

Khan KS, Wojdyla D, Say L, Gulmezoglu AM, Van Look PFA (2006) WHO analysis of causes of maternal death: a systematic review. *Lancet* 367: 1066-1074

Kikuchi T, Carbone DP (2007) Proteomics analysis in lung cancer: challenges and opportunities. *Respirology* 12: 22-8

Kikuchi Y, Kita T, Iwano I, Kuki E, Oomori K, Kizawa I (1989) Prediction of clinical course and recurrence of human ovarian cancer by several serum tumor markers. *Nippon Sanka Fujinka Gakkai Zasshi - Acta Obstetrica et Gynaecologica Japonica* 41: 69-76

Kumral A, Tuzun F, Yesilirmak D, Duman N, Ozkan H (2009) Role of epigenetic regulatory mechanisms in neonatal hypoxic-ischemic brain injury. *Medical Hypotheses* 72: 692-693

Lawn JE, Cousens S, Zupan J, Lancet Neonatal Survival S (2005) Neonatal survival 1 - 4 million neonatal deaths: When? where? why? *Lancet* 365: 891-900

Laws P, Li Z, Sullivan EA (2010) Australia's mothers and babies 2008. Perinatal statistics series no. 24. Cat. no. PER 50. , AIHW. (ed). Canberra

Listgarten J, Emili A (2005) Statistical and computational methods for comparative proteomic profiling using liquid chromatography-tandem mass spectrometry. *Mol Cell Proteomics* 4: 419-434

Meekins JW, Pijnenborg R, Hanssens M, McFadyen IR, van Asshe A (1994) A study of placental bed spiral arteries and trophoblast invasion in normal and severe pre-eclamptic pregnancies. *Br J Obstet Gynaecol* 101

Mihu D, Costin N, Mihu CM, Blaga LD, Pop RB (2008) C-reactive protein, marker for evaluation of systemic inflammatory response in preeclampsia. *Rev Med Chir Soc Med Nat Iasi* 112: 1019-25

Molloy MP, Brzezinski EE, Hang J, McDowell MT, VanBogelen RA (2003) Overcoming technical variation and biological variation in quantitative proteomics. *Proteomics* 3: 1912-9

Myatt L (2006) Placental adaptive responses and fetal programming. *J Physiol* 572

Norwitz ER (2006) Defective implantation and placentation: laying the blueprint for pregnancy complications. *Reprod Biomed Online* 13: 591-599

Parker MD, Chambers PA, Lodge JPA, Pratt JR (2008) Ischemia-reperfusion Injury and Its Influence on the Epigenetic Modification of the Donor Kidney Genome. *Transplantation* 86: 1818-1823

Patterson SD, Aebersold RH (2003) Proteomics: the first decade and beyond. *Nat Genet* 33 Suppl: 311-23

Pencina MJ, D'Agostino RB, Steyerberg EW Extensions of net reclassification improvement calculations to measure usefulness of new biomarkers. *Statistics in Medicine* 30: 11-21

Pencina MJ, D'Agostino RB, Vasan RS (2008) Evaluating the added predictive ability of a new marker: From area under the ROC curve to reclassification and beyond. *Statistics in Medicine* 27: 157-172

Pepe MS, Etzioni R, Feng Z, Potter JD, Thompson ML, Thornquist M, Winget M, Yasui Y (2001) Phases of bimarker development for early detection of cancer. *J Natl Cancer Inst* 93: 1054-1056

Rice GE, Edgell T, Autelitano DJ (2010) Evaluation of midkine and anterior gradient 2 in a multimarker panel for the detection of ovarian cancer. *Journal of Experimental & Clinical Cancer Research* 29: 62

Rice GE, Georgiou HM, Ahmed N, Shi G, Kruppa G (2006) Translational proteomics: Developing a predictive capacity - A review. *Placenta* 27: S76-S86

Rifai N, Ridker PM (2003) Population distributions of C-reactive protein in apparently healthy men and women in the United States: implication for clinical interpretation. *Clin Chem* 49: 666-9

Santos F, Dean W (2004) Epigenetic reprogramming during early development in mammals. *Reproduction* 127: 643-651

Shokry M, Bedaiwy MA, Fathalla MMF, Alsemary A, Elwakil S, Murphy A Maternal serum placental growth factor and soluble fms-like tyrosine kinase 1 as early predictors of preeclampsia. *Acta Obstetricia Et Gynecologica Scandinavica* 89: 143-146

Sucak A, Kanat-Pektas M, Gungor T, Mollamahmutoglu L Leptin levels and antihypertensive treatment in preeclampsia. *Singapore Medical Journal* 51: 39-43

Tissenbaum HA, Guarente L (2001) Increased dosage of a sir-2 gene extends lifespan in Caenorhabditis elegans. *Nature* 410: 227-30

Vidali G, Boffa LC, Bradbury EM, Allfrey VG (1978) Butyrate suppression of histone deacetylation leads to accumulation of multiacetylated forms of histones H3 and

H4 and increased DNase I sensitivity of the associated DNA sequences. *Proc Natl Acad Sci U S A* 75: 2239-43

Weaver IC, Cervoni N, Champagne FA, D'Alessio AC, Sharma S, Seckl JR, Dymov S, Szyf M, Meaney MJ (2004) Epigenetic programming by maternal behavior. *Nature neuroscience* 7: 847-54

WHO (2006) Promoting optimal fetal development: report of a technical consultation. *World Health Organization*

Zupan J, Aahman E, 2005 (2005) Perinatal mortality for the year 2000: estimates developed by WHO. Geneva: World Health Organization

3

Aqueous Extract of Human Placenta as a Therapeutic Agent

Piyali Datta Chakraborty[1] and Debasish Bhattacharyya[2,*]
[1]*Albert David Ltd, Kolkata,*
[2]*Division of Structural Biology and Bioinformatics,*
CSIR- Indian Institute of Chemical Biology, Kolkata,
India

1. Introduction

Traditional folk medicine makes good use of the flora and fauna of a region, including a number of mineral substances. These herbs and animals are used either whole or in part and made up in either simple or complicated preparations and have proved to be effective therapeutic remedies. Some of these medicinal substances of animal origin have been quite thoroughly studied with modern scientific methods, and their therapeutic properties have been confirmed although not always explained. Many others have yet to be subjected to scientific analysis and tests before their real value can be judged. Products of animal origin despite of their therapeutic values have been banned in many countries for the sake of sustainable development in addition to safeguard ecological balance.

It is known from traditional folk knowledge that the placenta, supporting the baby's growth and development in the mother's womb, contains a wide range of biologically active components. Research over decades has been uncovering more and more of these compounds. Indeed, it is claimed that the placenta is capable of producing just about any substance found in any organ of the body. This biochemical treasure house supplies the growing fetus with substances that the fetus itself cannot synthesize. Though a rich source of bioactive components unless recovered, placenta becomes a biomedical waste immediately after childbirth. Use of human placenta as a therapeutic agent, therefore, in no way hampers ecological balance rather promotes resource recovery from a designated biomedical waste. Since most of the natural products of medicinal value have a vast repertoire of potent biological components, there has been an increasing realization to shun synthetic and semi-synthetic medicines primarily because of their harmful side effects.

Research on human placental extract gained a momentum with the description of the preparation of its extract by Russian ophthalmologist Prof. V.P. Filatov. Prior to his research, there were no documents of therapeutic efficacy of the extract, though its use was popular in Europe and parts of Asia primarily China, Korea and Japan for over a century. Review of placenta therapy reveals its long usage from the days of distant past. Recent medical history

* Corresponding author

from 1912 showed that Filatov started research on grafting human corneas using the principle of transplantation of preserved material. He observed that when animal or vegetable tissues are isolated from the organism and subjected to the action of environmental factors that inhibit their vital processes, they undergo a biochemical readjustment. In consequence to this readjustment, the tissues develop substances that stimulate their vital processes. Filatov named these substances as *Biogenic stimulators* (Filatov, 1951). After many clinical experiments, Filatov was convinced that any tissue of human or animal origin could be used to obtain curative effect and this tissue may not necessarily correspond histologically to the tissue affected by the pathological process. He extended this principle to general medicine and confirmed that the process was just as valid for other human tissues. That is how the principle of therapeutic tissue was born (Filatov, 1955).

Placenta serves as a natural storehouse of many biologically active components with significant healing attributes (Tonello et al., 1996). Various extracts of placenta have been described, however, only an aqueous extract of fresh full term human placenta acts as a potent biogenous stimulator (Wu et al., 2003). Over a period of time, it has been demonstrated that only an aqueous extract of human placenta has effective therapeutic potential. The composition of the extracts depends on the method of its preparation and consequently, they show different therapeutic activities. Clinical efficacy of an aqueous extract of human placenta in wound healing is already established (Hong et al, 2010, Wu et al., 2003). Globally scientists are investigating on placenta as a total organ and they expect to discover new applications exploiting the potency of the organ and identify new compounds in near future. This aqueous extract finds importance owing to its ability in curing chronic non-healing wounds including post-surgical dressings and high degree of burn injuries (Wu et al., 2003).

Wound healing is a complicated interrelated process wherein the injured dermal and epidermal tissue is naturally regenerated. Though well regulated, the process of healing is susceptible to interruption or failure leading to the formation of chronic non-healing wounds. Factors which may contribute to this include diabetes, venous or arterial disease, old age and infection. Placental extract, ever since its usage has been shown to be clinically effective in healing normal as well as infected wounds (Shukla et al., 2004, Chakraborty et al., 2009). It is involved in almost every stage of healing. It is also used in wound dressings to speed up the process of recovery. Though clinically well-tested, emphasis is now being laid in understanding the bioactive components involved in the process of healing. Research on the extract has highlighted some important components that might play roles in this process while few more are yet to be identified. Once the active components are identified and a proper biochemical basis of their action is defined, these components may be used even for newer purposes (Chakraborty et al., 2009).

The way in which biological products are produced, controlled and administered requires necessary precautions. Unlike conventional pharmaceutical products, which are normally produced and controlled using reproducible chemical and physical techniques, biological products are manufactured by methods involving biological processes and materials, such as cultivation of cells or extraction of material from living organisms. These processes display inherent variability, so that the range and nature of by-products are also variable. This variability, commercially termed as batch variation, occurs to a higher degree in products of plant origin compared to those of animal origin. Thus in the manufacture of biological products for direct application to human, full adherence to GMP (Good Medical Practice) is necessary for all production steps, beginning with the starting material from which the active ingredients are produced (WHO, 1992).

For any drug to make its mark in the international market, certification from regulatory authority to ensure its safe use without side effects is compulsory. Exhaustive research to verify the pharmacological efficacy of the drugs derived from traditional medicine in pharmaceutical and biomedical arena is necessary. This would enable to confirm with ancient texts and to understand and verify how the specific pharmacological action of the drug is manifested. Research on the extract reveals ample opportunity for discovery of potent bioactive components whose precise mechanism of action is yet to be elucidated. In the present era of modern pharmaceutical and biomedical research, it has become necessary to verify the pharmacological effects of the drugs in order to check whether they correspond to the ancient texts and to study how the drugs work, and also to isolate the active principles that result in the specific pharmacological action of the extract. In this review, we aim to discuss the efficacy and the biochemical components present in the aqueous extract of human placenta, which has potent wound healing attributes.

2. Preparations of human placental extract

Placental extracts can be classified into two different types: aqueous extract and hydroalcoholic extract. The components present in the extract depend on the method of its preparation and are based on solubility of the components in respective solvent of extraction. Thus, an aqueous extract is likely to contain more polar molecules such as peptides/proteins, small organic components like amino acids, nucleotides, polydeoxyribonucleotides (PDRNs), carbohydrates and trace amount of lipids mostly bound to proteins which are comparatively soluble in aqueous medium. Likewise, various types of lipids may be present in hydroalcoholic extract (less polar and hydrophobic). Chemical analysis of the hydroalcoholic extract revealed the presence of glycosphingolipids, cholesterol, triglycerides, high density lipoproteins, carbohydrates, sialic acids and others, including amino acids, nucleotides, carotenes, vitamins, including small amount of low-molecular-weight proteins/peptides containing hydrophobic amino acid residues which are soluble in a less polar solvent.

Modern indigenous aqueous placental extract is prepared employing Filatov's procedure. The manufacturing procedure of the indigenous extract holding confidentiality of the proprietary terms is as follows: fresh placentae were stored in ice and portions were tested for HIV antibody and Hepatitis B surface antigen. Single hot and cold aqueous extractions were done after incubating dissected and minced placenta at 90^{0}C and 6^{0}C respectively. This was followed by sterilization of the extract under saturated steam (pressure 15-lbs/sq inch at 120^{0}C for 40 min). After filtration and addition of 1.5% (v/v) benzyl alcohol as preservative, ampoules were filled and sterilized once again under the said condition for 20 min. In the first sterilization, the extended duration of heat treatment essentially completed precipitation of a number of macromolecules like proteins. This is apart from adding safety margins to the temperature, time or both to destroy most resistant spore-producing species like *Clostridium tetani*. The terminal sterilization step was to maintain sterility of the products after they were filled and sealed in ampoules. Each milliliter of the drug was derived from 0.1 g of fresh placenta. A single batch was prepared from the pool of several placentae. The trade name of the extract is 'Placentrex'. Carried over bioactive components in the extract depends on the method of its preparation. As the extract is prepared by repeated sterilization process, it is expected that it may contain macromolecules in their degraded forms together with small bio-organic compounds such as amino acids, peptides, small sized polypeptides, nucleotides, small polynucleotide fragments etc. Only those molecules that are heat stable and are able to withstand high sterilization pressure will remain biologically active. The active components with significant biological activity have been discussed later on. Presence of various organic components gives the extract a yellowish tinge (Datta and Bhattacharyya, 2004a).

In India, several studies have been made on the drug used as wound healer. The extract is a potent biogenous stimulator and abundantly used as an efficient wound healer (Punshi, 1981). Broadly speaking, an aqueous extract of human placenta has the following actions in the body: it accelerates cellular metabolism providing the energy for the inflammatory response to occur. It also aids in absorption of exudates by controlling its formation, removal of unhealthy tissue by debridement and management of bacterial load that are required for good wound bed preparation (Hong et al., 2010). It stimulates tissue regeneration processes. Aqueous extract of placenta contain nucleotides like PDRNs and NADPH that are known for their regeneration effect (Nelson and Cox, 2000). In addition, it also supplements growth factors and small peptides that help in matrix formation and cell adhesion, thereby promoting wound healing as described in details later on.

The hydroalcolic extract of placenta is more effective for the treatment of vitiligo. The method of preparation of a hydroalcoholic extract of fresh human placenta meant for vitiligo treatment has been reported earlier (Pal et al., 1995). Such an extract from human placenta with efficient skin pigmenting activity has been developed based on experimental therapies. Glycosphingolipids, capable of inducing adhesion, spreading and motility of melanoma is present in the extract and therefore, may lead to skin pigmentation through induction of melanocytes (Pal et al., 2002).

3. Role of placental extract in wound healing

Wound healing is a very complex process that includes inflammation, cell migration, extracellular matrix deposition and cell maturation (Diegelmann and Evans, 2004). Several cytokines and growth factors are involved in inducing different cell types for healing. Extracellular matrixes such as collagen, laminin, and fibronectin are deposited in the dermis under the effects of fibroblasts in the later phase of healing. In the last phase, contraction of the dermis in full-thickness wounds and squamous differentiation of the keratinocytes on the surface of wounds concludes its maturation (Falanga, 2001). Among all the extracts of placenta that have been prepared, only the aqueous extract has been shown to have potent clinical efficacy in terms of healing. Aqueous extract from placenta is used as a licensed drug for wound healing under different trade names in India and overseas countries (Datta and Bhattacharyya, 2004a). This could be due the fact that the aqueous extract is a rich source of various bioactive peptides with tissue regeneration potential (Chakraborty and Bhattacharyya, 2005a; De et al., 2009). In addition, the extract also retains amino acids, nucleotides, polydeoxyribonucleotides and carbohydrates that might be responsible for wound healing. Most of the wound healers that are available in the market have antimicrobial (antibacterial or antifungal) properties but the potency of the extract lies in the fact that it not only reduces the inflammatory phase and microbial burden on the wound (Chakraborty and Bhattacharyya 2005b) but also help in cell migration (Gupta and Chottopadhyay, 2008), matrix formation and tissue regeneration thereby ensuring sequential uninterrupted healing. Placental extract plays a beneficial role as a topical agent in the management of chronic non-healing wounds. It is reported that the extract promotes fibrogenesis, neoangiogenesis and epithelialisation (Shukla et al., 2004). Globally, the extract is now accepted as an effective healer in burn injuries, chronic non-healing wounds, post surgical dressings, as well as bedsores (Chakraborty et al., 2009).

Clinical evaluation of the aqueous extract revealed that it has anti-inflammatory and anti-platelet aggregation activity. As reported the extract exhibits anti-inflammatory response probably either through inhibition/inactivation of chemical mediators or by directly modulating prostaglandin (PG) production by suppression of cyclooxygenase (COX). Kinins, chemical mediators of nonimmunological type of inflammation, have two membrane receptor B1 and B2, for their activities. It has been reported that in cotton pellet induced subacute inflammation model, the extract may act as inhibitor of the B1-receptor thereby exerting its anti-inflammatory effect. It also helps in activation of the clotting cascade by trauma which results in platelet activation, followed by aggregation. The clinical study of platelet aggregation reflects that this extract can either inhibit PGs synthesis pathway or 5-hydroxytryptamine (5-HT) release. In addition, an aqueous extract of human placenta has also shown to stimulate collagen synthesis *in vivo* in rats. The significant increase in tensile strength and tissue DNA in the animals given the extract (intra muscular) indicates it was associated with marked collagen synthesis. The cytoplasmic repairment was revealed from regeneration of protein in appreciable amount. The efficiency of formation of collagen depends mainly on the synthesis of hydroxyproline, which was also shown to be appreciably high in the i.m. treated rats with the extract. These evidences, as reported, were further supported by pictures of histopathological changes showing maximum accumulation of collagen fibrils and epithelialisation (Biswas et al., 2001).

Human and animal models show that placental extract has an immunostimulating action both at cellular and humoral levels. It probably increases IgG and IgM at the humoral level and total lymphokines at the cellular level. It also reports several advantages over antibiotics and chemotherapeutic agents in terms of antibacterial activity including vascularisation of wound environment and is free from side effects (Chakraborty et al., 2009).

The injectable form of placental extract was found to be very effective, inexpensive and excellent stimulant of granulation tissue, which is superior to the dressing of povidone iodine (Pati et al., 2001). Human placental dressing was found to be effective in clinical wound healing for chronic varicose ulcers (Burgos et al., 1989). Later, this finding was supported by Subramanian et al., 1990. The wound healing potency of the aqueous extract of placenta is thus clinically well established and a lot of evidences support these findings. However, the active components present and the molecular mechanisms that are involved in the healing process are yet to be defined. The variety of biological actions of aqueous extract of human placenta is a matter of increasing interest. Characterization of such extract by isolating the active components present in it and to determine their mechanism of action related to wound healing process is of utmost requirement. This is because scientific assessment of such extract is necessary for its better acceptance in medical practice with a more convincing approach.

4. Biochemical characterization and possible mechanism of action of the extract

Human placental extract manufactured by a proprietary extraction method using term human placenta as a raw material has potent therapeutic efficacy. Use of placental extract in different preparations under various trade names is a recommended worldwide practice. Developed from folk knowledge, the aqueous extract is used as a globally accepted licensed drug in post surgical dressings, as a healer in burn injuries and chronic wounds under different trade name in many countries including India (Chakraborty et al., 2009).

Isolating active components present in a biological extract is a natural propagation towards characterization of the drug. The contents present in the extract depend on the method of its preparation. An aqueous extract of placenta contains amino acids, peptides, glycosaminoglycans, lipids, polynucleotides (mainly polydeoxyribonucleotide fragments), vitamins, minerals etc. Some of them can be chemically or biologically synthesized but many of them can only be obtained by isolating them from a natural source. An aqueous extract of human placenta of potent therapeutic value is under research in terms of identifying the active components present and the biochemical basis of its mode of action. It was initiated at Indian Institute of Chemical Biology, Kolkata, India from 1999 and is still ongoing. The drug 'Placentrex' - manufactured by Albert David Ltd., Kolkata has been used for this purpose, which is used as wound healer from long back. The extract is prepared under relatively harsh conditions; as a result of which macromolecules are degraded generating low molecular weight bio-organic compounds e.g. amino acids, peptides, small sized polypeptides, nucleotides, small polynucleotide fragments etc. Owing to the presence of PDRNs, the spectral pattern of the extract corresponds mostly to that of DNA with a high absorption at 260 nm. Characterization of such extract by isolating the active components present in it and to determine their mechanism of action related to wound healing would be significant.

Major findings with its constituents include demonstration of minimal batch variation of the extract using conventional spectroscopic and chromatographic techniques like UV-VIS absorption spectra, FT-IR, TLC, HPTLC and HPLC and also by newly developed method for fingerprinting of multi-component drugs using fluorescence Excitation-Emission-Matrix (EEM) plots. Since there is no fingerprinting technique, which could be applied universally to separate different class of components, combination of different modes is used and upgradation of finger printing procedures is an active area of present research. Fluorescence spectroscopy has versatile application in chemistry and biochemistry. Modern versions of spectrofluorimeters are equipped with generation of three dimensional (3D) contour plots, also called EEM plots. where the z-axis represents emission intensity. Its advantage lies on presentation of chromophores having different excitation and emission patterns in a single profile. In analytical chemistry, it is frequently used in environmental and hydrological studies. Moreover, since wide excitation and emission zones are covered in a single profile, there is no scope of missing any newly emerged fluorophore in a batch. This safeguard is almost impossible to include in two-dimensional fluorescence emission profiles. A high degree of consistency between different batches of the drug was observed from EEM. Validity of these results from EEM was crosschecked by different spectroscopic and chromatographic modes (Datta and Bhattacharyya, 2004b). This consistency reflects standardization of the manufacturing process of the drug and also adherence of uniform placental composition irrespective of the nutritional status of mothers. Fluorescence spectroscopy has been shown to have capability of identifying the fluorophores in a complex multi-component biological system.

During characterization of the extract, a fluorophore has been detected which had excitation and emission properties similar to nicotinamide adenine dinucleotide, reduced form (NADH) and nicotinamide adenine dinucleotide phosphate, reduced form (NADPH). When excited at 340 nm, it results in fluorescence emission having maxima around 436 nm, which is fairly specific for NADH and NADPH. These are natural constituents of placenta and play important roles in different metabolic pathways including wound healing. NAD/NADH and NADP/NADPH are major redox-active 'electron storage' compounds. One or both of these 'redox pairs' is involved in every major biochemical pathway. They participate in the trafficking of electrons as 'reducing equivalents,' the electron packets that facilitate metabolism. Evidence of only free and bound NADPH (supplying as a substrate or cofactor for enzymes) were demonstrated using thin layer chromatography and reversed-phase HPLC. Since NADPH is known to regulate a number of phenomena related to wound healing, we have investigated its presence in different batches of the drug. Biological functionality of the fluorophore in the extract has been confirmed by enzymatic assay. It has been shown that NADPH in aging human skin cells increases synthesis of collagen involving filaggrin and keratin *in vitro* (Datta and Bhattacharyya 2004a).

The extract also has the ability for *in vitro* NO induction in mouse peritoneal macrophage and human peripheral blood mononuclear cells (PBMC). The aqueous extract has been investigated in terms of induction of NO by macrophages. It has been demonstrated that with an increase of NO production, concomitant decrease in NADPH present in the applied placental extract was observed, thereby indicating that the NADPH pool of placental extract is metabolized, further justifying the biological potency of this nucleotide in the extract (Chakraborty et al., 2006). It has been well documented that nitric oxide (NO) has multiple effects at the molecular, cellular and physiological level in wound healing. It promotes inflammatory mediation of repair mechanism and wound matrix development followed by remodeling. NO mediated cellular signaling possibly enhances wound repair by increasing tissue oxygen availability through angiogenesis. It is produced in macrophages by the enzyme inducible nitric oxide synthase (iNOS) during wound healing (Luo and Chen, 2005). It acts as a biological signaling and effector molecule capable of diffusing across membranes and reacting with a variety of targets. Once induced, production of NO within the tissue can induce an environment that is toxic to invading microorganism (Efron et al., 2000). It promotes inflammatory mediation of repair mechanism and wound matrix development followed by remodeling. The extract has also shown to induce interferon-γ (IFN-γ) production by macrophages (Chakraborty et al., 2006).

Anti-microbial property of the extract against a large number of pathological microorganisms related to prevention of secondary infections to wounds has also been demonstrated. The extract has an effective inhibitory role on the growth of different microbes particularly growth of clinically isolated bacteria, e.g. *E. coli* from urine and blood culture and *S. aureus* from pus cells. Drug resistant strains such as *E. coli DH5α Pet-16 AmpR and Pseudomonus aeruginosa CamR* were also significantly inhibited by the extract. The extract has both bacteriostatic and fungistatic activities. Dose-dependent response of the extract was observed. A mixture of polydeoxyribonucleotides (PDRNs) appears to be the causative agent. Partial protection of the wound from secondary microbial infection is thus indicated. Though the mechanism of such growth-inhibitory activities has not been studied, it is predicted that the PDRNs present in the extract enter the microbes and interfere with their replication machinery (Chakraborty and Bhattacharyya, 2005b).

An important finding was isolation and purification of a peptide of around 7.4 kDa from the extract. Derived partial amino acid sequence from mass spectrometric analysis showed its homology with human fibronectin type III. Under nondenaturing condition, it formed aggregate, the elution pattern of which was identical to that of fibronectin type III as confirmed by reverse-phase HPLC. Immuno-blot of the peptide showed strong cross reactivity with reference human fibronectin type III-$_C$. It draws special attention because its partial amino acid sequence showed homology with 10th type-III fibronectin peptide that also contains the 'RGD' signature sequence endowed with cell adhesion properties (Nath and Bhattacharyya, 2007). The importance of fibronectin in cutaneous wound healing is well documented as a general cell adhesion molecule by promoting the spread of platelets at the site of injury. It also helps in the adhesion and migration of neutrophils, monocytes, fibroblasts and endothelial cells into the wound region, and the migration of epidermal cells through the granulation tissue (Chakraborty and Bhattacharyya, 2005a).

Considering the importance of peptides in wound healing, the fraction was further characterized in terms of regulation of some enzyme activities related to repair mechanism. Primary investigation revealed that the drug stabilizes some serine proteases against their autodigestion by reversibly inactivating them, which enhances the efficiency of proteolytic enzymes thereby facilitates wound healing. Further it has been demonstrated that one or more peptides from human placental extract including fibronectin type III stabilize trypsin activity after strong association, which is reversible in nature. In presence of excess substrate, the conjugate is dissociated. Regulation of trypsin activity with prevention of autodigestion has been demonstrated in De *et al*, 2011.

As a working hypothesis, wound healing can be broadly categorized into three overlapping phases both in terms of time and space — cleansing or debridement, following which proliferation occurs to provide a platform for tissue regeneration and finally differentiation occurs. During debridement, extensive 'hydrolytic activity' ensures proper cleaning of the wounded tissue. The last two stages of healing require extensive 'synthetic activity' and minimal hydrolytic activity. Trypsin and similar proteolytic enzymes help in debridement and prevent keloid formation during wound healing and therefore regulation of its activity is an important criterion. Trypsin, chymotrypsin, collagenase, papain, bromelein etc were reported to be effective in wound healing as a debriding agent. These agents remove foreign bodies and necrotic tissues and reveals healthy, bleeding tissues so that the wound can heal (Buck and Phillips, 1970; Craig, 1975; Ramundo and Gray, 2009). Thus, it is expected that the peptide would have greater half-lives in the blood, as serine proteases form a major part of blood proteases. Proportionate mixing of 'Placentrex' with some proteolytic enzymes and subsequent evaluation of its efficacy in wound healing, may be another promising avenue of the future study leading to the development of an effective wound healer with debridement potential.

It remains questionable whether the proteins and peptides of the drug remain stable in human blood as the blood contains many proteases. There is an array of proteases in blood, which include thrombin, plasmin, Hageman factor, blood coagulation cascade enzymes etc. Though it is well known that blood proteases are quite specific about their substrates, the question of stability of the drug components remains an important issue from clinical point of view. It has been demonstrated by size exclusion HPLC that the peptide fraction of the drug remains unaffected in presence of plasma and serum proteases from human blood (Fig. 1). In reverse, it has also been demonstrated by gelatin zymography that the blood proteases remain unaffected after incubation for 48 hrs in presence of the placental peptide fraction (Fig. 2). However, protease-substrate interactions are not always guided by the specificity of the protease. One essential requirement for proteolysis is that the hydrolysable bond must be physically accessible to the catalytic site of the protease. Often proteins can survive proteolysis out of its compact globular structures under physiological conditions in presence of proteases. It is generally observed that any drug administered through intra venous or intra muscular remains active in circulation for a maximum period of 48 hours after which it is removed from circulation by metabolism or excretion. Thus the studies were restricted within 48 hrs.

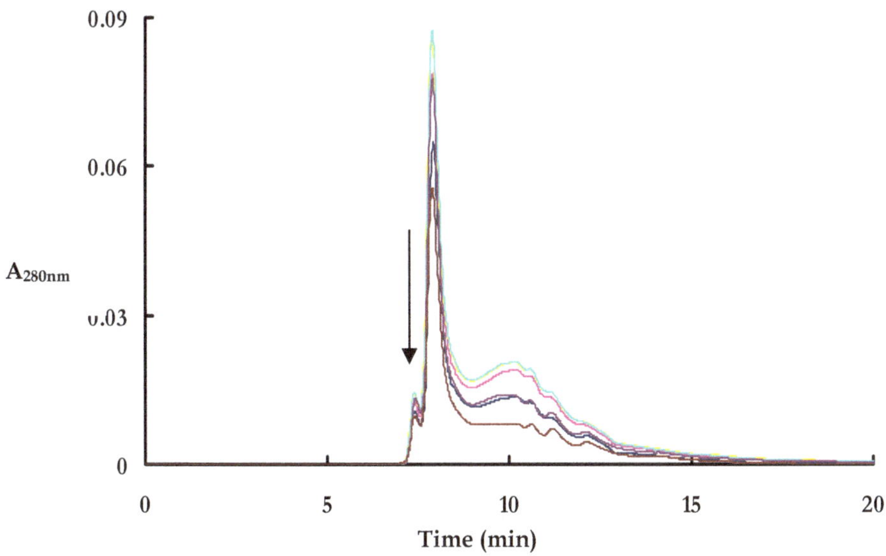

Fig. 1. Stability of the peptide fraction from placental extract in presence of blood protease (plasma) over 48 hr as observed from size exclusion HPLC using Waters Protein Pak 125 column (fractionation range 2-20 kDa). The sharp major peak corresponds to the unresolved peptide fractions of Mw 10-16 kDa while the second peak corresponds to elution of small bioorganic molecules. The overlapping profiles from top to bottom indicate samples of incubation time 0, 6, 18, 24, 48 hr respectively at 37°C. The loss of intensity appears to be due to partial precipitation of the peptides removed by centrifugation though there is no indication of multimer formation at the void volume of the column. The downward arrow indicates the void volume.

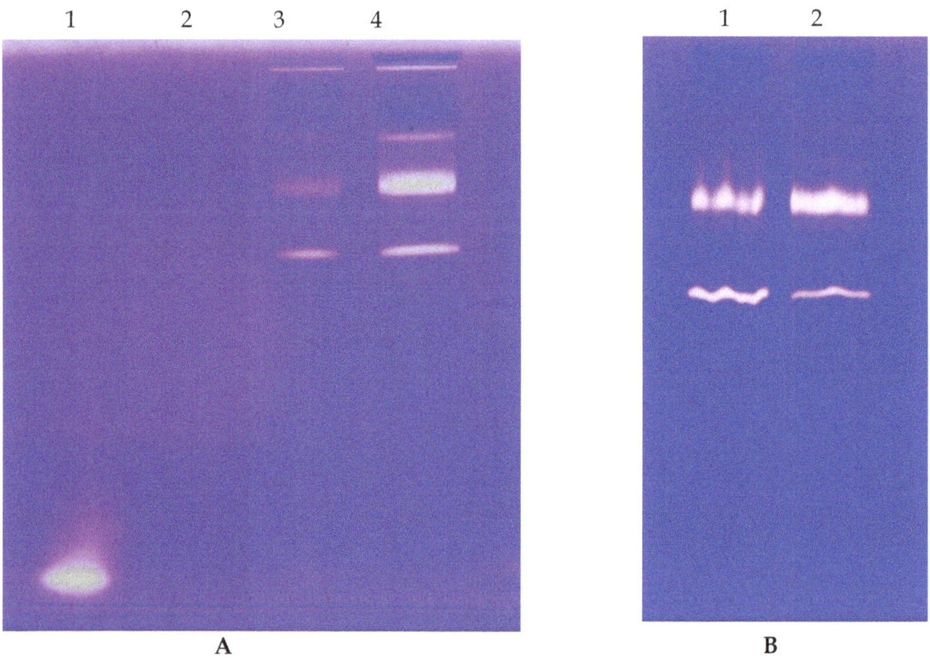

Fig. 2. Stability of blood proteases in presence of peptide fraction of human placental extract as observed by gelatin zymography. (A) Representing trypsin 0.75 ng (lane 1), buffer as control (lane 2), serum isolated from blood (lane 3) and plasma (lane 4), both were incubated for 48 hr with 10 μg/ml of peptide fraction of the placental extract. (B) Human serum (lane 1) and plasma (lane 2) as control.

As a part of the healing process, the body enters a hypermetabolic phase, where there is an increase in demand for carbohydrates. Cellular activity is fuelled by adenosine triphosphate (ATP), which is derived from glucose, providing the energy for the inflammatory response to occur. In addition to their role in metabolic process, carbohydrates are involved in cellular signaling as well as cell-cell interaction. While addressing roles of carbohydrates, interaction of lysozyme with the extract was investigated. The enzyme showed positive reactivity in a time and concentration dependent manner indicating that carbohydrate residues were present. Attempts are in progress to identify these residues by GC-MS in presence of reference sugars (unpublished observation).

This multifaceted character of the drug encourages further investigation following which the biochemical basis of its mode of action is likely to be highlighted.

5. Multiple therapeutic properties of aqueous extract of human placenta

Several clinical investigations and findings have been reported on effective therapeutic use of placental extract such as clinical evaluation in radiation-induced oral mucositis (Kaushal et al., 2001), restorative effects in X-ray-irradiated mice (Mochizuki and Kada, 1982), for the treatment of myopic and senile chorio-retinal dystrophies (Girotto and Malinverni, 1982), rheumatic arthritis (Rosenthal, 1982), osteoarthritis (Kim et al, 2010), skin diseases (Punshi, 1981), for prevention of recurring respiratory infections (Lo Polito, 1980), in the therapy of urticarias (Mittal, 1977), in therapy of children with asthmatic bronchitis (Vecchi et al., 1977), in atrophic rhinitis (Sinha et al, 1976), on hepatic drug metabolizing enzymes (Bishayee et al., 1995), in cerebral arteriosclerosis (Lafay 1965), in periodontal disease (Calvarano et al., 1989). Topical treatment of cervico-vaginal lesions using a placental extract with anticomplement activity (Sgro, 1978), local therapy of psoriasis (Lodi et al., 1986), treatment of vitiligo with topical melagenine (Suite and Quamina, 1991) has also been reported to be successful. A number of reports have been found on placental extract effective in arthritis (Yeom et al., 2003). Effectiveness of topical application of polydeoxiribonucleotide from human placenta in gynaecology has been documented (Bertone and Sgro, 1982). Post-irradiation cystitis improved by instillation of early placental extract in saline (Mićić and Genbacev, 1988) and placental extract injections in the treatment of loss of hair in women is also documented (Hauser, 1982). It was reported that aqueous human placental extract induced potentiation of morphine antinociception may have a clinical significance for the treatment of persistent or chronic pain (Gurgel et al., 2000). Clinical evaluation of the aqueous extract has shown that the drug acts as a potent wound healer with anti inflammatory and immunotropic effect. Placental extract has long been used as a cosmetic supplement for skin care and skin pigmentation (Pal et al., 2002). Recently it has been reported that menopausal symptoms and fatigue in middle-aged women improved after the treatment with the aqueous placental extract (Kong et al., 2008). It has been reported that an aqueous extract of human placenta was found to offer protection against established experimental visceral leishmaniasis in BALB/c mice and hamsters, whether the *Leishmania donovani* strain involved was one that was sensitive or resistant to pentavalent antimony. Based on the results of this pilot study, a further evaluation of the efficacy of human placental extract therapy, which may offer a cost-effective way of improving the treatment of antimony-resistant cases of visceral leishmaniasis, is being undertaken (Chakraborty et al., 2008).

Several studies have shown therapeutic use of other animal placenta also. Recent report shows that the protective effect of porcine placental extract in contact hypersensitivity is mediated by inhibition of the inflammatory responses and IgE production to modulate skin inflammation (Jash et al., 2011). Cow placental extract efficiently accelerates cell division and growth factor expression by raising the insulin-like growth factor (IGF-1) mRNA and protein level to increase hair follicle size and hair length in murine (Zhang et al., 2011). Bovine placental extract is capable of improving the tenderness of certain injuries that are relatively high in connective tissue, while avoiding myofibrillar protein hydrolysis (Phillips et al. 2000). An immunomodulatory peptide was isolated from aqueous extract of bovine placenta which showed no significant homology with other immunomodulatory peptides (Fang et al., 2007). Thus, the therapeutic potency of placental extract has earned global recognition.

6. Conclusion

Natural medicine continues to play an important role for prevention, alleviation and cure of diseases. In some part of the Western world, the use of traditional medicine has been largely lost. However, it is a widespread phenomenon in the developing countries where 80% of the population is still relying on traditional medicine for primary healthcare. Derived from folklore, human placental preparations show immense therapeutic value and can be safely used once it is ensured that the source is free from fatal infections like HIV, HBV, HCV and alike. The aqueous extract of human placenta is a scientifically proven potent wound healer. Characterization of active components present in different placental preparations and correlating them with their therapeutic actions are the promising avenue for future study. A fibronectin type III-like peptide present in the aqueous extract appears to be one of the key components for wound healing. It is known from the literature that this type of peptide inhibits tumor growth, angiogenesis and metastasis. Therefore, future work should include evaluation of human placental extract as anti-tumor agent. Identification of the possible signaling pathways for wound healing as well as other therapeutic properties of the placental peptide should receive immediate attention. Additional components identified include PDRN and NADPH. Further, yet unidentified peptides or small molecules might also be present in various preparations of the extract that might play roles in wound healing and related disorders. Identification of other biologically active components in the extract and their mechanism of action in terms of cellular signaling, which play significant role in wound healing also needs to be addressed.

7. Acknowledgement

Work was supported by a research grant from the drug house Albert David Ltd. Kolkata. We thank Ms. Debashree De (SRF, CSIR-New Delhi) and Ms. Anwesha Majumder (SRF, Albert David Ltd.) for their contribution in zymography and size exclusion HPLC experiments.

8. References

Bertone C, Sgro LC. Clinical data on topical application in gynaecology of polydeoxiribonucleotide of human placenta. *Int. J. Tissue React.* 1982; 4: 165-167.

Biswas TK, Auddy B, Bhattacharyya NP, Bhattacharyya S, Mukherjee B. Wound healing activity of human placental extract in rats. *Acta Pharmacol. Sin.* 2001; 22: 1113-1116.

Bishayee A, Banerjee AK, Chatterjee M. Effects of human placental extract on hepatic drug metabolizing enzyme. *Riv. Eur. Sci. Med. Farmacol.* 1995; 17: 19-26.

Buck JE, Phillips N. Trial of Chymoral in professional footballers. *Br J Clin Pract.* 1970; 24: 375-377.

Burgos H, Herd A, Bennett JP. Placental angiogenic and growth factors in the treatment of chronic varicose ulcers: preliminary communication. *J. Royal Soc. Med.* 1989; 82: 598–599.

Calvarano G, De Polis F, Sabatini G. Treatment with placental extract in periodontal disease. *Dent. Cadmos.* 1989; 57:85-86.

Chakraborty D, Basu JM, Sen P, Sundar S, Roy S. Human placental extract offers protection against experimental visceral leishmaniasis: a pilot study for a phase-I clinical trial. *Ann. Trop. Med. Parasitol.* 2008; 102: 21-38.

Chakraborty PD, Bhattacharyya D. Isolation of fibronectin Type III like peptide from human placental extract used as wound healer. *J. Chromatogr. B* 2005a; 818: 67-73.

Chakraborty PD, Bhattacharyya D. In vitro growth inhibition of microbes by human placental extract. *Curr. Sc.* 2005b; 88: 782-786.

Chakraborty PD, Bhattacharyya D, Pal S, Ali N. In vitro induction of nitric oxide by mouse peritoneal macrophages treated with human placental extract. *Int. Immunopharmacol.* 2006; 6: 100-107.

Chakraborty PD, De D, Bandyopadhyay S, Bhattacharyya D. Human aqueous placental extract as a wound healer. *J. Wound Care* 2009; 18: 462-467.

Craig RP. The quantitative evaluation of the use of oral proteolytic enzymes in the treatment of sprained ankles. *Injury* 1975; 6: 313-316.

Datta P, Bhattacharyya D. Spectroscopic and chromatographic evidences of NADPH in human placental extract used as wound healer. *J. Pharma. Biomed. Anal.* 2004a; 34: 1091-1098.

Datta P, Bhattacharyya D. Analysis of fluorescence excitation-emission matrix of multicomponent drugs: A case study with human placental extract used as wound healer. *J. Pharma. Biomed. Anal.* 2004b; 36: 211-218.

De D, Chakraborty PD, Bhattacharyya D. Analysis of free and bound NADPH in aqueous extract of human placenta used as wound healer. *J. Chromatogr. B.* 2009; 877: 2435

De D, Chakraborty PD, Bhattacharyya D. Regulation of trypsin activity by peptide fraction of an aqueous extract of human placenta used as wound healer. *J. Cell. Physiol.* 2011; 226: 2033-2040.

Diegelmann RF, Evans MC. Wound healing: an overview of acute, fibrotic and delayed healing. *Front. Biosci.* 2004; 9:283-289.

Efron DT, Most D, Barbul A. Role of nitric oxide in wound healing. *Curr. Opin. Clin. Nutr. Metab. Care* 2000; 3: 197–204.

Falanga V. Introducing the concept of wound bed preparation. *Int. Forum Wound Care* 2001; 16: 1-4.

Fang XP, Xia WS, Sheng QH, Wang YL. Purification and characterization of an immunomodulatory Peptide from bovine placenta water-soluble extract. *Prep. Biochem. Biotechnol.* 2007; 37: 173-184.

Filatov VP. Tissue therapy. *Med. Gen. Fr.* 1951; 11: 3-5.

Filatov VP. Tissue Therapy. Foreign Language Publishing House, Moscow; 1955.

Girotto G, Malinverni W. Use of placental extract for the treatment of myopic and senile chorio-retinal dystrophies. *Int. J. Tissue React.* 1982; 4: 169-172.

Gupta R, Chattopadhyay D. Glutamate is the chemotaxis-inducing factor in placental extracts. *Amino Acids* 2009: 37: 359-366.

Gurgel LA, Santos FA, Rao VS. Effects of human placental extract on chemical and thermal nociception in mice. *Eur. J. Pain* 2000; 4: 403-408.

Hauser GA. Placental extract injections in the treatment of loss of hair in women. *Int. J. Tissue React.* 1982; 4: 159-163.

Hong JW, Lee WJ, Hahn SB, Kim BJ, Lew DH. The effect of human placenta extract in a wound healing model. *Ann. Plast. Surg.* 2010; 65: 96-100.

Jash A, Kwon HK, Sahoo A, Lee CG, So JS, Kim J, Oh YK, Kim YB, Im SH. Topical application of porcine placenta extract inhibits the progression of experimental contact hypersensitivity. *J Ethnopharmacol.* 2011; 133; 654-662.

Kaushal V, Verma K, Manocha S, Hooda HS, Das BP. Clinical evaluation of human placental extract (placentrex) in radiation-induced oral mucositis. *Int. J. Tissue React.* 2001; 23: 105-110.

Kong MH, Lee EJ, Lee SY, Cho SJ, Hong YS, Park SB. Effect of human placental extract on menopausal symptoms, fatigue, and risk factors for cardiovascular disease in middle-aged Korean women. *Menopause* 2008; 15: 296-303.

Kim JK, Kim TH, Park SW, Kim HY, Kim S, Lee S, Lee SM. Protective effects of human placenta extract on cartilage degradation in experimental osteoarthritis. *Biol. Pharma. Bull.* 2010; 33: 1004-1010.

Luo JD,Chen AF, Nitric oxide: a newly discovered function on wound healing. *Acta pharmacol. Sin.* 2005; 26: 259-264.

Lo Polito F. Action of a human placenta extract used for prevention of recurring respiratory infections. *Minerva Pediatr.* 1980; 32: 261-266.

Lodi A, Cattaneo M, Betti R, Marmini A, Masnada MC. Local therapy of psoriasis with placental extract. *G. Ital. Dermatol. Venereol.* 1986; 121: XV-XVII.

Lafay J. Cerebral arteriosclerosis and placental extract. *Clinique* 1965; 60: 309-316.

Mittal KN. Role of placental extract in the therapy of urticarias. *Indian J. Dermatol.* 1977; 22: 117-120.

Mićić S, Genbacev O. Post-irradiation cystitis improved by instillation of early placental extract in saline. *Eur. Urol.* 1988; 14: 291-293.

Mochizuki H, Kada T. Restorative effects of human placenta extract in X-ray-irradiated mice. *J. Radiat. Res.* 1982; 23: 403-410.

Nath S, Bhattacharyya D. Cell adhesion by aqueous extract of human placenta used as wound healer. *Indian J. Exp. Biol.* 2007; 45: 732-738.

Nelson DL, Cox MM. Lehninger principles of biochemistry. 3rd ed. New York: Macmillan worth Publishers: 2000.

Pati S, Saumandal BK, Bhattacharyya AK, Saumandal P. Clinical evaluation of effect of dressing with placental extract (Inj Placentrex) in the treatment of infected wounds. *J. Obstet. Gynaecol.* (India) 2001; 51: 124-126.

Pal P, Roy R, Datta PK, Dutta AK, Biswas B, Bhadra R. Hydroalcoholic human placental extract: skin pigmenting activity and gross chemical composition. *Int. J. Dermatol.* 1995; 34: 61-66.

Pal P, Mallick S, Mandal SK, Das M, Dutta AK, Datta PK Bhadra R. Human placental extract: in vivo and in vitro assessments of its melanocyte growth and pigment-inducing activities. *Int. J. Dermatol.* 2002; 41: 760-767.

Punshi S K. Treatment of skin diseases with biogenous stimulator-placental extract. *Indian J. Dermatol.* 1981; 26: 11-13.

Phillips AL, Means WJ, Kalchayanand N, McCormick RJ, Miller KW. Bovine placental protease specificity toward muscle connective tissue proteins. *J. Anim. Sci.* 2000; 78: 1861-1866.

Ramundo J, Gray M. Collagenases for enzymatic debridement: A systematic review. *J Wound Ostomy Continence Nurs* 2009; 11: S4-S11.

Rosenthal M. The application of an extract of human placenta in the treatment of rheumatic affections. *Int. J. Tissue React.* 1982; 4: 147-151.

Shukla, V. K., Rasheed, M. A., Kumar, M., Gupta, S. K. and Pandey, S. S., A trial to determine the role of placental extract in the treatment of chronic non-healing wounds. *J. Wound Care*, 2004; 13: 177–179.

Sinha SN, Gupta SC, Samuel KC, Misra UC. Placental extract therapy in atrophic rhinitis. *Eye Ear Nose Throat Mon.* 1976; 55: 59-61.

Sgro LC, Topical treatment of cervico-vaginal lesions using a placental extract with anticomplement activity. *Minerva Ginecol.* 1978; 30: 671-682.

Subramanian T, Vijayarathinam P, Sathyavan V. Effects of placental dressing indolent ulcers. *J. Indian Med. Assoc.* 1990; 88: 314–316.

Suite M, Quamina DB. Treatment of vitiligo with topical melagenine, a human placental extract. *J. Am. Acad. Dermatol.* 1991; 24: 1018-1019.

Tonello G, Daglio M, Zaccarelli N, Sottofattori E, Mazzei M, Balbi A. Characterization and quantitation of the active polynucleotide fraction (PDRN) from human placenta, a tissue repair-stimulating agent. *J. Pharma. Biomed. Anal.* 1996; 14: 1555-1560.

Vecchi V, Faldella G, Paolucci G. Use of a human placental extract. Human placental S fraction or HRPS fraction in therapy of children with asthmatic bronchitis. *Minerva Pediatr.* 1977; 29: 1323-1330.

Wu CH, Chang GY, Chang WC, Hsu CT, Chen RS. Wound healing effects of porcine placental extracts on rats with thermal injury. *Br. J. Dermatol.* 2003; 148: 236 - 245.

WHO Expert Committee on Specifications for Pharmaceutical Preparations. Thirty-second report. Geneva, World Health Organization, 44-52 and 75-76 (1992) (WHO Technical Report Series, No. 823).

Yeom MJ, Lee HC, Kim GH, Shim I, Lee HJ, Hahm DH. Therapeutic effects of Hominis placenta injection into an acupuncture point on the inflammatory responses in subchondral bone region of adjuvant-induced polyarthritic rat. *Biol. Pharma. Bull.* 2003; 26: 1472-1477.

Zhang D, Lijuan G, Jingjie L, Zheng L, Wang C, Wang Z, Liu L, Mira L, Sung C. Cow placenta extract promotes murine hair growth through enhancing the insulin - like growth factor-1. *Indian J. Dermatol.* 2011; 56: 14-18.

Exploring the Human Term Placenta as a Novel Source for Stem Cells and Their Application in the Clinic

Celena Heazlewood[1,3*], Matthew Cook[1,3], Nina Ilic[2] and Kerry Atkinson[1,2,3]
[1]Mater Medical Research Institute, Level 3, Aubigny Place, Raymond Terrace, South Brisbane,
[2]Mater Adult Hospital, South Brisbane,
[3]University of Queensland, School of Medicine, Brisbane, Australia

1. Introduction

The human placenta is a fetomaternal organ, consisting of both fetal (amnion and chorion) and maternal (decidua) tissues (Parolini *et al.*, 2008). This complex organ begins to develop within a few days after fertilisation and is fundamental to the development and survival of the fetus throughout gestation. The placenta also acts as the lung, kidney and digestive system for the growing fetus and protects the fetus from infection throughout development (Parolini *et al.*, 2008).

The placenta is of interest to stem cell biologists since it is rich in stem cells and their progenitors. A stem cell is defined as a cell that has the ability to self renew and that can differentiate to progeny (daughter cells) of one or more of the germ layers. Stem cells are classified as either totipotent, pluripotent or multipotent. The most primitive stem cell, with the greatest ability to differentiate, is the totipotent cell of the zygote or first blastomere (Mitalipov and Wolf, 2009). This cell occurs from the first division of the zygote and has the ability to form an entire organism. Once these totipotent cells begin to divide, they give rise to the embryo and placenta. At the 32-cell stage of the embryo, known as the morula, the cells have lost their totipotency and are pluripotent (Mitalipov and Wolf, 2009, Witkowska-Zimny and Wrobel, 2011). These pluripotent cells contribute to all three germ layers in the developing embryo, the endoderm, mesoderm and ectoderm. Stem cells with limited differentiation ability are known as multipotent stem cells and can differentiate into a number of cell types within the same germ layer. Multipotent stem cells are committed to a particular organ or tissue and are the most mature stem cell type (Witkowska-Zimny and Wrobel, 2011).

1.1 Types of stem cells

1.1.1 Pluripotent stem cells

Embryonic stem (ES) cells derived from the inner cell mass of the very early embryo, are capable of giving rise to all three germ layers, and are pluripotent stem cells. Induced pluripotent stem cells (iPS) have many characteristics in common with ES, but are derived by re-programming adult stromal cells (Mitalipov and Wolf, 2009). As their name implies, they too are pluripotent and both types can divide indefinitely, and have the potential to develop benign teratomas consisting of tissues of all three germ layers. Regardless of this potential complication, neural cells differentiated from human ES cells are already in clinical trial (www.geron.com). The differentiated progeny of both ES and iPS cells (for example, neurons, cardiomyocytes, hepatocytes) are likely to be rejected by the immune system of an allogeneic recipient and the use of such progeny is likely to require administration of immune suppressive agents after their administration to prevent their immune-mediated rejection. Additionally, there are a number of ethical concerns particularly with the use of ES cells because of the inevitable destruction of the human embryo in the generation of ES cells. This concern does not apply to human iPS cells which can be generated from any postnatal human tissue, including those that are routinely disposed of, such as term placenta after safe delivery of the baby.

1.2 Multipotent stem cells

1.2.1 Haematopoietic stem cells

The best known example of a multipotent stem cell is the haematopoietic stem cell derived from the bone marrow, umbilical cord blood or mobilised peripheral blood. Less well-known is the fact that the placenta is an important source of HSC, at least during mid-gestation in the mouse (Gekas *et al.*, 2008, Gekas *et al.*, 2010). Haematopoietic stem cells (HSC) are the source of all blood cell types and continuously replenish the haematopoietic and immune systems throughout life. They are the best characterised adult stem cell and are the only stem or progenitor cells in routine clinical use today (Appelbaum, 2007). The transplantation of HSC is a potentially curative therapy for immunodeficiencies such as severe combined immune deficiencies, haematological malignancies such as leukaemia, myeloma, and myelodysplasia, and bone marrow failure syndromes such as severe aplastic anaemia. HSC transplantation (HSCT) was pioneered in the 1950s using bone marrow (BM) as the source of HSC, with the first successful allogeneic transplant performed in 1968. Mobilised peripheral blood (mPB) HSC, collected by apheresis, are now the most commonly used source of stem cells for HSC transplantation. However, both of these sources are restricted by the availability of a suitable human leukocyte antigen- (HLA-) matched related or unrelated living donor. The use of BM- or mPB- HSC from a matched unrelated donor or a partially mismatched family member has a higher incidence of potentially fatal, graft-versus-host disease (GVHD), a condition that occurs due to immune attack by donor leukocytes on recipient tissues. Umbilical cord blood (UCB) is now recognised as a promising alternative tissue source of HSC and it has some advantages over conventional sources since it is readily available and easy to collect. Most importantly, UCB can be used in transplants with less than optimal donor-recipient HLA-matching, thus providing broader access compared to BM- and mPB- HSC. The isolation and clinical applications of HSC derived from UCB will be discussed later in this chapter.

1.2.2 Mesenchymal stem cells

Another multipotent stem cell was discovered within the bone marrow by Friendenstein more than forty years ago (Friedenstein *et al.*, 1976). These cells are now commonly known as mesenchymal stem/stromal cells (MSC) and are cells that give rise to tissues of the mesodermal lineage, including bone, cartilage, muscle, tendons and adipose tissue. Their many advantages include their relative ease of isolation, expansion potential, stable phenotype and compatibility with different delivery methods and formulations (reviewed in "Therapeutic applications of mesenchymal stromal cells" (Brooke *et al.*, 2007)).

It is known that traditionally derived bone marrow (bm) MSC are a rare cell population (~0.001% of BM mononuclear cells) *in vivo*, resulting in a low MSC yield when isolated. Hence, *ex vivo* expansion is required to gain sufficient numbers for clinical applications. In general, MSC are isolated using a density gradient or cell lysis, after which the mononuclear cells are cultured in basal medium such as Dulbecco's modified Eagle's medium and 10 % - 20 % fetal calf serum (FCS) (Pittenger *et al.*, 1999, Mcbride *et al.*, 2003, Lodie *et al.*, 2002). Cells are subsequently maintained in culture for several days during which contaminating, non-adherent haematopoietic cells such as macrophages are depleted. Human MSC have a characteristic (but not unique) cell surface phenotype of $CD90^+$, $CD105^+$, $CD73^+$, $CD44^+$, HLA I^+, $CD45^-$, $CD34^-$ $CD11b^-$, HLA II^- (Pittenger *et al.*, 1999, Javazon *et al.*, 2003, Peister *et al.*, 2004). MSC are unique amongst nucleated mammalian cells in that they stimulate little allogeneic reactivity when administered to MHC-unmatched adult immune competent recipients, perhaps due to their lack, at least in the human, of expression of co-stimulatory cell surface molecules such as CD80 and CD86 (Weiss *et al.*, 2008, Wang *et al.*, 2009). Furthermore, they are actively suppressive of T cell, dendritic cell and B cell function (Weiss *et al.*, 2008, Wang *et al.*, 2009, Jiang *et al.*, 2005) and this is presumably linked to their ability to down-modulate exuberant inflammation, which can subsequently result in pathological remodeling and excessive fibrosis.

It has been proposed that current tissue culture methods used to expand MSC reduce multipotency and result in lower migratory/engraftment capacity of the expanded MSC. It has also been shown that humans and animals show a decreased rate of production of bone marrow mesenchymal stem and progenitor cells with increasing age (Caplan, 1994). Several studies have provided evidence of a strong correlation between age and the proliferative potential exhibited by MSC *in vitro* (Stenderup *et al.*, 2003, Bergman *et al.*, 1996, D'ippolito *et al.*, 1999). Thus, the progenitor pool may be depleted following extensive proliferation. Consequently, this results in a reduced ability to ensure regeneration after injury or disease depending on the age of the MSC (Ringe *et al.*, 2002). Such a decline in the quality of the cells is suboptimal for therapeutic application.

For these reasons, novel sources of MSC are now being investigated for clinical use in diseases in which the regenerative and immunomodulatory functions of MSC may be useful (Barlow *et al.*, 2008b, Chang *et al.*, 2006a, Jones *et al.*, 2007, Brooke *et al.*, 2009). A readily available and younger source that can be obtained by a non-invasive procedure, and which yields large numbers of MSC for *ex vivo* expansion would be an ideal alternative to adult bone marrow.

MSC derived from tissues normally disposed of, such as the term placenta and other gestational tissues that are fetal derived (In 'T Anker *et al.*, 2004, Yen *et al.*, 2005, Bailo *et al.*, 2004, Wulf *et al.*, 2004, De Coppi *et al.*, 2007) have been investigated to see if they fulfill these criteria. This chapter will describe various gestational tissue sources for human MSC as alternatives to bone marrow, the isolation of MSC from these sources and their application in the clinic.

2. The human term placenta

The human term placenta represents an attractive source of MSC due to its ready availability, its easy access without invasive procedures, and lack of the ethical issues that surround the use of embryonic stem cells. The placenta as a whole, represents both fetal (amnion and chorion) and maternal (decidua) components (Figure 1) and is vital for the development and survival of the fetus throughout gestation.

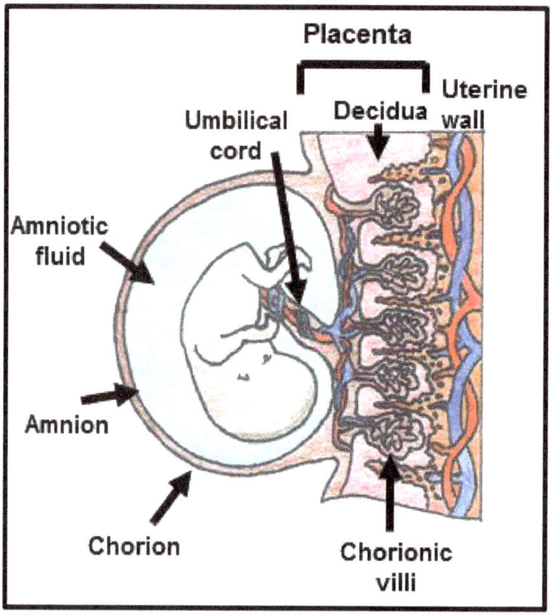

Fig. 1. A schematic diagram showing the developed human placenta. The diagram was adapted from the Merck Manual website. http://www.merckmanuals.com

Our group has isolated MSC from the whole placenta (amnion, chorion and decidua). Whole term placentas were collected from consenting healthy volunteer donors scheduled for elective Caesarean sections to minimise microbial contamination. Briefly, the whole placenta was cut into approximately 2 cm^2 pieces followed by enzymatic digestion using Collagenase Type 1 and DNase I. Ficoll density gradient or cell lysis was performed and cells placed in culture for *ex vivo* expansion. We found that human placental (hp) MSC differed to human bone marrow (hbm) MSC in proliferative capacity, with hbmMSC proliferating more slowly than hpMSC. Human pMSC were shown to be safe when administered into healthy mice at the same or higher dose than those currently used in clinical trials with hbmMSC (Barlow *et al.*, 2008a). Importantly, we also showed that the immune suppressive capacity of hpMSC to decrease T cell alloreactivity in mixed lymphocyte reaction (MLR) was equivalent to that of hbmMSC (Jones *et al.*, 2007). This thus suggested that human placenta is a potentially viable alternative source for human MSC and with this knowledge we are currently investigating placental-derived MSC in several human clinical trials (Brooke *et al.*, 2009).

3. Other gestational tissue sources of MSC

MSC derived from whole term placenta are of maternal origin (Barlow *et al.*, 2008a). Over the past decade much has been discovered about MSC in the developing fetal environment. Fetally-derived MSC are theoretically attractive because they generally have not been exposed to viruses and toxins, may contain less genetic abnormalities than adult tissue-derived MSC, and may have greater proliferative capacity and a greater retention of "stemness" memory. It has been suggested that they have properties intermediate between embryonic and adult stem cells (Guillot *et al.*, 2006). Thus, they may be a superior MSC source for clinical trials than the traditional source which is adult bone marrow.

This section will focus on the isolation of MSC from amniotic fluid (Mareschi *et al.*, 2009, Nadri and Soleimani, 2007, Roubelakis *et al.*, 2007), the amniotic membrane (Soncini *et al.*, 2007, Portmann-Lanz *et al.*, 2006, Diaz-Prado *et al.*, 2010), the chorion (chorion laeve and chorionic villi) (Soncini *et al.*, 2007, Portmann-Lanz *et al.*, 2006, Igura *et al.*, 2004, Poloni *et al.*, 2008), the decidua (Macias *et al.*, 2010, Aghajanova *et al.*, 2010), umbilical cord/Wharton's jelly (Mitchell *et al.*, 2003, Gonzalez *et al.*, 2010, Reinisch *et al.*, 2007, Petsa *et al.*, 2009) and umbilical cord blood (Mareschi *et al.*, 2001, Bieback *et al.*, 2004, Romanov *et al.*, 2003). This section will also discuss the isolation of haematopoietic stem cells from the umbilical cord blood and the application of these cells.

3.1 Amniotic fluid

Amniotic fluid helps protect the fetus throughout gestation. This unique environment allows the fetus to move freely within the uterus and protects the fetus from mechanical injury.

Amniocentesis is a diagnostic procedure that samples amniotic fluid from 14 weeks gestation until birth. This can be used to isolate amniotic fluid MSC (AF-MSC) for genetic screening purposes. It has been found that amniotic fluid contains a heterogeneous population of many cells including a large portion of epithelioid E-type cells, amniotic fluid-specific AF-type cells and fibroblast F-type cells (Witkowska-Zimny and Wrobel, 2011, Prusa and Hengstschlager, 2002). Although many cell types exist within the amniotic fluid, MSC have been found. It has been estimated that approximately 1% of cells in culture obtained from human amniocentesis are MSC. Only a few studies have successfully isolated single cell-derived MSC clones from amniotic fluid (Tsai *et al.*, 2004, De Coppi *et al.*, 2007, Antonucci *et al.*, 2009, Phermthai *et al.*, 2010, Witkowska-Zimny and Wrobel, 2011).

Amniotic fluid derived-MSC show typical MSC characteristics as well as expression of OCT4, a primitive stem cell marker (Roubelakis *et al.*, 2007). This suggests these cells may be more primitive than adult BM-MSC. Moreover, it has also been reported these cells have a high proliferative potential with over 250 population doublings without doubling time changes and can be differentiated into endodermal and ectodermal lineages *in vitro*. Although these properties seem theoretically more advantageous, it is debatable whether amniotic fluid is a practical and reliable source for generating MSC on a regular basis for clinical trials (Tsai *et al.*, 2004, De Coppi *et al.*, 2007, Antonucci *et al.*, 2009, Phermthai *et al.*, 2010, Witkowska-Zimny and Wrobel, 2011).

3.2 The amniotic membrane

The amnion is derived from the fetus and is the innermost membrane of the placenta. The amniotic membrane encases the amniotic fluid and fetus, and is highly flexible as it expands throughout gestation. It is a thin, avascular membrane and contains an epithelial cell layer and mesenchymal stromal cell layer. The amniotic epithelial cell layer is a single layer of flat, cuboidal and columnar cells in close contact with the amniotic fluid. The amnion epithelial cells are attached to a distinct basal lamina that is connected to the amniotic mesoderm (Blackburn, 2003, Parolini *et al.*, 2008). The amniotic mesoderm layer consists of macrophages and fibroblast-like mesenchymal cells (Parolini *et al.*, 2008). It is from this layer of the amniotic membrane that amniotic MSC (AMSC) can be isolated.

To isolate fetal-derived MSC-like cells from the amniotic membrane, enzymatic digestion is used. The amniotic membrane can be peeled from the chorionic membrane (Figure 1), washed until blood has been removed (until it appears almost translucent) and cut into smaller pieces. It is digested first using trypsin to remove the epithelial layer of cells and second, enzymatically digested to release the stromal cells. A ficoll density gradient or cell lysis can be performed and the mononuclear cells placed in culture. Similar to AF-MSC, these cells are fetally derived and exhibit similar characteristics to BM-MSC (Soncini *et al.*, 2007).

3.3 The chorion

The human chorion consists of the chorionic laeve (membrane), chorionic plate and chorionic villi. The chorionic laeve is the outer fetal membrane composed of layers of polygonal cells consisting of both mesoderm and trophoblast regions (Blackburn, 2003). The chorionic laeve is closely associated but not attached to the amniotic membrane and gives rise to the chorionic plate and villi. During development, the chorionic villi grow outwards into the endometrium to anchor at the decidua basalis (see below). This phenomenon occurs through dividing cytotrophoblasts and syncytiotrophoblasts and ultimately gives rise to a network of villi called the chorionic villi. Chorionic villi develop from the chorionic plate and stretch outwards (like finger-like projections) and attach to the decidua basalis to anchor the placenta in the uterus. The mesenchymal cells form a connective-tissue like support for the blood vessels growing into the villi and can also be found within this region.

To isolate fetal-derived MSC-like cells from the chorionic laeve, enzymatic digestion is suggested. The chorionic laeve is peeled from the amniotic membrane and cut at the chorionic plate. Similar to the amniotic membrane, the chorionic laeve is washed until blood clots have been removed and cut into smaller pieces. It is then digested using collagenase and DNase to release the stromal cells. A ficoll density gradient or cell lysis can be performed and the mononuclear cells placed in culture. Despite the chorionic laeve arising from the fetus, we have found from FISH and genotyping analyses from term chorionic membranes, that maternal cells are present in the cultured MSC population. It is predicted that this is a result of the decidua capularis (maternal derived) fusing to the chorionic leave early in pregnancy. Hence, we suggest that the chorionic laeve is not an optimal source for fetally derived MSC.

3.4 Chorionic villi

The chorionic villi are fetally derived and intercalates with the maternal decidua. It is responsible for the exchange of nutrients from the mother to the fetus. The chorionic villi are highly vascularised and consist of syncytiotrophoblasts, cytotrophoblasts and mesenchymal stromal cells. To isolate MSC, a diagnostic test, chorionic villus sampling, can be performed. This procedure is invasive to both mother and baby as it is performed *in utero*. Therefore, a less invasive method is to collect chorionic villi samples after birth (from term placenta). Due to the close interaction with maternal decidua, it is suggested that a dissecting microscope is used to mechanically separate fetal villi from maternal decidua. Despite these efforts, it can be a relatively ineffective method for isolating fetally derived cells with maternal cell contamination rapidly occurring in the cultured cell population. Hence, we do not recommend using this tissue source for isolating fetally derived MSC.

3.5 The decidua

After implantation of the blastocyst (~6-10 days post fertilisation), regional specialisation occurs within the endometrium to accommodate the developing embryo and placenta. The maternal decidua arises from this and forms 3 layers, decidua capularis, decidua basalis and decidua parietalis. The decidua capularis is adjacent to the embryo and fuses to the chorionic laeve as the embryo develops. At term this region of the decidua can not be distinguished from the chorion laeve. The decidua basalis is located between the myometrium and chorionic villi and can be difficult to distinguish. The decidua parietalis forms part of the uterine lining and is a better decidual source for isolating maternal MSC because it contains few invasive fetal cells (trophoblasts).

To obtain decidua parietalis, a suction or vacuum curettage of the uterine wall is used once the baby has been delivered. This is the most sterile technique but may cause complications to the mother such as post-natal uterine bleeding. The tissue is then digested and cells placed in culture.

3.6 Umbilical cord / Wharton's jelly

The life line that connects the fetus to the mother is the umbilical cord. The human umbilical cord allows vital nutrients and oxygen to be exchanged from the mother to the fetus. Within the umbilical cord are two arteries and one vein; these are surrounded by a gelatinous mucoid connective tissue known as Wharton's jelly. These tissues are derived from the extra-embryonic mesoderm, derived from the fetus (Witkowska-Zimny and Wrobel, 2011). The role of Wharton's jelly is to protect and insulate the umbilical cord vessels, and is composed of myofibroblast-like stromal cells, collagen fibers and proteoglycans. In 2003, primitive stem cell types were found to reside within the Wharton's jelly of the umbilical cord (Mitchell *et al.*, 2003). These cells are referred to as umbilical cord mesenchymal stromal/stem cells (UC-MSC).

There are several methods for the isolation of MSC from the umbilical cord. As with the isolation of whole marrow, the isolation of MSC from the umbilical cord includes enzymatic digestion of the tissue, followed by either a density gradient centrifugation or cell lysis. These cells can be isolated in large numbers, approximately 1.5x 10^6 cells/cm of the umbilical cord (Weiss *et al.*, 2005). It has been observed that UC-MSC proliferate faster than bmMSC and may be cultured for more than 80 population doublings with no indication of senescence or changes in morphology (Mitchell *et al.*, 2003).

3.7 Umbilical cord blood

The umbilical cord blood is known as a rich source for both MSC and HSC. MSC within the cord blood have been referred to as unrestricted somatic stem cells (USSC). However, there has been controversy over the efficiency and yield of USSC within the cord blood. It is proposed that possible explanations for the controversy involve the variability between donors, the isolation technique, and the use of different culture conditions by independent studies (Da Silva Meirelles *et al.*, 2008). Though the isolation of USSC from umbilical cord blood can be difficult, there have been some recent breakthroughs in attempts to optimise the isolation process. Flynn and colleagues (Bieback *et al.*, 2004, Chang *et al.*, 2006b, Flynn *et al.*, 2007, Kern *et al.*, 2006, Sparrow *et al.*, 2002) found the isolation process to be most efficient when the umbilical vein was cannulated and blood collected into a sterile bag containing either citrate phosphate dextrose or citrate-based anti-coagulant [0.6% acid citrate dextrose formula-A acid anti-coagulant and BSA (0.5% fraction V)], called ACD-A buffer (Flynn *et al.*, 2007, Mcguckin *et al.*, 2003). Once the umbilical cord blood has been collected it should be processed within 15 hours as USSC yield can decrease dramatically over time (Bieback *et al.*, 2004). Cord blood is processed using a ficoll density gradient and the mononuclear cells collected and placed in culture.

3.8 Isolation of HSC from the cord blood

The first successful UCB-derived HSCT was performed in 1989 by Gluckman and colleagues to treat a six year-old child with Fanconi anaemia (Gluckman *et al.*, 1989). Since then, UCB has become recognised as a promising alternative HSC source for HSCT. Some advantages that UCB has over bone marrow or mobilised peripheral blood from living donors is that it is readily available and available from cord blood banks throughout the world (Bradley and Cairo, 2005). Most importantly, UCB can be used in transplants with less than optimal donor-recipient HLA-matching, providing a broader application compared to BM and mPB. The reason behind this versatility is the immunologically naive nature of UCB which stems from its ontogenetic primitiveness compared to BM and mPB (Haylock and Nilsson, 2007).

UCB-derived HSC, and indeed all human HSC, are classically identified by cell surface expression of CD34, a cell surface glycoprotein (Andrews *et al.*, 1992, Okuno *et al.*, 2002, Osawa *et al.*, 1996). However, $CD34^+$ populations still contain a large population of committed progenitor cells with less than 1% of this population representing truly primitive HSC, as identified in transplantation assays (Wognum *et al.*, 2003). Thus, the CD34 marker is often used in combination with other markers such as Lin^-, $CD38^-$ and $CD90^+$ (Park *et al.*, 2008). In addition to these cell surface markers, other techniques have been developed to identify populations enriched for HSC based on some of the functional characteristics of these cells. These include dye exclusion due to efflux pumps of the fluorescent dyes Hoechst-33342 (Ho) and Rhodamine-123 (Rho) (Bertoncello *et al.*, 1988, Bertoncello and Williams, 2004, Goodell *et al.*, 1996, Li and Johnson, 1995, Schroeder, 2010, Wognum *et al.*, 2003). In the case of Ho, HSC actively pump the dye out of the cell and therefore can be fluorescently selected as $Ho^{-/low}$ (also known as side-population [SP] cells). Likewise, Rho is used to detect the low metabolic activity of HSC and they are identified as Rho^{low}. These techniques are used to both enrich and characterise HSC populations. However, the best and most accurate test of HSC quality is based on self-renewal potential and the ability to give rise to all cells of the haematopoietic lineage in an *in vivo* setting. This characteristic is assayed by measuring the ability of HSC to repopulate and contribute to haematopoiesis in lethally irradiated animals for long periods (usually greater than 3 months in mice).

While UCB has several advantages over BM and mPB as a HSC source, the application of UCB is limited by HSC yield. Consequently, the HSC dose (cells/kilogram) from a single cord is low for clinical transplantation. This is particularly evident in the adult setting, where multiple cords are often needed to permit a successful transplant. Therefore, there has been a strong focus in HSC expansion processes that may increase cell yield prior to transfusion.

4. Preclinical and clinical studies using cord blood HSC

Various culture methods have been proposed for both HSC expansion and for the production of mature cell end-products with clinical utility such as erythrocytes (particularly for trauma applications) and neutrophils (for neutropenia in the post-HSCT period). Historically, two main approaches have been taken towards achieving these aims.

1. Using *in vitro* culture systems supplemented with various combinations of haematopoietic growth factors.
2. Using a specific feeder cell monolayer to provide a supportive microenvironment.

This section will focus on HSC expansion techniques that use MSC as a supportive feeder layer and critique these in both pre-clinical and clinical settings.

The notion of using MSC to support HSC in culture arises from the HSC niche. Our understanding of the HSC niche has dramatically improved in the last three decades since Schofield first postulated the idea of a specialised micro-environment where stem cells exist (Schofield, 1978). This environment provides HSC with the necessary cues to maintain stem cell homeostasis by ensuring quiescence in a healthy state, or proliferation in the case of cytopenia or infection. These cues regulate HSC via cytokines, growth factors, extracellular matrix proteins, adhesion molecules and cell-cell interactions. Many of these signals are provided by the cells that make up the HSC niche, most notably those of the mesenchymal lineage. Thus, this innate supportive role characteristic of MSC has provided the basis for their use in *ex vivo* HSC expansion systems.

The most common source of MSC in MSC-HSC expansion systems is the BM. However, MSC have also been shown to be effective when sourced from other tissues including human placenta (Zhang *et al.*, 2004), umbilical cord (Bakhshi *et al.*, 2008, Huang *et al.*, 2007, Wang *et al.*, 2004) and adipose tissue (Nakao *et al.*, 2010). Recent papers have demonstrated that many of the specific cell-cell interactions between HSC and stromal cells are critical and may be essential for HSC regulation both *in vivo* (Steiner *et al.*, 2009) and *in vitro* (Jing *et al.*, 2010, Song *et al.*, 2010, Wagner *et al.*, 2008, Wagner *et al.*, 2007, Wein *et al.*, 2010). Indeed, a majority of studies have shown that cell-cell contact between HSC and MSC is essential for their *ex vivo* expansion. There is also evidence that the most primitive HSC directly interact with stromal cells (Song *et al.*, 2010, Zhang *et al.*, 2006). Although, MSC may provide growth factors themselves, one disadvantage of this technique, at least in the human system, is that the co-cultures still require additional supplementation with growth factor cocktails (Andrade *et al.*, 2010, Da Silva *et al.*, 2005, Mcniece *et al.*, 2004).

Clinical trials using co-culture expanded HSC are few in number. The proprietary Replicell technology developed by Aastrom Biosciences Inc. was shown to be feasible but not definitively effective in enhancing myeloid, erythroid or platelet engraftment in the clinical setting (Jaroscak *et al.*, 2003, Pecora *et al.*, 2001). The system uses stromal co-cultures while also providing a continuous supply of culture medium containing fetal calf serum, horse serum, PIXY321 (a GM-CSF/IL-3 fusion protein), flt3 (FL) and erythropoietin (EPO) (Stiff *et al.*, 2000). One of the most comprehensive co-culture clinical trials has recently been initiated by the company Mesoblast PTL using a BM-derived multipotent progenitor cell (an MSC-like cell) product to expand UCB cells. As with clinical trials using cytokine-expanded HSC, the study transfused one unmanipulated UCB unit together with one 14-day expanded unit. Expansion using this method enhanced neutrophil recovery by 14 days and the grafts were shown to elicit less GVHD compared to that of published reports using unmanipulated UCB transplants (Mesoblast ASX announcement, 06 Nov 2009, www.mesoblast.com) (Kelly *et al.*, 2009). While long-term follow up results are yet to be reported, it will be interesting to determine whether the therapeutic value of the expanded unit is purely short-term myeloid support, as is the case in the Delaney's cytokine-mediated expansion trial (Delaney *et al.*, 2010), or whether the expanded unit also provides durable long-term engraftment.

5. Manufacturing process of human placental-derived MSC under GMP conditions, quality assurance and regulatory considerations

In this section we discuss the manufacturing processes that are required for using current good manufacturing practice (cGMP), quality assurance and regulatory considerations when conducting clinical trials with placenta-derived mesenchymal stem cells in Australia.

We have chosen to utilise term human placental-derived mesenchymal stem/stromal cells (hpMSC) for a series of clinical trials. Placentas obtained during elective term Caesarean sections were used as our source for hpMSC manufacture in order to minimise the risk of microbial contamination, a major concern with *ex vivo* expansion of cells for therapeutic use.

With no need to MHC-match the donor to the intended recipient, hpMSC from a single manufacturing campaign can be utilised in numerous clinical trials and for number of patients (Brooke *et al.*, 2009). However, hpMSC manufacture currently represents a complex, specialised, time-consuming and labour-intensive exercise (Ilic *et al.*, 2011). At present MSC manufacture requires an "open" system due to the multiple steps required for isolation and expansion of MSC from placenta. Although class II safety cabinets or clean rooms can be utilised, the extended period of expansion (up to 6 weeks in our process) introduces the risk of microbial contamination. We have utilised extensive in-process and end-product testing prior for release of product for clinical use to minimise these risks (Ilic *et al.*, 2011).

The Code of Good Manufacturing Practice (cGMP) standard (or its close equivalent) is applied across the entirety of the hpMSC manufacturing process, including acquisition of the starting cell population (placental tissue), isolation of cells, processing, storage and transport. A Quality Management System (QMS) is required to provide support for the manufacturing process based on the International Organization for Standardization (ISO) standard requirements.

The new Biologicals Framework was established recently by the Therapeutic Goods Administration (TGA) in Australia (http://www.tga.gov.au/industry/btb.htm). Its purpose is to improve the regulation of human tissue and cellular therapies and provide improved clarity by applying different levels of pre-market regulation to biological products based on the risks associated with the use of each product. According to the Biologicals Framework, hpMSC are categorised as Class 3 products. As a result, any trial utilising hpMSC (Class 3 product) can be conducted under the TGA's Clinical Trial Notification (CTN) Scheme. The CTN scheme is designed to combine rapid approval of clinical trial protocols with ongoing monitoring and supervision by a Human Research Ethics Committee (HREC) acting in accordance with nationally agreed guidelines developed by the Australian National Health and Medical Research Council (NHMRC). It is important to note that the TGA does not review any data relating to the trial under this scheme. The Human Research Ethics Committee (HREC) reviewing a new clinical trial protocol utilising hpMSC must have sufficient experience among committee members in order to effectively review the protocol ensuring that the proposed trial has scientific validity, and that participants' rights and well-being are protected according to the Australian National Health and Medical Research Council's National Statement on Ethical Conduct in Human Research 2007, the Declaration of Helsinki and International Conference on Harmonisation Good Clinical Practice ICH GCP(CPMCP/ICH/135/95).

Along with the study protocol, a Participant Information Sheet and Consent Form (PISCF) and other supporting documents including an Investigators Brochure is submitted for review by the HREC and the TGA, and is used by study personnel to facilitate their understanding of the key features of the protocol, in particular, the dosing and methods of administration of the hpMSC.

5.1 Pre-manufacturing and quality management

All hpMSC donors are subject to screening requirements according to the AusCord (Australian National Network of Umbilical Cord Blood Banks and Cord Blood Collection Centres) Guide to Selection of Mothers and Cord Blood Donors. Prior to the collection of the placenta, the donating mother undergoes screening serology for infectious disease markers and completes an in-depth medical questionnaire (as per AusCord Guidelines). The same process is repeated at 180 days after placental donation and information is sought about the health of the baby to identify if any medical conditions have been identified that may exclude the donated placenta.

An operational unit provides support to advanced clinical research based upon high level cell manipulation, such as *ex vivo* expansion of hpMSC, through its Quality Management System. Our Quality Management System comprises the organisational structure, procedures, processes and resources that control quality activities within the operational unit. It is defined in a series of policy statements in the Quality Manual and it is implemented through Standard Operating Procedures. Standard Operating Procedures (SOPs) are used to ensure that work having an effect on service and product quality, either directly or indirectly, is carried out in a consistent and satisfactory manner. Clear and effective procedures are developed and maintained by relevant staff. Procedures are regularly reviewed for accuracy, relevance and consistency with the policies, requirements of the relevant standards, guidelines and best practices.

5.2 Manufacturing

The placenta is obtained from healthy mothers undergoing elective Caesarean sections with their full informed consent prior to delivery. The placenta is subsequently double bagged, placed in a cool box and transferred to our manufacturing facility for processing. Our protocol for the isolation of MSC from placenta utilises a GMP grade collagenase-based digestion of tissue which has been dissected and washed to remove blood before isolation of cells. After digestion, large particulate matter is removed by low speed centrifugation and cell suspensions are collected and filtered into fresh tubes using 70 μm filters. The cells are then pelleted by centrifugation, resuspended and erythrocytes are subjected to rapid lysis with water. The cells are washed with Hank's Balanced Salt Solution (HBSS) and the final cell pellet is resuspended in Dulbecco's Modified Eagle Medium (DMEM-LG), 25% fetal calf serum (FCS), and 50 μg/ml gentamycin. Cells are initially seeded into eight T175 cm^2 tissue culture flasks and cultured in a humidified incubator at 37°C, 5% CO_2. A scheme of the production schedule is shown in Figure 2.

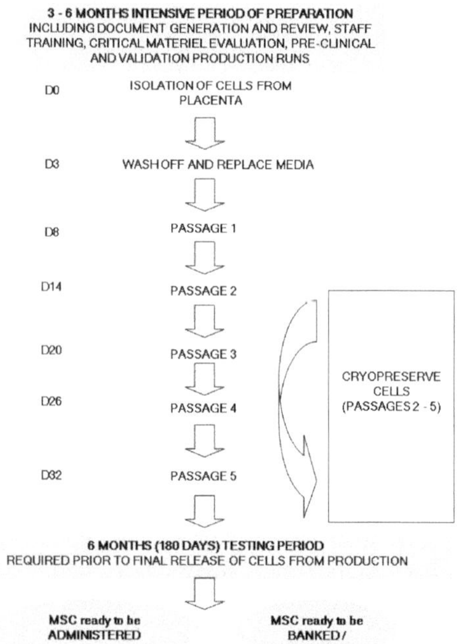

Fig. 2. Human placenta-derived MSC manufacturing flow diagram. D, day of manufacturing process

5.3 Release criteria

Prior to placenta donation, the mother must fulfil the criteria in the health questionnaire and undergo screening serology testing for infectious disease markers, the results of which must be negative. At day 180, a health questionnaire for both mother and baby are performed and both must be satisfactory. The mother's infectious disease markers are repeated and, again, must be negative (Table 1). In addition, for the cryopreserved cells to be available for subsequent use in a clinical trial, the following release criteria must be met: MSC passages (P) zero to five (P0-P5) must be sterile after 14 days microbiology culture; the MSC must be greater than 70% viable (using Trypan Blue exclusion); MSC purity is determined by flow cytometry, and must be >85% $CD73^+$, >85% $CD105^+$, and <1% $CD45^+$. A normal karyotype analysis must be demonstrated on MSC from P2 - P5; Gram stain (P2-P5) must be negative; mycoplasma testing (P2-P5) must be negative, and endotoxin testing (P2- P5) must show a level of < 2 EU/ml (Table 1).

Test Completed	Pre-donation Screening	P0	P1	P2	P3	P4	P5	Day 180**
Gram stain	N/A	N/A	N/A	Required	Required	Required	Required	N/A
Sterility	N/A	N/A	N/A	Required	Required	Required	Required	N/A
Mycoplasma	N/A	N/A	N/A	Required	Required	Required	Required	N/A
Endotoxin	N/A	N/A	N/A	Required	Required	Required	Required	N/A
FACS phenotype	N/A	N/A	N/A	Required	Required	Required	Required	N/A
Karyotype	N/A	N/A	N/A	Required	Required	Required	Required	N/A
Donor serology*	Required	N/A	N/A	N/A	N/A	N/A	N/A	Required
Donor health questionnaire	Required	N/A	N/A	N/A	N/A	N/A	N/A	Required

* For infectious disease markers. ** Donor/mother and the baby follow-up. N/A = Not applicable. P = Passage.

Table 1. Human placenta-derived MSC Quality Control Testing used by the Stem Cell Biology, Regenerative Medicine and Stem Cell-based anti-Cancer Therapeutics Group, MHS/MMRI, Brisbane, Australia.

6. Placental-derived MSC in the clinic

6.1 Application in clinical trials

Clinical trials of MSC therapy in humans have shown promising results in several clinical settings. Many patients have now received MSC by intravenous infusion for multiple clinical indications world-wide. A search on ClinicalTrails.gov listed a total of 192 MSC clinical studies in July 2011, including 171 studies with their status indicated. Clinical diseases treated to date have included acute graft-versus-host disease (GVHD) following allogeneic HSC transplantation, Crohn's disease, insulin-dependent diabetes mellitus and renal transplantation (Kebriaei and Robinson, 2011). The tissue repair capability of MSC is also being investigated in clinical trials for cardiac muscle repair after acute myocardial infarction, congenital bone disorders such as osteogenesis imperfecta, severe bone fractures, meniscal tears and liver repair in patients with cirrhosis. Studies have also been carried out using MSC to treat various metabolic disorders, ischemic stroke and neurological disorders.

Currently, four clinical trials using bone marrow-derived MSC are completed or in progress in Australia. Our group was the first to conduct clinical trials with human placenta-derived MSC. We are currently conducting three clinical trials using hpMSC and have four additional clinical trials in preparation.

6.2 Phase I clinical trial of hpMSC co-transplanted with umbilical cord blood transplants

In 2007, we submitted a HREC application for our first Phase I clinical trial, which was a multicentre, open label dose-escalation study of volunteer unrelated, MHC-unmatched placenta-derived MSC in recipients of unrelated umbilical cord blood HSC transplants. In this setting it was hypothesised that the transplanted MSC would support engraftment of HSC and reduce the frequency and severity of graft-versus-host disease (GVHD). The total time from submission of the application until final approval was 1 year. During this time, a request was made by our institutional HREC for an external audit to be conducted on the manufacturing processes outlined in the study protocol. This was performed by the Australian Red Cross Blood Service (ARCBS) and a two-way clinical trial agreement was established between the two participating hospitals. This agreement included an appropriate indemnification for each of the participating sites and ensured reporting of any adverse events related to the administration of the hpMSC.

6.2.1 Course of clinical trial

One day after the completion of pre-transplant myeloablative conditioning with cyclophosphamide and total body irradiation, a 20 year old Caucasian male with acute myeloid leukemia in second remission was given 1.20×10^8 human placental MSC (1×10^6/kg) intravenously. These were suspended in 30 ml and infused over 7 min using a 200 µm in-line filter. No adverse events were noted. Five hours later the patient received two cord blood units. Post-thaw, the total nucleated cell dose from the two cord blood units was 3.6×10^7/kg and the total $CD34^+$ cell dose was 1.2×10^5/kg. The MSC were MHC-unmatched with both the recipient and the two cord units. The MSC donor serology tests were negative for cytomegalovirus (CMV), as were the two cord blood donors (Brooke *et al.*, 2009).

6.2.2 Post-transplant clinical course

Cyclosporine and mycophenylate mofetil were used as prophylaxis for graft-versus-host diseases (GVHD). The patient developed Strepotococcus viridans septicemia on day 7 post-transplant and was treated accordingly. Subsequently, the patient developed a skin rash on day 14 and the skin biopsy was consistent with acute GVHD and resolved with treatment. Neutrophil engraftment with an absolute neutrophil count > 500/µl occurred at day 38. CMV reactivation occurred at day 45 and the patient was treated with ganciclovir. However, at day 52 staphylococcal bacteremia occurred with the subsequent development of fever, fluid overload, respiratory distress and hypoxia. On day 68 the patient died of respiratory failure, thought due to interstitial pneumonitis. The patient did not become platelet-independent by the time of his death and the treating physicians did not consider any of the post-transplant complications to be related to the MSC infusion (Brooke *et al.*, 2009).

6.2.3 Lessons learned from this trial

One patient was enrolled in this study and later died from pneumonitis related to CMV reactivation. It is important to note that the donor of the hpMSC was CMV-negative prior to the collection of the placenta and again at the follow-up screening period. This particular study did not yield significant clinical results. Unfortunately, this particular study has now been closed as umbilical cord blood transplants are no longer being performed in adults at the specific hospitals involved.

However, it did highlight some of the impracticalities in incorporating the manufacturing protocol within a given clinical trial protocol. As a result, a new manufacturing protocol was established in 2009. This manufacturing protocol allowed us to continue manufacturing hpMSC independent of a clinical trial and therefore established a master cell bank of hpMSC. This protocol was approved by our institutional HREC under the provision that any clinical trial utilising the hpMSC as the investigational product was to be reviewed by the Human Research Ethics Committee.

6.3 Phase I clinical trial of hpMSC in patients with idiopathic pulmonary fibrosis

In 2010 we initiated a phase I study to evaluate the potential role of placenta-derived MSC in the treatment of idiopathic pulmonary fibrosis (IPF). MSC represent an attractive and novel therapeutic agent for lung diseases, as the lungs are the first site in which MSC lodge after intravenous injection (Figure 3). IPF is a relatively common chronic, fibrosing lung disease of unknown aetiology that results in severe, refractory and progressive breathlessness. MSC have theoretical benefits to patients with IPF because of their immunomodulatory capacity to decrease fibrosis. It is possible that any therapeutic role for MSC in this disease will be mediated by their ability to remodel extracellular matrix, or their ability to suppress the immune response through contact-dependent and soluble mediators, or both.

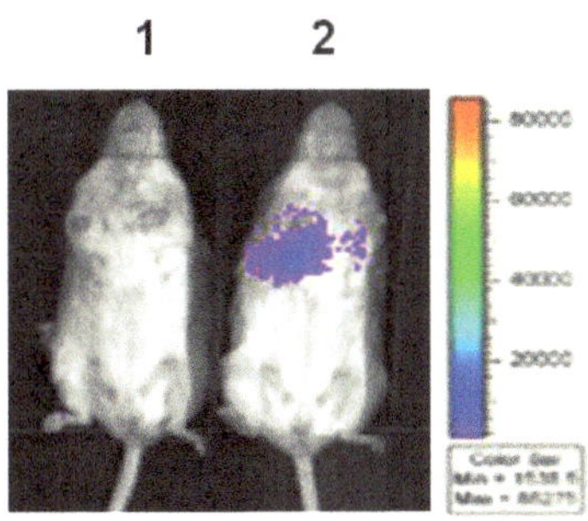

Fig. 3. *In vivo* luciferase activity of MSC after intravenous injection. Images were taken 38 min after injection with an exposure period of 10 min. Mouse 1: No cells administered (negative control), Mouse 2: 1 x 10^6 MSC transgenic for luciferase.

6.3.1 Course of clinical trial and monitoring

Our hpMSC were transported in a dry shipper to the participating hospital where they were thawed and infused intravenously. This is another Phase I study (since we regard hpMSC as a "first-in-man" reagent that need to be investigated in a Phase I trial for each different patient population) to assess the safety of hpMSC in IPF patients, as well as to perform an MSC dose-escalation study, with the approval of the Data Safety Monitoring Committee to initiate the second dose-cohort. The first 4 patients receive 1 x 10^6 MSC/kg and the second 4 patients receive 2 x 10^6 MSC/kg. To date 3 patients have been infused in Cohort 1 without any adverse events due to the hpMSC. Specifically, no serious adverse events relating to infusional toxicity or ectopic tissue formation have been reported. Instructions for monitoring for infusional toxicity are represented in Table 2. Infusional toxicity is defined as any one of the criteria observed in Table 2 at any time within the 4-hr post-infusion period.

Vital Sign	**Measurement**
Systolic Blood Pressure (mmHg)	< 90 > 180 > 25% decrease > 25% increase
Diastolic Blood Pressure (mmHg)	< 50 > 100 > 25% decrease > 25% increase
Heart Rate (bpm)	< 60 > 110 > 25% decrease > 25% increase
Body Temperature (°F)	> 101.5 > 2° decrease > 2° increase

Table 2. Monitoring for infusional toxicity

6.3.2 Lessons learned from this trial

Thus far, human placenta-derived MSC appear safe with no adverse events noted after intravenous infusion. If safety is confirmed in this Phase I trial we will proceed to a Phase II trial powered for efficacy.

6.4 Phase I clinical trial of hpMSC for Achilles tendinopathy

In 2011 we initiated our first study in the treatment of chronic refractory tendinopathy. Tendinopathy is a common condition associated with pain and tendon dysfunction. Tendinopathy often occurs in young, active adults. As life expectancy increases, so does the incidence of tendinopathy. This in turn will place large costs on the health system budget. The initial management of all tendinopathies is usually conservative and includes activity modification, medication, injections and exercises. If prolonged disability occurs, surgical treatment is considered which is expensive and involves periods of immobilisation. Current treatment is relatively ineffective, as tendons have a poor capacity to repair themselves. Therefore, stem cell therapies have been extensively researched in preclinical models as a possible treatment.

Several animal studies have shown that MSC can repair the tendon defect, and regenerate the tendinopathic tissue (Nourissat *et al.*, 2010, Chen *et al.*, 2009, Lim *et al.*, 2004). It may be that the main mechanism of MSC repair in this case is to enable differentiation into tenocytes. The biomechanics of the resulting tendon can be improved further by applying mechano-stimulation (e.g. exercise). This regenerative technique has not shown any complications in the published preclinical animal studies and seems a promising treatment in man.

6.4.1 Course of clinical trial

This is a phase I, open-label, single centre, non-randomized dose-escalation evaluation of the safety and feasibility of MSC treatment for patients diagnosed with refractory Achilles tendinopathy. Up to nine patients will be enrolled in the study. All patients will receive ultrasound-guided precision intratendinous injection of hpMSC into their damaged Achilles tendon. Injections will occur at least 4 weeks after the previous patient so that any early adverse effects from the previous hpMSC application can be closely monitored and assessed, both clinically and via diagnostic power doppler ultrasound examination.

There will be 3 cohorts, each with 3 patients, to assess the safety of the MSC dose. The first cohort of 3 patients will receive a single dose of 1.0×10^6 placenta-derived MSC (1.0 ml of solution containing 1.0×10^6 MSC per ml) each. The next cohort of 3 patients will receive 4.0×10^6 MSC (1.0 ml of solution containing 4.0×10^6 MSC per ml) each. The final cohort of 3 patients will receive 1.6×10^7 MSC (1.0 ml of solution containing 1.6×10^7 MSC per ml) each. An interim safety analysis will be carried out by the Data Safety Management Committee (DSMC) after each group of 3 has received their individual injection. This will occur following the 4 week post injection assessment, of the third member of each group. Should no serious adverse events be documented due to, or likely due to, the MSC injection, the subsequent group will receive a local guided precision injection at the next ascending dose.

The injection phase of the study will take at least 9 months to complete. Therefore, from this clinical trial, there will be data to show if intra-tendinous injection of MSC is a safe treatment of otherwise treatment-refractory Achilles tendinopathy.

6.4.2 Post-injection clinical course

The primary purpose of this trial is to provide evidence of the safe delivery of intra-tendinous injection of MSC. This will be assessed at 2 days post injection (via telephone), 2 weeks, 4 weeks, 10 weeks and 26 weeks and will include ultrasound assessment of the tendon (after 4, 10 and 26 weeks).

The second purpose is to measure the possible effectiveness of MSC in reducing the chronic morbidity associated with Achilles tendinopathy after 4, 10 and 26 weeks after intratendinous injection. Evidence for improvement in ultrasound and power doppler ultrasound assessment of tendon structure will include the following parameters: (i) tendon thickness (sagittal plane), (ii) echogenicity, (iii) discontinuity, (iv) neovascularisation and (v) other abnormalities.

6.4.3 Expected outcomes

It is proposed MSC may offer a safe and highly cost effective treatment for chronic refractory tendinopathy, which could increase population activity levels, improve quality of life, and minimise dependence on costly long term medication and allied health treatments. MSC-initiated tendon regeneration could reduce the requirement for surgical treatments, thereby reducing the risks and costs of surgery and post-operative immobility. MSC injections also have the potential to augment and accelerate orthopaedic surgical tendon repair, either intraoperatively or by percutaneous injection, and offer an alternative treatment for individuals in whom tendon surgery has failed or is not possible.

To the best of our knowledge, this is the first trial of the use of allogeneic placenta-derived mesenchymal stem cells in the treatment of chronic refractory tendinopathy. Although we have chosen to use MSC derived from whole placenta for our current clinical trials, we are currently conducting research that explores the possibility of more advantageous MSC residing within the placenta. It is hypothesised that fetal MSC derived from the term placenta may have different biological properties from maternal MSC, given the differences in age at the time of their development. Such differences may have implications in the potential use of MSC as therapeutic agents. Therefore, this research may prove to be useful for choosing the optimal gestational product MSC for our future clinical trial program.

7. Conclusion/summary

Human gestational tissues show great promise as alternative stem cell sources. They are readily available and provide a basically unlimited supply of donor tissue for generating both MSC, and in the case of cord blood, HSC therapeutic products.

8. Acknowledgements

This work was made possible by a postgraduate research scholarship from the University of Queensland and grants from the Inner Wheel of Australia, the Queensland Academy of Sports, Prince Charles Hospital, Brisbane, The Flack Foundation, The Mater Foundation and The Australian Stem Cell Foundation.

9. References

Aghajanova, L., Horcajadas, J. A., Esteban, F. J. & Giudice, L. C. (2010) The bone marrow-derived human mesenchymal stem cell: potential progenitor of the endometrial stromal fibroblast. *Biol Reprod,* 82, 1076-87.

Andrade, P. Z., Dos Santos, F., Almeida-Porada, G., Da Silva, C. L. & Jm, S. C. (2010) Systematic delineation of optimal cytokine concentrations to expand hematopoietic stem/progenitor cells in co-culture with mesenchymal stem cells. *Mol Biosyst,* 6, 1207-15.

Andrews, R. G., Bryant, E. M., Bartelmez, S. H., Muirhead, D. Y., Knitter, G. H., Bensinger, W., Strong, D. M. & Bernstein, I. D. (1992) CD34+ marrow cells, devoid of T and B lymphocytes, reconstitute stable lymphopoiesis and myelopoiesis in lethally irradiated allogeneic baboons. *Blood,* 80, 1693-701.

Antonucci, I., Iezzi, I., Morizio, E., Mastrangelo, F., Pantalone, A., Mattioli-Belmonte, M., Gigante, A., Salini, V., Calabrese, G., Tete, S., Palka, G. & Stuppia, L. (2009) Isolation of osteogenic progenitors from human amniotic fluid using a single step culture protocol. *BMC Biotechnol,* 9, 9.

Appelbaum, F. R. (2007) Hematopoietic-cell transplantation at 50. *N Engl J Med,* 357, 1472-5.

Bailo, M., Soncini, M., Vertua, E., Signoroni, P. B., Sanzone, S., Lombardi, G., Arienti, D., Calamani, F., Zatti, D., Paul, P., Albertini, A., Zorzi, F., Cavagnini, A., Candotti, F., Wengler, G. S. & Parolini, O. (2004) Engraftment potential of human amnion and chorion cells derived from term placenta. *Transplantation,* 78, 1439-48.

Bakhshi, T., Zabriskie, R. C., Bodie, S., Kidd, S., Ramin, S., Paganessi, L. A., Gregory, S. A., Fung, H. C. & Christopherson, K. W., 2nd (2008) Mesenchymal stem cells from the Wharton's jelly of umbilical cord segments provide stromal support for the maintenance of cord blood hematopoietic stem cells during long-term ex vivo culture. *Transfusion,* 48, 2638-44.

Barlow, S., Brooke, G., Chatterjee, K., Price, G., Pelekanos, R., Rossetti, T., Doody, M., Venter, D., Pain, S., Gilshenan, K. & Atkinson, K. (2008a) Comparison of human placenta- and bone marrow-derived multipotent mesenchymal stem cells. *Stem Cells Dev,* 17, 1095-107.

Barlow, S., Brooke, G., Chatterjee, K., Price, G., Pelekanos, R., Rossetti, T., Doody, M., Venter, D., Pain, S., Gilshenan, K. & Atkinson, K. (2008b) Comparison of Human Placenta- and Bone Marrow-Derived Multipotent Mesenchymal Stem Cells. *Stem Cells and Development,* in press.

Bergman, R. J., Gazit, D., Kahn, A. J., Gruber, H., Mcdougall, S. & Hahn, T. J. (1996) Age-related changes in osteogenic stem cells in mice. *J Bone Miner Res,* 11, 568-77.

Bertoncello, I., Hodgson, G. S. & Bradley, T. R. (1988) Multiparameter analysis of transplantable hemopoietic stem cells. II. Stem cells of long-term bone marrow-reconstituted recipients. *Exp Hematol,* 16, 245-9.

Bertoncello, I. & Williams, B. (2004) Hematopoietic stem cell characterization by Hoechst 33342 and rhodamine 123 staining. *Methods Mol Biol,* 263, 181-200.

Bieback, K., Kern, S., Kluter, H. & Eichler, H. (2004) Critical parameters for the isolation of mesenchymal stem cells from umbilical cord blood. *Stem Cells,* 22, 625-34.

Blackburn, S. (2003) *Maternal, Fetal, & Neonatal Physiology: A Clincal Perspective,* Saunders: An Imprint of Elsevier Science.

Bradley, M. B. & Cairo, M. S. (2005) Cord blood immunology and stem cell transplantation. *Hum Immunol,* 66, 431-46.

Brooke, G., Cook, M., Blair, C., Han, R., Heazlewood, C., Jones, B., Kambouris, M., Kollar, K., Mctaggart, S., Pelekanos, R., Rice, A., Rossetti, T. & Atkinson, K. (2007) Therapeutic applications of mesenchymal stromal cells. *Semin Cell Dev Biol,* 18, 846-58.

Brooke, G., Rossetti, T., Pelekanos, R., Ilic, N., Murray, P., Hancock, S., Antonenas, V., Huang, G., Gottlieb, D., Bradstock, K. & Atkinson, K. (2009) Manufacturing of human placenta-derived mesenchymal stem cells for clinical trials. *Br J Haematol,* 144, 571-9.

Caplan, A. I. (1994) The mesengenic process. *Clin Plast Surg,* 21, 429-35.

Chang, C. J., Yen, M. L., Chen, Y. C., Chien, C. C., Huang, H. I., Bai, C. H. & Yen, B. L. (2006a) Placenta-derived multipotent cells exhibit immunosuppressive properties that are enhanced in the presence of interferon-gamma. *Stem Cells,* 24, 2466-77.

Chang, Y. J., Tseng, C. P., Hsu, L. F., Hsieh, T. B. & Hwang, S. M. (2006b) Characterization of two populations of mesenchymal progenitor cells in umbilical cord blood. *Cell Biol Int,* 30, 495-9.

Chen, X., Song, X. H., Yin, Z., Zou, X. H., Wang, L. L., Hu, H., Cao, T., Zheng, M. & Ouyang, H. W. (2009) Stepwise differentiation of human embryonic stem cells promotes tendon regeneration by secreting fetal tendon matrix and differentiation factors. *Stem Cells,* 27, 1276-87.

D'ippolito, G., Schiller, P. C., Ricordi, C., Roos, B. A. & Howard, G. A. (1999) Age-related osteogenic potential of mesenchymal stromal stem cells from human vertebral bone marrow. *J Bone Miner Res,* 14, 1115-22.

Da Silva, C. L., Goncalves, R., Crapnell, K. B., Cabral, J. M., Zanjani, E. D. & Almeida-Porada, G. (2005) A human stromal-based serum-free culture system supports the ex vivo expansion/maintenance of bone marrow and cord blood hematopoietic stem/progenitor cells. *Exp Hematol,* 33, 828-35.

Da Silva Meirelles, L., Caplan, A. I. & Nardi, N. B. (2008) In search of the in vivo identity of mesenchymal stem cells. *Stem Cells,* 26, 2287-99.

De Coppi, P., Bartsch, G., Jr., Siddiqui, M. M., Xu, T., Santos, C. C., Perin, L., Mostoslavsky, G., Serre, A. C., Snyder, E. Y., Yoo, J. J., Furth, M. E., Soker, S. & Atala, A. (2007) Isolation of amniotic stem cell lines with potential for therapy. *Nat Biotechnol,* 25, 100-6.

Delaney, C., Heimfeld, S., Brashem-Stein, C., Voorhies, H., Manger, R. L. & Bernstein, I. D. (2010) Notch-mediated expansion of human cord blood progenitor cells capable of rapid myeloid reconstitution. *Nat Med,* 16, 232-6.

Diaz-Prado, S., Muinos-Lopez, E., Hermida-Gomez, T., Rendal-Vazquez, M. E., Fuentes-Boquete, I., De Toro, F. J. & Blanco, F. J. (2010) Multilineage differentiation potential of cells isolated from the human amniotic membrane. *J Cell Biochem,* 111, 846-57.

Flynn, A., Barry, F. & O'brien, T. (2007) UC blood-derived mesenchymal stromal cells: an overview. *Cytotherapy,* 9, 717-26.

Friedenstein, A. J., Gorskaja, J. F. & Kulagina, N. N. (1976) Fibroblast precursors in normal and irradiated mouse hematopoietic organs. *Exp Hematol,* 4, 267-74.

Gekas, C., K, E. R. & H, K. a. M. (2008) Isolation and analysis of hematopoietic stem cells from the placenta. *J Vis Exp.*

Gekas, C., Rhodes, K. E., Van Handel, B., Chhabra, A., Ueno, M. & Mikkola, H. K. (2010) Hematopoietic stem cell development in the placenta. *Int J Dev Biol,* 54, 1089-98.

Gluckman, E., Broxmeyer, H. A., Auerbach, A. D., Friedman, H. S., Douglas, G. W., Devergie, A., Esperou, H., Thierry, D., Socie, G., Lehn, P. & Et Al. (1989) Hematopoietic reconstitution in a patient with Fanconi's anemia by means of umbilical-cord blood from an HLA-identical sibling. *N Engl J Med,* 321, 1174-8.

Gonzalez, R., Griparic, L., Umana, M., Burgee, K., Vargas, V., Nasrallah, R., Silva, F. & Patel, A. (2010) An efficient approach to isolation and characterization of pre- and postnatal umbilical cord lining stem cells for clinical applications. *Cell Transplant,* 19, 1439-49.

Goodell, M. A., Brose, K., Paradis, G., Conner, A. S. & Mulligan, R. C. (1996) Isolation and functional properties of murine hematopoietic stem cells that are replicating in vivo. *J Exp Med,* 183, 1797-806.

Guillot, P. V., O'donoghue, K., Kurata, H. & Fisk, N. M. (2006) Fetal stem cells: betwixt and between. *Semin Reprod Med,* 24, 340-7.

Haylock, D. N. & Nilsson, S. K. (2007) Expansion of umbilical cord blood for clinical transplantation. *Curr Stem Cell Res Ther,* 2, 324-35.

Huang, G. P., Pan, Z. J., Jia, B. B., Zheng, Q., Xie, C. G., Gu, J. H., Mcniece, I. K. & Wang, J. F. (2007) Ex vivo expansion and transplantation of hematopoietic stem/progenitor cells supported by mesenchymal stem cells from human umbilical cord blood. *Cell Transplant,* 16, 579-85.

Igura, K., Zhang, X., Takahashi, K., Mitsuru, A., Yamaguchi, S. & Takashi, T. A. (2004) Isolation and characterization of mesenchymal progenitor cells from chorionic villi of human placenta. *Cytotherapy,* 6, 543-53.

Ilic, N., Brooke, G., Murray, P., Barlow, S., Rossetti, T., Pelekanos, R., Hancock, S. & Atkinson, K. (2011) Manufacture of clinical grade human placenta-derived multipotent mesenchymal stromal cells. *Methods Mol Biol,* 698, 89-106.

In 'T Anker, P. S., Scherjon, S. A., Kleijburg-Van Der Keur, C., De Groot-Swings, G. M., Claas, F. H., Fibbe, W. E. & Kanhai, H. H. (2004) Isolation of mesenchymal stem cells of fetal or maternal origin from human placenta. *Stem Cells,* 22, 1338-45.

Jaroscak, J., Goltry, K., Smith, A., Waters-Pick, B., Martin, P. L., Driscoll, T. A., Howrey, R., Chao, N., Douville, J., Burhop, S., Fu, P. & Kurtzberg, J. (2003) Augmentation of umbilical cord blood (UCB) transplantation with ex vivo-expanded UCB cells: results of a phase 1 trial using the AastromReplicell System. *Blood,* 101, 5061-7.

Javazon, E., Tebbets, J., Beggs, K., Sena-Esteves, M., Campagnoli, C., Radu, A. & Flake, A. (2003) Isolation, expansion and characterisation of murine adult bone marrow derived mesenchymal stem cells. *Blood,* 102, 180B-181B.

Jiang, X. X., Zhang, Y., Liu, B., Zhang, S. X., Wu, Y., Yu, X. D. & Mao, N. (2005) Human mesenchymal stem cells inhibit differentiation and function of monocyte-derived dendritic cells. *Blood,* 105, 4120-6.

Jing, D., Fonseca, A. V., Alakel, N., Fierro, F. A., Muller, K., Bornhauser, M., Ehninger, G., Corbeil, D. & Ordemann, R. (2010) Hematopoietic stem cells in co-culture with mesenchymal stromal cells - modelling the niche compartments in vitro. *Haematologica,* 95, 542-50.

Jones, B. J., Brooke, G., Atkinson, K. & Mctaggart, S. J. (2007) Immunosuppression by placental indoleamine 2,3-dioxygenase: a role for mesenchymal stem cells. *Placenta,* 28, 1174-81.

Kebriaei, P. & Robinson, S. (2011) Treatment of graft-versus-host-disease with mesenchymal stromal cells. *Cytotherapy,* 13, 262-8.

Kelly, S. S., Sola, C. B., De Lima, M. & Shpall, E. (2009) Ex vivo expansion of cord blood. *Bone Marrow Transplant,* 44, 673-81.

Kern, S., Eichler, H., Stoeve, J., Kluter, H. & Bieback, K. (2006) Comparative analysis of mesenchymal stem cells from bone marrow, umbilical cord blood, or adipose tissue. *Stem Cells,* 24, 1294-301.

Li, C. L. & Johnson, G. R. (1995) Murine hematopoietic stem and progenitor cells: I. Enrichment and biologic characterization. *Blood,* 85, 1472-9.

Lim, J. K., Hui, J., Li, L., Thambyah, A., Goh, J. & Lee, E. H. (2004) Enhancement of tendon graft osteointegration using mesenchymal stem cells in a rabbit model of anterior cruciate ligament reconstruction. *Arthroscopy,* 20, 899-910.

Lodie, T. A., Blickarz, C. E., Devarakonda, T. J., He, C., Dash, A. B., Clarke, J., Gleneck, K., Shihabuddin, L. & Tubo, R. (2002) Systematic analysis of reportedly distinct populations of multipotent bone marrow-derived stem cells reveals a lack of distinction. *Tissue Eng,* 8, 739-51.

Macias, M. I., Grande, J., Moreno, A., Dominguez, I., Bornstein, R. & Flores, A. I. (2010) Isolation and characterization of true mesenchymal stem cells derived from human term decidua capable of multilineage differentiation into all 3 embryonic layers. *Am J Obstet Gynecol,* 203, 495 e9-495 e23.

Mareschi, K., Biasin, E., Piacibello, W., Aglietta, M., Madon, E. & Fagioli, F. (2001) Isolation of human mesenchymal stem cells: bone marrow versus umbilical cord blood. *Haematologica,* 86, 1099-100.

Mareschi, K., Rustichelli, D., Comunanza, V., De Fazio, R., Cravero, C., Morterra, G., Martinoglio, B., Medico, E., Carbone, E., Benedetto, C. & Fagioli, F. (2009) Multipotent mesenchymal stem cells from amniotic fluid originate neural precursors with functional voltage-gated sodium channels. *Cytotherapy,* 11, 534-47.

Mcbride, C., Gaupp, D. & Phinney, D. G. (2003) Quantifying levels of transplanted murine and human mesenchymal stem cells in vivo by real-time PCR. *Cytotherapy,* 5, 7-18.

Mcguckin, C. P., Pearce, D., Forraz, N., Tooze, J. A., Watt, S. M. & Pettengell, R. (2003) Multiparametric analysis of immature cell populations in umbilical cord blood and bone marrow. *Eur J Haematol,* 71, 341-50.

Mcniece, I., Harrington, J., Turney, J., Kellner, J. & Shpall, E. J. (2004) Ex vivo expansion of cord blood mononuclear cells on mesenchymal stem cells. *Cytotherapy,* 6, 311-7.

Mitalipov, S. & Wolf, D. (2009) Totipotency, pluripotency and nuclear reprogramming. *Adv Biochem Eng Biotechnol,* 114, 185-99.

Mitchell, K. E., Weiss, M. L., Mitchell, B. M., Martin, P., Davis, D., Morales, L., Helwig, B., Beerenstrauch, M., Abou-Easa, K., Hildreth, T., Troyer, D. & Medicetty, S. (2003) Matrix cells from Wharton's jelly form neurons and glia. *Stem Cells,* 21, 50-60.

Nadri, S. & Soleimani, M. (2007) Comparative analysis of mesenchymal stromal cells from murine bone marrow and amniotic fluid. *Cytotherapy,* 9, 729-37.

Nakao, N., Nakayama, T., Yahata, T., Muguruma, Y., Saito, S., Miyata, Y., Yamamoto, K. & Naoe, T. (2010) Adipose Tissue-Derived Mesenchymal Stem Cells Facilitate Hematopoiesis In Vitro and In Vivo. Advantages Over Bone Marrow-Derived Mesenchymal Stem Cells. *Am J Pathol.*

Nourissat, G., Diop, A., Maurel, N., Salvat, C., Dumont, S., Pigenet, A., Gosset, M., Houard, X. & Berenbaum, F. (2010) Mesenchymal stem cell therapy regenerates the native bone-tendon junction after surgical repair in a degenerative rat model. *PLoS One,* 5, e12248.

Okuno, Y., Iwasaki, H., Huettner, C. S., Radomska, H. S., Gonzalez, D. A., Tenen, D. G. & Akashi, K. (2002) Differential regulation of the human and murine CD34 genes in hematopoietic stem cells. *Proc Natl Acad Sci U S A,* 99, 6246-51.

Osawa, M., Hanada, K., Hamada, H. & Nakauchi, H. (1996) Long-term lymphohematopoietic reconstitution by a single CD34-low/negative hematopoietic stem cell. *Science,* 273, 242-5.

Park, C. Y., Majeti, R. & Weissman, I. L. (2008) In vivo evaluation of human hematopoiesis through xenotransplantation of purified hematopoietic stem cells from umbilical cord blood. *Nat Protoc,* 3, 1932-40.

Parolini, O., Alviano, F., Bagnara, G. P., Bilic, G., Buhring, H. J., Evangelista, M., Hennerbichler, S., Liu, B., Magatti, M., Mao, N., Miki, T., Marongiu, F., Nakajima, H., Nikaido, T., Portmann-Lanz, C. B., Sankar, V., Soncini, M., Stadler, G., Surbek, D., Takahashi, T. A., Redl, H., Sakuragawa, N., Wolbank, S., Zeisberger, S., Zisch, A. & Strom, S. C. (2008) Concise review: isolation and characterization of cells from human term placenta: outcome of the first international Workshop on Placenta Derived Stem Cells. *Stem Cells,* 26, 300-11.

Pecora, A. L., Stiff, P., Lemaistre, C. F., Bayer, R., Bachier, C., Goldberg, S. L., Parthasarathy, M., Jennis, A. A., Smith, A. K., Douville, J., Chen, B., Armstrong, R. D., Mandalam, R. K. & Preti, R. (2001) A phase II trial evaluating the safety and effectiveness of the AastromReplicell system for augmentation of low-dose blood stem cell transplantation. *Bone Marrow Transplant,* 28, 295-303.

Peister, A., Mellad, J. A., Larson, B. L., Hall, B. M., Gibson, L. F. & Prockop, D. J. (2004) Adult stem cells from bone marrow (MSCs) isolated from different strains of inbred mice vary in surface epitopes, rates of proliferation, and differentiation potential. *Blood,* 103, 1662-8.

Petsa, A., Gargani, S., Felesakis, A., Grigoriadis, N. & Grigoriadis, I. (2009) Effectiveness of protocol for the isolation of Wharton's Jelly stem cells in large-scale applications. *In Vitro Cell Dev Biol Anim,* 45, 573-6.

Phermthai, T., Odglun, Y., Julavijitphong, S., Titapant, V., Chuenwattana, P., Vantanasiri, C. & Pattanapanyasat, K. (2010) A novel method to derive amniotic fluid stem cells for therapeutic purposes. *BMC Cell Biol*, 11, 79.

Pittenger, M. F., Mackay, A. M., Beck, S. C., Jaiswal, R. K., Douglas, R., Mosca, J. D., Moorman, M. A., Simonetti, D. W., Craig, S. & Marshak, D. R. (1999) Multilineage potential of adult human mesenchymal stem cells. *Science*, 284, 143-7.

Poloni, A., Rosini, V., Mondini, E., Maurizi, G., Mancini, S., Discepoli, G., Biasio, S., Battaglini, G., Berardinelli, E., Serrani, F. & Leoni, P. (2008) Characterization and expansion of mesenchymal progenitor cells from first-trimester chorionic villi of human placenta. *Cytotherapy*, 10, 690-7.

Portmann-Lanz, C. B., Schoeberlein, A., Huber, A., Sager, R., Malek, A., Holzgreve, W. & Surbek, D. V. (2006) Placental mesenchymal stem cells as potential autologous graft for pre- and perinatal neuroregeneration. *Am J Obstet Gynecol*, 194, 664-73.

Prusa, A. R. & Hengstschlager, M. (2002) Amniotic fluid cells and human stem cell research: a new connection. *Med Sci Monit*, 8, RA253-7.

Reinisch, A., Bartmann, C., Rohde, E., Schallmoser, K., Bjelic-Radisic, V., Lanzer, G., Linkesch, W. & Strunk, D. (2007) Humanized system to propagate cord blood-derived multipotent mesenchymal stromal cells for clinical application. *Regen Med*, 2, 371-82.

Ringe, J., Kaps, C., Burmester, G. R. & Sittinger, M. (2002) Stem cells for regenerative medicine: advances in the engineering of tissues and organs. *Naturwissenschaften*, 89, 338-51.

Romanov, Y. A., Svintsitskaya, V. A. & Smirnov, V. N. (2003) Searching for alternative sources of postnatal human mesenchymal stem cells: candidate MSC-like cells from umbilical cord. *Stem Cells*, 21, 105-10.

Roubelakis, M. G., Pappa, K. I., Bitsika, V., Zagoura, D., Vlahou, A., Papadaki, H. A., Antsaklis, A. & Anagnou, N. P. (2007) Molecular and proteomic characterization of human mesenchymal stem cells derived from amniotic fluid: comparison to bone marrow mesenchymal stem cells. *Stem Cells Dev*, 16, 931-52.

Schofield, R. (1978) The relationship between the spleen colony-forming cell and the haemopoietic stem cell. *Blood Cells*, 4, 7-25.

Schroeder, T. (2010) Hematopoietic stem cell heterogeneity: subtypes, not unpredictable behavior. *Cell Stem Cell*, 6, 203-7.

Soncini, M., Vertua, E., Gibelli, L., Zorzi, F., Denegri, M., Albertini, A., Wengler, G. S. & Parolini, O. (2007) Isolation and characterization of mesenchymal cells from human fetal membranes. *J Tissue Eng Regen Med*, 1, 296-305.

Song, Y., Bahnson, A., Hall, N., Yu, H., Shen, H., Koebler, D., Houck, R., Xie, Y. & Cheng, T. (2010) Stem cell traits in long-term co-culture revealed by time-lapse imaging. *Leukemia*, 24, 153-61.

Sparrow, R. L., Cauchi, J. A., Ramadi, L. T., Waugh, C. M. & Kirkland, M. A. (2002) Influence of mode of birth and collection on WBC yields of umbilical cord blood units. *Transfusion*, 42, 210-5.

Steiner, D., Gelovani, J., Savoldo, B., Robinson, S. N., Decker, W. K., Brouard, N., Najjar, A., Xing, D., Yang, H., Li, S., Marini, F., Zweidler-Mckay, P. A., Bollard, C. M., Shpall, E. J., Dotti, G. & Simmons, P. J. (2009) Noninvasive bioluminescent imaging demonstrates long-term multilineage engraftment of ex vivo-expanded CD34-selected umbilical cord blood cells. *Stem Cells*, 27, 1932-40.

Stenderup, K., Justesen, J., Clausen, C. & Kassem, M. (2003) Aging is associated with decreased maximal life span and accelerated senescence of bone marrow stromal cells. *Bone*, 33, 919-26.

Stiff, P., Chen, B., Franklin, W., Oldenberg, D., Hsi, E., Bayer, R., Shpall, E., Douville, J., Mandalam, R., Malhotra, D., Muller, T., Armstrong, R. D. & Smith, A. (2000) Autologous transplantation of ex vivo expanded bone marrow cells grown from small aliquots after high-dose chemotherapy for breast cancer. *Blood,* 95, 2169-74.

Tsai, M. S., Lee, J. L., Chang, Y. J. & Hwang, S. M. (2004) Isolation of human multipotent mesenchymal stem cells from second-trimester amniotic fluid using a novel two-stage culture protocol. *Hum Reprod,* 19, 1450-6.

Wagner, W., Wein, F., Roderburg, C., Saffrich, R., Diehlmann, A., Eckstein, V. & Ho, A. D. (2008) Adhesion of human hematopoietic progenitor cells to mesenchymal stromal cells involves CD44. *Cells Tissues Organs,* 188, 160-9.

Wagner, W., Wein, F., Roderburg, C., Saffrich, R., Faber, A., Krause, U., Schubert, M., Benes, V., Eckstein, V., Maul, H. & Ho, A. D. (2007) Adhesion of hematopoietic progenitor cells to human mesenchymal stem cells as a model for cell-cell interaction. *Exp Hematol,* 35, 314-25.

Wang, J. F., Wang, L. J., Wu, Y. F., Xiang, Y., Xie, C. G., Jia, B. B., Harrington, J. & Mcniece, I. K. (2004) Mesenchymal stem/progenitor cells in human umbilical cord blood as support for ex vivo expansion of CD34(+) hematopoietic stem cells and for chondrogenic differentiation. *Haematologica,* 89, 837-44.

Wang, M., Yang, Y., Yang, D., Luo, F., Liang, W., Guo, S. & Xu, J. (2009) The immunomodulatory activity of human umbilical cord blood-derived mesenchymal stem cells in vitro. *Immunology,* 126, 220-32.

Wein, F., Pietsch, L., Saffrich, R., Wuchter, P., Walenda, T., Bork, S., Horn, P., Diehlmann, A., Eckstein, V., Ho, A. D. & Wagner, W. (2010) N-cadherin is expressed on human hematopoietic progenitor cells and mediates interaction with human mesenchymal stromal cells. *Stem Cell Res,* 4, 129-39.

Weiss, M. L., Anderson, C., Medicetty, S., Seshareddy, K. B., Weiss, R. J., Vanderwerff, I., Troyer, D. & Mcintosh, K. R. (2008) Immune properties of human umbilical cord Wharton's jelly-derived cells. *Stem Cells,* 26, 2865-74.

Weiss, M. L., Medicetty, S., Bledsoe, A. R., Rachakatla, R. S., Choi, M., Merchav, S., Luo, Y., Rao, M. S., Velagaleti, G. & Troyer, D. (2005) Human Umbilical Cord Matrix Stem Cells: Preliminary Characterization and Effect of Transplantation in a Rodent Model of Parkinson's Disease. *Stem Cells.*

Witkowska-Zimny, M. & Wrobel, E. (2011) Perinatal sources of mesenchymal stem cells: Wharton's jelly, amnion and chorion. *Cell Mol Biol Lett,* 16, 493-514.

Wognum, A. W., Eaves, A. C. & Thomas, T. E. (2003) Identification and isolation of hematopoietic stem cells. *Arch Med Res,* 34, 461-75.

Wulf, G. G., Viereck, V., Hemmerlein, B., Haase, D., Vehmeyer, K., Pukrop, T., Glass, B., Emons, G. & Trumper, L. (2004) Mesengenic progenitor cells derived from human placenta. *Tissue Eng,* 10, 1136-47.

Yen, B. L., Huang, H. I., Chien, C. C., Jui, H. Y., Ko, B. S., Yao, M., Shun, C. T., Yen, M. L., Lee, M. C. & Chen, Y. C. (2005) Isolation of multipotent cells from human term placenta. *Stem Cells,* 23, 3-9.

Zhang, Y., Chai, C., Jiang, X. S., Teoh, S. H. & Leong, K. W. (2006) Co-culture of umbilical cord blood CD34+ cells with human mesenchymal stem cells. *Tissue Eng,* 12, 2161-70.

Zhang, Y., Li, C., Jiang, X., Zhang, S., Wu, Y., Liu, B., Tang, P. & Mao, N. (2004) Human placenta-derived mesenchymal progenitor cells support culture expansion of long-term culture-initiating cells from cord blood CD34+ cells. *Exp Hematol,* 32, 657-64.

Part 2

Placental Toxicology, Infection, and Complicated Pregnancies

5

Placental Toxicology of Pesticides

Gladis Magnarelli and Natalia Guiñazú
IDEPA-CONICET, Universidad Nacional del Comahue, Argentina

1. Introduction

The placenta used to be regarded as an organ protecting the fetus from exposure to toxic chemicals. However, we now know that xenobiotics can cross through the placenta and enter the fetal blood stream (Barr et al., 2007). In addition, some toxicants may accumulate in the placenta and potentially affect its development or function. Therefore, understanding how the placenta affects xenobiotics, and conversely, what the latter do to the placenta, should provide a basis for the use of this organ as a tool to investigate and predict some aspects of developmental toxicity (Myllynen et al., 2005). In this sense, the placenta is a key tool for biomonitoring xenobiotic exposure. Furthermore, it provides a large sample for analysis and is the most accessible and readily available component of the triad mother-infant-placenta. The cumulative effects of pregnancy-related events are shown by the placenta, which also reflects the intrauterine environment, and may be examined to a degree that is usually impossible in the infant. A critical issue for placenta toxicological analysis is the availability and appropriate use of biomarkers, as these provide measures of the exposure, toxic effects and individual susceptibility to toxicants. However, as epidemiological studies cannot resolve all the confounding factors, further experiments are also necessary. Thus, *in vitro, in vivo* and *ex vivo* models have been used in attempts to elucidate the toxicology of the toxicants occurring in the human placenta. Nevertheless, these approaches have their limitations. Despite having common physiological functions, placentas from different species are not homogeneous in their morphology, transport or metabolism of xenobiotics, thereby making it difficult to obtain a good representative model of the human placenta (Prouillac & Lecoeur, 2010). Moreover, changes in the placental function due to chemical exposure may also depend on the gestational period in which this occurs. Consequently, little research has been carried out into the biochemical and molecular toxicity of xenobiotics in human placenta.

Among the toxicants, pesticides are the only chemicals which have been intentionally introduced into the environment. Experimental approaches have established that exposure to pesticides during embryonic development influences the F1 generation. Furthermore, it has been noted that the epigenetic actions of pesticides may act on a gestating mother to influence subsequent (F1-F4) generations (Anway & Skinner, 2006).

Human environmental exposure to pesticides during the gestational period is associated with adverse reproductive outcomes (Arbuckle et al., 2001; Triche & Hossain, 2007), spontaneous miscarriage (Figa-Talamanca, 2006; Pathak, 2010) low birth weight (Figa-

Talamanca et al., 2006; Lopez-Espinosa et al., 2007; Triche & Hossain, 2007) and intrauterine growth retardation (Levario-Carrillo et al., 2004a). The association of maternal pesticide exposure with an increased risk of urogenital malformations (Fernandez et al., 2007) and impaired reproductive development (Andersen et al., 2008) has also been reported.

Organochlorine pesticides (OC) are persistent and ubiquitous environmental contaminants, with commercial-grade DDT (bis[4-chlorophenyl]-1,1,1-trichloroethane) being one of the most commonly used in history (Cohn et al, 2010). The majority of OC have been restricted or banned in industrialized nations, and their contamination levels have either been reduced or are expected to decline in the future. However, since OC are the most lipophilic pesticides in nature and have long half lives of months, or even years, they tend to accumulate in the adipose tissues and then biomagnify through the food chain, thus creating a persistent exposure risk to humans (Pathak et al., 2010). In fact, nearly all people have measurable levels of DDT-related compounds in their blood or tissue samples. In addition, DDT is still used in developing countries, and many others are currently preparing to reintroduce DDT in vector control to prevent disease (van den Berg, 2009). Therefore, OC exposure may occur not only through the ingestion of residues in the diet but also via inhalation and dermal absorption.

One of the most important classes of chemicals actively applied to the environment is the cholinesterase-inhibiting organophosphates (OP). Almost every person is, or has been, exposed to OP insecticides in their home, work or environment (Casida & Quistad, 2004), with pesticide exposure arising from living next to treated areas or in agricultural regions, as well as from house and yard pesticide treatment. The direct ingestion of residues in the diet or through secondary ingestion of contaminated house dust/soil, or from hand-to-mouth contact, inhalation of vapors or aerosols, or dermal absorption following contact with the skin, may represent other entry vias. Although the dermal and inhalation exposure pathways are likely to dominate in occupational exposure to pesticides, ingestion is likely to be the predominant pathway in the exposure of ordinary people (Eaton et al., 2008).

2. How the placenta affects pesticides

The transfer of molecules between the maternal and fetal circulation occurs across the endothelial-syncytial membrane of the placenta. Moreover, the placenta interferes with chemical delivery to the fetus, by expressing active membrane transporters and xenobiotic metabolism enzymes. The regulation of these enzymes and transporters and the effects of genetic polymorphisms on their functions may have important implications in fetal and placental exposure to xenobiotics and their potential toxicities (Prouillac & Lecoeur, 2010).

2.1 Placental incorporation and accumulation of pesticides

OP and OC are non-polar pesticides that can cross the placental microvillus brush border membrane by passive diffusion, with the rate of their incorporation into this compartment being determined by their physicochemical properties, such as lipid solubility and their toxicokinetic characteristics (elimination half-life in the mother, protein binding, lipid sequestration, and metabolism in maternal and placental compartments).

OC are the highest lipophilic but the poorest metabolized pesticides. Therefore, when exposure takes place, they are accumulated preferentially in the adipose tissue. In fact, dosimetry of *p,p'*-dichlorodiphenyldichloroethylene (*p,p'*-DDE, a metabolite of DDT) in the tissue of pregnant rats after oral intoxication, demonstrated that *p,p'*-DDE levels in the placenta were almost four times lower than in the maternal adipose tissue (You et al., 1998). A redistribution of OC storage may occur during late gestation, when there is an enhanced maternal adipose tissue lipolytic activity. Consequently, lipid storage is movilized and OC enter the maternal blood circulation and reach the placenta. Although no clear and precise model for the bioaccumulation of OC has yet been developed, it is known that some OC metabolites selectively accumulate in the placenta, thereby suggesting a tissue specific metabolic activity. The OC levels in human placenta and paired breast milk samples from Danish and Finnish samples were studied by Shen et al. (2007). As expected by their differential lipid content, the milk samples had higher levels of OC than the placenta. In agreement, when the distribution of the OC levels in the maternal, placental and fetal compartments was analyzed in a Spanish population, the concentration of endosulfan I and II in female adipose tissue was similar to that in breast milk, but higher than that of the placenta or cord blood. In contrast, the polar metabolites endosulfan diol and endosulfan sulfate were more frequently found in the placenta and cord blood (Cerrillo et al., 2005).

Unlike OC pesticides, the OP pesticides are rapidly metabolized and excreted. A study of the toxicokinetics and the placental transfer of a single low dermal dose of labeled [^{14}C]-methyl parathion administered to pregnant rats, showed that at 96 h the urine contained 91 % of the administered dose. The placenta was demonstrated to be a poor barrier against methyl parathion, resulting in an extensive placental transfer. However, the values of relative residence with respect to the maternal plasma (which reflects OP tissue relative exposure), revealed that among the studied compartments (maternal liver, kidney, brain, placenta and fetus) the placenta exhibited the highest levels, suggesting that this organ functions as a temporary depot (Abu-Qare et al., 2000).

Radiolabeled [^{14}C]-chlorpyrifos, administered intravenously to pregnant rats in a single injection at various gestational ages, was used to investigate the distribution of chlorpyrifos and the metabolite 3,5,6-trichlorpyridinol (TCPy) in the mother and the fetus. Radioactivity and TCPy were identified in all tissues five minutes after dosing. Also, in the matrix studied (maternal blood, liver, brain, and placenta, and fetus), the maximum concentration was found in the maternal liver, with the levels in the fetus and in the placenta only being marginally lower (Abdel-Rahman et al., 2002).

Considering the above information together, it is clear why there exists information about OC residue levels in human placenta whereas there is a lack of information about OP residues. Nevertheless, recognized OP targets, such as acetylcholinesterase (AChE) and carboxilesterase (CaE), may be used as reference biomarkers in order to evaluate OP placenta exposure (see 2.3.1.2).

2.2 Placental extrusion of pesticides

Interest in the ability of the placenta to reduce the passage of drugs has increased since Lankas et al. (1998), reported carrier-mediated transport of xenobiotics in the placenta by the ATP-binding cassette (ABC) transporters in this organ. Depending on their location, some of these proteins can act as efflux pumps, thereby expelling xenobiotics from the placenta to the maternal plasma (Prouillac et al., 2009).

A number of efflux transporters, including multidrug resistance proteins (ABCB1/P-gp), multidrug resistance associated proteins (MRP1-3 and 5) and breast cancer resistance protein (BCRP), are present in the syncytiotrophoblast. Studies using preterm placenta suggest that transporter expression varies with gestation (Sun et al., 2006; Aleksunes et al., 2008). BCRP expression in the placenta peaks at mid-gestation, with P-gp progressively decreasing and MRP2 progressively increasing with gestational age. The differential expression over the course of pregnancy possibly provides a compensatory mechanism for the protection of the fetus at different gestational stages (Mao, 2008), and xenobiotic transporters in fetal membranes may provide an additional route to protect the fetus against chemicals (Aleksunes et al., 2008).

ABCB1/P-gp, located in the microvillous membrane (Atkinson et al., 2003), preferentially transports hydrophobic compounds, such as pesticides, and also weakly basic compounds (Mao, 2008). Consistent with a protective role that limits exposure of the fetus to xenobiotics, Lankas et al. (1998) showed that the absence of P-gp expression increases pesticide avermectine content in the placenta.

ABC transporter polymorphism can produce interindividual variations in the toxicokinetics of foreign compounds in the feto-placental unit. However, it is still unclear whether specific ABCB1 or ABCG2 genotypes are risk factors for teratogenicity/fetotoxicity (Vanderlelie et al, 2008) or placental toxicity.

Several pesticides, including methoxychlor (OC) and fenitrothion (OP) are substrates for human MRP1 (Tribull et al., 2003). MRP2 is expressed in the syncytiotrophoblast, whereas MRP1 and MRP3 are expressed in both the blood vessel endothelia and in the syncytiotrophoblast (St-Pierre et al., 2000), with MRP5 being expressed in the basal membrane of the syncytiotrophoblasts and around fetal vessels (Macias et al., 2009).

In addition, pesticides may affect the ATP-efflux transporters function and expression. The interaction of methoxychlor and fenitrothion, with ABCC1 modulating the transport of physiological substrates has been demonstrated (Sharom, 2008). Also, low exposure to diazinon (OP) increased P-gp expression in the small intestine (Lecoeur et al., 2006). However, there is a lack of information about whether these types of interactions occur in the placenta.

2.3 Placental pesticide metabolism

2.3.1 Detoxifying enzymes

There is little contribution made by placental biotransformation in the conversion of xenobiotics into potential metabolites. Furthermore, compared to the liver, the role of placental metabolism is minor (Pasanen, 1999).

2.3.1.1 Phase I metabolism

Phase I reactions include monooxygenations, oxidations, reductions, hydrolyses and epoxide hydration, with all of these, except reductions, introducing a polar group to the molecule. The vast majority of compounds metabolized in phase I are processed by the microsomal cytochrome P450 monooxygenases (CYPs), which may generate metabolites (such as oxon) that are more neurotoxic than the parent compound (OP). Several CYPs, including CYP1, CYP2 and CYP3, have been isolated from the placenta. The members and quantity of the CYPs vary as a function of placental development, length of gestation and maternal health status (Hakkola et al., 1996a; 1996b), with the expression of human CYPs declining during gestation from the first to the second and third trimesters (Syme et al., 2004). However, not all CPYs are functional in human placenta, and the full spectrum of phase I enzyme expression, activity and developmental changes remains to be defined. For instance, although expression of CYP3A4 (mRNA and protein) has been demonstrated in the placenta, several marker substrates are not metabolized, suggesting that this enzyme is not functional. CYP1A1 is in fact the only CYP whose function and inducibility have been unquestionably demonstrated in the placenta (Vanderlelie et al., 2008).

Because OPs are esters of phosphoric or phosphotioic acid, they are susceptible to hydrolysis by A-esterases (calcium-dependent hydrolases also called paraoxonases). Their substrates are parent compounds having the P=O group or the oxon metabolites of the parent pesticides, with the hydrolysis being able to destroy the anti-cholinesterase activity of these compounds and being a potentially significant route of detoxification. However, although A-esterases display a low affinity for many compounds, they have high affinity for certain other compounds, such as chlorpyrifos-oxon and diazinon-oxon. In addition, carboxylesterases (CaEs) hydrolyze carboxylic acid esters, which are rarely encountered within the OP pesticides. Nevertheless, CaEs are still important contributors to the stoichiometric detoxication of many oxons, even those that have a low affinity for the A-esterases. Another serine esterase that detoxifies oxons stoichiometrically is the acetylcholinesterase (AChE). However, because this detoxication is stoichiometric and not catalytic, it is saturable and may have a limited efficacy if the OPs are present at high concentrations (Tang et al., 2006).

In summary, due to the variety in the types of atoms and groups present in OP (acids, alcohols, esters and ethers), many phase I reactions are possible, with the most prominent reactions being oxidation and hydrolysis (Tang et al., 2006). Also, by having an active, albeit restricted metabolic capacity, the placenta might convert certain OP to their oxon forms (Gupta, 2007). In fact, we found a significant inhibition (about 40 %) of CaE activity in placentas from women living in agricultural areas exposed to OP (Vera, unpublished results). Related to this, considering that CaE are known to catalyse the biotransformation of pyrethroids (Godin et al., 2006), a decrease in CaE activity in the placenta may have a toxicological significance in women exposed to pesticide mixtures.

With regard to the OC metabolism, it is known that epoxidation/hydroxylation mediated by CYPs are involved in the alicyclic OC metabolism, while DDT dehydrochlorinase (the enzyme transforming DDT to DDE) occurs in the cell soluble fraction (Rose & Hodgson, 2004). However, no information about these biotransformations in the placenta is currently available.

2.3.1.2 Phase II reactions

The phase II metabolism conjugates water-soluble moieties, such as glucuronic acid, sulfate and glutathione (GSH), among other groups, to xenobiotic metabolites. In addition to phase I enzymes, the placenta also expresses phase II conjugating enzymes, for example glutathione-S transferase (GST) isoforms, epoxide hydrolase, N-acetyl transferase, sulfotransferases and UDP-glucuronosyl transferase isoforms. As GST catalyzes the conjugation of biologically active electrophiles to GSH, it appears that placental GST plays a role in protecting the fetus against electrophiles or oxidative stress (Vanderlelie et al., 2008). Xenobiotic exposure, however, may affect the detoxification pathways. During OP desulfuration, activated sulfur atoms are formed that bind irreversibly to the specific CYP isoforms that catalyze the reaction, resulting in a time-dependent decrease in the enzymatic activity. Also, OP may down-regulate CYP mRNA, as was demonstrated in liver and testis of rats intoxicated with OP profenofos (Moustafa et al., 2008). It has been established that DDE induces CYP2B and CYP3A enzymes and selected conjugation enzymes in liver (You, 2004). Furthermore, enzyme induction by xenobiotics may increase the clearance of endogenous steroids, and hence produce endocrine disruption, which is a matter of great concern. However, there is no information yet available about these potential associations in the placenta.

3. How pesticides affect the placenta

3.1 Endocrine disruption

An endocrine disrupter (ED) is an exogenous chemical substance or a mixture of substances which alters the structure or function (s) of the endocrine system. EDs act by interfering directly with natural hormones, since they are not only able to interact with various hormone receptors, but can also interfere with the synthesis, transport, metabolism and elimination of hormones (Mnif et al., 2011). Many chemicals that have been identified as EDs are pesticides. Nuclear compartmentalization of these compounds, insertion into membranes and chemical stress production may be associated with deleterious consequences on the endocrine system.

3.1.1 Effects on aromatase

The placenta is the main organ responsible for estrogen synthesis in pregnant women. CYP19 aromatase (ArM), the enzyme that catalyzes the conversion of the androgens androstenedione (A-dione) and testosterone to estrogens, has been proposed to be an important molecular target of ED chemicals (Figure 1). ArM, a complex comprised of P450-aromatase and NADH-cytochrome P450 reductase, is an inducible enzyme whose expression is tightly regulated. ArM is located in the microvilli surface, in the the lateral plasma membrane, and in the endoplasmic reticulum in the syncytiotrophoblast of the placenta (Nagamuna et al., 1990).

Several *in vitro* assays have been used for studying ArM as a potential target of pesticides inducing endocrine disruption. Some studies were conducted on human placental JEG-3 cells, which are morphologically similar to their cells of origin (i.e. the trophoblast of the normal first trimester) and provide a cell model to study the placental function (Tremblay et al., 1999). Since regulation of ArM expression in these cells is the same as in the placenta, JEG-3 cells have been proposed to be a valuable tool for the assessment of potential steroidogenesis disruption. ArM activity was found to decrease by incubation with the OCs lindane (γHCH) and heptachlor (Laville et al., 2006), with a significant association between γHCH levels in female blood and recurrent miscarriages also being reported (Pathak et al., 2010). These findings could be related to alterations in estradiol levels, since this hormone plays a critical role in the maintenance of primate pregnancy (Albrecht et al., 2000), with its synthesis depending on ArM activity. In contrast, the OCs aldrin, chlordane, endosulfan and methoxychlor were reported to induce ArM activity in JEG-3 cells (Laville et al., 2006). Considering that an increased level of estradiol in the syncytiotrophoblast may have an impact on testicular descent (Hadˇziselimović et al., 2000), and that an association of congenital cryptorchidism with trans-chlordane levels in breast milk has been reported (Damgaard et al., 2006), it now remains to be determined if the increasing incidence of this reproductive abnormality is associated with trans-chlordane induced up regulation of placental ArM.

Exposure of placental explants to two isomers of DDT (*o,p*´-DDT and *p,p*'-DDT) and their metabolites (*o,p*'-DDE and *p,p*'-DDE) caused reductions in estradiol secretion due to a direct action on ArM activity and expression (Wójtowicz et al., 2007a). However, different effects (stimulatory after short-term and inhibitory after long-term exposure) of these compounds were observed on progesterone secretion. In addition, both short- and long-term exposure to these compounds caused decreased hCG (human chorionic gonadotrophin) secretion, a crucial hormone for pregnancy maintenance, suggesting the existence of a local axis between the steroid hormones and hCG in the placenta (Wójtowicz et al., 2007b; 2008).

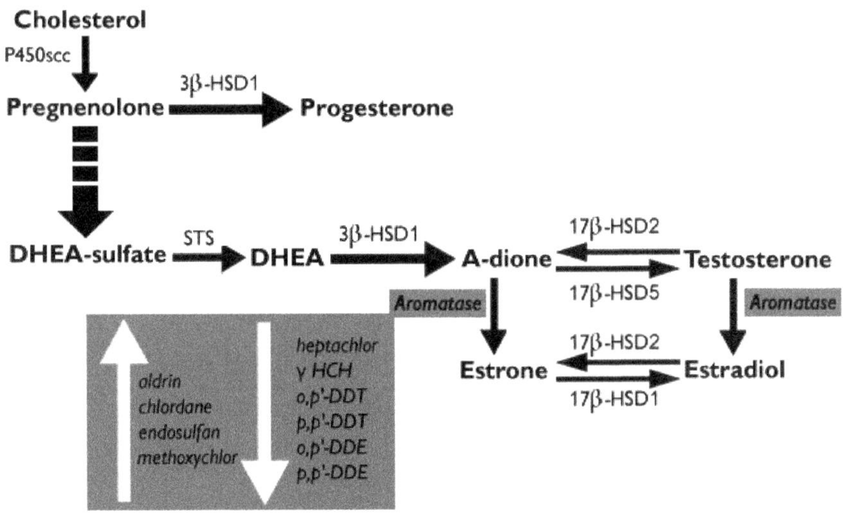

Fig. 1. Estrogen synthesis and OC effects on human placental aromatase

As these authors used concentrations covering the range of OC levels present in the serum of pregnant women, they proposed that these hormonal imbalances could influence the pregnancy outcome. It should be noted that *p,p*'-DDE is currently a dominant pollutant found in the placenta of different populations and *o,p*'-DDT has also been detected in samples of various populations (Lopez-Espinosa et al., 2007; Shen et al., 2005). With respect to OP, there is no available information concerning the OP effect on ArM in the placenta.

3.1.2 Other potential mechanisms involved in endocrine disruption

As shown in Table 1, several authors have studied other possible targets of pesticides affecting the placenta, which could also be associated with endocrine disruption. It has been established that OC may bind hormone receptors, with *o,p*'-DDT being the most estrogenic component of the DDT complex, and having a relative binding affinity to estrogen receptors (ER) of 2.9 x 10^{-3} relative to 17-β estradiol. In the case of the *p,p'*-DDE isomer, it is anti-androgenic with an inhibitive binding to the androgen receptor (AR), and has a relative binding affinity of 3.1 x 10^{-3} relative to dihydrotestosterone (Rogan & Chen, 2005). Considering the persistent exposure of placental tissues to these DDT isomers and that various cellular components of human placenta express ER (in the form of either ERα or ERβ) (Bukovsky et al., 2003) as well as AR (Hsu, 2009), then wider implications in terms of their potential role in endocrine disruption may be postulated.

An appropriate intracellular Ca^{2+} concentration is necessary for blastocyst implantation and proper placental development and function, with recent studies having pointed out that alterations in Ca^{2+} homeostasis can lead to placental pathologies such as pre-eclampsia and intrauterine growth restriction (Baczyk et al., 2011). The effects of the exposure of trophoblastic cells to methoxychlor and *p,p'*-DTT in comparison with exposure to estradiol and diethylstilbestrol (DES), were studied to test the hypothesis that cellular Ca^{2+} handling is a target for these EDs. Treatment with DDT, methoxychlor, DES, or estradiol increased the cellular Ca^{2+} uptake, and the expression of trophoblast-specific human Ca^{2+} binding protein (HCaBP) was down-regulated by both methoxychlor and DDT. In addition, treatment with methoxychlor, DDT, and DES inhibited cell proliferation, induced apoptosis, and suppressed the expression of several trophoblast differentiation marker genes. These results strongly suggest that the trophoblast Ca^{2+} handling functions are endocrinally modulated, and that their alteration by EDs, such as methoxychlor and DDT, constitutes a possible pathway for these agents to produce harmful effects on the placental function and fetal development (Derfoul et al., 2003).

Target	Pesticide	Reported"/ potential effect	References
Phosphoinositides metabolism and PI-4 kinase activity	heptachlor *o, p´*-DDT	Lactogen release disruption	Souza et al. (2005)
PKC activity	heptachlor *o, p´*-DDT	hCG secretion disruption	Magnarelli et al. (2009)
PKA activity	*o, p´*-DDT	hCG secretion disruption	Magnarelli et al. (2009)
Ca^{2+} uptake and expression of trophoblast-specific human Ca^{2+} binding protein	methoxychlor *o, p´*-DDT	Estrogen-like effects*	Derfoul et al. (2003)

Table 1. Other targets associated with pesticide ED in placenta

We have previously reported that a significant increase was produced in protein kinase A (PKA) activity by *in vitro* incubations of human placental villi homogenates with *o-p'* DDT, whereas the protein kinase C (PKC) activity was reduced by heptachlor and *o-p'* DDT (Magnarelli et al., 2009). These differential effects on kinase activities may be associated with the oxidative stress produced by the pesticides. Experimental evidence has demonstrated that the sensitivity of PKA isoforms to oxygen radicals may vary, depending upon the type of oxygen free radicals produced and the antioxidant system present, both of which are tissue-dependent (Dimon-Gadal et al., 1998). Also, PKC is under a complex redox regulation and shows different responses to oxidative stress depending on the PKC isoform (Poli et al., 2004). Since placental human gonadotropin-releasing hormone (GnRH) transduction signaling couples with both the PKC and PKA pathways (Cheng et al., 2000), the *o,p*'-DDT effects observed may contribute to the impairment of hCG secretion reported by Wójtowicz et al. (2008).

We also studied the placenta phosphoinositide (PI) metabolism as a potential target of pesticide action. PI-mediated signaling plays an essential role in normal morphogenesis and placental function, as was demonstrated in knock out mice by Nakamura et al. (2005). Also, PI- signaling has been associated with lactogen release (Petit et al., 1989) and fibroblast growth factor activation of phospholipase C in the human placenta (Ferriani et al., 1994). *In vitro* incubations of cell-free homogenates showed that different patterns of lipid phosphorylation were produced by OP and OC. However, both types of pesticides affected the post-membrane supernatant of PI 4-kinase, a key enzyme in PI metabolic pathway. A biphasic effect on membrane and nuclear PI4-kinase activity was seen with heptachlor (OC), with the strongest effect being found with *o-p*'-DDT on nuclear PI4-kinase activity, while substantial changes were also observed in membrane fractions (Souza et al., 2004).

3.2 Oxidative stress

Pregnancy is characterized by a strictly regulated physiological increase in the oxidative processes in the mother and the fetus, which is determined by the rise in oxygen consumption and by the use of some reactive oxygen species (ROS) in cellular processes. These ROS include: superoxide radical, hydrogen peroxide and hydroxyl radical, among other molecules. Both a short or a long term lack of anti-oxidant/pro-oxidant balance provokes oxidative stress. ROS excess may cause disorders in protein synthesis and enzyme activity, as well as changes in the synthesis and activity of hormones and cell membrane receptors, and also damage to the DNA. Moreover, these alterations can produce cellular loss of function and apoptosis, thereby affecting the normal course of pregnancy (Corria Osorio & Cruz Manzano, 2009). In fact, oxidative stress in the placental tissues is an essential pathogenic factor of premature delivery miscarriage (Prokopenko et al., 2006) and pre-eclampsia (Vanderlelie et al., 2005).

Placental oxidative stress may directly or indirectly lead to oxidative stress in the maternal circulation. It was reported that the concentration of maternal plasma cell-free fetal DNA was positively correlated with the concentration of urinary 8-OHdG (8-hydroxydeoxyguanosine, an oxidized nucleoside of DNA), and plasma isoprostane (prostaglandin-like compounds formed *in vivo* from the free radical-catalyzed peroxidation of essential fatty acids) at 26 to 30 weeks of gestation. These cell-free fetal DNAs were most likely derived from the placenta, which then entered maternal circulation during the process of deportation of the syncytiotrophoblastic microparticles, with this event possible leading to activation of maternal neutrophils and subsequent production of ROS. Alternatively, both the increase in maternal oxidative stress and the breakdown of the syncytial surface might be caused by a common insult to the placenta, i.e. oxidative damage induced by ischemia-reperfusion (Hung et al., 2010). Interestingly, pesticides are capable of inducing oxidative stress by enzymatic conversion to secondary reactive products and/or ROS, by depletion of antioxidant defenses, as well as by impairment of antioxidant enzyme functions (Franco et al., 2009). Another way that ROS generation occurs, as described in OP toxicity, is through high energy consumption coupled with oxidative phosphorylation (Lukaszewicz-Hussain, 2010). Preliminary *in vitro* studies in our laboratory with chlorpyrifos treated JEG-3 cells showed that cell viability and the content of GSH (a reducing agent of antioxidant defense) was significantly reduced. However, the pretreatment of JEG-3 cells with the antioxidant N-Acetylcisteine was able to revert these effects, suggesting that oxidative stress was the mechanism of injury (Chiapella et al., unpublished). Also, OC (endrin and γHCH) were demonstrated to be capable of inducing oxidative stress in fetal and placental tissues in mice after the administration of teratogenic doses of these pesticides (Hassoun & Stohs, 1996).

Oxidative stress is a complex phenomenon to investigate in pesticide exposed populations. Several toxicants, such as metals, carbon monoxide, dioxin, radiations, polychlorinated biphenils, polycyclic aromatic hydrocarbons (Lukaszewicz-Hussain, 2010) and cigarette smoke (Menon et al., 2011) have been identified as producers of pro-oxidant conditions in several tissues and must therefore be considered to be confounding factors when oxidative stress is studied as a probable consequence of pesticide exposure

3.3 Proliferation/death imbalance

Apoptosis is one of the major forms of cell death, in which the cell designs and executes the program of its own death, with this process being important in normal placental development. Trophoblast apoptosis increases in normal placentas as gestation proceeds, and its concurrent appearance with cell proliferation reflects the growth and remodeling of the placenta. These two processes work together to maintain the placental tissue homeostasis. Apoptosis may be initiated by the death receptor pathways or intrinsically by the mitochondria pathway (Straszewski-Chavez et al., 2005). Also, excessive ROS production may lead to cellular dysfunction and culminate in cell death, with the ROS produced during oxidative stress having been shown to initiate signaling cascades and lead to apoptosis (Yuan et al., 2008).

The mechanism of chlopyrifos (OP) induced citotoxicity was investigated in the trophoblast JAR cell line, which is less differentiated than the JEG-3 cell line but has a higher proliferation rate. Apoptosis was only partially mediated through activation of caspase system, and surprisingly, the p38 MAPK signaling pathway was involved in protection against chlorpyrifos-induced toxicity. In addition, among the genes known to regulate apoptosis, Bcl-2, DKN2A, MTA2, TEK and TWIST1 were down regulated, while FAS, TNFα, ITGB1 and ITGA4 were up-regulated. These authors concluded that apoptosis was not dependent on FAS/TNF signaling, activation of caspases or the inhibition of AChE (Saulsbury et al., 2008). In agreement, results from our laboratory indicate that incubation of the JEG-3 cell line with chlorpyrifos or phosmet (OP) induces cell death as a consequence of apoptosis induction, and that JEG-3 cells may be more tolerant to chlorpyrifos toxicity than JAR cells (Guiñazú et al, unpublished observations). Differential susceptibility to chlorpyrifos in these two cell lines may be explained, at least in part, by the fact that the transcription factor HNF1α (hepatic nuclear factor 1α) is expressed ten times more in JAR than in JEG-3 cells (Serrano et al., 2007), with this transcription factor playing an important role in CYP regulation. Although the involvement of CYPs in OP-induced apoptosis in neuronal cells has been previously reported (Kashyap et al., 2011), it is still not clear whether OP metabolism by CYPs and the induction of oxidative stress are implicated in trophoblast cell death.

OC and ROS generation have been described to interfere with various signaling pathways, including MAPKs. In fact, all MAPK cascades are known to be activated in response to oxidant injury (Martindale & Holbrook, 2002), and they can therefore have an impact on cell survival and death. Wojtowics et al. (2007b) demonstrated that *p,p'*-DDT and *p,p'*-DDE could act as both pro-apoptotic or anti-apoptotic factors, depending on the isomer type and concentration, with a small concentration of all these compounds tending to decrease the caspase-3 activity (Wojtowics et al, 2007b). Derfoul et al. (2003) reported that *p,p'*-DDT inhibited JEG-3 cell proliferation, induced apoptosis and suppressed the expression of several of the marker genes responsible for trophoblast differentiation.

Serine-threonine kinases and transcription factors play important roles in the progression of the cell cycle. Experiments on mouse trophoblast stem cells and the human placental cell line HTR demonstrated that less than half of serine-threonine kinases and transcription factors have a higher level of phosphorylation at the M phase than at the interphase (Liu et al., 2004). Using *in vitro* homogenate villi incubations, we showed that total serine/threonine kinase activity was increased by 10 μM heptachlor and *o-p'* DDT in a particulate fraction (Magnarelli et al., 2009). Since insufficient trophoblast proliferation is one of the causes for loss of embryos, this result may appear controversial with the reported effects about OC reproductive outcomes. However, the understanding of the mechanisms underlying trophoblast injury by pesticides requires an integrated vision of all the molecular targets involved.

3.4 Impairment of the mitochondrial function

Oxidative phosphorylation, the primary process by which the energy derived from the catabolism of fuels is used to synthesize ATP, occurs in the mitochondria. It has been recognized that the mitochondria has homeostatic functions in metabolic cell signaling, ion homeostasis, regulation of cell morphology, multiplication and apoptosis. The mitochondrias of the human placenta are not only involved in the production of ATP. Mitochondrias of the syncthiotrophoblast are the main source of progesterone, whose synthesis requires the delivery of cholesterol to the inner mitochondrial membrane, in order to convert mitochondrial cholesterol to pregnenolone by CYP_{scc} (Tuckey et al., 2004).

The mitochondrial membranes may be the site of toxic effects of lipophilic pesticides. Because the mitochondria is a ROS source and is an organelle enriched with polyunsaturated fatty acids, the impairment of the mitochondrial function may increase ROS production and lipoperoxides. Some pesticides directly affect the mitochondrial electron transfer chain, which leads to a further increased formation of damaging ROS and nitrogen free radicals (Gomez et al., 2007). The effects of OP (parathion, dichlorvos) and OC (dieldrin and DDE) on the mitocondrial function have been studied in diverse experimental systems, and have identified ROS generation and the inhibition of the electron transport chain complexes, along with ATP-synthase and phosphate transporters, to be the primary mechanisms of action. Depending on the pesticide and concentration used, reduced mitochondrial membrane potential, decreased respiratory control and ADP/O ratio, and initiation of the apoptotic cascade have been observed (Binukumar et al., 2010; Gomez et al., 2007).

We have recently studied the citotrophoblast mitochondria (CM) and the sincytiotrophoblast mitochondria (SM) isolated from term placentas of women living in agricultural areas exposed to OP. On comparing exposed samples to unexposed ones, the complex I and complex III activities were reduced in both CM and SM. In addition, there was less placental progesterone content (Rivero et al., unpublished results). Alterations in the phospholipid composition were also observed in SM (Vera et al., unpublished results).

3.5 Immune imbalance

The concept that maternal immunity is not in a baseline resting state and is ignorant of the antigens in the invading embryo, is somewhat counterintuitive and requires our reassessment of maternal-fetal immune interactions (Nagamatsu et al., 2010). Immune components play a crucial role during pregnancy by synthesizing and releasing many of the cytokines which contribute to gestation maintenance. Hence, abnormal activation of immune components may be associated with pregnancy complications. Related to this, it has been proposed that cytokines form a self-generating network, a minor increase in key proinflammatory cytokines may eventually invoke terminal events that trigger preterm birth (Bryant-Greenwood et al., 2009). In the early stages of pregnancy, cytokines are involved in embryo implantation, the regulation of trophoblast invasion, as well as immunoregulatory functions (Bowen et al., 2002; McEwan et al., 2009, Naruse et al., 2010, Van Mourik et al., 2009). Then, later on in pregnancy, the cytokines play a role in the initiation of labour (Bowen et al., 2002). Thus, cytokine balance is relevant during pregnancy, in the early stages during blastocyst implantation and also in placental development (Chaouat et al. 2007; Moffett & Loke 2006; Schäfer-Somi, 2003).

Despite it has been demonstrated that OP may alter the cytokine balance (Duramad et al., 2006; Oostingh et al., 2009), few studies have analyzed whether pesticides can produce cytokine imbalance locally at the placenta. Saulsbury et al. (2008) showed that incubation of the JAR trophoblast cell line with chlorpyrifos induces the transcription of the transforming necrosis factor alpha (TNFα). Results from our laboratory also indicate that the incubation of JEG-3 cells with chlorpyrifos or phosmet induces the production of TNFα, mRNA and protein (Guiñazú et al, unpublished observations).

Only limited information is available regarding the production of IL-13 by gestational tissues. Low levels of IL-13 mRNA have been detected in first trimester chorionic villi (Bennett et al., 1999; Dealtry et al., 1998). In addition, IL-13 mRNA has also been identified in placental trophoblasts at all stages of gestation, whereas IL-13 immunoreactivity within the placenta was restricted to between 16 and 27 weeks (Williams et al., 2000). Increased levels of IL-13 have been identified as the dominant effector cytokine of fibrosis in several experimental models of fibrosis (Wynn, 2008). Moreover, results from our laboratory suggest that maternal environmental exposure to OP may regulate cytokine synthesis in the placenta, since the expression of IL-13 mRNA was only found in placentas from women living in rural areas where these pesticides are intensively applied (Bulgaroni et al., unpublished results). Concerning OC exposure, increased placental *p,p*'-DDE was associated with a significant increase in the cord plasma IL-13. Furthermore, both the cord plasma IL-4/ IFN-γ and IL-13/IFN-γ ratios were significantly positively associated with the placental p,p'-DDE concentration (Brooks et al, 2007).

3.6 Alterations in the cholinergic system

Although the placenta is a tissue without innervations, it contains all the components of the cholinergic system. Koshakji et al. (1974) demonstrated that placental acetylcholine (ACh) varies with gestational age, reaching a peak at 20-22 weeks of gestation and declining toward term. This developmental pattern is paralleled by the activity of choline acetyltransferase (ChaT), suggesting that the placental cholinergic system may be involved in regulating the developmental processes relevant to placental growth. Multiple muscarinic receptor (mAChR) subtypes and all subtypes of the nicotinic receptor (nAChR) alfa subunit are present in the placenta (Bhuiyan et al., 2006; Lips et al., 2005), with ACh appearing to be an important placental signaling molecule that, through the stimulation of nAChR, controls the uptake of nutrients, blood flow and fluid volume in the placental vessels, and also vascularisation during placental development. As placenta ChAt expression overlaps that of eNOS (endotelial nitric oxide synthase), it has been hypothesized that the locally produced ACh may stimulate eNOS vía a Ca^{2+}-dependent mechanism. Studies using the trophoblast BeWo cell line have provided evidence that ACh acts via mAChR on the trophoblast cell membrane to modulate NO (nitric oxide) in an estrogen-dependent manner (Bhuiyan et al., 2006). The expression of mAChR receptor in placenta showed a decrease after OP exposure in rats (González-García et al., 2006), suggesting that the related placental cholinergic functions might be affected (Table 2).

Level of effect	**Human OP environmental exposure**	**Rat OP exposure (sublethal doses)**
Molecular	Up-regulation of the AChE expression	Down regulation of mAChR expression
Biochemical	Increased AChE activity	Decrease AChE activity
Morphological	Increased placental maturity index and deposition of fibrinoid material Atypical villi	Trophoblast degenerated cells Extensive areas of fibrosis

Table 2. Molecular and biochemical effects on the cholinergic system and morphological changes in placenta associated with human and experimental OP exposure.

The AChE is active in the syncytiotrophoblast, cytotrophoblast cells, endothelial cells and the media of fetal blood vessels of the human placenta (Hahn et al., 1993). As cited above, AChE inhibition is associated with OP and also with carbamate pesticide exposure (Gil & Pla, 2001). However, differential effects on AChE placental activity have been observed (Table 2). A single cutaneous dose of OP decreased placental AChE activity in rats (Abu-Qare & Abou-Donia, 2001) whereas when the activity of placental AChE in residents of rural communities exposed to OP was studied, the average AChE activity obtained in placentas collected during the pulverization season was significantly higher than in those collected during the non-pulverization period (Souza et al., 2005). This latter result was later confirmed in two biomonitoring assays performed in our laboratory in subsequent years on the same population. We postulate that as a consequence of the transient elevation of ACh levels produced by AChE inhibition, the expression of genes located in the "cholinergic locus" may be stimulated. In fact, an up-regulation of the AChE expression was detected in some of the samples analyzed (Vera et al., unpublished results).

In summary, the above findings demonstrate that the placental cholinergic system is a sensitive target of OP exposure, with potential consequences on the placenta development and function.

3.7 Alterations in placental morphology

Placental morphology was studied in pregnant rats exposed orally to the OP methylparathion (technical formulation) in *ad libitum* fed and restricted diet animals. The main effects of methylparathion treatment were an increase in the vascular congestion at the labyrinth area, a remarkable internalization of material by trophoblast giant cells of the junctional area, an increase in the population of decidual and trophoblast degenerated cells, more extensive areas of fibrosis and haemorrage in the decidua, and the persistence of nucleated red cells in the fetal circulation. There was also a rise in the number of phagosomic vacuoles per cell in rats exposed to methylparathion, with the authors suggesting that the increased phagocytosis may have been a consequence of the clearence of dead and degenerated cells (Levario-Carrillo et al., 2004). Interestingly, these authors also reported that the placentas of women environmentaly exposed to methylparathion showed microinfarctions, microcalcifications and an increased deposition of fibrinoid material, along with a larger proportion of atypical characteristics of villi, such as bullous and balloon-like formations with non-homogeneous surfaces and other areas devoid of microvilli (Levario Carrillo et al., 2001).

Placental maturity is characterized by an increase in the number of terminal villi, a reduction in the thickness of epithelial plates and the development of blood vessels. However, placental maturation involves metabolic and endocrine processes that are still poorly understood. Acosta-Maldonado et al. (2009) performed a morphometric analysis on placentas derived from women living in rural areas exposed to anti-cholinesterasic pesticides. The placenta maturity index (PMI) was calculated by dividing the number of epithelial plates by their thickness in mm^2 of the placental parenchyma. In the full-term placentas of women not exposed to pesticides, the PMI was similar in both regions, despite the fact that the development of the capillaries and sinusoids was greater in the central area. However, in placentas from women exposed to pesticides, the PMI was greater in the central region than in peripheral areas. These results suggest that exposure to pesticides may affect the homogeneity of the maturity of the placental tissue. Although the mechanisms underlying the effect of pesticides on maturity of placental tissue in a region-dependent manner are not known at present, it has been suggested that the ACh concentration may be related to the development of the terminal villi and/or blood vessels, and in this way plays a role in the maturity of the placenta. Therefore, disruption of the cholinergic system might precede the observed morphological alterations (Table 2).

3.8 Challenges and future directions

Microarray technology and bioinformatics can reveal changes in gene expression profiling simultaneously across thousand of genes. This provides expression profiles that can be used to predict outcomes and thus helps to elucidate the mechanisms of toxicity. The agreement between *in vivo* observations and gene expression findings demonstrates the ability of genomics to accurately categorize chemicals, identify toxic mechanisms of action, and predict subsequent pathological responses (Martin et al., 2007), as well as identifying unexpected molecular targets. Information about gene expression arrays can be complemented by metabolomics (which may reveal target and off-target toxicities) and proteomics (a research field currently undergoing rapid development, involving the analysis of protein level alterations, and post-translational modifications and function). The main advantage of using these technologies derives from the global approach to understanding the mechanisms involved in toxicology, with these techniques being able to characterize not only novel chemicals but also complex mixtures. However, both are costly and the interpretation and application of the findings requires adequate databases in order to define the range of genes affected by chemicals and those indicative of critical health effects. In this sense, a comparative toxicogenomic data base was recently developed as a tool to investigate the impact of environmental chemicals on human health (Davis et al., 2009). Moreover, novel chemical-protein associations which had not been previously predicted may now be obtained (Audouze et al., 2010).

Because of the central role that the placenta has in fetal and maternal physiology and development, there is the possibility that variations in placental gene expression patterns might be linked to important abnormalities in maternal or fetal health, or even to effects in later life. DNA microarray analyses of gene expression patterns in samples of amnion, chorion, umbilical cord, and sections of villus parenchyma from human placentas of healthy pregnancies have revealed a rich and diverse picture of molecular variation in the placenta, with interindividual differences in the expression patterns of villous parenchyma and systematic differences among the maternal, fetal, and intermediate layers being found (Sood et al., 2006). Although the effects of several environmental toxicants on gene expression have been investigated in human full-term placentas (Huuskonen et al., 2008), there is still a lack of information about pesticide effects on gene expression patterns, metabolites and protein levels.

4. Conclusions

The placenta is a target organ for toxicity originating from persistent and rapidly metabolized and excreted pesticides. The above findings strengthen the view that pesticide-induced damaged in the placenta may contribute to the occurrence of reproductive and developmental adverse effects in humans. Endocrine disruption is one of the most established and identified mechanisms, which possibly underlies deleterious OC reproductive effects, whereas the cholinergic system is a sensitive and specific target of OP effects. In addition, oxidative stress is a complex phenomenon that needs to be studied in order to evaluate how pesticides might interfere with human reproduction. As humans are exposed to multiple pesticides, the understanding of the molecular events associated with pesticide exposure is particularly complex. Microarray technology may help to elucidate the mechanisms of mixture toxicity and thus provide the basis for defining new prevention and treatment strategies in order to improve reproductive outcomes.

5. Acknowledgments

The authors thank student Diego Potás for the figure design, and Dr. Paul David Hobson, native speaker, for revision of the manuscipt.

6. References

Abdel-Rahman, A.; Blumenthal, G.; Abou-Dia, S.; Fouad, A.; Abdel-Monem A. & Abou-Donia, M. (2002). Pharmacokinetic profile and placental transfer of a single intravenous injection of [^{14}C] chlorpyrifos in pregnant rats. *Archives of Toxicology*, Vol.76, No.8, pp.452-459, ISSN 0340-5761.

Abu-Qare, A.W. & Abou-Donia, M.B. (2001). Inhibition and recovery of maternal and foetal cholinesterase enzyme activity following a single cutaneous dose of methyl parathion and diazinon alone and in combination, in pregnant rats. *Journal of Applied Toxicology*, Vol.21, No.4, pp. 307-316, ISSN 0260-437X.

Abu-Qare, A.W.; Abdel-Rahman, A.; Kishk, A.M. & Abou-Donia, M. (2000). Placental transfer and pharmcokinetic of a single dermal dose of [^{14} C] methyl parathion rats. *Toxicological Science*, Vol.53, No.1, pp.5-12, ISSN 1096-6080.

Acosta-Maldonado, B.; Sánchez-Ramírez, B.; Reza-López, S. & Levario-Carrillo, M. (2009). Effects of Exposure to Pesticides Turing Pregnancy on Placental Maturity and Weight of Newborns: A Cross-Sectional Pilot Study in Women from the Chihuahua State, Mexico. *Human and Experimental Toxicology*, Vol.28, No.8, pp 451-459, ISSN 0960-3271

Albrecht, E.; Graham,A. & Gerald P. (2000). The role of estrogen in the maintenance of primate pregnancy. *American Journal of Obstetrics and Gynecology*,Vol.182, No.2, pp. 432-438, ISSN 0002-9378.

Aleksunes, L.; Cui, Y. & Klaasen, C. (2008). Prominent Expression of Xenobiotic Efflux Transporters in Mouse Extraembryonic Fetal Membranes Compared with Placenta, *Drug Metabolism and Disposition*, Vol.36, No.9, pp. 1960-1970, ISSN 0090-9556.

Andersen, H.; Scmidt, I.; Grandjean, P.; Jensen,T.; Budtz-Jorgensen, E.; Kjaerstad, M.; Baelun, J.; Nielsen, J.; Skakkebaek, N. & Main, K. (2008). Impaired reproductive development in sons of women occupationally exposed to pesticides during pregnancy. *Environmental Health Prespectives*, Vol.116, No.4, pp. 566-572, ISSN 0091-6765.

Anway, M. D. & Skinner, M. K. (2006). Epigenetic Transgenerational Actions of Endocrine Disruptors , *Endocrinology*, Vol.147, No.6, pp 43-49, ISSN 0013-7227.

Arbuckle, T.; Lin, Z. & Mery, S. (2001). A exploratory analysis of the effect of pesticide exposure on the risk of spontaneous abortion in an Ontario farm population. *Environmental Health Prespectives*, Vol.109, No.8, pp. 851-857, ISSN 0091-6765.

Atkinson, D.; Greenwood, S.; Sibley, C.; Glazier, J. & Fairbairn, L. (2003). Role of MDR1 and MRP1 in Trophoblast Cells, Elucidated using Retroviral Gene Transfer. *American Journal of Physiology- Cell Physiology*, Vol.285, No. 3, pp. 584-591, ISSN 0363-6143.

Audouze, K.; Juncker, A. S.; Roque, F.; Krysian-Baltyn, K.; Weinhold, N.; Taboureau, O.; Jensen, T. S. & Brunak, S. (2010). Deciphering Diseases and Biological Targets for Environmental Chemicals using Toxicogenomics Networks. *PLoS Computational Biology*, Vol.6, No.5, pp. 1-11, ISSN 1553-734X.

Baczyk, D.; Kingdom, J. & Uhlén, P. (2011). Calcium signaling in placenta. *Cell Calcium*,Vol.49, No.5, pp. 350-356, ISSN 0143-4160.

Barr, D.; Bishop, A. & Needham, L. (2007). Concentrations of xenobiotic chemicals in the maternal-fetal unit. *Reproductive Toxicology*, Vol.23, No.3, pp. 260-266, ISSN 0890-6238.

Bennett, W.A.; Lagoo-Deenadayalan, S.; Whitworth, N.S.; Stopple, J.A.; Barber, W.H.; Hale, E.; Brackin, M.N. & Cowan, B.D. (1999). First-trimester human chorionic villi express both immunoregulatory and inflammatory cytokines: a role for interleukin-

10 in regulating the cytokine network of pregnancy. *American Journal of Reproductive Immunology*, Vol.41, No.1, pp. 70-78, ISSN 1600-0897.

Bhuiyan, B.; Murad, F. & Fant, M. (2006). The placental cholinergic system: localization to the cytotrophoblast and modulation of nitric oxide. *Cell Communication and Signaling*, Vol.4, No.4, ISSN 1478-811X.

Binukumar, B.; Bal, A.; Kandimalla, R.; Sunkaria, A. & Dip Gill, K. (2010). Mitochondrial energy metabolism impairment and liver dysfunction following chronic exposure to dichlorvos. *Toxicology*, Vol.270, No.2-3, pp. 77-84, ISSN 0300-483X.

Bowen, J.M; Chamley, L.; Mitchell, M.D & Keelan, J.A. (2002). Cytokines of the placenta and extra-placental membranes: biosynthesis, secretion and roles in establishment of pregnancy in women. *Placenta*, Vol.**23**, No.4, pp. 239–256, ISSN 0143-4004.

Brooks, K.; Hasan, H.; Samineni; S.; Gangur, V. & Karmaus, W. (2007). Placental p,p'-dichlorodiphenyldichloroethylene and cord blood immune markers. *Pediatric Allergy and Immunology*, Vol.18, No.7, pp. 621-624, ISSN 0905-6157.

Bryant-Greenwood, G.D.; Yamamoto, S.Y.; Sadowsky, D.W.; Gravett, M.G. & Novy, M.J. (2009). Relaxin stimulates interleukin-6 and interleukin-8 secretion from the extraplacental chorionic cytotrophoblast. *Placenta*, Vol.30, No.7, pp 599-606, ISSN 0143-4004.

Bukovsky, A.; Caudle, M.; Cekanova, M.; Fernando, R.; Wimalasena, J.; Foster, J.; Henley, D. & Elder, R. (2003). Placental expression of estrogen receptor beta and its hormone binding variant–comparison with estrogen receptor alpha and a role for estrogen receptors in asymmetric division and differentiation of estrogen-dependent cells. *Reproductive Biology and Endocrinology*, Vol.1, No.36, pp. 1-21, ISSN 1477-7827.

Casida, J. &. Quistad, G. (2004). Organophosphate Toxicology: Safety Aspects of Nonacetylcholinesterase Secondary Targets. *Chemical Research in Toxicology*, Vol.17, No.8, pp. 983-992, ISSN 0893-228X.

Cerrillo, I.; Granada, A.; López-Espinosa, M.J.; Olmos, B.; Jiménez, M.; Caño, A.; Olea, N. & Olea-Serrano, M.F. (2005). Endosulfan and its Metabolites in Fertile Women, Placenta, Cord Blood, and Human Milk. *Environmental Research*, Vol.98, No.2, pp. 233-239, ISSN 0013-9351.

Cheng, K.W.; Nathwani, P.S. & Leung, P.C. (2000). Regulation of human gonadotropin-releasing hormone receptor gene expression in placental cells. *Endocrinology*, Vol.141, No.7, pp. 2340-9, ISSN 0013-7227.

Chaouat, G.; Dubanchet, S. & Ledée, N. (2007). Cytokines: Important for implantation? *Journal of Assisted Reproduction and Genetics*, Vol.24, No.11, pp. 491-505, ISSN 1058-0468.

Cohn, B.; Cirillo, P. & Christianson, R. (2010). Prenatal DDT Exposure and Testicular Cancer: A Nested Case-Control Study. *Archives of Environmental & Occupational Health*, Vol.65, No.3 , pp.127-134, ISSN 1933-8244.

Corria Osorio, J. & Cruz Manzano, E. (2009). Balance between Reactive Species and Antioxidant Systems in a Normal Pregnancy. *Revista Cubana de Obstetricia y Ginecología*, Vol.35, No.2, pp.1-10, ISSN 0138-600X.

Damgaard, I.; Skakkebæk, N.; Toppari, j.; Virtanen, H.; Shen, H.; Schramm K.; Petersen, J.; Jensen,T. &. Main, K. (2006). Persistent Pesticides in Human Breast Milk and Cryptorchidism. *Environmental Health Perspectives*, Vol.114, No.7, pp. 1133–1138, ISSN 0091-6765.

Davis, A.P.; Murphy, C.G.; Saraceni-Richards, C.A.; Rosenstein, M.C.; Wiegers, T.C. & Mattingly, C.J. (2009). Comparative Toxicogenomics Database: a Knowledgebase and Discovery Tool for Chemical-Gene-Disease Networks. *Nucleic Acids Research*, Vol.37, pp. D786-792, ISSN 0305-1048.

Dealtry, G.B.; Clark, D.E.; Sharkey, A.; Charnock-Jones, D.S. & Smith, S.K. (1998). Expression and localization of the Th2-type cytokine interleukin-13 and its receptor in the placenta during human pregnancy. *American Journal of Reproductive Immunology*, Vol.40, No.4, pp. 283-290, ISSN 1600-0897.

Derfoul, A.; Lin, F.J.; Awumey, E.M.; Kolodzeski, T.; Hall, D.J. & Tuan, R.S. (2003). Estrogenic endocrine disruptive components interfere with calcium handling and differentiation of human trophoblast cells. *Journal of Cellular Biochemistry*, Vol.89, No.4, pp. 755-770, ISSN 1097-4644.

Devrim, E.; Tarhan, I.; Ergüder, I.B. & Durak, I. (2006). Oxidant/Antioxidant Status of Placenta, Blood, and Cord Blood Samples From Pregnant Women Supplemented With Iron. *Reproductive Sciences*, Vol.13, No. 7, pp. 502-505 ISSN 1933-7191.

Dimon-Gadal, S.; Gerbaud, P.; Keryer, G.; Anderson, W.; Evain-Brion, D. & Raynaud, F. (1998). In Vitro Effects of Oxygen-derived Free Radicals on type I and type II cAMP-dependent Protein Kinases. *Journal of Biological Chemistry*, Vol.273, No.35, pp. 22833-22840, ISSN 0021-9258.

Duramad, P.; Tager, I.B.; Leikauf, J.; Eskenazi, B. & Holland, N.T. (2006). Expression of Th1/Th2 cytokines in human blood after in vitro treatment with chlorpyrifos, and its metabolites, in combination with endotoxin LPS and allergen Der p1. *Environmental Health Perspectives*, Vol.114, No.12, pp. 1916-1922, ISSN 0091-6765.

Eaton, D.; Daroff, R.; Autrup, H.; Bridges, J.; Buffler, P.; Costa, L.; Coyle, J.; McKhann, G.; Mobley, W.; Nadel, L.; Neubert, D.; Schulte-Hermann, R. & Spencer, P. (2008). Review of the Toxicology of Chlorpyrifos With an Emphasis on Human Exposure and Neurodevelopment. *Criticals Reviews in Toxicology*, Vol.38, No.s2, pp. 1-125, ISSN 1040-8444.

Fernandez, M.F.; Molina-Molina, J.M.; Lopez-Espinosa, M.J.; Freire, C.; Campoy, C.; Ibarluzea, J.; Torne, P.; Pedraza, V. & Olea, N. (2007). Biomonitoring of Environmental Estrogens in Human Tissues. *International Journal of Hygiene and Environmental Health* , Vol.210, No.3- 4, pp. 429-432, ISSN 0960-3123.

Ferriani, R.A.; Aluned, A.; Sharkey, A. & Smith, S.K. (1994). Colocalization of Acidic and Basic Fibroblast Growth Factor (FGF) in Human Placenta and the Cellular Effects of bFGF in Trophoblast Cell Line JEG-3. *Growth Factors*, Vol.10, No.4, pp. 259-268, ISSN 0897-7194.

Figa-Talamanca, I. (2006). Occupational Risk Factors and Reproductive Health of Women. *Occupational Medicine*, Vol.56, No.8, pp. 521-531, ISSN 0962-7480.

Franco, R.; Sánchez-Olea, R.; Reyes-Reyes, E.M. & Panayiotidis, M.I. (2009). Enviromental Toxicity, Oxidative Stress and Apoptosis: Ménage à Trois. *Mutation Research*, Vol.674, No.1-2, pp. 3-22, ISSN 1383-5718.

Gil, F. & Pla, A. (2001). Biomarkers as biological indicators of xenobiotic exposure- Review. *Journal of Applied Toxicolicology*,Vol.21, No. 4, pp. 245-255, ISSN 0260-437X.

Godin, S.J.; Scollon, E.J.; Hughes, M.F.; Potter, P.M.; DeVito, M.J. & Ross, M.K. (2006). Species differences in the in vitro metabolism of deltamethrin and fenvalerate:

differential oxidative and hydrolytic metabolism by humans and rats. *Drug Metabolism Disposition*, Vol.24, No.10, pp. 1764-1771, ISSN 0090-9556.

Gomez, C.; Bandez, M. & Navarro A. (2007). Pesticides and Impairment of Mitochondrial Function in Relation with the Parkinsonian Syndrome. *Frontiers in Bioscience*, Vol.12, pp. 1079-1093, ISSN 1039-9946.

González-García, B.; Levario-Carrillo, M.; Ramos-Martínez, E.; Arévalo-Gallegos, S.; Infante-Ramírez, R.; Olave-Arreola, M.E.; González-Horta, C. & Sánchez-Ramírez, B. (2006). Muscarinic Cholinergic Receptor Expresión in Placenta From Rats Exponed to Methyl Parathion. *Placenta*, Vol.27, No.1 A56, ISSN 0143-4004.

Gupta R. (2007). Placental toxicity. In: *Veterinary Toxicology, basic and clinical principles*, Gupta Ramesh C. (Ed.), pp 245 -262. Elsevier Academic press, ISBN: 978-0-12-370467-2 NY, USA.

Had˘ziselimović, F.; Geneto, R. & Emmons, L.R. (2000). Elevated placental estradiol: a possible etiological factor of human cryptorchidism. ***The Journal of Urology***, Vol.164, No.5, pp. 1694-1695, ISSN 0022-5347.

Hahn, T.; Desoye, G.; Lang, I. & Skofitsch, G. (1993). Location and activities of acetylcholinesterase and butyrylcholinesterase in the rat and human placenta. *Anatomy and Embryology*,Vol.188, No.5, pp. 435-440, ISSN 0340-2061.

Hakkola, J.M.; Pasanen, J.; Hukkanen, O.; Pelkonen, J.; Mäenpää, R.J.; Edwards, A.R.; Boobis & Raunio, H. (1996a). Expression of xenobiotic- metabolizing cytochrome P450 forms in human full-term placenta. *Biochememical Pharmacoly*, Vol.51, No. 4, pp. 403-411, ISSN 0006-2952

Hakkola, J.; Raunio, H.; Purkunen, R.; Pelkonen, O.; Saarikoski, S.; Cresteil, T. & Pasanen, M. (1996b). Detection of cytochrome P450 gene expression in human placenta in first trimester of pregnancy. *Biochememical Pharmacoly*, Vol.52, No.2, pp. 379–383, ISSN0006-2952.

Hassoun, E.A. & Stohs, S.J. (1996). TCDD, endrin and lindane induced oxidative stress in fetal and placental tissues of C57BL/6J and DBA/2J mice. *Comparative Biochemistry and Physiology C: Comparative Toxicology & Pharmacology*, Vol.115, No.1, pp. 11-18, ISSN 1532-0456.

Hsu, T.Y. (2009). Expression of androgen receptor in human placentas from normal and preeclamptic pregnancies. *Taiwanese Journal of Obstetrics and Gynecology*, Vol.48, No.3, pp. 262-267, ISSN 1028-4559.

Hung, T.; Lo, L.; Chiu, T.; Li, M.; Yeh, Y.; Chen, S. & Hsieh, T. (2010). A Longitudinal Study of Oxidative Stress and Antioxidant Status in Women with Uncomplicated Pregnancies throughout Gestation. *Reproductive Sciences*, Vol.17, No.4, pp.401-409. ISSN 1933-7191.

Huuskonen, P.; Storvik, M.; Reinisalo, M.; Honkakoski, P.; Rysä, J.; Hakkola, J. & Pasanen, M. (2008) Microarray Analysis of the Global Alterations in the Gene Expression in the Placentas From Cigarette-smoking Mothers. *Clinical Pharmacology & Therapeutics*, Vol. 83, No. 4, pp 542-550, ISSN 0009-9236.

Kashyap MP, Singh AK, Kumar V, Tripathi VK, Srivastava RK, Agrawal M, Khanna VK, Yadav S, Jain SK, Pant AB. (2011). Monocrotophos induced apoptosis in PC12 cells: role of xenobiotic metabolizing cytochrome P450s. *PLoS One*, Vol.6, No.3, pp. e17757, ISSN 1932-6203 (Electronic).

Koshakji, R.P.; Sarstry, B.V. & Harbison, R.D. (1974). Studies on the levels and nature of cholinesterase in human and mosuse placenta. *Research Communications in Chemical Pathology and Pharmacology*, Vol.9, No.1, pp. 181-184, ISSN 0034-5164.

Lankas, G.; Wise, L.; Cartwright, M.; Pippert, T. & Umbenhauer, D. (1998). Placental P-glycoprotein Deficiency enhances Susceptibility to Chemically Induced Birth Defects in Mice. *Reproductive Toxicology*, Vol.12, No.4, pp. 457-463, ISSN 0890-6238.

Laville, N.; Balaguer, P.; Brion, F.; Hinfray, N.; Casellas, C.; Porcher, J. M. & Aït-Aïssa, S. (2006). Modulation of Aromatase Activity and mRNA by various selected Pesticides in the Human Choriocarcinoma JEG-3 Cell Line. *Toxicology*, Vol. 228, pp. 98-108, ISSN 0300-483X.

Lecoeur, S.; Videmann, B. & Mazallon, M. (2006). Effect of organophosphate pesticide diazinon on expression and activity of intestinal P-glycoprotein. *Toxicology Letters*, Vol.**161,** No. 3, pp. 200-209, ISSN 0378-4274.

Levario-Carrillo, M.; Feria-Velasco, A.; De Celis, R.; Ramos-Martínez, E.; Córdova-Fierro, L. & Solís, F.J. (2001). Parathion, a cholinesterase-inhibiting plaguicide induces changes in tertiary villi of placenta of women exposed: a scanning electron microscopy study. *Gynecologic and Obstetric Investigation*, Vol.52, No.4, pp. 269-275, ISSN: 0378-7346.

Levario-Carrillo, M.; Amato, D.; Pstrosky-Wegman, P.; González- Horta, C.; Corona, Y. & Sanin, L.H. (2004a). Relation between pesticide exposure and intrauterine growth retardation. *Chemosphere*, Vol.55, No.10, pp. 1421-1427, ISSN 0045-6535.

Levario-Carrillo, M.; Olave, M.E.; Corral, D.C.; Alderete, J.G.; Gagioti, S.M. & Bevilacqua, E. (2004b). Placental morphology of rats prenatally exposed to methyl parathion. *Experimental and Toxicologic Pathology*. Vol.55, No.6, pp. 489-496, ISSN 0940-2993.

Lips, K.S. & Brüggmann, D. (2005). Nicotinic acetylcholine receptors in rat and human placenta. *Placenta*, Vol.26, No.10, pp. 735-746, ISSN 0143-4004.

Liu, J.; Puscheck, E.E.; Wang, F.; Trostinskaia, A.; Barisic, D.; Maniere, G.; Wygle, D.; Zhong, W.; Rings, E. & Rappolee, D. (2004). Serine-threonine Kinases and Transcription Factors Active in Signal Transduction are Detected at High Levels of Phosphorylation during Mitosis in Preimplantation Embryos and Trophoblast Stem Cells. *Reproduction*, Vol.128, No. 5, pp. 643-654, ISSN 1470-1626.

Lopez-Espinosa, M.J; Granada, A.; Carreno, J.; Salvatierra, M.; Olea-Serrano, F. & Olea, N. (2007). Organochlorine Pesticides in Placentas from Southern Spain and Some Related Factors. *Placenta*, Vol.28, No.7, pp. 631- 638, ISSN 0143-4004.

Lukaszewicz-Hussain, A. (2010). Role of Oxidative Stress in Organophosphate Insecticide Toxicity - Short review. *Pesticide Biochemistry and Physiology*, Vol.98, No.2, pp. 145-150, ISSN 0048-3575.

Macias, R.; Marin, J. J. & Serrano, M. A. (2009). Excretion of biliary compounds during intrauterine life. *World Journal of Gastroenterology*, Vol.21, No.15, pp. 817–828, ISSN 1007-9327.

Magnarelli, G.; Souza, M.S & P. de D' Angelo, A. M. (2009). Heptachlor and op´DDT effects on protein kinase activities associated with human placenta particulated fractions. *Journal of Biochemical and Molecular Toxicology*, Vol.23, No.3, pp. 185-192, ISSN 1095-6670.

Mansour, S.A. (2004) Pesticide Exposure-Egyptian Scene. *Toxicology*, Vol. 198, No. 1-3, pp. 91-115, ISSN 0300-483X.

Mao Q. (2008). BCRP/ ABCG2 in the Placenta: Expression, Function and Regulation, *Pharmaceutical Research,* Vol.25, No.6, pp.1244-1255, ISSN 0724-8741.

Martin, M.T.; Brennan, R.J.; Hu, W.; Ayanoglu, E.; Lau, C.; Ren, H.; Wood, C. R.; Corton, J.C.; Kavlock, R.J. & Dix, D.J. (2007). Toxicogenomic Study of Triazole Fungicides and Perfluoroalkyl Acids in Rat Livers Predicts Toxicity and Categorizes Chemicals Based on Mechanisms of Toxicity. *Toxicological Sciences,* Vol.97, No. 2, pp. 595-613, ISSN 1096-6080.

Martindale, J.L. & Holbrook, N.J. (2002). Cellular response to oxidative stress: Signaling for suicide and survival. *Journal of Cellular Physiology,* Vol.192, No.1, pp.1-15, ISSN 0021-9541.

McEwan, M.; Lins, R.J.; Munro, S.K.; Vincent, Z.L.; Ponnampalam, A.P. & Mitchell, M.D. (2009). Cytokine regulation during the formation of the fetal–maternal interface: focus on cell–cell adhesion and remodeling of the extra-cellular matrix. *Cytokine and Growth Factor Reviews,.* Vol.**20**, No.3, pp. 241–249, ISSN 1359-6101.

Menon, R.; Fortunato, S.J.; Yu, J.; Milne, G.L.; Sanchez, S.; Drobek, C.O.; Lappase, M. & Taylor R.N. (2011). Cigarette Smoke Induces Oxidative Stress and a Poptosis in Normal Term Fetal Membranes. *Placenta,* Vol.32, No.4, pp. 317-322, ISSN 0143-4004.

Mnif, W.; Hassine, A.; Bouaziz, A.; Bartegi, A.; Thomas, O. & Roig, B. (2011). Effect of Endocrine Disruptor Pesticides: A Review. *International Journal of Environmental Research and Public Health,* Vol.8, No. 6, pp. 2265-2303, ISSN 1660-4601.

Moffett, A. & Loke, C. Immunology of placentation in eutherian mammals. (2006). *Nature Reviews Immunology,* Vol. 6, No.8, pp. 584-594, ISSN 1474-1733.

Moustafa, G.; Ibrahim, Z.; Ahmed, M.; Ghoneim, M.; Sakamoto, K.; Ishizuka, M. & Fujita, S. (2008). Downregulation of Male-specific Cytochrome P450 by Profenofos. *Japanese Journal of Veterinary Research,* Vol.56, No. 2, pp. 109-118, ISSN 0047-1917.

Myllynen, P.; Pasanen, M. & Pelkonen, O. (2005). Human placenta: a human organ for developmental toxicology research and biomonitoring. *Placenta,* Vol.26,No. 5, pp. 361-371, ISSN 0143-4004.

Nagamatsu, T. & Schust, D.J. (2010). The immunomodulatory roles of macrophages at the maternal-fetal interface. *Reproductive Sciences.* Vol. 17, No. 4, pp 209-218. ISSN: 1933-7191.

Nagamuna, H.; Ohtani, H.; Harada, N. & Nagura, H. (1990). Immunoelectron Microscopic Localization of Aromatase in Human Placenta and Ovary using Microwave Fixation. *Journal of Histochemistry and Cytochemistry,* Vol.38, pp 1427-1432, ISSN 0022-1554.

Nakamura, Y.; Hamada, Y.; Fujiwara, T.; Enomoto, H.; Hiroe, T.; Tanaka, S.; Nose, M.; Nakahara, M.; Yoshida, N.; Takenawa, T. & Fukami, K. (2005). Phospholipase C-δ1 and -δ3 are Essential in the Trophoblast for Placental Development. *Molecular and Cellular Biology,*Vol.25 , No.24 , pp. 10979-10988, ISSN 0270-7306.

Naruse, K.; Innes, B.A.; Bulmer, J.N.; Robson, S.C.; Searle, R.F. & Lash, G.E. (2010). Secretion of cytokines by villous cytotrophoblast and extravillous trophoblast in the first trimester of human pregnancy. *Journal of Reproductive Immunology.* Vol. 86, No. 2, pp 148-150. ISSN: 0165-0378

Oostingh, G.J.; Wichmann, G.; Schmittner, M.; Lehmann, I. & Duschl, A. (2009). The cytotoxic effects of the organophosphates chlorpyrifos and diazinon differ from their immunomodulating effects. *Journal of Immunotoxicology*, Vol.6, No.2, pp. 136-145, ISSN, 1547-691X.

Pasanen, M. (1999). The expression and regulation of drug metabolism in human placenta. *Advanced Drug Delivery Reviews*, Vol.38, No.1, pp. 81-97, ISSN 0169-409X.

Pathak, R.; Mustafa, M.D.; Ahmed, R.; Tripathi, A.; Guleria, K. & Banerjee, B.D. (2010). Association between recurrent Miscarriages and Organochlorine Pesticide Levels. *Clinical Biochemistry*, Vol. 43, No.1-2, pp. 131-135, ISSN 0009-9120.

Petit, A.; Guillen, G.; Tence, M.; Jard, S.; Gallo-Payet, N.; Bellabaraba, D.; Lehoux, J. G. & Belisle, S. (1989). Angiotensin II Stimulates both Inositol Phosphate Production and Human Placental Lactogen Release from Human Trophoblast Cells. *Journal of Clinical Endocrinology and Metabolism*, Vol.69, No. 2, pp. 280-286, ISSN 0021-972X.

Poli, G.; Leonarduzzi, G.; Biasi, F. & Chiarpotto, E. (2004). Oxidative Stress and Cell Signalling. *Current Medicinal Chemistry*, Vol.11, No. 9, pp. 1023-1042, ISSN 0929-8673.

Prokopenko, V.M.; Partsalis, G.K. & Burmistrov, S.O. (2006). The Gluthaione-Dependent System of Placenta Antioxidant Defense in Miscarriage. *Human Physiology*, Vol.32, No.2, pp 197-199, ISSN 0362-1197.

Prouillac, C.; Videmann, B.; Mazallon, M. & Lecoeur, S. (2009). Induction of cells differentiation and ABC transporters expression by a myco-estrogen, zearalenone, in human choriocarcinoma cell line (Be Wo). *Toxicology*, Vol.263, No.3, pp. 100-107. ISSN 0300-483X.

Prouillac C. & Lecoeur S. (2010). The Role of the Placenta in Fetal Exposure to Xenobiotics: Importance of Membrane Transporters and Human Models for Transfer Studies. *Drug Metabolism and Disposition*, Vol.38, No. 10, pp. 1623-1635, ISSN 0090-9556.

Rogan, W. & Chen, A. (2005). Health Risks and Benefits of Bis(4-Chlorophenyl)-1,1,1-trichloroethene (DDT). *Lancet*, Vol.366, pp. 763-773, ISSN 0140-6736.

Rose, R.L. & Hodgson, E. (2004). Metabolism of Toxicants, In: *A textbook of Modern Toxicology, Third Edition*, Ernest Hodgson Edit., pp111-148, ISBN 0-471-26508-X John Willey and Sons Inc.USA.

Saulsbury, M.D.; Heyliger, S.O.; Wang, K. & Round D. (2008). Characterization of chlorpyrifos-induced apoptosis in placental cells. *Toxicology*, Vol.244, No.2-3, pp. 98-110, ISSN 0300-483X.

Schäfer-Somi, S. (2003). Cytokines during early pregnancy of mammals: a review. *Animal Reproduction Science*. Vol.75, No.1-2, pp. 73-94, ISSN 0378-4320.

Serrano, M.A.; Macias, R.I.; Briz, O.; Monte, M.J.; Blazquez, A.G.; Williamson, C.; Kubitz, R. & Marin, J.J. (2007). Expression in human trophoblast and choriocarcinoma cell lines, BeWo, Jeg-3 and JAr of genes involved in the hepatobiliary-like excretory function of the placenta. *Placenta*. Vol. 28, No. 2-3, pp. 107-117. ISSN: 0143-4004.

Sharom, F.S. (2008). ABC multidrug transporters: structure, function and role in chemoresistance. *Pharmacogenomics*, Vol.9, No.1, pp. 105-127, ISSN 1462-2416.

Shen, H.; Main, K.M.; Kaleva, M.; Virtanen, H.; Damggard, I.N.; Haavisto, A.M.; Kaleva, M.; Boisen, K.A.; Schmidt, I.M.; Chellakooty, M.; Skakkebaek, N.E.; Toppari, J. & Schramm, K. W. (2007). From mother to child: Investigation of Prenatal and postnatal exposure to persistent bioaccumulating toxicants using breast milk and placenta biomonitoring. *Chemosphere*, Vol.67, pp. S256-S262, ISSN 0045-6535.

Shen, H.; Main, K.M.; Kaleva, M.; Virtanen, H.; Haavisto, A. M.; Skakkebaek, N.E.; Toppari, J. & Schramm, K. W. (2005). Prenatal Organochlorine Pesticides in Placentas from Finland: Exposure of Male Infants born 1997-2001. *Placenta,* Vol.26, No.6 , pp. 512-514, ISSN 0143-4004.

Sood, R., Zehnder, J.L.; Druzin, M.L. & Brown, P.O. (2006). Gene expression patterns in human placenta. *Proceedings of the National Academy of Sciences,* Vol.103, No.14, pp. 5478-5483, ISSN 0027-8424.

Souza, M.S.; Magnarelli, G.; Rovedatti, M.G.; Santa Cruz, S. & Pechén de D`Angelo, A.M. (2005). Prenatal Exposure to Pesticides: Analysis of Human Placental Acetylcolinesterase, Glutathione-S-transferase and Catalase as biomarkers of effect. *Biomarkers,* Vol.10, No.5, pp.376-389, ISSN 1354-750X.

Souza, M.S.; Magnarelli de Potas, G. & Pechen de D´Angelo, A.M. (2004). Organophosphorus and organochlorine pesticides affect human placental phosphoinositides metabolism and PI-4 kinase activity. *Journal of Biochemical and Molecular Toxicology,* Vol. 18, pp. 30-36, ISSN 1095-6670.

St-Pierre, M.V.; Serrano, M.A.; Macias, R.I.; Dubs, U.; Hoechli, M.; Lauper, U.; Meier, P.J. & Marin, J.J. (2000). Expression of members of the multidrug resistance protein family in human term placenta. *American Journal of Physiology- Regulatory Integrative and Comparative Physiol*ogy, Vol.279, No.4, pp. R1495-1503, ISSN 0363-6119.

Straszewski-Chavez, S.L.; Abrahams, V.M. & Mor, G. (2005). The role of apoptosis in the regulation of trophoblast survival and differentiation during pregnancy. *Endocrine Reviews,* Vol.26, No.7, pp. 877-97, ISSN 0163-769X.

Sun, M.; Kingdom, J.; Baczyk, D.; Lye, S. J.; Matthews, S. G. & Gibb, W. (2006). Expression of the Multidrug Resistance P-Glycoprotein, (ABCB1 Glycoprotein) in the Human Placenta Decreases with Advancing Gestation. *Placenta,* Vol.27, No.6, pp. 602-609, ISSN 0143-4004.

Syme, M.R.; Paxton, J.W. & Keelan, J.A. (2004). Drug Transfer and Metabolism by the Human Placenta. *Clinical Pharmacokinetics,* Vol.,No.8, pp. 487-514, ISSN 0312-5963.

Tang, J.; Rose, R.L.; & Chambers, J.E. (2006). Metabolism *of* organophosphorus and carbamate pesticides. In: *Toxicology* of *Organophosphate and Carbamate Compounds*. Gupta, R.C. (Ed.*),* pp. 127–143, Elsevier Academic Press, ISBN 13:978-012-088523-7, London.

Tremblay, J.; Hardy, D.B.; Pereira, L.E. & Yang, K. *(*1999*).* Retinoic acid stimulates the expression of 11beta-hydroxysteroid dehydrogenase type 2 in human choriocarcinoma JEG-3 cells. *Biology of Reproduction,* Vol *60,* pp. *541*–545, ISSN 0006-3363.

Tribull, T.E.; Bruner, R.H. & Bain, L.J. *(*2003).The multidrug resistance-associated protein 1 transports methoxychlor and protects the seminiferous epithelium from injury. *Toxicology Letters*; Vol.142, No1-2, pp. 61-70, ISSN0378-4274.

Triche, E.W. & Hossain, N. Environmental factors implicated in the causation of adverse pregnancy outcome. *(*2007*). Seminars in Perinatology,* Vol.31, No.4, pp. 240-242, ISSN 0146-0005.

Tuckey, R.; Bose, H.; Czerwionka, I. & Miller, W. (2004). Molten Globule Structure and Steroidogenic Activity of N-218 MLN64 in Human Placental Mitochondria. *Endocrinology,* Vol.145, No.4, pp. 1700-1707, ISSN 0013-7227.

van den Berg, H. (2009). Global Status of DDT and Its Alternatives for Use in Vector Control to Prevent Disease. *Environmental Health Perspectives*, Vol.117, pp. 1653-1663, ISSN 0091-6765.

van Mourik, M.S.M.; Macklon, N.S. & Heijnen, C.J. (2009). Embryonic implantation: cytokines, adhesion molecules, and immune cells in establishing an implantation environment. *Journal of Leukocyte Biology*, Vol.**85,** No.1, pp. 4–19, ISSN 0741-5400.

Vanderlelie, J.; Venardos, K.; Clifton, V.L.; Gude, N.M.; Clarke, F.M. & Perkins A.V. (2005). Increased Biological Oxidation and Reduced Anti-oxidant Enzyme Activity in Pre-eclamptic Placentae. *Placenta*, Vol.26, No.1, pp. 53-58, ISSN 0143-4004.

Vanderlelie, J.; Gude, N. & Perkins, A.V. (2008). Antioxidant Gene Expression in Preeclamptic Placentae: A Preliminary Investigation. *Placenta*, Vol.29, No.6, pp. 519-522, ISSN 0143-4004.

Williams, T.J.; Jones, C.A.; Miles, E.A.; Warner, J.O. & Warner, J.A. (2000). Fetal and neonatal IL-13 production during pregnancy and at birth and subsequent development of atopic symptoms. *Journal of Allergy and Clinical Immunology*, Vol.105, No.5, pp. 951-959, ISSN 0091-6749.

Wójtowicz, A.K.; Milewicz, T. & Gregoraszczuk, E. (2007a). DDT and its Metabolite DDE Alter Steroid Hormone Secretion in Human Term Placental Explants by Regulation of Aromatase Activity. *Toxicology Letters*, Vol.173, pp. 24-30, ISSN 0378-4274.

Wójtowicz, A.K.; Augustowska, K. & Gregoraszczuk, E.L. (2007b). The short- and long-term effects of two isomers of DDT and their metabolite DDE on hormone secretion and survival of human choriocarcinoma JEG-3 cells. *Pharmacological Reports*, Vol.59, No.2, pp. 224-32, ISSN 1734-1140.

Wójtowicz, A.K.; Milewicz, T. & Gregoraszczuk, E. (2008). Time-dependent action of DDT (1,1,1-trichloro-2,2-bis(*p*-chlorophenyl)ethane) and its metabolite DDE (1,1-dichloro-2,2-bis(*p*-chlorophenyl)ethylene) on human chorionic gonadotropin and progesterone secretion. *Gynecological Endocrinology*,Vol.24, No.1, pp. 54-58, ISSN 0951-3590.

Wynn, T.A. (2008). Cellular and molecular mechanisms of fibrosis. *The Journal of Pathology*, Vol.214, No.2, pp. 199-210, ISSN 1096-9896.

You, L. (2004). Steroid Hormone Biotransformation and Xenobiotic Induction of Hepatic Steroid Metabolizing Enzymes. *Chemico-Biological Interactions*, Vol.147, pp. 233-246, ISSN 0009-2797.

You, L.; Casanova, M.; Archibeque-Engle, S.; Sar, M.; Fan, L. & Heck, H. (1998). Impaired Male Sexual Development in Perinatal Sprague-Dawley and Long-Evans Hooded Rats Exposed in Utero and Lactationally p,p'-DDE. *Toxicological Sciences*, Vol.45, pp. 162-173, ISSN 1096-6080.

Yuan, B.; Ohyama, K.; Bessho, T.; Uchide, N. & Toyoda, H. (2008). Imbalance between ROS production and elimination results in apoptosis induction in primary smooth chorion trophoblast cells prepared from human fetal membrane tissues. *Life Sciences*, Vol. 82, No. 11-12, pp. 623-630, ISSN 0024-3205.

6

Placental Infection by Trypanosome Cruzi, the Causal Agent of Congenital Chagas´ Disease

Cintia Diaz-Luján[1], Maria Fernanda Triquell[1], Luciana Mezzano[1] and Ricardo E. Fretes[1,2,*]
[1]*Placenta and Chagas Laboratory, Cell Biology, Histology and Embryology Department, Medicine Faculty, Universidad Nacional Córdoba, Cordoba,*
[2]*IICSHUM and Cathedra of Histology, Embryology and Genetic, Health Department, Universidad Nacional La Rioja, La Rioja, Argentina*

1. Introduction

Placenta is a transitory organ which simultaneously separate and connect mother and fetus. It has the major importance in the nutrition of fetus, scavenger waste products from fetus, secretion of hormones and immunological factors, allowing fetus to grow in a sea of maternal immunologic environment and regulating mother metabolism. Also, placenta protects fetus to some infectious agents. It has been described that placental barrier is effective to avoid viral, bacterial and protozoan fetal infections, such as Cytomegalovirus, Lysteria monocytogenes and Trypanosoma cruzi (Dolcini et al., 2008; Leopardi et al., 1994; Robbins et al., 2010).

Placenta has evolved allowing an independent life to mother. Human placenta is discoidal, villous and hemochorial in structure (Benirschke et a., 2006) meaning it has a particular structure which is not shared with other commonly species employed in biomedical research such as mice. The monkey great apes have similar placenta to human but it is expensive and also needs a special environment and protection of rare species. Guinea pig has a hemochorial placenta similar to human and it would be necessary to study deeper this specie in relation to transmission of infectious agent from mother to fetus at least in Chagas transmission.

To study human placental invasion by infectious agents, such as Trypanosoma cruzi, researchers have three possible models, the culture of either isolated trophoblast or chorionic villi explants in interaction with the parasite, or perfusion of placental cotyledons in an extracorporeal system, or to analyze the organ from chagasic women obtained at the end of pregnancy. The aim of this chapter is to study mechanisms and processes of the interaction between placental barrier and the causal agent of Chagas´disease, the *Trypanosoma cruzi*, mainly *in vitro* systems. Most of the studies with human placenta were done in *in vitro* systems approximately the last 15 years.

---

* Corresponding author

2. Chagas´disease: some aspects

Chagas´disease was first described by Carlos Chagas a little more than 100 years ago. He described the causal agent, the vectorial transmission and reservoirs and the clinical manifestations in humans, that is the complete cycle of the disease. Also, Chagas suggested the congenital transmission. Carlos Chagas was nominated twice to the Nobel Prize, but never (unfairly) obtained it (Clayton, 2010).

Chagas disease is an enzootic condition in Latin America, caused by the protozoan Trypanosoma cruzi, an obligated intracellular parasite which is transmitted to human by different ways. The most common and important of those ways is by the feces of an infected triatomine which defecate while feeding. Congenital transmission is another important route by which the parasite infects the fetus or the new born, implying in utero or perinatal transmission. This review aimed on transplacental transmission of T. cruzi.

The disease has an acute stage mainly seen in children with no symptoms, or mild symptoms or evident ones, such as fever, swelling of lymph nodes, conjunctivitis and skin lesions (Kierszenbaum 2007, Teixeira et al. 2006). It has been also described, myocarditis, encephalitis and meningitis. Death is a rare condition in this period. All symptoms and signals cede spontaneously and patients pass to the indeterminate period of the disease. Approximately 12 million of individuals, who are coursing this stage, are positive to specific serological tests and neither have symptoms and signs of the disease nor ECG and X ray abnormalities, but they are reservoirs for T. cruzi. Approximately one third of all of these individuals develop chronic Chagas disease, 20 to 30 years later to acquire it. Chronic Chagas disease is associated to cardiomyopathy or digestive disorders. Dead is associated with this stage of the disease.

3. Congenital Chagas transmission (CCT)

3.1 Definition

The transmission of live T. cruzi from a chagasic pregnant woman to the fetus implies that the new born has the parasite in his/her tissues at the moment of delivery. To consider a congenital case, it should fulfill the following conditions: Mother should be positive for T. cruzi and also new born should have T. cruzi in their tissues at delivery. Congenital Chagas should be diagnosed detecting parasites in infants at delivery or later or detecting own antibodies against parasite antigens discarding blood transfusion or vectorial transmission.

The congenital transmission has been described in pregnant women coursing the acute and the indeterminate stages of the disease, even though the incidence of positive transmission were higher when mother was in the acute period with high parasitemias (see 5. Survival of T. cruzi in the placental environment) (Schijman 2007). Thus, the amount of parasites could be an important risk factor for CCT.

Positive pregnant women may transmit the parasite to one or all siblings, or to jump a gestation. However, family clustering has been described, and siblings of a congenital case are at high risk that merits testing for Chagas in them (Sanchez-Negrete et al. 2005). Frequently, positive children born to chagasic mothers are asymptomatics (Moya et al. 1979). However, approximately half of the infected new borns depict clinical signs of congenital Chagas disease (Sanchez-Negrete et al. 2005, Torrico et al. 2004). Clinical manifestation might appear at delivery, or days or weeks later (Freilij et al. 1994). There is an association between premature births and low birth weight with CCT (Azogue 1985, Bittencourt 1992, Sanchez-Negrete et al. 2005) and they should be considered as risk factors. The condition of chagasic in the mother does not have any consequence on the uninfected infant (Shijman 2007). It is controversial if sex participates as risk factor, even though it seems there are more males than females congenitally infected with T. cruzi (Bittencourt 1992, Carlier and Truyens 2010, Torrico et al. 2004).

3.2 Epidemiological importance of congenital infection by T. cruzi

The prevalence of Chagas´ disease in pregnant women in South America ranges between 4% to 64,4% with 0.1% to 7% of these transmitting the infection to their newborns (Romero 2011, WHO 2007). There were 1136 congenital T. cruzi reported cases from 1994 to 2001. According to Gurtler et al, (2003) there were more cases than the reported ones; and the estimated for these authors was of 6.3 expected cases per each reported case. So, the real situation in Argentina, at least in those 8 years was of 7157 new cases in Argentina. As it was reported that congenital transmissions was cluster in families, so brothers of congenital children are in risk, drawing a very serious picture for Chagas transmission in endemic countries due to congenital T. cruzi transmission.

Congenital transmission has already surpassed the number of vector-mediated acute cases by a factor of 10 in Argentina (Gurtler et al 2003). This form of transmission constitutes an increasing public health problem and is responsible for the urbanization and spreading of the disease to non endemic areas, such as cities of Latin America, United States of America and Europe (Schijman, 2007; Clik Lambert, 2008). The permanence of high prevalence of chagasic pregnant women in some cities of Latin America is worsening the situation.

3.3 Possible routes by which T. cruzi reaches the fetus

Congenital transmission of T. cruzi has been well documented (Freilij et al., 1995, Schijman 2007). Although this form of transmission was first suggested one hundred years ago by Carlos Chagas, the precise route by which the parasite reaches the fetus has not yet been elucidated, if there was only one.

The chorionic villous offers the major surface for interaction between mother and fetus, therefore is one of the possible routes that *Trypanosoma cruzi* employs to infect the placenta leading to the congenital Chagas´ disease. It was described the villous trophoblast as being the first barrier that T. cruzi must cross in order to reach the offspring (Bittencourt, 1992, Schijman, 2007). But, Fernandez-Aguilar (2005) and Moya et al. (1979), studying placentas from chagasic mothers, found parasites at the chorionic plate but do not describe parasites at the chorionic villi. These authors therefore suggested that the route by which T. cruzi accesses the fetus is by hematogenous route through the marginal sinus, spreading into the chorionic plate rather than by the trophoblast.

It was also described that the genital canal at birth could be another route of connatal transmission (Schijman 2007). A possible fourth route for T. cruzi congenital transmission could be through transfusion of blood from mother to fetus in the uterus (Bianchi and

Romero, 2003, Vernochet et al., 2007), mechanism that has not been either studied or described yet to the best of our knowledge.

4. Influence of strains of T. cruzi in the congenital transmission

Strains of T. cruzi have been involved in different clinical forms of Chagas' disease (Dutra et al. 2005, Zingales et al. 1999), thus implicating a different genetic population in tissue tropism, replication and virulence, and in consequences in disease outcome (Dutra et al., 2005; Macedo et al., 2004; Mejía and Triana, 2005). Maternal conditions, strains of T. cruzi and immunological competence of the placenta, might all participate in the congenital Chagas' disease transmission. Whether strains of T. cruzi contribute to congenital infection is a matter of controversy. Andrade (1982) found that three different strains of T. cruzi had differential tropism to placenta in mice. Epidemiological studies showed geographical differences in the incidence and clinical forms of congenital Chagas' disease (Bittencourt, 1992). These data may indicate that different T. cruzi strains and/or host individuality participate, as suggested by the occurrence of family clustering of congenital Chagas disease (Sanchez-Negrete et al, 2005, Schijman 2007). Virreira et al (2006) and Burgos et al., (2007) concluded that congenital transmission of T. cruzi is not associated with genetic polymorphism of T. cruzi. Recently, Burgos et al. (2007) described that TcIId is the most prevalent lineage found in pregnant women both in those who transmit and also in those who did not transmit congenitally to their babies and Virreira et al. (2006) found TcIIb, TcIId and TcIIe in blood in the umbilical cord, indicating there is not a specific strain of T. cruzi implicated in congenital transmission. However, Solana et al. (2002) described biological differences among subpopulations of T. cruzi in experimental vertical transmission. Furthermore, experimentally in *in vitro* co-cultures of explants of chorionic villi incubated with trypomastigotes of two strains of T. cruzi, it was showed that there are biological differences between both strains, surviving more one of the strain with respect to the other (Triquell et al. 2009). The survival of specific strain in the placental environment could be more important than parasitemia itself to amplify possibilities of infection of the placental tissue. Differential susceptibility of different strains of the parasite in the intervillous space might explain those cases of high parasitemia of the mother but without congenital infection. Andrade et al. (1972) in experimental infections found that the level of parasitemia was lower in the two strains of T. cruzi associated with human congenital transmission.

The data presented above depict a picture of differences between biological behavior (Andrade et al. 1972, Lujan et al. 2004) and molecular characterization of different populations of T. cruzi (Burgos et al., 2007, Virreyra et al. 2006). On one hand different populations of T. cruzi have different biological behavior but there is not a specific DTU of T. cruzi associated to CCT. These differences merit further investigation in this area, considering individual factors specific to each chagasic pregnant woman (Torrico et al., 2004).

5. Survival of T. cruzi in the placental environment

It was demonstrated that trophoblasts and/or other chorionic villi cells produce various immunological agents such as hormones, cytokines, nitric oxide and nitrogen and oxygen derivatives products (Benirschke et al. 2006, Haugel-de-Mouzon and Guerre-Millo 2006). Some of these are also released to the intervillous space. This aspect concomitantly with maternal low blood flow in the intervillous space where T. cruzi might be present in chagasic pregnant women, open the possibility that the parasite could be damaged and consequently the parasitemia could be reduced or cleaned out of the intervillous space. The low flow of the mother blood in the intervillous space might allow the parasiticidal agents to destroy the parasite cell limiting the placental invasion by T. cruzi.

The presence and quantity of parasite cells in the intervillous space seems to be an important matter in the congenital transmission of T. cruzi. In the acute stage of the disease, the pregnant women have intense and persistent parasitemia (Carlier and Truyens 2010, Freilij et al. 1995, Schijman 2007). The rate of T. cruzi transmission from mother to fetus is increased when pregnant women coursed an acute stage of the infection, as was described by Moretti et al. (2005), and reviewed by Freilij et al. (1994), Carlier and Truyens (2010), Bittencourt (1976) and Shijman (2007). Also, in experimental infection, high parasitemia worsen mating and pregnancy outcome, with high resorptions of fetuses (Mjihdi et al. 2002, Mjihdi et al. 2004, Solana et al. 2009). These results are independent of the strains of the mice and of the parasite given that Mjihdi et al. (2002) employed BALB/c mice infected with Tehuantepec population of T. cruzi, while Solana et al. (2009) employed C3H/HcN mice with K98 clone derived from the CA-I strain of T. cruzi, obtaining similar results.

There were few publications analyzing the survival of T. cruzi in the placental environment. This aspect was studied by Triquell et al. (2009) in *in vitro* experiments employing chorionic villi explants. In this work authors employed the whole placental barrier co-cultured with two populations of the T. cruzi, one was the laboratory maintained tulahuen strain and the other was isolated from a congenitally acquired new born. To study the effect of placental environment upon T. cruzi cell, authors employed two different strategies. In one of them, parasites were collected at the end of co-cultures placental explants - trypomastigotes and their viability were quantified. The population of T. cruzi obtained from a congenital case had a significantly higher survival rate than the tulahuen population of T. cruzi when parasites were incubated with chorionic villi explants but there was no difference in their survival between both populations when parasites were incubated with Vero cells as control. In the other strategy, authors collected culture media from placental explants and Vero cells (as control) and then treated trypomastigotes for 1h at 37°C with those media and also with fresh medium as control. Again, culture media from placental explants affect both strains of T. cruzi, eventhough there were more viable parasites of the congenital strain of T. cruzi. These results indicate that the placental environment alters the viability of the parasite cell and that there is a different behavior of different populations of T. cruzi in that environment. This aspect is evidently related to the permanence of the parasite in the intervillous space.

Another interesting aspect still poorly analyzed is referred to the time that T. cruzi remains in the intervillous space. There is a work that indirectly analyzed this aspect employing a placental perfusion model (Shippey et al. 2005). After the spiral arteries cross the basal plate, the maternal blood is poured into the intervillous space where circulates around the villi outside of the endothelium of the maternal vascular system (Brenishke, 2006). Then, blood return to the basal plate where veins drain the maternal blood into de general circulation of the mother. Differences between arterial-venous pressure is the force by which the maternal blood flows within placenta (Bernishke, 2006). According to a radioangiographic study, maternal blood fills rapidly the centers of the villous trees and then spreads slowly toward the centrifugal subchorial and peripheral zones. Due the form of the intervillous space as narrow clefts (Bernishke 2006), maternal blood circulates slowly within placenta, allowing T. cruzi to interact with placental barrier in chagasic pregnant women. So the question is how much time the T. cruzi cell is able to stay in the intervillous space interacting with trophoblast? Shippey et al. (2005) used placental perfusion model to study transplacental passage of the causal agent of Chagas disease. A solution containing a great mass of trypomastigotes of T. cruzi (approximately 10^7 cells) was injected as a bolus through the maternal perfusate flow. Authors have not informed the strain of T. cruzi they employed. After the bolus infusion of parasites, the fetal and maternal circulations were maintained with sterile saline solution till 2 hs. The PCR (polymerase chain reaction) to detect T. cruzi DNA in the fetal and maternal effluents indicated presence of the parasite at 30 min, 60 min and 90 min only in the maternal one and was negative (there was not parasite DNA) in the fetal effluent. These data implicate that T. cruzi remains within placenta after several flows of sterile saline perfusion and also that there was not any passage to fetal circulation despite the great mass of parasites injected. This result acquires importance due the differential survival that different strains of T. cruzi have in the placental environment and the similar infectivity that these strains of the parasite have upon the placental tissue (Triquell et al. 2009). Thus, the biological characteristics of the parasite may play a role in the permanence of T. cruzi in the placental environment and it could be more important than the reproduction rate within the placental tissue.

6. Infection and survival of Trypanosoma cruzi in the placental tissue

6.1 Mechanism of infection

Trypanosoma cruzi which could be present in the maternal blood in the intervillous space, cross the trophoblastic barrier, the first placental line of defense or other placental tissues deprived of trophoblastic defenses. The trypomastigotes into the stromal of chorionic villi (the second placental line of defense) and/or chorionic plate constituted by connective tissue fibers and cells such as fibroblasts, myofibroblasts and macrophages (Hofbauer cells), can further multiplicate within such cells if that have not been destroyed by mesenchymal phagocytic cells. The parasite formed nest o pseudocysts which once rupture, releases new motile parasites. Sequential infection of other cells, finally infecting myocytes and endothelial cells of fetal vessels in villous chorion, chorionic plate and gain access to fetal circulation and infect the fetus causing the congenital form of the disease (Bittencourt 1976, 1992; Carlier 2005; Fernandez Aguilar et al 2005). Some authors believe that the trypomastigote have to find a lesion in the trophoblast in order to penetrate the placental tissue (Bittencourt 1963) because trophoblast may conform a barrier to T. cruzi infection. Histopathological analysis of placentas to brazilian infected women showed placental inflammation with villitis and areas of trophoblast destruction or necrosis which induced to release inflammatory cytokines such as TNF-α and production of local inflammatory mediators. These factors can induce a rupture of the trophoblastic barrier facilitating fetal infection (Redline 2004).

The invasion mechanism of the protozoan parasite T. cruzi was originally assumed to be similar to the many bacterial pathogens which mobilize the actin cytoskeleton of host cells in a phagocytosis-like process (Galan and Bliska 1996). Works studying in vivo invasion revealed a gradual accumulation of host cell lysosomes at the parasite entry site, and progressive fusion of these lysosomes with the plasma membrane as invasion proceeded into several cell types (Andrews 1995, Sibley and Andrews 2000, Tan and Andrews 2002). Morphometric and cytochemical analyses have demonstrated increased lysosomes in placentas of women with Chagas disease (Fretes and Fabro 1995)..

The cortical actin cytoskeleton acts as a barrier for lysosome recruitment and fusion. However not polymerized actin was detected around T. cruzi containing intracellular vacuoles and invasion was significantly enhanced by disruption of host cell microfilaments (Tardieux et al 1992). Sartori et al. (2003) have observed in cultures of explants of placental villi in vitro that the parasite induced disassembly of the cortical actin cytoskeleton, and authors proposed this is a step in the T. cruzi invasion mechanism into placental cells that allowing lysosomes to access to the plasma membrane, and to form the parasitophorous vacuole. Fusion of lysosomes with the plasma membrane is required for parasite entry into several cell types and that the process is triggered by elevations in intracellular free Ca^{2+} concentration (Burleigh and Andrews 1998). T. cruzi might be taking advantage of Ca^{2+}-regulated lysosomal exocytosis in the repair of plasma membrane lesions (Redddy et al. 2001) for cell invasion.

The specific signaling pathway and mechanisms for T. cruzi entry into placental cells is still not well understood. In order to understand the process, Calderón and Fabro (1983) studied the interaction between syncytial plasma membranes from the human placenta and from the parasites; they found modifications of membrane lipids and proteins of the villi trophoblast. Also modifications in trophoblast enzymatic activity and in chorionic villi have been described (Fretes and Fabro, 1990; Fretes and Fabro, 1994; Fretes and Fabro, 1995). Placental alkaline phosphatase (PLAP) is a trophoblast plasma membrane protein and has been proposed to have a pathogenetic role in the congenital chagas disease. PLAP activity decreased in women with Chagas disease and is related to congenital transmission (Sartori et al, 1997) and also is modified in placental villi cultured with T. cruzi (Sartori et al 2002, Fretes and Fabro 1990). PLAP anchored to the cell membrane lipid layer by a glycosylphosphatidylinositol (GPI) molecule participates in the process of T. cruzi invasion into placental syncitiothrophoblast cells by hydrolysis of the GPI molecule (Bertello et al 2000). Activation of tyrosin kinase proteins increase cytosolic calcium and rearrangement actin filaments of the host cells (Shijman 2007). Treatment of microvilli with phospholipase C before engagement by T. cruzi hinders parasite invasion into placental trophoblast (Sartori et al 2002), probably altering the placental alkaline phosphatase.

6.2 Placental areas of parasite invasion

The trophoblast according to Rassi (1958) and Carlier (2010) constitutes a potential barrier to penetration of T. cruzi (Bittencourt 1976; Carlier and Truyens 2010). The histopatological analyses of placentas from congenital cases display intense villitis with parasites in villous trophoblast as well as in villous stromal cells (Bittencourt 1976; Bittencourt 1988; Drut and Araujo 2000). However in other studies villitis was uncommon and parasites were not o hardly identified in trophoblast (Moya et al 1979; Azogue et al 1985; Carlier 2005). Also the parasite was described in the trophoblast but the fetus was free of infection (Bittencourt 1992). Some in vitro studies mention that trophoblastic cells are easily infected by T. cruzi (Sartori et al 2002; Shippey et al 2005) but other authors show low multiplication rate of the parasite and the incapacity of T. cruzi to produce a sustainable infection in the normal chorionic villous explants in vitro (Luján et al 2004, Triquell et al. 2009). The different results might be referred to different number of parasites employed by researchers, as was demonstrated by Duaso et al. (2010) and also to different strains of *T. cruzi*.

Parasite was found in placental areas deprived from trophoblast at chorionic plate and amastigotes were seen within membranes of amniotic epithelium a fact that may suggest the presence of trypomastigotes in the amnionic liquid in association with chorionitis (Moya et al 1979; Azogue 1985; Carlier 2005; Fernandez Aguilar et al 2005). Biopsies in placentas from infected newborns showed high density of parasites at the level of marginal zone (Carlier 2005) eluding as a consequence, the defenses of the trophoblast (Lujan et al. 2004).

6.3 Survival of T. cruzi in the placental tissue: mechanisms of resistance

Considering the lower congenital transmission incidence and also the report of uninfected infants with parasitized trophoblast of chorionic villi (Freillij et al 1994; Bittencourt 1992), it argues for the efficacy of the placenta to control the T. cruzi infection.

Previous analysis involves lysosomes in the T. cruzi invasion into host cells, and also in Chagas parasite destruction (Carvalho and de Souza 1989; Milder and Kloetzel 1980). Fretes and Fabro (1995) described increasing lysosomes and acid phosphatase activity in chagasic placentas without congenital transmission, suggesting that lysosomes population are involved in the processes of placental infection and human congenital transmission of Chagas disease. Modifications of enzymatic activity in the trophoblast and in chorionic villi have been described (Fretes and Fabro, 1990a; Fretes and Fabro, 1990b; Fretes and Fabro, 1994; Fretes and Fabro, 1995). Furthermore, it was demonstrated that normal human placental lysosome subfraction and its supernatant subfractions of normal placentas have deleterious effects upon the *T. cruzi* in in vitro placental cell-free system (Frank et al., 2000).

In this way it was determined an absence of productive infection of *T. cruzi* into normal chorionic villi in an experimental system of chorionic villi explants co-cultured with the parasite in contrast to susceptible cells such as VERO cells (Luján et al. 2004). These findings may be in accordance with pathological results found in chagasic placentas, where parasites are found in placental chorionic villi but newborns are free of parasites without congenital transmission (Bittencourt 1992).

All of these data were obtained employing an *in vitro* system of chorionic villi explants co-cultured with infective forms of the T. cruzi, as have been previously successfully employed with bacteria, virus and protozoan (Poliotti. et al 2002). The experimental system employed is very similar to the real situation in the uterus where placental villi are floating in the intervillous space bathed by the mother´s blood which could contain T. cruzi in the pregnant chagasic woman.

Which are the possible mechanisms involved in the control of productive infection of T. cruzi in chorionic villi and protective function of the placenta? Placentas express eNOS and iNOS (endothelial and inducible nitric oxide synthases respectively) and produce a large amount of Nitric Oxide (NO) (Conrad 1995; Myatt et al 1993, Soorana et al 1999) which has been implicated as parasiticidal agent to microorganisms, including *T. cruzi* (Villalta1998, Gobert 2000). The causal agent of Chagas disease is affected by NO, according to in vitro and in vivo studies in cardiomyocytes (Fichera et al 2004).

According to Triquell et al. (2009) eNOS transcription and protein expression was significantly higher when parasites were present in in vitro experimental system. Also, the level of NO in the placental environment contains deleterious NO levels to *T. cruzi* (Triquell et al. 2009, Villalta et al. 1998), with two strains of *T. cruzi* behaving differently in this environment. Although there are several immunological mechanism to eliminate the intracellular pathogens as NO, parasites have elaborated a variety of strategies to escape of the immune response and to make possible their survival and replication in the host. Some parasites modulate the production of several toxic molecules synthesized by the immnune system. Interestingly, it has been described that some parasites were able to escape to deleterious NO due to the arginase induction (Stempin and Cerban, 2007). Consequently, only certain strain of the parasite may produce a sustainable infection and offer the subsequent possibility of infecting the fetus in pregnant women with Chagas disease. So, at this time, by contrast with information collected in experimental murine model (Solana et al., 2002) there is no clear evidence of a relationship between T. cruzi genotype and congenital infection in humans (Shijman 2007, Burgos 2007).

The capacity of each placenta to produce deleterious agents in the placental environment, the different susceptibility of strains of *T. cruzi* in this deleterious medium (Triquell et al. 2009), the low capacity of the parasite to induce a reproductive infection in chorionic villi (Lujan et al. 2004), as well as the possibility that different placental cells types have differential susceptibility to be infected by T. cruzi (work that is on going in our lab) can modulate the success of transplacental transmission for congenital Chagas disease via chorionic villi route.

7. Association of placental infection by T. cruzi with other pathological conditions

7.1 Chagas placental alterations and associated pathologies

It is thought that congenital Chagas´ disease is a product of a complex interaction among the maternal immunological or nutritional status, obstetrical history, maternal stage of disease, placental factors, and the characteristics of the parasite, such as the strain of T. cruzi or the parasitic load (Bittencourt 1992; Carlier, 2005; Burgos, et al 2007), but none of these factors have been conclusively demonstrated yet (Moretti et al, 2005).

During pregnancy, there is an increased susceptibility to certain autoimmune diseases and intracellular infections (Guilbert, et al 1993; Lin et al, 2005), like Acquired Immune Deficiency Syndrome (AIDS) (Derrien et al, 2005), infections associated with AIDS (Margono et al, 1994), malaria (Gamain, et al 2006), toxoplasmosis (Biedermann, 1995), etc. The restructured placental barrier possibly facilitates the invasion of diverse pathogens. In addition to T. cruzi, other congenital diseases caused by parasites have also been described, among which Plasmodium falciparum, the agent responsible for causing malaria, (Rogerson, et al, 2007; Desai et al, 2007), schistosoma (Friedman et al, 2007), Toxoplasma gondii (Biedermann, 1995; Correa et al, 2007) and Trypanosoma brucei (Rocha et al, 2004) are of importance (Kemmerling et al, 2010).

7.2 Chagas, Diabetes and Hiperglycemia

Diseases caused by protozoa have been reported to be associated with nutritional deficiencies, wasting and diabetes. An association between human T. cruzi infection and obesity and diabetes, has been suspected and there has been general belief, that the incidence of diabetes may be increased in the chagasic population (Nagajyothi et al, 2009).

Pancreas is one of the organs affected in Chagas´ disease. Patients with this disease have plasma pancreatic glucagon and pancreatic polypeptide levels reduced (Long et al, 1980), lower insulin activity (Guariento et al, 1994), and morphometric and morphologic alterations of pancreatic ganglia and islets (Saldanha et al, 2001). Hyperglycemia and abnormal glucose tolerance tests observed in some patients with chronic Chagas' disease suggest the possibility of morphological changes in pancreatic islets and/or denervation (dos Santos et al, 1999; Saldanha et al, 2001). The observed morphometric and morphologic alterations are consistent with functional changes in the pancreas, including glycemia and insulin disturbances (Saldanha et al, 2001).

Experimental infections in hamsters caused pancreatitis, erratic blood glucose levels and a tendency to hypoinsulinemia (Dos Santos et al, 2004). Diabetes in pregnancy is associated with serious abnormalities in the hormonal and metabolic milieu, and in the maternal and fetal blood supply. These changes are likely to initiate structural and biochemical alterations in placental tissue, which may in turn be related to disturbances in placental functions and metabolic performances (Vannini, 1994; Garner, 1995; Desoye & Shafrir, 1996). On the other hand, different authors have reported that diabetics have an increased susceptibility to a variety of infectious agents (Plouffe et al, 1978, Casey J, Sturm 1982). The course of parasitic diseases such as malaria (Tulbert & McGhee, 1960), schistosomiasis (Mahmoud, 1979) and trypanosomiasis (Tanowitz et al, 1988) has been studied in diabetic animals.

Hyperglycemia has been previously observed to increase the morbidity and mortality of murine T. cruzi infection (Tanowitz et al, 1988). While T. cruzi infection causes hypoglycemia which correlates with mortality, hyperglycemia is associated with increased parasitemia and mortality (Nagajyothi et al, 2009). It has also been observed that women with the chronic cardiac form of Chagas' disease have diabetes mellitus and disturbances in the regulation of glycemic level at a higher frequency than normal controls, probably due to reduced activity of the parasympathetic system (dos Santos et al, 1999). But, according to the analysis of the bibliography, there is not any study analyzing an association between pregnant women affected with both Chagas´ disease and diabetes with congenital transmission or with the effect on the new born. Furthermore, there is no marker for placental or fetus infection in Chagas´ disease (Mezzano et al, 2012).

T. cruzi crosses the placental barrier and infects the fetus, causing the congenital form of the disease (Bittencourt, 1976). In order to understand the mechanism used by the parasite to cross this barrier, the interaction between syncytiotrophoblast plasma membranes from the human placenta and the parasite was previously studied, with modifications in lipid and protein patterns from trophoblast membranes being found (Calderón, Fabro, 1983). However, the mechanism by which the parasite infects the placenta as well as the effects upon the protein contents of the placental barrier is still not well understood.

Due the effect of the Chagas parasite on some proteins located at the lipid raft of chorionic villi trophoblast (Fretes RE, de Fabro 1990; Priotto et al, 2009); as well as in trophoblast lipids (Fabro AE, Calzolari, 1990), it was analyzed the possible modification of the main glucose transporter located at the syncytiotrophoblast, the GLUT1 protein, produced by placental T. cruzi infection. These experiments showed that GLUT1 protein expression was significantly diminished in normal placental villi cultured under high glucose concentration in vitro infected with T. cruzi, compared to controls (Mezzano et al, 2012).

It was reported that T. cruzi causes disorganization of the basal membrane of the trophoblast and the stroma of the chorionic villi, in in vitro experiments (Duaso et al, 2010). Similar changes were registered in human placental explants cultured under high glucose concentration, so, both conditions hyperglycemia and T. cruzi infection can modify the stroma of the human chorionic villi (Mezzano et al, 2012).

Furthermore, T. cruzi produces plasmatic membrane modifications, by altering their lipid (Fabro AE, Calzolari 1990, Calderón RO, Fabro 1983) and protein components, such as Placental Alkaline Phosphatase (Sartori et al, 2003; Lin et al, 2004; Lin et al, 2005; Mezzano et al, 2005, Fretes RE, Fabro 1990, Sartori et al, 2005), and Glut1 protein (Mezzano et al, 2012). On the other hand, we observed in our laboratory, that Gamma glutamyltranspeptidase, another enzyme present in the placenta's brush border, is not affected in cells co-cultured with T. cruzi (Priotto et al, 2009), suggesting that the parasite affects molecules inserted in lipid microdomains of the membrane, as PLAP (Salamon et al, 2005) and GLUT1 (Sakyo et al, 2007). As the hyperglycemia characteristic of diabetes mellitus also affects these membrane components, it was suggested that both the parasite and the high glucose conditions could have been provoking, by different ways, a lower placenta efficacy as a barrier against infections (Mezzano et al, 2012). Reduced GLUT1 expression observed in placental cultures with parasites could imply a down-regulated GLUT1 activity in pregnant women with Chagas´ disease. If this disease is causing damage to pancreas islets (Long et al, 1980; Guariento et al, 1994; Saldanha et al, 2001), or happens together with a previous diabetic condition, the adverse effects of reduced GLUT1 activity may be exacerbated. As a consequence, it is of importance to perform a systematic study analyzing new born from pregnant women who have both conditions diabetes and Chagas (Mezzano et al, 2012).

It has been described that chorionic villi in vitro has low susceptibility to infection by T. cruzi in normal D-glucose concentration (Luján et al, 2004, Triquell et al, 2009). Nagajyothi et al. (2010) have been studied the effects of hyperglycemia on T. cruzi infection rekindled by the increased incidence of obesity and diabetes mellitus, which have the potential to worsen the disease, in areas where T. cruzi infection is endemic. In recent years, there have been several studies indicating that diabetes and obesity may be more common in the population of individuals at risk for T. cruzi infection (dos Santos et al, 1999; Guariento et al, 1993; oliveira et al, 1993; Geraix et al, 2007; Nagajyothi et al, 2009; Nagajyothi et al. 2011; Saldanha et al, 2001).

7.3 Chagas and HIV

The reactivation of T. cruzi infection is observed in individuals who undergo immunosuppressive therapy for malignancies and organ transplantation as well as in individuals with human immunodeficiency virus (HIV) infection and AIDS (Tanowitz et al, 2009; Sartori et al, 2007; Vaidian et al, 2004; Barcán et al, 2005).

HIV and parasitic infections interact and affect each other mutually. Whereas HIV infection may alter the natural history of parasitic diseases, impede rapid diagnosis or reduce the efficacy of antiparasitic treatment, parasitoses may facilitate the infection with HIV as well as the progression from asymptomatic infection to AIDS. There are data on known interactions for malaria, leishmaniasis, Human African Trypanosomiasis, Chagas' disease, onchocerciasis, lymphatic filariasis, schistosomiasis and intestinal helminthiases. The common immunopathogenetic basis for the deleterious effects of parasitic diseases may have on the natural history of HIV infection seems to be a particular type of chronic immune activation and a preferential activation of the T helper (Th)2 type of help. Control of parasitic diseases should complement the tools currently used in combating the HIV pandemic (Harms and Feldmeier, 2002).

While for Human African Trypanosomiasis, as well as for onchocerciasis and lymphatic filariasis there is little evidence for an interaction with HIV as yet, T. cruzi clearly behaves as an opportunistic agent in the presence of HIV infection (Harms and Feldmeier, 2002). In analogy to the mechanisms in Leishmania/HIV co-infections, the ongoing immunosuppression allows T. cruzi to multiply, particularly in the chronic stage of Chagas´ disease (Perez-Ramirez et al. 1999). Clinically, it may be difficult to differentiate Chagas' disease reactivation as a consequence of HIV infection and chronic chagasic disease. However, reactivation of Chagas' disease in HIV-positive individuals is always associated with high parasitaemia, while in chronic disease, parasitaemia is very low and can only be detected by xenodiagnosis (Perez-Ramirez et al, 1999). Treatment of T. cruzi infection in HIV-positive individuals is recommended to be started early in the reactivation process when irreversible alterations have not yet occurred (Sartori et al, 1998).

Almeida and col. (2010) studied the prevalence of Chagas' disease among HIV seropositive patients, registering that the prevalence of co-infected subjects was 1.3% (Almeida et al, 2010). Dolcini and col. (2008) demonstrated that the presence of an intracellular pathogen, such as T. cruzi, is able to impair HIV-1 transduction in an in vitro system of human placental histocultures. Direct effects of the parasite on cellular structures as well as on cellular/viral proteins essential for HIV-1 replication might influence viral transduction in this model. Nonetheless, additional mechanisms including modulation of cytokines/chemokines at placental level could not be excluded in the inhibition observed. Further experiments need to be conducted in order to elucidate the mechanism(s) involved in this phenomenon. Therefore, coinfection with T. cruzi may have a deleterious effect on HIV-1 transduction and thus could play an important role in viral outcome at the placental level (Dolcini et al 2008).

Maternal viral load and immunological status are the main factors that determine the risk of HIV- Mother-to-child transmission (MTCT) (Bongertz 2001; Scarlatti, 2004). Other risk factors are coinfections of the mother (WHO/UNAIDS 1999, Hotez etal, 2006), an important issue since world regions with the highest prevalence of HIV-1 infection are also affected by other infections. Thus, HIV positive pregnant women are usually infected with other pathogens, and such placental coinfections may have consequences on mother to child transmission of the pathogens.

Data from HIV-T.cruzi coinfected patients indicated reactivation of parasite infection with exacerbation of clinical signs and unusual clinical manifestations (Ferreira MS, Borges 2002; Harms G, Feldmeier, 2002; Sartori et al, 2002; Sartori et al, 2007). Even if no evidence exist of coinfection in the mothers, MTCT of both pathogens with severe outcome for the children (Freilij H, Altcheh , 1995) and congenital transmission of T. cruzi without confirmation of HIV-1 MTCT (Nisida et al, 1999) were reported. However, little is known about interaction of both pathogens on an in vitro cellular or ex vivo tissue model.

As a result of the significant burden of the HIV pandemics in resource-poor regions, a number of potential epidemiological, biological, and clinical interactions between HIV and other tropical pathogens gained relevance and need to be studied. The interactions between HIV and tropical infectious agents are complex. Each pathogen has the potential to alter the epidemiology, natural history, and/ or response to therapy of the other pathogens (Karp & Auwaerter, 2007); therefore, it is unpredictable to establish the outcome of such coinfections.

In Latin America, one of the most significant endemic protozoonoses is Chagas' disease, and several clinical studies from HIV-T. cruzi coinfected patients have been reported (Ferreira MS, Borges 2002; Harms G, Feldmeier, 2002; Sartori et al, 2002; Sartori et al, 2007). MTCT is one way of transmission shared by both pathogens. The exact mechanisms involved in MTCT of both pathogens are not clear. Hence, the study of their interaction at the placental level is critical for designing strategies that abolish MTCT. In in vitro culture system of term placental histocultures, as well as in the trophoblast cell line BeWo, it was demonstrated that acute coinfection with T. cruzi and HIV-1 pseudotyped virus decreases HIV-1 replication. This is the first report about interaction of these pathogens at the placental level (Dolcini et al, 2008).

A great impairment of HIV-1 replication was observed in coinfection with viable T. cruzi trypomastigotes purified from mouse blood (BT). Moreover, when other source of viable trypomastigotes was used, such as those grown in cell culture (CT), the same effect on HIV-1 replication was observed. In all cases, hCG secretion was measured in histoculture supernatants and no significant differences were observed between control, viral infection, or treatment with trypomastigotes. These results indicate that placental tissue remains viable and that parasite impairment of HIV-1 replication was not associated with direct cell toxicity caused by T. cruzi. Previous data indicate that the parasite induces rearrangement of cortical cytoskeleton of syncytiotrophoblast with actin microfilament depletion during human placental invasion (Sartori et al, 2003). Considering that after entering the cell, the HIV-1 virion interacts initially with actin filaments which assist binding to microtubules and transport to the nuclear periphery (Warrilow and Harrich, 2007), modifications in trophoblast cytoskeleton might impair viral replication at an early phase in the case of active T.cruzi invasion. However, the inhibition of HIV replication seems to be caused not only by viable trypomastigotes but also by soluble factors shed by the parasite, either from BT or CT (Dolcini et al, 2008).

Dolcini et al. (2008) evaluated whether the parasite or its soluble products were able to modify the placental environment. In fact, many soluble factors, including cytokines and hormones, with regulatory activities are essential for establishing and maintaining pregnancy (Saito, 2000; Bowen, 2002). HIV-1 and antiretroviral treatment in pregnant women have an impact on the pattern of placental soluble factors (Faye et al, 2007; Pornprasert 2006). Little is known about the changes in human fetal-maternal interface in T. cruzi infection (Dolcini et al, 2008).

8. Conclusion

Spreading of Chagas to non-endemic cities of the world due mainly to congenital Chagas transmission put this form of the disease in one of the top public health problem, needing more attention for researchers, epidemiologists and governmental officials. There are still many questions not answered yet that need more support to elucidate them. Data from chorionic villi-resistance to T. cruzi could lead to obtain mechanisms that lead to prevention of fetal infection.

9. Acknowledgments

This work was supported by SECyT-National University of Córdoba; SECyT-National University of La Rioja; MINCyT-Córdoba (PID 48).

10. References

Almeida EA, Lima JN, Lages-Silva E, Guariento ME, Aoki FH, Torres-Morales AE, Pedro RJ., 2010. Chagas' disease and HIV co-infection in patients without effective antiretroviral therapy: prevalence, clinical presentation and natural history. Trans R Soc Trop Med Hyg 104(7):447-452.

Andrade SG, da Silva AA, Carvalho ML, Figueira RM. 1972. Behavior of a strain of Trypanosoma cruzi in hosts with low resistance. Rev Inst Med Trop Sao Paulo 14:154-161.

Andrade SG. 1982. The influence of the strain of Trypanosoma cruzi in placental infections in mice. Trans. R. Soc. Trop. Med. Hyg 76: 123–128.

Andrews NW., 1995. Lysosome recruitment during host cell invasión by Trypanosoma cruzi. Trens Cell Biol. 5: 133-137.

Azogue E, La Fuente C, Darras C., 1985. Congenital Chagas' disease in Bolivia: epidemiological aspects and pathological findings. Trans R Soc Trop Med Hyg. 79(2):176–180.

Barcán L, Lunaó C, Clara L, Sinagra A, Valledor A, De Rissioí AM, Gadanoá A, García MM, de Santibañes E, Riarte R., 2005. Transmission of T. cruzi infection via liver transplantation to a nonreactive recipient for Chagas' disease. Liver Transpl 11:1112–1116.

Benirschke K, Kaufmann P, Baergen RN. 2006. Pathology of the Human Placenta. Springer Science + Business Media, New York.

Bertello LE, Alves MJ, Coli W, de lederkeremer RM., 2000. Evidence for phospholipase from Trypanosoma cruzi active on phosphatidylinositol and inositolphosphoceramide. Biochem J. 45 (Pt 1):7-84.

Bianchi DW, Romero R. 2003. Biological implications of bi-directional fetomaternal cell traffic. J Matern Fetal Neonatal Med 14: 123-129.

Biedermann K, Flepp M, Fierz W, Joller-Jemelka H, Kleihues P. ,1995. Pregnancy, immunosuppression and reactivation of latent toxoplasmosis. J Perinat Med 23(3): 191-203.

Bittencourt AL, Barbosa HS, Rocha T, Sodre I, Sodre A., 1972. Incidence of congenital transmission of Chagas' disease in premature births in the Maternidade Tsylla Balbino (Salvador, Bahia). Rev Inst Med Trop Sao Paulo. 14: 131–134.

Bittencourt AL, Barbosa HS, Santos I, Ramos MEA., 1974. Incidência da transmissâo congênita da doenças de Chagas em partos a termo. Rev Inst Med Trop S Paulo, 16: 197-199.

Bittencourt AL, Barbosa HS., 1972. Incidencia da transmissâo congênita da doenças de Chagas em partos a termo. Rev Inst Med Trop S Paulo, 14: 257-259.

Bittencourt AL., 1963. Chagasic placentitis and congenital transmission of Chagas' disease. Rev Inst Med Trop Sao Paulo. 5: 62-67.

Bittencourt AL., 1976. Congenital Chagas disease. Am J Dis Child. 130: 97-103.

Bittencourt AL., 1988. American trypanosomiasis (Chagas' disease). In: Parasitic Infection in Pregnancy and the Newborn (Macleod C, editor). Oxford: Oxford Medical Publication.62-86.

Bittencourt AL., 1988. Parasitic infection in pregnancy and the newborn. American trypanosomiasis (Chagas´disease). American trypanosomiasis (Chagas´disease). Oxford Med. Publ Oxford. 62 -86.

Bittencourt AL., 1992. Possible risk factors for vertical transmission of Chagas´s disease. Rev Inst Med Trop. San Pablo, 34: 403-408.

Bittencourt, A., 1985 Doença de Chagas congenital como un problema de saúde pública, Ann. Soc. Belge. Med. Trop. 65(1), 103-106.

Bittencourt, A., Barbosa, H., 1972 Importancia do estudo do feto macerado para o diagnostico da forma congenita doenca de Chagas, Revista de Instituto Medico Tropical de Sao Paulo. 14(6), 260-263.

Bongertz V., 2001. Vertical human immunodeficiency virus type 1 (HIV-1) transmission: a review. Mem Inst Oswaldo Cruz 96:1-14.

Bowen JM, Chamley L, Keelan JA, Mitchell MD., 2002. Cytokines of the placenta and extra-placental membranes: roles and regulation during human pregnancy and parturition. Placenta 23:257-273.

Brenière, S., Bailly, M., Carrasco, R., Carlier, I. 1983 Transmission transplacentaire des anticorps anti-Trypanosoma cruzi, Cah. ORSTOM, ser., Ent. Méd. Et Parasitol, 21(3), 139-140.

Burgos JM, Altcheh J, Bisio M, Duffy T, Valadares HM, Seidenstein ME, Piccinali R, Freitas JM, Levin MJ, Macchi L, Macedo AM, Freilij H, Schijman AG., 2007. Direct molecular profiling of minicircle signatures and lineages of Trypanosoma cruzi bloodstream populations causing congenital Chagas disease. Int J Parasitol 37(12): 1319-1327.

Burleigh, B.A., and N.W. Andrews. 1998. Signaling and host cell invasion by by Ca2+-regulated exocytosis of lysosomes. Cell. 106:157-169.

Calderón RO, Fabro SP de., 1983. Trypanosoma cruzi: Fusogenic ability of membranes from cultured epimastigotes in interaction with human syncytiotrophoblast. Exp Parasitol 56: 169-179.

Carlier Y. 2005. Factor and mechanisms involved in the transmission and development of congenital infection whit Trypanosoma cruzi. Rev Soc Bras Med Trop. 38 (Suppl 2): 105-107.

Carlier, Y., Truyens, C., 2010. Modes of transmission: Maternal- fetal transmission of Trypanosome cruzi. In: Telleria, J., Tibayrenc, M., eds. American Tripanosomiasis. Chagas disease one hundred years of research. Philadelphia: Elsevier inc. 539-581.

Carvalho TMU, de Souza W., 1989. Early events related with the behaviour of Trypanosoma cruzi within and endocytic vacuole in mouse peritoneal macrophages. Cell Struc Funct. 14:383-392.

Casey J, Sturm CJr., 1982. Impaired response of lymphocytes from non-insulin dependent diabetes to staphage lysate, and tetanus antigen. J Clin Microbiol 15:109-114.

Clayton J., 2010. Chagas disease 101. NATURE 465: S4-S5.

Click Lambert R, Kolivras KN, Resler LM, Brewster CC, Paulson SL. 2008. The potential for emergence of Chagas disease in the United States. Geospat Health 2 (2): 227-39.

Conrad KP.,1995. Nitric oxide and parasitic disease. Adv Parasitol. 37: 1-56.

Correa D, Canedo-Solares I, Ortiz-Alegria LB, Caballeroortega H, Rico-Torres CP., 2007. Congenital and acquired toxoplasmosis: diversity and role of antibodies in different compartments of the host. Parasite Immunol 29(12): 651-660.

Delgado M, Santos-Buch C., 1978. Transplacental transmission and fetal parasitosis of Trypanosoma cruzi in outbret white Swiss mice. Am J trop Med Hyg, 27:1108-1115.

Derrien M, Faye A, Dolcini G, Chaouat G, Barre-Sinoussi F, Menu E., 2005. Impact of the placental cytokine-chemokine balance on regulation of cell-cell contact-induced human immunodeficiency virus type 1 translocation across a trophoblastic barrier in vitro. J Virol. 79(19): 12304-12310.

Desai M, Ter Kuile FO, Nosten F, Mcgready R, Asamoa K, Brabin B, Newman RD., 2007. Epidemiology and burden of malaria in pregnancy. Lancet Infect Dis 7(2): 93-104.

Desoye G and Shafrir E., 1996. The human placenta in diabetic pregnancy. Diabetes reviews 4(1):70-89.

Dolcini GL, Solana ME, Andreani G, Celentano AM, Parodi LM, Donato AM, Elissondo N, González Cappa SM, Giavedoni LD and L Martínez Peralta., 2008. Trypanosoma cruzi (Chagas' disease agent) reduces HIV-1 replication in human placenta. Retrovirology 5:53.

Dos Santos VM, Da Cunha SF, Texeira VD, Monteiro JP, Dos Santos JA, Dos Santos TA, Dos Santos LA, Da Cunha DF., 1999. [Frequency of diabetes mellitus and hyperglycemia in chagasic and non-chagasic women]. Rev Soc Bras Med Trop 32(5): 489-96.

Dos Santos VM, de Lima MA, Cabrine-Santos M, de Stefani Marquez D, de Araújo Pereira G, Lages-Silva E, Ramírez LE., 2004. Functional and histopathological study of the pancreas in hamsters (Mesocricetus auratus) infected and reinfected with Trypanosoma cruzi. Parasitol Res 94(2): 125-133.

Dos Santos VM, Teixeira Vde P, da Cunha DF, da Cunha SF, Monteiro JP, dos Santos JA, dos Santos TA, dos Santos LA., 1999. Pancreatic anatomopathologic changes in chronic chagasic women. Preliminary data. Arq Gastroenterol 36(3):127-132.

Drut R, Araujo MO, 2000. Image analysis of nucleomegalic cells in Chagas disease placentitis. Placenta. 21: 280-282.

Duaso J, Rojo G, Cabrera G, Galanti N, Bosco C, Maya JD, Morello A, Kemmerling U., 2010. Trypanosoma cruzi induces tissue disorganization and destruction of chorionic villi in an ex vivo infection model of human placenta. Placenta 31(8):705-711.

Dutra WO, Rocha MO, Teixeira MM. 2005. The clinical immunology of human Chagas disease. Trends Parasitol 21: 581-587.

Fabro AE, Calzolari G., 1990. Increase of lipids in human chagasic placentas: cytochemical and biochemical study. Rev Fac Cienc Med Univ Nac Córdoba 48:25-32.

Faye A, Pornprasert S, Mary JY, Dolcini G, Derrien M, Barre-Sinoussi F, Chaouat G, Menu E., 2007. Characterization of the main placental cytokine profiles from HIV-1-infected pregnant women treated with anti-retroviral drugs in France. Clin Exp Immunol 149:430-439.

Fernandez- Aguilar S, Lambot MA, Torrico F, Alonso Vega C, Cordoba M, Suarez E, et al., 2005. Placental lesions in human Trypanosoma cruzi infection. Rev Soc Bras Med Trop. 38 (suppl 2): 84-86.

Ferreira MS, Borges AS., 2002. Some aspects of protozoan infections in immunocompromised patients- a review. Mem Inst Oswaldo Cruz 97:443-457.

Fichera LE, Albareda MC, Laucella SA, Postan M., 2004. Intracellular growth of Trypanosoma cruzi in cardiac myocytes is inhibited by cytokine-induced nitric oxide release. Infect Immun. 72: 359-363.

Frank MF, Sartori MJ, Asteggiano C, Lin S, Fabro SPde, Fretes RE., 2000. The effect of placental subfractions on Trypanosoma cruzi. Exp Mol Pathol. 69: 144-151.

Freilij H, Altcheh J, 1995. Congenital Chagas´disease: Diagnostic and Clinical aspects. 1995. Clin Infect Dis 21: 551-555.

Freilij H, Altcheh J. Storino R. 1994. Chagas congénito. En Storino R, Milei J, eds. Enfermedad de Chagas. 1era. Ed. Buenos Aires, Doyma SA., 1994: 267-278.

Fretes RE, de Fabro SP. 1990. Trypanosoma cruzi: modification of alkaline phosphatase activity induced by trypomastigotes in cultured human placental villi. Rev Inst Med Trop Sao Paulo 32(6): 403-408.

Fretes RE, Fabro SP de., 1990. Human chagasic placental localization of enzymes associated to syncytiotrophoblast membrane. Comun Bio.l 9: 51-59.

Fretes RE, Fabro SP, 1995. In vivo in vitro analysis of lysosomes and acid pgosphatase activity in human chagasic placentas. Exp Mol Pathol 63: 153-160.

Fretes RE, Fabro SPde, 1994. Aumento de células de Hofbauer en placentas humanas cocultivadas in vitro con Trypanosoma cruzi. Rev Fac Cienc Méd Córdoba 52: 5.

Friedman JF, Mital P, Kanzaria HK, Olds GR, Kurtis JD., 2007. Schistosomiasis and pregnancy. Trends Parasitol 23(4): 159-164.

Galan JE, Bliska JB., 1996. Cross-talk betwen bacterial pathogens and their host cells. Annu rev Cell Dev Biol. 12: 1221-1134.

Gamain B, Smith Jd, Viebig Nk, Gysin J, Scherf A., 2007. Pregnancyassociated malaria: parasite binding, natural immunity and vaccine development. Int J Parasitol 37(3-4): 273-283.

Garner P. 1995. Type 1 diabetes mellitus and pregnancy. Lancet 346: 157-161.

Geraix J, Ardisson LP, Marcondes-Machado J, Pereira PC., 2007. Clinical and nutritional profile of individuals with Chagas disease. Braz J Infect Dis 11:411–414.

Gobert AP, Daulouede S, Lepoivre M, Boucher JL, Vincendeau P., 2000. L-Arginine availability modulates local nitric oxide production and parasite killing in experimental trypanosomiasis. Infect Immunol. 68: 4653-4657.

Guariento ME, Olga E, Muscelli A, Rocha Gontijo JA., 1994. Chronotropic and blood pressure response to oral glucose load in Chagas' disease. Sao Paulo Med J 112(3): 602-606.

Guariento ME, Saad MJ, Muscelli EO, Gontijo JZ., 1993. Heterogenous insulin response to an oral glucose load by patients with the indeterminate clinical form of Chagas' disease. Braz J Med Biol Res 26: 491–495.

Guilbert L, Robertson SA, Wegmann TG., 1993. The trophoblast as an integral component of a macrophage-cytokine network. Immunol Cell Biol 71 (Pt 1): 49-57.

Gürtler RE, Segura EL, Cohen JE. 2003. Congenital transmission of Trypanosoma cruzi infection in Argentina. Emerg Infect Dis. 9: 29-32.

Harms G, Feldmeier H., 2002. HIV infection and tropical parasitic diseases - deleterious interactions in both directions? Trop Med Int Health 7:479-488.

Haugel-de-Mouzon S, Guerre-Millo M. 2006. The placenta cytokine network and inflammatory signals. PLACENTA 27: 794-798.

Hotez PJ, Molyneux DH, Fenwick A, Ottesen E, Ehrlich Sachs S, Sachs JD. 2006. Incorporating a rapid-impact package for neglected tropical diseases with programs for HIV/AIDS, tuberculosis, and malaria. PLoS Med 3:e102.

Karp CL, Auwaerter PG., 2007. Coinfection with HIV and tropical infectious diseases. I. Protozoal pathogens. Clin Infect Dis 45:1208-1213.

Kemmerling U, Bosco C and N Galanti., 2010. Infection and invasion mechanisms of Trypanosoma cruzi in the congenital transmission of Chagas' disease: A proposal. Biol Res 43: 307-316.

Kierszenbaum F. 2007. Mechanisms of pathogenesis in Chagas disease. Acta Parasitologica 52: 1-12.

Leopardi O, Colecchia M, Dedè A, Ghione M. 1994. Histopathologic findings in CD1 albino mice infected with Plasmodium berghei in pregnancy. Experimental model for pathology of the feto- placental unit in malaria. Pathologica 86: 284-290.

Lin S, Sartori MJ, Mezzano L, de Fabro SP., 2004. Epidermal growth factor (EGF) in the human placental infection with Trypanosoma cruzi. Placenta 25:283-286.

Lin S, Sartori MJ, Mezzano L, de Fabro SP., 2005. Placental alkaline phosphatase (PLAP) enzyme activity and binding to IgG in Chagas' disease. Placenta 26:789-795.

Long RG, Albuquerque RH, Prata A, Barnes AJ, Adrian TE, Christofides ND, Bloom SR.,1980. Response of plasma pancreatic and gastrointestinal hormones and growth hormone to oral and intravenous glucose and insulin hypoglycaemia in Chagas's disease. Gut 21(9): 772-7.

Luján C, Triquell MF, Sembaj A, Guerrero CE, Fretes RE. 2004. The Chorionic villous from normal human Placenta limits productive infection of Trypanosoma cruzi in vitro. Exp Parasitol 108: 176-181.

Macedo AM, Machado CR, Oliveira RP, Pena SDJ. 2004. Trypanosoma cruzi: genetic structure of populations and relevance of genetic variability to the pathogenesis of Chagas disease. Mem. Inst. Oswaldo Cruz 99: 1–12.

Mahmoud A., 1979. Host-parasite relationship in Schistosoma mansoni in the mutation diabetic mouse (db/db). Am J Trop Med Hyg 28: 286-290.

Margono F, Mroueh J, Garely A, White D, Duerr A, Minkoff HI.,1994. Resurgence of active tuberculosis among pregnant women. Obstet Gynecol 83(6): 911-914.

Mejía AM, Triana O. 2005. Genetic variability of Trypanosoma cruzi in blood and organs of infected mice determined by LSSP-PCR. Biomedica 25: 76-86.

Mezzano L, Repossi G, Fretes RE, Lin S, Sartori MJ, de Fabro SP., 2012. In Vitro Infection of Trypanosoma cruzi Causes Decrease in Glucose Transporter Protein-1 (GLUT1) Expression in Explants of Human Placental Villi Cultured under Normal and High Glucose Concentrations. Journal of Tropical Medicine, Volume 2012, Article ID 969243, 8 pages.

Mezzano L, Sartori MJ, Lin S, Repossi G, de Fabro SP., 2005. Placental alkaline phosphatase (PLAP) study in diabetic human placental villi infected with Trypanosoma cruzi. Placenta 26(1):85-92.

Milder R, Kloetzel J., 1980. The development of Trypanosoma cruzi in macrophages in vitro. Interaction with lysosomes and host cell fate. Parasitol. 80: 139-145.

Mjihdi A, Lambot MA, Stewart IJ, Detournay O, Noel JC, Carlier Y, .. et al. 2002. Acue Trypanosoma cruzi infection in mouse induces infertility or placental parasite invasion and ischemic necrosis associated with massive fetal loss. Am J Pathol 161: 673-680.

Mjihdi A, Truyens C, Detournay O, carlier Y. 2004. Systemic and placental productions of tumor necrosis factor contribute to induce fetal mortality in mice acutely infected with Trypanosoma cruzi. Exp Parasitol 107: 58-64.

Moretti E, Basso B, Castro I, Carrizo Paez M, Chaul M, Barbieri G, Canal Feijoo D, Sartori MJ, Carrizo Paez R., 2005. Chagas' disease: study of congenital transmission in cases of acute maternal infection. Rev Soc Bras Med Trop 38(1):53-55.

Moya P, Villagia L, Risco JJ. Enfermedad de Chagas congénita. Hallazgos anatomopatológicos en placenta y cordón umbilical. Rev Fac Cienc Med Univ (Cordoba).1979; 37: 21.

Myatt L, Brockman DE, Eis ALW, Pollock JS., 1993. Immunohistochemical localization of nitric oxide synthase in the human placenta. Placenta. 14: 487-495.

Nagajyothi F, Desruisseaux MS, Jelicks LA, Machado FS, Chua S, Scherer PE, Tanowitz HB., 2009. Perspectives on adipose tissue, chagas disease and implications for the metabolic syndrome. Interdiscip Perspect Infect Dis. 2009:824324.

Nagajyothi F, Desruisseaux MS,Weiss LM, Chua S, Albanese C, Machado FS, Esper L, Lisanti MP, Teixeira MM, Scherer PE, Tanowitz HB., 2009. Chagas disease, adipose tissue and the metabolic syndrome. Mem Inst Oswaldo Cruz 104(1):219–225.

Nagajyothi F, Zhao D, Machado FS, Weiss LM, Schwartz GJ, Desruisseaux MS, Yang Z, Factor SM, Huan H, Albanese C, Teixeira MM, Scherer PE, Chua Jr SC, Tanowitz HB., 2010. Crucial Role of the Central Leptin Receptor in Murine Trypanosoma cruzi (Brazil Strain) Infection. Journal of Infectious Diseases 202(7):1104-1113.

Nagajyothi F, Weiss LM, Silver DL, Desruisseaux MS, Scherer PE, Herz J, Tanowitz HB., 2011. Trypanosoma cruzi utilizes the host low density lipoprotein receptor in invasion. PLoS Negl Trop Dis 5(2):e953.

Nisida IV, Amato Neto V, Braz LM, Duarte MI, Umezawa ES,. 1999. A survey of congenital Chagas' disease, carried out at three health institutions in Sao Paulo City, Brazil. Rev Inst Med Trop Sao Paulo 41:305-311.

Ogilvy-Stuart AL, Beardsall K., 2010. Management of hyperglycaemia in the preterm infant. Arch Dis Child Fetal Neonatal 95(2):F126-131.

Oliveira LC, Juliano Y, Novo NF, Neves MM., 1993. Blood glucose and insulin response to intravenous glucose by patients with chronic Chagas' disease and alcoholism. Braz J Med Biol Res 26:1187–1190.

Perez-Ramirez L, Barnabe C, Sartori , Sartori AMC, Ferreira MS, Tolezao JE, Nunes EV, Burgarelli MK, Silva AC, Shikanai-Yasuad MA, Lima JN, Da Cruz AM, Oliveira OC, Guilhereme C, Bastrenta B & Tibayrenc M.,1999. Clinical analysis and parasite genetic diversity in human immunodeficiency virus/Chagas disease coinfection in Brazil. American Journal of Tropical Medicine and Hygiene 61, 198–206.

Plouffe J, Silva J Jr, Fekety R, Allen J., 1978.Cell mediated immunity in diabetes mellitus. Infect & Immun 21:425-429.

Poliotti BM, Gnall-Sazenski S, Laughlin TS, Miller RK., 2002. Inhibitory effects of human chorionic gonadotropin (hCG) preparations on HIV infection of human placenta in vitro. Placenta. 23: 102-106.

Pornprasert S, Faye A, Mary JY, Dolcini G, Leechanachai P, Chaouat G, Ngo N, Barre-Sinoussi F, Menu E., 2006. Down modulation of TNFalpha mRNA placental expression by AZT used for the prevention of HIV-1 mother-to-child transmission. Placenta 27:989-995.

Priotto S, Sartori MJ, Repossi G, Valentich MA., 2009. Trypanosoma cruzi: participation of cholesterol and placental alkaline phosphatase in the host cell invasion. Exp Parasitol 122(1):70-73.

Rassi A, Borges C, Koeberle F, De Paula OH., 1958. Sobre a transmissao congênita da doenca de Chagas. Rev Goiania Med. 4: 319-332.

Reddy, A., E. Caler, Andrews NW. 2001. Plasma membrane repair is mediated by calcium2 regulated exocytosis of the lysosome. Cell 106: 157-169.

Redline RW., 2004. Placental inflamation. Semin Neonatol. 9: 265-274.

Robbins JR, Skrzypczynska KM, Zeldovich VB, Kapidzic M, Bakardjiev AI 2010. Placental Syncytiotrophoblast Constitutes a Major Barrier to Vertical Transmission of Listeria monocytogenes. PloS Pathogens 6: e1000732.

Rocha G, Martins A, Gama G, Brandao F, Atouguia J., 2004. Possible cases of sexual and congenital transmission of sleeping sickness. Lancet. 17;363(9404): 247.

Rogerson SJ, Hviid L, Duffy PE, Leke RF, Taylor DW., 2007. Malaria in pregnancy: pathogenesis and immunity. Lancet Infect Dis 7(2): 105-117.

Romero M, Postigo J, Schneider D, Chippaux JP, Santalla JA, Brutus L., 2011. Door-to-door screening as a strategy for the detection of congenital Chagas disease in rural Bolivia. Trop Med Int Health 16: 562-569.

Saito S., 2000. Cytokine network at the feto-maternal interface. J Reprod Immunol 47:87-103.

Sakyo T, Naraba H, Teraoka H, Kitagawa T., 2007. The intrinsic structure of glucose transporter isoforms Glut1 and Glut3 regulates their differential distribution todetergent-resistant membrane domains in nonpolarized mammalian cells. FEBS J 274(14):3753.

Salamon Z, Devanathan S, Alves ID, Tollin G., 2005. Plasmon-waveguide resonance studies of lateral segregation of lipids and proteins into microdomains (rafts) in solid-supported bilayers. J Biol Chem 280(12):11175-11184.

Saldanha JC, Dos Santos VM, Dos Reis MA, Da Cunha DF, Teixeira VPA., 2001. Morphologic and morphometric evaluation of pancreatic islets in chronic Chagas' disease. Rev Hosp Clin Fac Med Sao Paulo 56(5): 131-138.

Sanchez Negrete O, Mora MC, Basombrio MA. 2005. High prevalence of congenital Trypanosoma cruzi infection and family clustering in Salta, Argentina. Pediatrics 115: e668-e672.

Sartori AM, Caiaffa-Filho HH, Bezerra RC, do SGC, Lopes MH, Shikanai- Yasuda MA., 2002. Exacerbation of HIV viral load simultaneous with asymptomatic reactivation of chronic Chagas' disease. Am J Trop Med Hyg 67:521-523.

Sartori AM, Ibrahim KY, Nunes Westphalen EV, Braz LM, Oliveira OC Jr, Gakiya E, Lopes MH, Shikanai-Yasuda MA., 2007. Manifestations of Chagas disease (American trypanosomiasis) in patients with HIV/AIDS. Ann Trop Med Parasitol 101:31-50.

Sartori AM, Shikanai-Yasuda MA, Amato V & Lopes MH., 1998. Follow-up of 18 patients with human immunodeficiency virus infection and chronic Chagas'disease, with reactivation of Chagas' disease causing cardiac disease in three patients. Clinical Infectious Diseases 26, 177-179.

Sartori MJ, Lin S, Frank FM, Malchiodi EL, de Fabro SP., 2002 Role of placental alkaline phosphatase in the interaction between human placental trophoblast and Trypanosoma cruzi. Exp Mol Pathol. 72(1): 84-90.

Sartori MJ, Lin S, Fretes RE, Ruiz Moreno L, Goldemberg L, de Fabro SP, 1997. Alkaline Phosphatase activity in plasma of pregnant chagasic patients. Rev Fac Cien Med Univ Nac Cordoba. 55(1-2): 5-8.

Sartori MJ, Mezzano L, Lin S, Muñoz S, Fabro SP de., 2003. Role of Placental Alkaline Phosphatase in the internalization of trypomastigotes of Trypanosoma cruzi into HEp2 cells. Trop Med & Int Health 8: 832-839.

Sartori MJ, Pons P, Mezzano L, Lin S, Fabro SP de., 2003. Trypanosoma cruzi Infection Induces Microfilament Depletion in Human Placenta Syncytiotrophoblast. Placenta 24: 767-771.

Sartori MJ, Pons P, Mezzano L, Lin S, Repossi G, Fabro SP de., 2005. Componentes celulares y fosfatasa alcalina placentaria en la infección por T. cruzi. Revista da Sociedade Brasileira de Medicina Tropical, 38 (II): 87-91.

Scarlatti G. 2004. Mother-to-child transmission of HIV-1: advances and controversies of the twentieth century's. AIDS Rev 6:67-78.

Schijman AG., 2007. Congenital Chagas disease. In: Congenital and other related infectiou diseases of the newborn, Elsevier, DOI 10.1016/S0168-7069(06)13012-8.

Shippey SH, Zahn CM, Cisar M, Wu TJ, Satin AJ. 2005. Use of placental perfusion model to evaluate transplacental passage of Trypanosoma cruzi. Am J Obstet Gynecol 192: 586-591.

Sibley LD, Andrews NW. 2000. Cell invasion by un-palatable parasite. Traffic 1: 100-106.

Solana ME, Celentano AM, Tekiel V, Jones M, Gonzalez Cappa SM. 2002. Trypanosoma cruzi: effect of parasite subpopulation on murine pregnancy outcome. J. Parasitol 88: 102-106.

Solana ME, Alba Soto CD, Fernandez MC, Poncini CV, Postan M, Gonzalez Cappa SM. 2009. Reductoin of parasite levels in blood improves pregnancy outcome during experimental Trypanosoma cruzi infection. Parasitology 136: 627-639.

Sooranna SR, Oteng-Ntim E, Meah R, Ryder TA, Bajoria R., 1999. Characterization of human placental explants:morphological, biochenical and physiological studies using first and third trimester placenta. Human Reproduction. 2 (14):536-541.

Stempin CC, Cerban FM., 2007. Macrophagos e inducción de arginasa como mecanismo de evasión de parásitos. Medicina (Buenos Aires). 67: 737-746.

Tafuri WL, Reis E, Nunan B, 1984. Doença de Chagas congênita: Estudo clínico-patlógico de um caso com sobrevida de seis meses. Rev Inst Med Trop Sao Paulo. 15: 322-330.

Tan H, Andrews W., 2002. Don´t to knock-the cell invasión strategy of Trypanosoma cruzi. TRENDS Parasitol. 18 (10).

Tanowitz HB, Amole B, Hewlett D, Wittner M., 1988. Trypanosoma cruzi infection in diabetic mice. Trans R Soc Trop Med Hyg 82(1): 90-93.

Tanowitz HB, Machado FS, Jelicks LA, et al. Perspectives on Trypanosoma cruzi-induced heart disease (Chagas disease). Prog Cardiovasc Dis 2009; 51:524-539.

Tardieux P, Webster P, Ravesloot J, Boron W, Lunn JA, Heuser JE , Andrews NW., 1992. Lysosome recruitment and fusion are early events required for Trypanosome invasion of mammalian cells. Cell, 71: 1117-1130.

Teixeira ARL, Nascimento RJ, Sturm NR, 2006. Evolution and pathology in Chagas disease - A Review. Mem Inst Oswaldo Cruz 101: 463-491.

Torrico F, Alonso.Vega C, Suarez E, Rodriguez P, Cruz-Torrico M, Dramaix M, Truyens C, Carlier Y. 2004. Am J Trop Med Hyg 70: 201-209.

Triquell MF, Díaz-Luján C, Freilij H, Paglini P, Fretes RE., 2009.Placental infection by two subpopulations of Trypanosoma cruzi is conditioned by differential survival of the parasite in a deleterious placental medium and not by tissue reproduction. Transactions Royal Society Tropical Medicine and Hygiene 103: 1011-1018.

Tulbert M and McGhee R., 1960. The effect of alloxan diabetes on Plasmodium berghei infection in albino rats. J Parasitol 46: 552-558.

Vaidian AK, Weiss LM, Tanowitz HB., 2004. Chagas' disease and AIDS. Kinetoplastid Biol Dis 3:2.

Vannini P., 1994. Pregnancy in diabetes: physiopathological aspects. Minerva Endocrinol 19: 45-50.

Vernochet C, Caucheteux SM, Kanellopoulos-Langevin C 2007. Bi-directional cell trafficking between mother and fetus in mouse placenta. Placenta 28: 639-649.

Villalta F, Zhang Y, Bibb KE, Kappes JC, Lima MF, 1998. The cysteine-cysteine family of chemokines RANTES, MIP-1α and MIP-1β induce trypanocidal activity in human macrophages via nitric oxide. Infect Immun. 10: 4690-4695.

Virreira M, Alonso-Vega C, Solano M, Jijena J, Brutus L, Bustamante Z et al. 2006. Congenital Chagas disease in Bolivia is not associated with DNA polymorphism of *Trypanosoma cruzi*. Am. J. Trop. Med. Hyg 75: 871–879.

Warrilow D, Harrich D., 2007. HIV-1 replication from after cell entry to the nuclear periphery. Curr HIV Res 5:293-299.

WHO/UNAIDS.,1999. HIV in pregnancy: a review. WHO/CHS/RHT/ 99.15, UNAIDS/99.35E.

WHO Reporte del grupo de trabajo científico sobre la enfermedad de Chagas 2007. TDR/GTC/06 World Health Organization.

Zingales B, Stolf BS, Souto RP, Fernandes O, Briones MR. 1999. Epidemiology, biochemistry and evolution of Trypanosoma cruzi lineages based on ribosomal RNA sequences. Mem Inst Oswaldo Cruz 94 Suppl 1:159-164.

7

Protein Expression of Aryl Hydrocarbon Receptors in Human Placentas from Mild Preeclamptic and Early Pregnancies

Ke-hong Hao[1], Qian Zhou[2], Qi-zhi He[3], Jing Zheng[4,*] and Kai Wang[2,*]
[1]*Department of Obstetrics, Shanghai First Maternity and Infant Hospital, Tongji University School of Medicine, Shanghai,*
[2]*Clinical and Translational Research Center, Shanghai First Maternity and Infant Hospital, Tongji University School of Medicine, Shanghai,*
[3]*Department of Pathology, Shanghai First Maternity and Infant Hospital, Tongji University School of Medicine, Shanghai,*
[4]*Department of Obstetrics and Gynecology, Perinatal Research Laboratories, University of Wisconsin, Madison, WI,*
[1,2,3]*P.R. China*
[4]*USA*

1. Introduction

The aryl hydrocarbon receptor (AhR), a ligand-dependent transcription factor, mediates a variety of biological processes [[1]]. AhR is a classic receptor for environmental toxicants/carcinogens such as 2,3,7,8-tetrachlorodibenzo-p-dioxin (TCDD) and 3-methylcholanthrene (3MC). Upon binding to these ligands, AhR could adversely affect embryonic and fetal growth as well as male and female reproduction [[1],[2]]. For instance, prenatal exposure to TCDD may cause fetotoxicity, delayed puberty, decreased sperm count, and reduced fertility [[2]]. Interestingly, AhR knockout in mice can also lead to similar adverse phenotypes in the reproductive system (e.g., impaired implantation and pregnancy) [[3]-[6]]. Thus, these data clearly indicate the physiological roles of AhR in implantation and pregnancy.

Preeclampsia is a life threatening complication of pregnancy, accounting for almost 10-15% of pregnancy-associated deaths and one of the major causes of iatrogenic prematurity among newborns [[7]]. The pathogenesis of preeclampsia is thought to act at three levels, defective placentation, placental ischemia, and endothelial cell dysfunction.

Protein expression of AhR has been identified in the placentas of many mammalian species including mouse and rabbit [[8],[9]]. Human placentas also contained high density of specific binding sites for TCDD as compared with rat and mouse livers, implying high AhR expression in human placentas [[10]]. This was confirmed by the observation that human

---

[*] Corresponding Author

placentas had highest levels of AhR mRNA among many human organs including lung, liver, heart, brain, and kidney [[11]]. Recently, we have also reported that AhR protein is highly expressed in term human placentas, although no difference in AhR protein levels was detected between normal (N) and severe preeclamptic (sPE) placentas [[12]]. However, the information on AhR protein expression in mild preeclamptic (mPE) and first trimester placentas was still lacking. Herein, we examined the AhR protein expression in term human placentas from women with N and mPE pregnancies as well as in first trimester placentas using immunohistochemistry and Western blotting.

2. Materials and methods

2.1 Tissue collection

Term placentas were obtained immediately after cesarean section delivery from women with N (n = 14) and mPE (n = 10) pregnancies as described [[12],[13]]. The first trimester placentas (n = 12) were obtained from women with induced abortion at gestation time of 6-8 weeks. Collection of placentas was approved by the Ethics Committee of Shanghai First Maternity and Infant Hospital, Tongji University School of Medicine. Written informed consent to participate in the study was obtained from each patient. Preeclampsia was defined according to the guideline of USA National Institutes of Health publication No. 00-3029 [[14]]. The mPE was defined as onset of hypertension during late pregnancy with systolic and diastolic blood pressure more than 140 / 90 mmHg on at least two occasions and urinary protein more than 0.3g / 24h. All of the study subjects didn't have any medication during gestation. They were free of major diseases and substance abuse. Smokers were excluded. Patients' ages were similar between N and mPE pregnancies. There was no significant difference in gestation ages and fetal weights between N and mPE pregnancies (see table 1). Placental tissues under the chorionic and basal plates were dissected (~10 g each), snap-frozen and quickly stored in liquid nitrogen for Western blotting. Additional placental tissues from first trimester (n = 5) and term placentas (n = 5), and mPE placentas (n = 5) were fixed overnight at 4°C using 4% paraformaldehyde in 10 mM PBS and embedded them in paraffin for immunohistochemistry.

Characteristics	Normal (n = 14)	Mild PE (n = 10)	P value ($p \leq 0.05$)
Patient ages (yr)	24 ± 1.2	25±1.8	NS
Gestation ages (wk)	39 ± 0.2	38 ± 0.6	NS
Fetal weights (g)	3414 ± 80.3	2966 ± 130.2	NS

Data are expressed as means ± SEM, $p \leq 0.05$ is considered statistically significant

Table 1. The characteristics of women from normal and mPE pregnancies.

2.2 Immunohistochemistry

Immunolocalization of AhR in placental tissues was visualized by indirect observation via the avidin:biotinylated-peroxidase complex method (Vector Laboratories, Burlingame, CA) as described [[12],[13]]. Tissue sections (5 µm thick) were deparaffinized and dehydrated, followed by incubating the sections in a 10 mM citrate buffer solution (pH 6.0) in a microwave for 10 min for antigen retrieval. Then the tissue sections were immersed in 3%

H_2O_2 in methanol for 10 min in order to quench endogenous peroxidase activity. After blocking the non-specific binding sites with 1% horse serum albumin, the sections were incubated with a rabbit AhR antibody (1:500; BIOMOL International, Plymouth Meeting, PA) for 1 h and a biotinylated mouse anti-rabbit antibody (ABC kit; Vector Laboratories) for 30 min. The specific immunoreactivity was visualized by 3-amino-9-ethylcarbazole (AEC, Vector Laboratories). The tissue sections were lightly counter-stained with Harris Modified Hematoxylin (Fisher Scientific, Pittsburgh, PA). Additional adjacent tissue sections as negative controls were incubated with the same dilution of preimmune rabbit IgG as the primary antibody.

2.3 Western blotting

Western blotting was carried out as described [[12],[13]]. Placental tissues were pulverized in liquid nitrogen using a mortar and pestle, followed by prepared in RIPA lysis buffer (50 mM HEPES, 0.1 M NaCl, 10 mM EDTA, 4 mM sodium pyrophosphate, 10 mM sodium fluoride, 2 mM sodium orthovanadate [pH 7.5]; 1 mM phenyl methyl sulfonyl fluoride [PMSF], 1% Triton X-100, 5 μg/ml leupeptin, 5 μg/ml aprotinin), and further lyzsed by sonication. After centrifugation, the supernatant was saved and protein concentrations in supernatants were determined by BCA kit.

The protein samples (40 μg) were subjected to electrophoresis on 10% SDS-PAGE gels, followed by electrically transferring to polyvinylidene difluoride membranes. The membranes were incubated with the AhR antibody (1:2000; BIOMOL) and then reprobed with a GAPDH (1:5000; KANGCHEN, Shanghai, China) antibody as a loading control. Membranes were reacted with ECL reagents (Amersham Biosciences, Piscataway, NJ). Protein bands on the membranes were visualized by exposuring them to chemiluminescence films. The immunoreactive signals were analyzed by densitometry. The optical density (OD) value was measured by the Image-J imaging analysis software (US National Institutes of Health; Bethesda, MD).

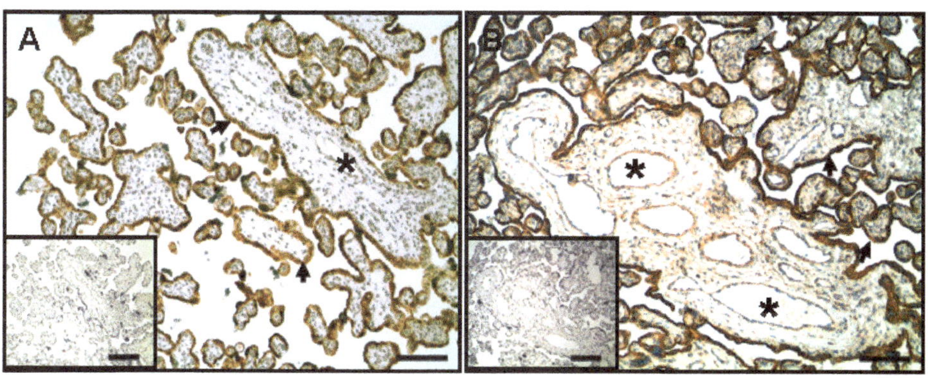

Fig. 1. Immunolocalization of AhR in human placentas from women with normal and mPE pregnancies. The adjacent tissues sections were incubated either with a rabbit AhR antibody (4 μg/ml) or preimmune rabbit IgG (4 μg/ml; in inserts). Reddish color indicates positive staining for AhR. Representative images from N (A) and mPE (B) pregnancies are shown. Arrows heads, syncytiotrophoblasts; asterisk, lumen of blood vessels. *Bar*, 100 μm.

2.4 Statistics procedures

Data for the AhR protein levels were analyzed using the Student's t-test (SigmaStat; Jandel Co., San Rafael, CA); $*p \leq 0.05$ were considered to be statistically significant.

3. Results

3.1 AhR protein localization and expression in N and mPE placentas

Positive reddish staining for AhR was observed primarily in syncytiotrophoblasts in N and mPE placentas. There was also moderate staining in endothelial cells from large blood vessels (Fig. 1A and 1 B) as described ([12]). The protein levels of AhR in N and mPE placentas were further determined by Western blotting (Fig. 2). The AhR band was detected at ~95 kDa (Fig. 2A) as previously reported in many species including human [[12],[15]]. The AhR protein levels in mPE placentas were approximately 5.6 fold higher ($p \leq 0.05$) than those in N placentas (Fig. 2B).

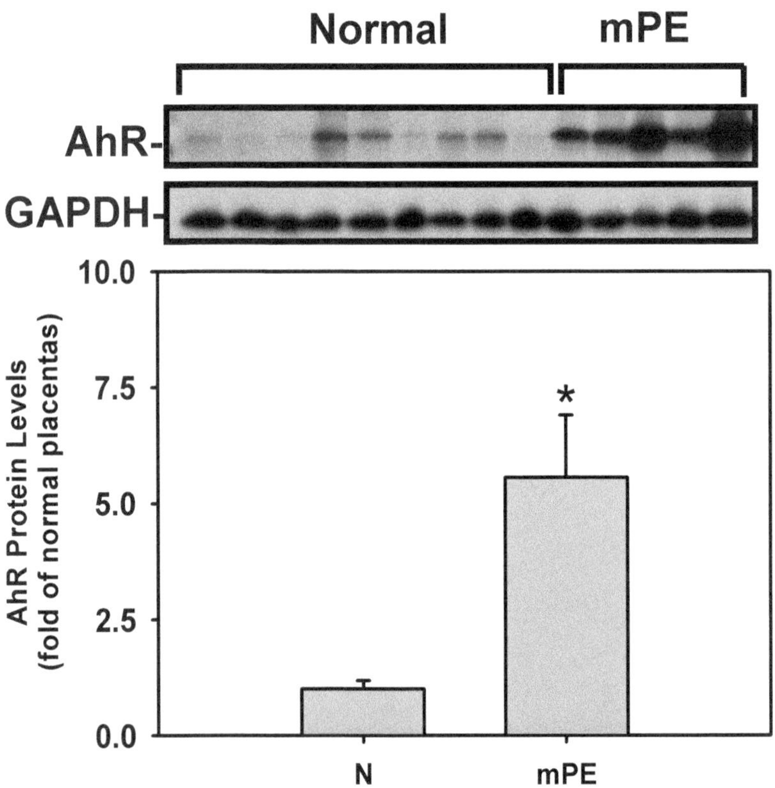

Fig. 2. Western blot analysis for AhR in human placentas from women with N and mPE pregnancies. Human placentas were obtained from N (n = 14) and mPE (n = 10) pregnancies. Representative Western blot images are shown for AhR and GAPDH. Data normalized to GAPDH are expressed as means ± SEM fold of N placentas. *Differs ($p \leq 0.05$) from the N placentas.

3.2 Protein expression of AhR in first trimester placentas

Similar to term plancentas, AhR was also mainly immunolocalized in syncytiotrophoblasts in first trimester placental villi (Fig. 3A). However, in contrast to term placentas, moderate positive AhR staining was observed in capillaries within first trimester placental villi (Fig. 3B), suggesting the possible roles of AhR in mediating placental endothelial functions including angiogenesis during human early pregnancy. Western blot analysis indicated that overall AhR protein levels in term placentas were ~ 2.2 fold higher ($p \leq 0.05$) than those in first trimester placentas (Fig. 4).

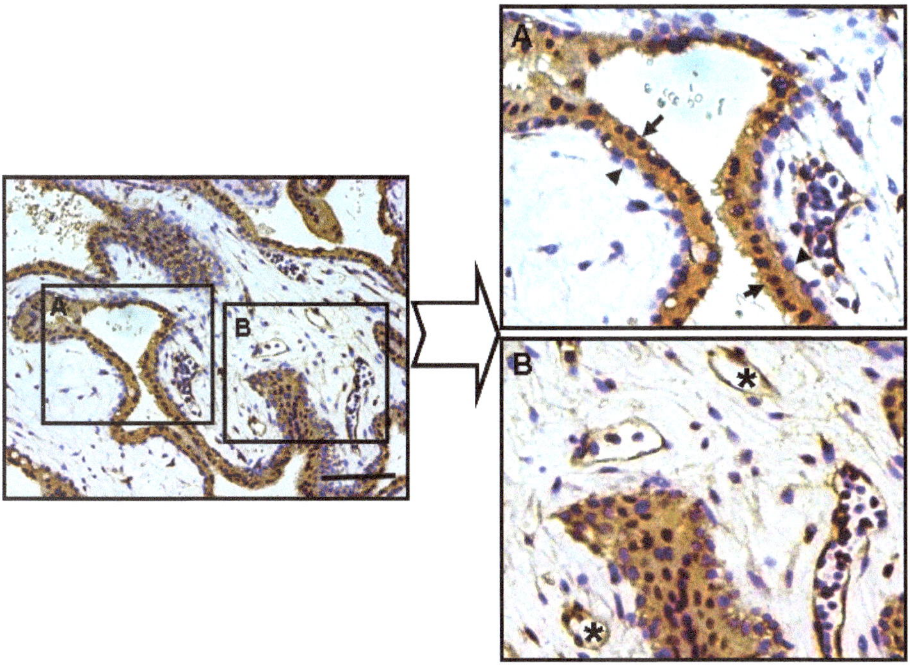

Fig. 3. Immunolocalization of AhR in human first trimester placentas. Reddish color indicates positive staining for AhR. Representative images from first-trimester placentas are shown. Arrow heads, syncytiotrophoblasts; arrows, cytotrophoblasts; asterisk, lumens of blood vessels. *Bar,* 100 μm.

4. Disscusion

In the current study, we have described the expression and localization of AhR protein in human term placentas from N and mPE preeclamptic pregnancies as well as in human first trimester placentas using immunohistochemistry and Western blot analyses. It is the first, as far as we know, to report that higher AhR protein levels were associated with mPE, while much higher AhR protein levels were expressed in term placentas as compared to first trimester placentas. Another major finding of the current study was that intense AhR staining was detected primarily in syncytiotrophoblasts in both first trimester and term placentas. Interestingly, moderate AhR expression was observed in capillary endothelial

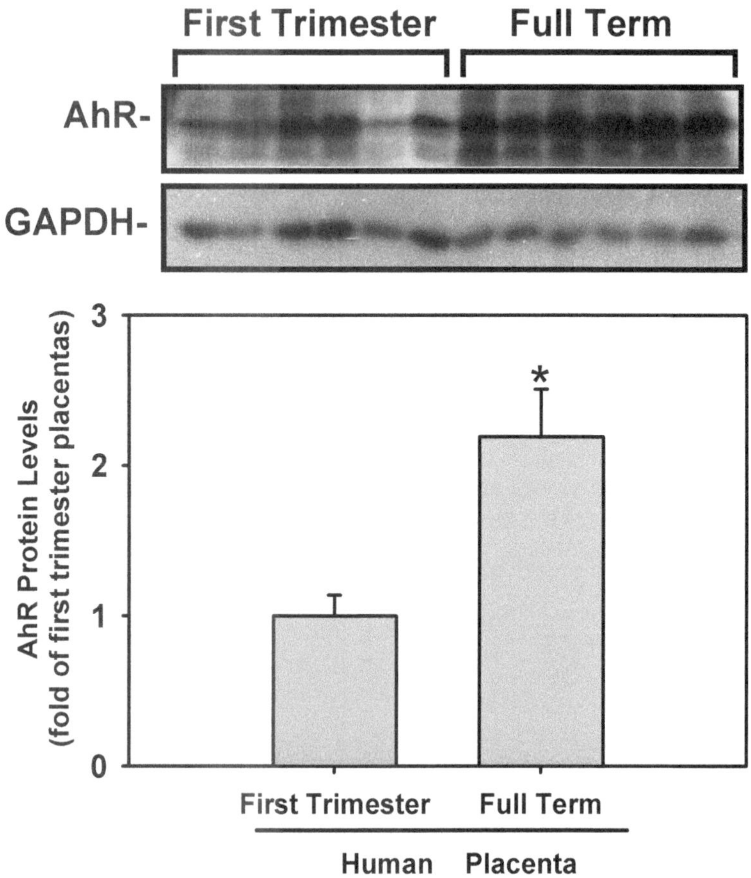

Fig. 4. Western blot analysis for AhR in human first trimester and full term placentas. First trimester (n = 12) placentas were obtained from women with induced abortion at 5 to 8 weeks of gestation without any complications. Representative Western blots are shown for AhR and GAPDH. Data normalized to GAPDH are expressed as means ± SEM fold of first trimester placentas. *Differs ($p \leq 0.05$) from first trimester placentas.

cells within villi in the first trimester, but not term placentas (the current study and [12]). These findings suggest that AhR might play a critical role in mediating syncytiotrophoblast function, particularly in mPE and term placentas. The distinct distribution patterns of AhR protein in different placental vasculatures (capillaries vs. large blood vessels) during early and late pregnancies also imply that AhR might differentially mediate placental endothelial functions. For example, AhR may actively mediate placental angiogenesis at early pregnancy and placental vasodilatation during late pregnancy.

The expression of AhR mRNA and protein has been reported in the placenta of many mammalians including mouse and rabbit [[8],[9]]. We have also reported the AhR protein expression in the term human placenta from N and sPE pregnancies using Western blot analysis [[12]]. The current study further showed the AhR protein expression in mPE and early pregnant placentas. Interestingly, the higher AhR protein levels were associated with mPE, while our previous work detected similar levels of AhR protein in normal term and sPE placentas [[12]]. Although mechanisms underlying such differential AhR protein expression between mPE and sPE placentas remain to be elucidated, it is possible that such differences might attribute to the shorter gestation ages in sPE than mPE pregnancies since women with sPE were much more likely to suffer premature delivery. This is also in line with our present observation that placental AhR protein levels were much lower in early pregnancy than those in term pregnancy. These data also support the notion that the pathogenesis of mPE and sPE may not be completely the same as proposed previously [[15]]. Moreover, the higher protein levels of AhR could be potentially used as a marker for predicting mPE when in conjunction with other clinical diagnoses.

Our current observations that AhR protein was mainly present in the cytoplasm and nuclei of syncytiotrophoblasts, but not in cytotrophoblast cells in both first trimester and full term placentas were in agreement with recent findings by Stejskalova et al [[16]], suggesting that AhR might predominantly act on syncytiotrophoblasts during human pregnancy. The exact roles of AhR in syncytiotrophoblasts are currently unclear. However, given that syncytiotrophoblasts are terminally differentiated cells and are also responsible for producing many types of steroid and peptide hormones. It is possible that AhR might dynamically mediate syncytiotrophoblast differentiation and placental hormonal synthesis, particularly during late pregnancy, to support pregnancy and embryo/fetal development in uteri as AhR null female mice have difficulties to do so [[6],[7]]. In addition, higher AhR protein levels in term placentas than early pregnant placentas also suggest that the former might be more sensitive to AhR ligands' stimulation regardless if these ligands are derived from exogenous or endogenous sources [[17],[18]].

In conclusion, together with the recent findings of endogenous AhR ligands produced by human and animals [[17],[18]], the current data strongly support the notion that AhR plays important physiological roles in mediating normal differentiation and development of cytotrophoblast as well as placental endothelial cells to maintain successful pregnancy.

5. Acknowledgments

This work was supported, in part, by US NIH grants HL64703 and HD38843 (JZ), National Natural Science Foundation of China (No. 39970579, KW), and Shanghai Natural Science Foundation (No.11ZR1428700, KW)

6. References

[1] Hernandez-Ochoa, I., B.N. Karman, and J.A. Flaws, The role of the aryl hydrocarbon receptor in the female reproductive system. Biochem Pharmacol, 2009. 77(4): p. 547-59.

[2] Peterson, R.E., H.M. Theobald, and G.L. Kimmel, Developmental and reproductive toxicity of dioxins and related compounds: cross-species comparisons. Crit Rev Toxicol, 1993. 23(3): p. 283-335.

[3] Fernandez-Salguero, P.M., et al., Lesions of aryl-hydrocarbon receptor-deficient mice. Vet Pathol, 1997. 34(6): p. 605-14.
[4] Benedict, J.C., et al., Physiological role of the aryl hydrocarbon receptor in mouse ovary development. Toxicol Sci, 2000. 56(2): p. 382-8.
[5] Abbott, B.D., et al., Adverse reproductive outcomes in the transgenic Ah receptor-deficient mouse. Toxicol Appl Pharmacol, 1999. 155(1): p. 62-70.
[6] Hernandez-Ochoa, I., et al., The ability of the aryl hydrocarbon receptor to regulate ovarian follicle growth and estradiol biosynthesis in mice depends on stage of sexual maturity. Biol Reprod, 2010. 83(5): p. 698-706.
[7] Page, N.M., The endocrinology of pre-eclampsia. Clin Endocrinol (Oxf), 2002. 57(4): p. 413-23.
[8] Kitajima, M., et al., Expression of the arylhydrocarbon receptor in the peri-implantation period of the mouse uterus and the impact of dioxin on mouse implantation. Arch Histol Cytol, 2004. 67(5): p. 465-74.
[9] Tscheudschilsuren, G., et al., Expression of the arylhydrocarbon receptor and the arylhydrocarbon receptor nuclear translocator during early gestation in the rabbit uterus. Toxicol Appl Pharmacol, 1999. 160(3): p. 231-7.
[10] Manchester, D.K., et al., Ah receptor in human placenta: stabilization by molybdate and characterization of binding of 2,3,7,8-tetrachlorodibenzo-p-dioxin, 3-methylcholanthrene, and benzo(a)pyrene. Cancer Res, 1987. 47(18): p. 4861-8.
[11] Dolwick, K.M., et al., Cloning and expression of a human Ah receptor cDNA. Mol Pharmacol, 1993. 44(5): p. 911-7.
[12] Jiang, Y.Z., et al., Expression of aryl hydrocarbon receptor in human placentas and fetal tissues. J Histochem Cytochem, 2010. 58(8): p. 679-85.
[13] Chung, J.Y., et al., Differential expression of vascular endothelial growth factor (VEGF), endocrine gland derived-VEGF, and VEGF receptors in human placentas from normal and preeclamptic pregnancies. J Clin Endocrinol Metab, 2004. 89(5): p. 2484-90.
[14] Report of the National High Blood Pressure Education Program Working Group on High Blood Pressure in Pregnancy. Am J Obstet Gynecol, 2000. 183(1): p. S1-S22.
[15] Gregg, A.R., Hypertension in pregnancy. Obstet Gynecol Clin North Am, 2004. 31(2): p. 223-41, v.
[16] Stejskalova, L., et al., Aryl hydrocarbon receptor (AHR) and aryl hydrocarbon nuclear translocator (ARNT) expression in human and rat placentas and transcription activity in human trophoblast cultures. Toxicol Sci, 2011.
[17] Song, J., et al., A ligand for the aryl hydrocarbon receptor isolated from lung. Proc Natl Acad Sci U S A, 2002. 99(23): p. 14694-9.
[18] Nguyen, L.P. and C.A. Bradfield, The search for endogenous activators of the aryl hydrocarbon receptor. Chem Res Toxicol, 2008. 21(1): p. 102-16.

8

Mechanism of Congenital Chagas Disease: Effective Infection Depends on the Interplay Between *Trypanosoma cruzi* and the Different Tissue Compartments in the Chorionic Villi of the Human Placenta

Juan Duaso, Christian Castillo and Ulrike Kemmerling
Institute for Biomedical Sciences, Faculty of Medicine, University of Chile, Chile

1. Introduction

American trypanosomiasis, or Chagas disease, a zoonosis caused by *Trypanosoma cruzi* (*T. cruzi*), is endemic in Latin America and ten million people are estimated to be infected (Araújo et al 2009, World Health Organization (WHO), 2010). In the past decades, Chagas disease has been increasingly detected in other non-endemic countries such as Canada, the United States of America, Australia, Japan and in Europe. The presence of Chagas disease outside Latin America is the result of population mobility, notably migration, but also from travelers returning from Latin America and in adopted children (Schmunis, 2007). Subsequent transmission occurs through transfusion, transplantation or vertical routes. More than 10 000 deaths are estimated to occur annually from Chagas disease; its incapacitating effects and mortality are ones of the biggest public-health problems in Latin America. The 10-year mortality rate may range from 9% to 85%, depending on the extent of the cardiac damage induced by the parasite (WHO, 2010).

Chagas disease manifests first with an acute phase, lasting for about 2 months, characterized by high parasitaemia. Most cases are asymptomatic or present nonspecific symptoms. Then, it turns into a chronic phase, the parasites hiding in target tissues, especially in the heart and digestive muscles (WHO, 2010) and in case of pregnancy, also in the placenta (Bittencourt, 1976). During the chronic phase, different clinical manifestations may be observed: 1) the cardiac form; 2) the digestive form, particularly enlargement of the esophagus and the colon; and 3) a mixed form (cardiac plus digestive) (Rassi, 2006).

2. Congenital Chagas disease

Congenital *T. cruzi* infection is associated with premature labor, low birth weight, and stillbirths (Altemani et al, 2000; Bittencourt, 1976; Shippey et al, 2005). Serologic prevalence among pregnant women may reach 80%, and rates of congenital infection vary from 1-21% (Blanco et al, 2000; Burgos et al, 2007; Kirchhoff, 1999; Shippey et al, 2005; Torrico et al,

2005). In Chile, in two of the endemic regions (IV and V regions), the congenital transmission rate of the parasite is 8.4% (Jercic et al, 2010). WHO/PAHO has considered that the number of infected woman at fertile age is of approximately 1.809.000 and that 14.400 neonates are being infected at year (WHO, 2006).

During congenital transmission, the parasite reaches the fetus by crossing the placental barrier (Carlier and Truyens, 2010; Duaso et al, 2010; Kemmerling et al, 2010). The fact that only a percentage of the infected mothers transmit parasites to their fetuses raises the question of the ability of the placenta as well as the immunological status of mother and fetus/newborn to impair the parasite transmission. Therefore, it is thought that congenital Chagas disease is product of a complex interaction between the parasite, the maternal and fetus/newborn immune responses and placental factors (Burgos et al, 2007; Kemmerling et al, 2010).

2.1 The parasite

T. cruzi is a haemophlagelated protozoan of the *Kinetoplastida* Order and *Trypanosomatidae* family (Chagas, 1909). The parasite biological cycle includes three cellular forms characterized by the relative positions of the flagellum, kinetoplast, and nucleus (Prata, 2001): 1) Trypomastigotes: Approximately 20 μm in length and sub terminal kinetoplast. They constitute the non-replicative, mammalian infecting cellular form that is found in the blood and in the posterior intestine of triatomids. In mammals, this is the cellular form that disseminates infection through blood. 2) Epimastigotes: Also 20 μm in length with a kinetoplast anterior to the nucleus. They represent the multiplying parasite form in the triatomid intestine. 3) Amastigotes: Approximately 2 μm in diameter, rounded, with no emergent flagellum. It multiplies within the mammalian host cells, forming "nests", until they rupture after several cell divisions. Before their release from the host cells, amastigotes differentiate into trypomastigotes that invade the blood stream; they may then enter any other nucleated cell. Epimastigotes can be grown in axenic cultures while amastigotes grow in cultured mammalian cells, releasing trypomastigotes that can be harvested to perform *in vitro* assays.

T. cruzi display great biological, biochemical and genetic diversity, therefore different strains of the parasite have been identified and classified into six discrete typing units (DTU) (Telleria et al, 2010; Zingales et al, 2009). *T. cruzi* strains corresponding to different DTUs might have relevant consequences on congenital transmission and fetal/neonatal pathology. Nevertheless, different parasite strains identified in congenitally infected children correspond to the same strain identified in the mother, that is the predominantly *T. cruzi* lineage in the respective geographic region (Carlier and Truyens, 2010). There is no clear evidence that a relationship between *T. cruzi* strains and congenital infection in humans exists. Nevertheless, parasitaemia is associated with the risk of congenital transmission. Thus, a high parasitaemia, as in acute infection, correlates with a higher transmission rate (around 50%). In chronic infected patients, with very low parasitaemia, the transmission rate is between 1-21% (Brutus et al, 2010; Moretti et al, 2005). Though appearing a low rate of infection, chronically infected pregnant women represent a high risk of maintenance of Chagas disease both in endemic and non endemic areas.

2.2 Mother and fetus/newborn immune response

The immune system is fundamental to protect the mother against the environment and to prevent damage to the fetus. During pregnancy the maternal immune system is characterized by a reinforced network of cellular and molecular recognition, communication, trafficking and repair; it raises the alarm to maintain the well-being of the mother and the fetus. On the other side, the fetus provides a developing active immune system that will modify the way the mother responds to the environment, providing a uniqueness of the immune system responses during pregnancy (Mor and Cardenas, 2010).

A crucial factor to stop, limit, or permit the development of fetal/neonatal infection relates to the capacity of the mother and fetus/newborn to mount innate and/or specific immune response(s) against pathogens. Clinical studies have shown a strong association between intrauterine infections and pregnancy disorders such as abortion, preterm labor, intrauterine growth retardation and pre-eclampsia (Koga and Mor, 2010). As described above, congenital *T. cruzi* infection is associated with some of these pathologies (Altemani et al, 2000; Bittencourt, 1976; Carlier and Truyens, 2010; Shippey et al, 2005).

Production of pro-inflammatory cytokines can be observed in uninfected babies born to infected mothers (Carlier and Truyens, 2010). Contrarily, the levels of inflammation markers and activation of NK cells are rather low in congenitally infected newborns (Hermann et al, 2010). These data highly suggest a protective role of such innate defenses in an uninfected newborn from infected mothers. On the other side, maternal *T. cruzi*-specific IgG antibodies play protective roles in mothers and in fetuses when antibodies are transferred through the placenta (Breniere et al, 1983) and also may contribute to a reduction in parasitaemia (Carlier and Truyens, 2010).

2.3 Placenta

The placenta is the principal site for the exchange of nutrients and gases between the mother and fetus. This organ plays an important role in hormone, peptide, and steroid synthesis necessary for a successful pregnancy (Moore and Perseaud, 2004). The human placenta is classified as a hemochorial villous placenta in which the free chorionic villi, formed by the trophoblast and the villous stroma, are the functional units. The trophoblast contacts maternal blood in the intervillous space and is separated by a basal lamina from the villous stroma, which is connective tissue containing the vascular endothelium, fibroblasts and macrophages (Bernischke et al, 2006). Trophoblast, basal *laminae* and villous stroma with the endothelium of fetal capillaries form the placental barrier that must be crossed by different pathogens, including *T. cruzi,* to infect the fetus during vertical transmission (Carlier and Truyens, 2010; Duaso et al, 2010; Kemmerling et al, 2010) (**Figure 1**).

Placentas from mother with acute Chagas disease (high parasitaemia) show severe histopathological changes, such as extensive necrosis, inflammatory infiltrate and amastigote nests (Altemani et al, 2000). Contrarily, placentas from mother with chronic Chagas disease do not present necrotic foci and inflammatory infiltrate. Although parasite antigens can be visualized in the villous stroma, the typical amastigote nests are not present (Duaso et al, 2011b). In accordance with these results, in *ex vivo* infected placental explants although parasite antigens and DNA can be detected (Al Khan et al, 2011; Duaso et al, 2010; Luján et al, 2004), amastigote nests are not observed. Only few individual parasites can be detected. These evidences suggest that anti-parasite mechanisms may exist in the placental tissue of women suffering chronic Chagas disease.

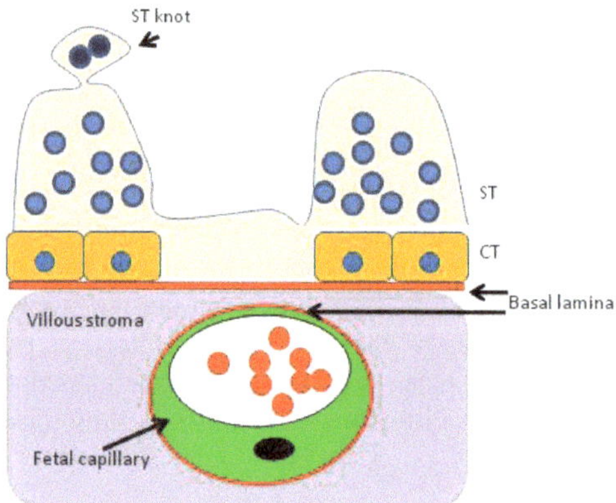

The placental barrier is composed of syncytiotrophoblast (ST) with ST knots, cytotrophoblast (CT), fetal connective tissue of the villous stroma, fetal capillary and basal lamina between villous stroma and trophoblast as well as around fetal endothelium.

Fig. 1. Human placental barrier

3. *Trypanosoma cruzi* interaction with the trophoblast

The major constituent of the human placenta is the trophoblast, the first cell lineage that develops before any embryonic tissue arises. Between morula and blastocyst stages, the trophoblast lineage forms a cover around the early embryo (the embryoblast) (Bernischke et al, 2006; Huppertz and Borges, 2008). The human trophoblast differentiates into two major subtypes (Drewlo et al, 2008; Huppertz and Gauster, 2010; Huppertz and Borges, 2008): a) Cells that invade maternal uterine tissue and differentiate into the *extravillous trophoblast*, and b) Cells that remain within the placenta and differentiate into the *villous trophoblast* forming the epithelial cover of the placental villi and constituting part of the placental barrier (Bernischke et al, 2006; Kemmerling et al, 2010) (see **Figure 1**). The *villous trophoblast* is composed of two cellular layers: the *syncytiotrophoblast* (ST) and the *cytotrophoblast* (CT). The CT displays high proliferative properties, whereas the differentiated ST loses its generative capacity and is no longer able to proliferate. The ST is a multinucleated layer that forms the outer surface of placental villi and comes into direct contact with maternal blood (Bernischke et al, 2006; Huppertz and Borges, 2008). This cell layer is a typical syncytium with plasma membranes only on the apical and basal sides. The ST is continuous and normally uninterrupted, covering all villous trees of the human placenta. It is generated and maintained through syncytial fusion by incorporation of CT cells (Bernischke et al, 2006; Huppertz, 2010).

During congenital infection the first fetal cells exposed to the parasite are those of the syncytiotrophoblast. In human chorionic villi infected *ex vivo* the parasite induces detachment and destruction of this tissue layer (Duaso et al, 2010). Other pathogen like cytomegalovirus (Chan and Gilbert, 2006), *Plasmodium falciparum* (Maubert et al, 1997) and *Toxoplasma gondii* (Abbasi et al, 2003) also induce syncytiotrophoblast damage.

The trophoblast, as covering epithelia, forms a physical barrier to pathogens. On the other hand, the epithelial turnover has been considered part of the innate immune system (Janeway and Traver, 2004) due to the fact that pathogens, prior to cell invasion, must attach to the surface of cells. As these cells are continuously eliminated, the attached pathogens are removed with them.

Trophoblast turnover: Trophoblast turnover implies precise orchestration of different cellular processes that include cell proliferation of the CT, differentiation (meaning the syncytial fusion by incorporating CT cells into a non replicative ST and differentiation of CT cells previous fusion with the ST) and cell death (Berniscke et al, 2006; Huppertz, 2010). Cell death in the trophoblast manifests by formation of apoptotic ST knots which are released into the maternal blood. The apoptotic knots counterbalance the continuous incorporation of CT cell into the ST (Berniscke et al, 2006).

Cell proliferation: As previously reviewed and described above, cells of the CT are the only ones showing capacity for cell proliferation (Berniscke et al, 2006). Importantly, growth, expansion and maintenance of the ST throughout pregnancy depend mainly on the continuous incorporation of CT cells into the ST (Berniscke et al, 2006; Huppertz, 2010). Therefore cell proliferation of CT is fundamental for the trophoblast turnover in health and disease. We identified an increase in cell proliferation in the CT upon infection of villous explants with *T. cruzi*, particularly in cells beneath the areas where the ST is detached and destroyed (**Figure 2**).

Cell differentiation in the trophoblast: Trophoblast fusion is dependent on and regulated by multiple factors such as fusion proteins, proteases and cytoskeletal proteins as well as cytokines, hormones and transcription factors (Huppertz 2010; Huppertz and Gauster, 2011). Some of these factors, considered as trophoblast "differentiation markers" or "fusion markers", are the following:

a. *Syncytin family proteins*: Syncytins are fusogenic proteins encoded by envelope genes (*env* genes) of the human endogenous retrovirus (HERV)-W (Syncytin-1), (HERV)-FRD (Syncytin-2), and (HERV)-P(b) (Syncytin-3;) (Ruebner et al, 2010). HERVs contribute to genome plasticity, protect the host against infection with related pathogenic and exogenous retroviruses, and play a vital role in the development of the placenta (Black et al, 2010). Knock down of syncytin-1 inhibited syncytialization of primary trophoblasts (Gauster et al, 2009).
b. *Transcription factors*: Glial cell missing-1 (GCM1), a placenta-specific transcription factor, regulates transcription via two GCM1 binding sites upstream the 5'-long terminal repeat of the syncytin-1 gene (Huppertz and Borges, 2008; Yu et al, 2002). GCM1 is expressed in highly differentiated CT cells (Baczyk et al, 2004; Huppertz and Borges, 2008).
c. *Other membrane proteins*: Presence of gap junctions is considered as a prerequisite for trophoblast syncytialization (Gauster et al, 2009). Inhibition of connexin 34 expression by antisense techniques impairs cell fusion in primary trophoblast cultures (Frendo et al, 2003).

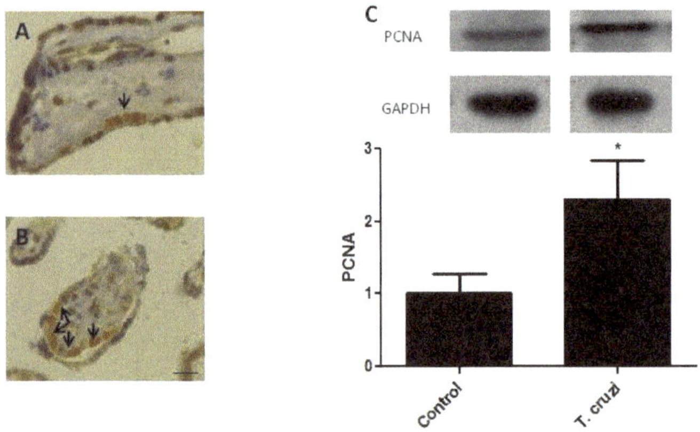

Human chorionic villi incubated with 1 x 10^5 trypomastigotes DM28c strain for 24 hours (**B**) show increase in PCNA immunoreactivity compared to control tissue (**A**). In control (**A**, arrow) and *ex vivo* infected chorionic villi (**B**, arrows) PCNA immunoreactivity can be observed. Note that PCNA immunoreactivity is increased in cells beneath syncythiotrophoblast detachment (arrows). Chorionic villi were processed for routine immunohistochemistry and Antigen-Antibody complex was stained with DAB. Bar scale: 20 μm.
In (C) upper panel a representative western blot for PCNA detection is shown. The bar graphs under the Western blots represent the ratios, normalized with respect to control values, of PCNA over GAPDH. Values represents means ±SD, $p \leq 0.5$, n=3.

Fig. 2. *T. cruzi* induces cell proliferation in the trophoblast

Cell differentiation and apoptosis: In the trophoblast, cell differentiation and apoptotic cell death are closely related (Huppertz and Gauster, 2010). While seemingly paradoxical, there are strong evidences that initiator caspases, especially caspase-8, are involved not only in apoptosis but in differentiation processes in diverse cell types and tissues. Some examples are the enucleation processes during terminal differentiation of erythrocytes (Carlile et al, 2004) and keratinocytes (Denecker et al, 2008) as well as other differentiation processes such as monocytes into macrophages (Sordet et al, 2002) or formation of myotubes in striated skeletal muscle tissue (Fernando et al, 2002).

Programmed cell death in the trophoblast presents most, but not all, of the classic features of apoptosis (Bernischke, 2006; Huppertz and Gauster, 2010). The most remarkable difference between "classic apoptosis" and "trophoblast apoptosis" is that the latter is a prolonged form of apoptosis (3-4 weeks) (Bernischke, 2006). The following data suggests that this prolonged form of apoptosis drives, at least partially, the stages of trophoblast differentiation and turnover:

a. Initiation stages of apoptosis are responsible for the CT cell exit from the cell cycle and for its entrance into the differentiation pathway (Bernischke, 2006; Huppertz et al, 2002). The matador/Bcl-2 ovarian killer (Mtd/Bok) regulates human trophoblast apoptosis and proliferation. The main isoform of Mtd/Bok associated with trophoblast proliferation is Mtd-L, the full-length isoform, which preferentially is localized in the nuclear compartment in proliferating cells, whereas during apoptosis it switched localization to the cytoplasm where it is associated with mitochondria. Mtd-L expression in proliferating cells co-localized with cyclin E1, a G_1/S phase cell cycle regulator (Ray et al, 2010).

b. Caspase 8 is activated in highly differentiated CT just prior to fusion and escorts the fusing cell content including the nucleus into the ST; interestingly, it has not been found in proliferating CT cells (Black et al, 2010; Huppertz and Gauster, 2010; Huppertz and Borges, 2008).
c. Activation of caspase-8 induces phosphatidylserine "flip", which is a key signal for syncytial fusion (Huppertz and Gauster, 2010; Huppertz and Gauster, 2011) and for cell death by apoptosis (Savill, 1998). Highly differentiated CT cells display the flip of phosphatidylserine without any signs of apoptosis (Huppertz et al, 1998; Rote et al, 2010). Furthermore, it has been demonstrated that the phosphatidylserine flip is also required for fusion of trophoblast-derived BeWo choriocarcinoma cells (Lyden et al, 1993).
d. Caspase-8 is responsible for cytoskeleton rearrangement previous to cell fusion (Rote el al, 2010) by cleaving α-fodrin (Huppertz and Gauster, 2011). α-fodrin belongs to the spectrin protein family of sub-membranous cytoskeletal proteins that carry binding sites for phosphatidylserine. The spectrin network maintains the curvature of the plasma membrane and its degradation affects membrane curvature facilitating fusion (Martens and McMahon, 2008). The expression of α-fodrin is diminished in highly differentiated CT and is entirely missing in the ST (Huppertz and Gauster, 2011).
e. Upon syncytial fusion, excess expression of apoptosis inhibitors like bcl-2 and mcl-1 blocks further progression of the apoptosis cascade for 3 to 4 weeks (Bernischke, 2006; Huppertz et al, 1998; Huppertz and Gauster, 2011).

Interestingly, diverse pathogens, including *T. cruzi,* induce apoptosis in the placenta, especially in the trophoblast (Duaso et al, 2011a).

Regulation of trophoblast differentiation: Cytokines and growth factors derived from the maternal and fetal environment are involved in regulating trophoblast turnover (Gauster et al, 2009). Epidermal growth factor (EGF) (Morrish et al, 1987), colony-stimulating factor (CSF) (Garcia-Lloret et al, 1994), granulocyte-macrophage colony stimulating factor (GM-CSF), leukemia-inhibitory factor (LIF) (Yang et al, 2003), transforming growth factor (TGF)-α and vascular endothelial growth factor (VEGF) (Crocker et al, 2001; Gauster et al, 2009) induce syncytialization of CT and secretion of human chorionic gonadotropin (hCG) as well as of human placental lactogen (hPL). Interestingly, hCG secreted by the ST can act in an autocrine manner to increase syncytium formation (Shi et al, 1993; Yang et al, 2003). The secretion of hCG and hPL are the main biochemical markers of trophoblast differentiation *in vitro* (Drewlo et al, 2008). In contrast, tumor necrosis factor (TNF)-a (Leisser et al, 2006) as well as transforming growth factor (TGF)-β impaired syncytium formation in chorionic villi explants *in vitro* and inhibited secretion of hCG and hPL (Morrish et al, 1987; Huppertz and Gauster, 2011).

Trophoblast and inflammatory response: Expression of all 10 described TLRs, as well as of various co-receptors and accessory proteins, has been described in the human placenta (Koga and Mor, 2010). TLRs 1-2 and 4-6 are membrane receptors while TLRs 3 and 9 are cytoplasmic receptors and recognize extracellular and intracellular signals, respectively.

Following ligation, the majority of TLRs recruit the intracellular signaling adapter protein, myeloid differentiation factor 88 (MyD88), leading to a subsequent kinase cascade, which triggers the activation of NFκB pathway, with resultant generation of an inflammatory response. TLR3 and TLR4 can also signal in a MyD88-independent manner (Yamamoto et al, 2003). This signaling occurs through an adapter protein Toll/IL-1 receptor domain-containing adaptor inducing IFN-b (TRIF), which not only activates the NFκB pathway, but also results in the phosphorylation of IFN regulatory factor-3 (IRF-3). This alternative pathway generates a response associated with the production of type I IFNs and IFN-inducible genes (Hemmi et al, 2000; Koga and Mor, 2010). The expression of TLR varies during pregnancy, but TLR-2, TLR-4 (Ma et al, 2006) as well as TLR 9 (Komine-Aizawa, 2008) are expressed in human term placenta and recognize *T. cruzi*. The principal *T. cruzi* mediated TLR activation is induced by members of GPI-anchored mucins located on *T. cruzi* trypomastigote surface that activates TLR-2 and by CpG-rich parasite DNA that activates TLR-9 (DosReis, 2011; Tarleton, 2007). The most important cytokines secreted after TLR-2, -4 and -9 activation are IL-1α, IL-6, IL-8 and TNF-α. TLR-4 also mediates the production of IFN-β (Koga and Mor, 2010). Interestingly, activation of TLR-2 also induces activation of caspase 8 (Abrahams and Mor, 2005), an enzyme that is fundamental in apoptotic cell death as well as in trophoblast differentiation (see above).

4. *Trypanosoma cruzi* interaction with the villous stroma

To reach fetal capillaries, the parasite must cross the villous stroma. The villous stroma is a connective tissue that contains mesenchymal cells, fibroblasts and macrophages inserted in the extracellular matrix (ECM).

T. cruzi invades preferentially macrophages and fibroblasts, both present in the villous stroma. However, during tissue invasion the parasite not only must internalize into the cells but also have to deal with the ECM.

The basal lamina, a specialized structure of ECM molecules located between trophoblast and the fetal connective tissue, is one barrier that the parasite must cross. *T. cruzi* presents surface molecules, such as gp85 (Marino et al, 2003) and gp83 (Nde et al, 2006) glycoproteins that bind to laminin and fibronectin (Marino et al, 2003; Nde et al, 2006) and to sulfated glycosamineglicans such as heparan sulphate (Lima et al, 2002). We have previously shown that the parasite induces a decrease of glycosylated molecules of the basal lamina, specifically laminin and heparan sulphate (Duaso et al, 2010; Duaso et al 2011b).

Collagen IV, other basal lamina components, is also destroyed by the parasite, as evidenced by the decrease in the immunoreactivity of this macromolecule. The decrease in immunoreactivity could also be explained by a change in the epitope as a result of this binding. Interestingly, fibronectin, another principal basal lamina component, is not altered during *ex vivo* infection. The selective destruction of the basal lamina could be part of the mechanism of connective tissue invasion, after an effective epithelial infection.

Basal lamina is also present between the fetal endothelium and the connective tissue. This basal lamina is the last barrier that any pathogen should cross to reach fetal circulation. As expected, *T. cruzi* trypomastigotes induce a similar decrease of laminin and heparan sulphate in the basal lamina located around the fetal capillaries, as compared to that observed in the basal lamina beneath the trophoblast (Duaso et al, 2010).

Collagen IV is an exception to this since no change is observed. Possibly, the destruction of collagen IV around fetal endothelium is not necessary for the parasite invasion of fetal capillaries or occurs at a later time (Duaso et al, 2010). In other studies, an increase of laminin expression in cardiac tissue has been reported (Scharfstein and Morrot, 1999; Marino et al, 2003). The increase of laminin expression could be induced by the parasite, which needs to attach to ECM molecules for cellular invasion (Marino et al, 2003). The silencing of the laminin gene inhibits cell invasion of the *T. cruzi* (Nde et al, 2006). The parasitic protease cruzipain degrades collagen IV and fibronectin, exposing epitopes to which *T. cruzi* binds (Scharfstein and Morrot, 1999), facilitating also the binding to laminin and consequently the cell invasion. On the other hand, the breakdown of the ECM facilitates the penetration of the parasite through basal lamina and connective tissue of villous stroma.

Between the trophoblast and fetal capillaries, the fetal connective tissue is another important barrier for the parasite. *Ex vivo* infection of human chorionic villi induces a severe collagen I disorganization as seen by Picrosirius red-hematoxylin staining (Duaso et al, 2010). The same effect can be observed in placentas from woman with chronic Chagas disease (Duaso et al, 2011b). The collagen I degradation is probably due to the presence of cruzipain that degrades this type of ECM component (Scharfstein and Morrot, 1999). In other tissue, specifically the lamina propria of seminiferous tubules in mice, *T. cruzi* infection also induces collagen I disorganization (Carvalho et al, 2009). Other enzymes which may participate in collagen I destruction are the metalloproteinases MMP-2 and MMP-9. These proteases are induced by *T. cruzi* in the myocardium of mice with acute Chagas´disease; and its inhibition reduces myocarditis and improves survival during the acute phase of infection (Gutiérrez et al, 2008). Preliminary studies of our laboratory indicates that the parasite increase the activity of the MMP-2 and MMP-9. Collagen I constitute a basic component of the tri-dimensional network of ECM, formed by different types of collagen and elastic fibers, proteoglycans and glycoproteins. If the "basic skeleton" of the ECM is destroyed, the normal conformation of ECM is disorganized, a condition which may facilitate the mobilization of the parasite inside the tissue to its target. Additionally, it has been proposed that ECM alterations produced by the parasite's presence not only promote its motility in tissues and its entrance into cells, but also alter the presence of cytokines and chemokines, which in turn permits *T. cruzi* to modulate and escape both the inflammatory response and the immune response (Marino et al, 2003; Duaso et al, 2010; Duaso et al, 2011b).

5. Conclusion

T. cruzi induces trophoblast destruction and detachment, selective disorganization of the basal lamina and of collagen I in the connective tissue of villous stroma and apoptosis in the chorionic villi. These results suggest that the penetration of this parasite in the placenta is a consequence of its proteolytic activity on the basal lamina and on the connective tissue. Together with the induction of apoptosis these may be part of the mechanisms of infection and tissue invasion by this parasite.

6. Acknowledgment

This study was supported by grants 11080166 and 1120230 (to UK) from FONDECYT and CONICYT-PBCT Anillo ACT 112, Chile.

7. References

Abbasi, M.; Kowalewska-Grochowska, K.; Bahar, M. A.; Kilani, R. T.; Winkler-Lowen, B. & Guilbert, L. J. (2003), Infection of placental trophoblasts by Toxoplasma gondii, *The Journal of Infectious Diseases,* Vol.188, No.4, (August 2003), pp.608-616.

Abrahams, V. M. & Mor, G. (2005), Toll-like receptors and their role in the trophoblast, *Placenta, Vol.*26, No.7, (August 2005), pp.540-547.

Al-Khan, A.; Aye, I. L.; Barsoum, I.; Borbely, A.; Cebral, E.; Cerchi, G.; Clifton, V. L.; Collins, S.; Cotechini, T.; Davey, A.; Flores-Martin, J.; Fournier, T.; Franchi, A. M.; Fretes, R. E.; Graham, C. H.; Godbole, G.; Hansson, S. R.; Headley, P. L.; Ibarra, C.; Jawerbaum, A.; Kemmerling, U.; Kudo, Y.; Lala, P. K.; Lassance, L.; Lewis, R. M.; Menkhorst, E.; Morris, C.; Nobuzane, T.; Ramos, G.; Rote, N.; Saffery, R.; Salafia, C.; Sarr, D.; Schneider, H.; Sibley, C.; Singh, A. T.; Sivasubramaniyam, T. S.; Soares, M. J.; Vaughan, O.; Zamudio, S. & Lash, G. E. (2011), IFPA Meeting 2010 Workshops Report II: Placental pathology; trophoblast invasion; fetal sex; parasites and the placenta; decidua and embryonic or fetal loss; trophoblast differentiation and syncytialisation, *Placenta, Vol.*32, Suppl2, (October 2010), pp.90-99, Santiago Chile, October 2010.

Altemani, A. M.; Bittencourt, A. L. & Lana, A. M. (2000), Immunohistochemical characterization of the inflammatory infiltrate in placental Chagas disease: a qualitative and quantitative analysis, *The American Journal of Tropical Medicine and Hygiene, Vol.*62, No.2, (February 2000), pp.319-324.

Araújo, A.; Jansen, A. M.; Reinhard, K. & Ferreira, L. F. (2009), Paleoparasitology of Chagas disease–a review, *Memórias Do Instituto Oswaldo Cruz, Vol.*104, Suppl 1,(July 2009), pp.9-16.

Baczyk, D.; Satkunaratnam, A.; Nait-Oumesmar, B.; Huppertz, B.; Cross, J. C. & Kingdom, J. C. P. (2004), Complex patterns of GCM1 mRNA and protein in villous and extravillous trophoblast cells of the human placenta, *Placenta, Vol.*25, No.6, (July 2004), pp.553-559.

Breniere, S.F., Bailly, M., Carrasco, R., Carlier, Y., (1983). Transmission transplacentaire des anticorps anti-Trypanosoma cruzi.,Cah. O. R. S. T. O. M., Ser. Ent. *Med. Parasitol.* Vol. 21,No.3, pp.139-140.

Benirschke, K. & Kaufmann, P. (2000), *Pathology of the human placenta,* (Fifth edition), Springer, New York USA.

Bittencourt, A. L. (1976), Congenital Chagas disease, *American Journal of Diseases of Children (1960)* , Vol.130, No.1, (January 1976), pp.97-103.

Black, S. G.; Arnaud, F.; Palmarini, M. & Spencer, T. E. (2010), Endogenous retroviruses in trophoblast differentiation and placental development, *American Journal of Reproductive Immunology,* Vol.64, No.4, (October 2010), pp.255-264.

Blanco, S. B.; Segura, E. L.; Cura, E. N.; Chuit, R.; Tulián, L.; Flores, I.; Garbarino, G.; Villalonga, J. F. & Gürtler, R. E. (2000), Congenital transmission of Trypanosoma cruzi: an operational outline for detecting and treating infected infants in north-western Argentina, *Tropical Medicine & International Health: TM & IH,* Vol.5, No.4, (April 2000), pp.293-301.

Brutus, L.; Castillo, H.; Bernal, C.; Salas, N. A.; Schneider, D.; Santalla, J.-A. & Chippaux, J.-P. (2010), Detectable Trypanosoma cruzi parasitemia during pregnancy and delivery as a risk factor for congenital Chagas disease, *The American Journal of Tropical Medicine and Hygiene,* Vol.83, No.5, (November 2010), pp.1044-1047.

Burgos, J. M.; Altcheh, J.; Bisio, M.; Duffy, T.; Valadares, H. M. S.; Seidenstein, M. E.; Piccinali, R.; Freitas, J. M.; Levin, M. J.; Macchi, L.; Macedo, A. M.; Freilij, H. & Schijman, A. G. (2007), Direct molecular profiling of minicircle signatures and lineages of Trypanosoma cruzi bloodstream populations causing congenital Chagas disease, *International Journal for Parasitology,* Vol.37, No.12, (October 2007), pp.1319-1327.

Carlier Y and Truyens C. (2010) Maternal-Fetal Transmission of Trypanosoma cruzi. In: *American Trypanosomiasis Chagas Disease One Hundred years of Research* Telleria and Tibayrenc, (First Edition), pp. 539-581, Elsevier Inc. New York USA.

Carlile, G. W.; Smith, D. H. & Wiedmann, M. (2004), Caspase-3 has a nonapoptotic function in erythroid maturation, *Blood,* Vol.10311, (June 2004), pp.4310-4316.

Carvalho, L. O. P.; Abreu-Silva, A. L.; Hardoim, D. d. J.; Tedesco, R. C.; Mendes, V. G.; da Costa, S. C. G. & Calabrese, K. d. S. (2009), Trypanosoma cruzi and myoid cells from seminiferous tubules: interaction and relation with fibrous components of extracellular matrix in experimental Chagas disease, *International Journal of Experimental Pathology,* Vol.90, No.1, (February 2009), pp.52-57.

Chan, G. & Guilbert, L. J. (2006), Ultraviolet-inactivated human cytomegalovirus induces placental syncytiotrophoblast apoptosis in a Toll-like receptor-2 and tumour necrosis factor-alpha dependent manner, *The Journal of Pathology,* Vol.210, No.1, (September 2006), pp.111-120.

Crocker, I. P.; Strachan, B. K.; Lash, G. E.; Cooper, S.; Warren, A. Y. & Baker, P. N. (2001), Vascular endothelial growth factor but not placental growth factor promotes trophoblast syncytialization in vitro, *Journal of the Society for Gynecologic Investigation,* Vol.8, No.6, (November 2001), pp.341-346.

Denecker, G.; Ovaere, P.; Vandenabeele, P. & Declercq, W. (2008), Caspase-14 reveals its secrets, *The Journal of Cell Biology,* Vol.180, No.3, (February 2008), pp.451-458.

DosReis, G. A. (2011), Evasion of immune responses by Trypanosoma cruzi, the etiological agent of Chagas disease, *Brazilian Journal of Medical and Biological,* Vol.44, No.2, (February 2011), pp.84-90.

Drewlo, S.; Baczyk, D.; Dunk, C. & Kingdom, J. (2008), Fusion assays and models for the trophoblast, *Methods in Molecular Biology,* Vol.475, No 2, pp.363-382.

Duaso, J.; Rojo, G.; Cabrera, G.; Galanti, N.; Bosco, C.; Maya, J. D.; Morello, A. & Kemmerling, U. (2010), Trypanosoma cruzi induces tissue disorganization and destruction of chorionic villi in an ex vivo infection model of human placenta, *Placenta,* Vol.31,No.8, (August 2010), pp.705-711.

Duaso, J.; Rojo, G.; Jaña, F.; Galanti, N.; Cabrera, G.; Bosco, C.; López-Muñoz, R.; Maya, J. D.; Ferreira, J. & Kemmerling, U. (2011), Trypanosoma cruzi induces apoptosis in ex vivo infected human chorionic villi, *Placenta,* Vol.32, No.5, (May 2011), pp.356-361.

Duaso, J.; Yanez, E.; Castillo, C.; Galanti, N.; Cabrera, G.; Corral, G.; Maya, JD.; Zulantay, I.; Apt, W. & Kemmerling, U. (2011), Reorganization of extracellular matrix in placentas from women with asymptomatic Chagas disease: Mechanism of parasite invasion, or local placental defense?, *Journal of Tropical Medicine,* 2012;2012:758357

Fernando, P.; Kelly, J. F.; Balazsi, K.; Slack, R. S. & Megeney, L. A. (2002), Caspase 3 activity is required for skeletal muscle differentiation, *Proceedings of the National Academy of Sciences of the United States of America,* Vol.99, No.17, (August 2002), pp.11025-11030.

Frendo, J.-L.; Cronier, L.; Bertin, G.; Guibourdenche, J.; Vidaud, M.; Evain-Brion, D. & Malassine, A. (2003), Involvement of connexin 43 in human trophoblast cell fusion and differentiation, *Journal of Cell Science,* Vol.116, No.Pt 16, (August 2003), pp.3413-3421.

Garcia-Lloret, M. I.; Morrish, D. W.; Wegmann, T. G.; Honore, L.; Turner, A. R. & Guilbert, L. J. (1994), Demonstration of functional cytokine-placental interactions: CSF-1 and GM-CSF stimulate human cytotrophoblast differentiation and peptide hormone secretion, *Experimental Cell Research,* Vol.214, No.1, (September 1994), pp.46-54.

Gauster, M.; Moser, G.; Orendi, K. & Huppertz, B. (2009), Factors involved in regulating trophoblast fusion: potential role in the development of preeclampsia, *Placenta,* Vol.30 Suppl A, (March 2009), pp.49-54.

Gutierrez, F. R. S.; Lalu, M. M.; Mariano, F. S.; Milanezi, C. M.; Cena, J.; Gerlach, R. F.; Santos, J. E. T.; Torres-Dueñas, D.; Cunha, F. Q.; Schulz, R. & Silva, J. S. (2008), Increased activities of cardiac matrix metalloproteinases matrix metalloproteinase (MMP)-2 and MMP-9 are associated with mortality during the acute phase of experimental Trypanosoma cruzi infection, *The Journal of Infectious Diseases,* Vol.197, No.10, (May 2008), pp.1468-1476.

Hemmi, H.; Takeuchi, O.; Kawai, T.; Kaisho, T.; Sato, S.; Sanjo, H.; Matsumoto, M.; Hoshino, K.; Wagner, H.; Takeda, K. & Akira, S. (2000), A Toll-like receptor recognizes bacterial DNA, *Nature,* Vol.408, No.6813, (December 2000), pp.740-745.

Hermann, E.; Berthe, A.; Truyens, C.; Alonso-Vega, C.; Parrado, R.; Torrico, F.; Carlier, Y. & Braud, V. M. (2010), Killer cell immunoglobulin-like receptor expression induction on neonatal CD8(+) T cells in vitro and following congenital infection with Trypanosoma cruzi, *Immunology,* Vol.129, No.3, (March 2010), pp.418-426.

Huppertz, B. (2010), IFPA Award in Placentology Lecture: Biology of the placental syncytiotrophoblast-myths and facts, *Placenta,* Vol.31 Suppl, pp.75-81, , Santiago Chile, October 2010.

Huppertz, B.; Frank, H. G.; Kingdom, J. C.; Reister, F. & Kaufmann, P. (1998), Villous cytotrophoblast regulation of the syncytial apoptotic cascade in the human placenta, *Histochemistry and Cell Biology,* Vol.110, No.5, (November 1998), pp.495-508.

Huppertz, B. & Borges, M. (2008), Placenta trophoblast fusion, *Methods in Molecular Biology,* Vol.475, pp.135-147.

Huppertz, B. & Gauster, M. (2011), Trophoblast fusion, *Advances in Experimental Medicine and Biology,* Vol.713, 81-95.

Huppertz, B.; Kaufmann, P. & Kingdom, J. (2002), Trophoblast Turnover in Health and Disease, *Fetal and Maternal Medicine Review,* Vol.13, No.02, pp.103-118.

Janeway, C. (2005), *Immunobiology: the immune system in health and disease,* Garland Science, New York.

Jercic, M. I.; Mercado, R. & Villarroel, R. (2010), Congenital Trypanosoma cruzi infection in neonates and infants from two regions of Chile where Chagas disease is endemic, *Journal of Clinical Microbiology,* Vol.48, No.10, (October 2010), pp.3824-3826.

Kemmerling, U.; Bosco, C. & Galanti, N. (2010), Infection and invasion mechanisms of Trypanosoma cruzi in the congenital transmission of Chagas disease: a proposal, *Biological Research,* Vol.43, No.3, pp.307-316.

Kirchhoff, L. V. (1993), American trypanosomiasis (Chagas disease)–a tropical disease now in the United States, *The New England Journal of Medicine,* Vol.329, No.9, (August 1993), pp.639-644.

Koga, K. & Mor, G. (2010), Toll-like receptors at the maternal-fetal interface in normal pregnancy and pregnancy disorders, *American Journal of Reproductive Immunology (New York, N.Y.: 1989)* , Vol.63, No.6, (June 2010), pp.587-600.

Komine-Aizawa, S.; Majima, H.; Yoshida-Noro, C. & Hayakawa, S. (2008), Stimuli through Toll-like receptor (TLR) 3 and 9 affect human chorionic gonadotropin (hCG) production in a choriocarcinoma cell line, *The Journal of Obstetrics and Gynaecology Research,* Vol.34, No.2, (April 2008), pp.144-151.

Lima, A. P. C. A.; Almeida, P. C.; Tersariol, I. L. S.; Schmitz, V.; Schmaier, A. H.; Juliano, L.; Hirata, I. Y.; Müller-Esterl, W.; Chagas, J. R. & Scharfstein, J. (2002), Heparan sulfate modulates kinin release by Trypanosoma cruzi through the activity of cruzipain, *The Journal of Biological Chemistry,* Vol.277, No.8, (February 2002), pp.5875-5881.

Luján, C. D.; Triquell, M. F.; Sembaj, A.; Guerrero, C. E. & Fretes, R. E. (2004), Trypanosoma cruzi: productive infection is not allowed by chorionic villous explant from normal human placenta in vitro, *Experimental Parasitology,* Vol.108, No.3-4, (November 2004), pp.176-181.

Lyden, T. W.; Ng, A. K. & Rote, N. S. (1993), Modulation of phosphatidylserine epitope expression by BeWo cells during forskolin treatment, *Placenta,* Vol.14, No.2, (March 1993), pp.177-186.

Marino, A. P. M. P.; Silva, A. A.; Pinho, R. T. & Lannes-Vieira, J. (2003), Trypanosoma cruzi infection: a continuous invader-host cell cross talk with participation of extracellular matrix and adhesion and chemoattractant molecules, *Brazilian Journal of Medical and Biological* , Vol.36, No.8, (August 2003), pp.1121-1133.

Maubert, B.; Guilbert, L. J. & Deloron, P. (1997), Cytoadherence of Plasmodium falciparum to intercellular adhesion molecule 1 and chondroitin-4-sulfate expressed by the syncytiotrophoblast in the human placenta, *Infection and Immunity,* Vol.65, No.4, (April 1997), pp.1251-1257.

Moore, K. L. & Persaud, T. V. N. (2003), *The developing human: clinically oriented embryology,* (Eighth edition), Saunders, Barcelona España.

Mor, G. & Cardenas, I. (2010), The immune system in pregnancy: a unique complexity, *American Journal of Reproductive Immunology,* Vol.63, No.6, (June 2010), pp.425-433.

Moretti, E.; Basso, B.; Castro, I.; Carrizo Paez, M.; Chaul, M.; Barbieri, G.; Canal Feijoo, D.; Sartori, M. J. & Carrizo Paez, R. (2005), Chagas disease: study of congenital transmission in cases of acute maternal infection, *Revista Da Sociedade Brasileira De Medicina Tropical,* Vol.38, No.1, (January 2005), pp.53-55.

Morrish, D. W.; Bhardwaj, D.; Dabbagh, L. K.; Marusyk, H. & Siy, O. (1987), Epidermal growth factor induces differentiation and secretion of human chorionic gonadotropin and placental lactogen in normal human placenta, *The Journal of Clinical Endocrinology and Metabolism,* Vol.65, No.6, (December 1987), pp.1282-1290.

Nde, P. N.; Simmons, K. J.; Kleshchenko, Y. Y.; Pratap, S.; Lima, M. F. & Villalta, F. (2006), Silencing of the laminin gamma-1 gene blocks Trypanosoma cruzi infection, *Infection and Immunity,* Vol.74, No.3, (March 2006), pp.1643-1648.

Prata, A. (2001), Clinical and epidemiological aspects of Chagas disease, *The Lancet Infectious Diseases,* Vol.1, No.2, (Sepember 2001), pp.92-100.

Rassi, Anis, J.; Rassi, A.; Little, W. C.; Xavier, S. S.; Rassi, S. G.; Rassi, A. G.; Rassi, G. G.; Hasslocher-Moreno, A.; Sousa, A. S. & Scanavacca, M. I. (2006), Development and validation of a risk score for predicting death in Chagas heart disease, *The New England Journal of Medicine,* Vol.355, No.8, (August 2006), pp.799-808.

Ray, J. E.; Garcia, J.; Jurisicova, A. & Caniggia, I. (2010), Mtd/Bok takes a swing: proapoptotic Mtd/Bok regulates trophoblast cell proliferation during human placental development and in preeclampsia, *Cell Death and Differentiation,* Vol.17, No.5, (May 2010), pp.846-859.

Rote, N. S.; Wei, B.-R.; Xu, C. & Luo, L. (2010), Caspase 8 and human villous cytotrophoblast differentiation, *Placenta,* Vol.31, No.2, (February 2010), pp.89-96.

Ruebner, M.; Strissel, P. L.; Langbein, M.; Fahlbusch, F.; Wachter, D. L.; Faschingbauer, F.; Beckmann, M. W. & Strick, R. (2010), Impaired cell fusion and differentiation in placentae from patients with intrauterine growth restriction correlate with reduced levels of HERV envelope genes, *Journal of Molecular Medicine (Berlin, Germany)* , Vol.88, No.11, (November 2010), pp.1143-1156.

Savill, J. (1998), Apoptosis. Phagocytic docking without shocking, *Nature,* Vol.392, No.6675, (April 1998), pp.442-443.

Scharfstein, J. & Morrot, A. (1999), A role for extracellular amastigotes in the immunopathology of Chagas disease, *Memórias Do Instituto Oswaldo Cruz,* Vol.94 Suppl 1, pp.51-63.

Schmunis, G. A. (2007), Epidemiology of Chagas disease in non-endemic countries: the role of international migration, *Memórias Do Instituto Oswaldo Cruz,* Vol.102 Suppl 1, (October 2007), pp.75-85.

Shi, Q. J.; Lei, Z. M.; Rao, C. V. & Lin, J. (1993), Novel role of human chorionic gonadotropin in differentiation of human cytotrophoblasts, *Endocrinology,* Vol.132, No.3, (March 1993), pp.1387-1395.

Shippey, Stuart H, 3r.; Zahn, C. M.; Cisar, M. M.; Wu, T. J. & Satin, A. J. (2005), Use of the placental perfusion model to evaluate transplacental passage of Trypanosoma cruzi, *American Journal of Obstetrics and Gynecology,* Vol.192, No.2, (February 2005), pp.586-591.

Sordet, O.; Rébé, C.; Plenchette, S.; Zermati, Y.; Hermine, O.; Vainchenker, W.; Garrido, C.; Solary, E. & Dubrez-Daloz, L. (2002), Specific involvement of caspases in the differentiation of monocytes into macrophages, *Blood,* Vol.100, No.13, (December 2002), pp.4446-4453.

Tarleton, R. L. (2007), Immune system recognition of Trypanosoma cruzi, *Current Opinion in Immunology,* Vol.19, No.4, (August 2007), pp.430-434.

Telleria, J.; Biron, D. G.; Brizard, J.-P.; Demettre, E.; Séveno, M.; Barnabé, C.; Ayala, F. J. & Tibayrenc, M. (2010), Phylogenetic character mapping of proteomic diversity shows high correlation with subspecific phylogenetic diversity in Trypanosoma cruzi, *Proceedings of the National Academy of Sciences of the United States of America,* Vol.107, No.47, (November 2010), pp.20411-20416.

Torrico, F.; Castro, M.; Solano, M.; Rodriguez, P.; Torrico, M.-C.; Truyens, C. & Carlier, Y. (2005), Effects of maternal infection with Trypanosoma cruzi in pregnancy development and in the newborn infant, *Revista Da Sociedade Brasileira De Medicina Tropical,* Vol.38 Suppl 2, pp.73-76.

World Health Organization (2006), Estimación cuantitativa de la enfermedad de Chagas en las Americas. In: *OPS/HDM/CD/* 425-06, Retrieved from <www.bvsops.org.uy/pdf/chagas19.pdf>.

World Health Organization (2010), First report on neglected tropical diseases: *working to overcome the global impact of neglected tropical diseases,* Retrieved from <http://whqlibdoc.who.int/publications/2010/9789241564090_eng.pdf>.

Yamamoto, M.; Sato, S.; Hemmi, H.; Hoshino, K.; Kaisho, T.; Sanjo, H.; Takeuchi, O.; Sugiyama, M.; Okabe, M.; Takeda, K. & Akira, S. (2003), Role of adaptor TRIF in the MyD88-independent toll-like receptor signaling pathway, *Science (New York, N.Y.)*, Vol.301, No.5633, (August 2003), pp.640-643.

Yang, M.; Lei, Z. M. & Rao, C. V. (2003), The central role of human chorionic gonadotropin in the formation of human placental syncytium, *Endocrinology,* Vol.144, No.3, (March 2003), pp.1108-1120.

Yu, C.; Shen, K.; Lin, M.; Chen, P.; Lin, C.; Chang, G.-D. & Chen, H. (2002), GCMa regulates the syncytin-mediated trophoblastic fusion, *The Journal of Biological Chemistry,* Vol.277, No.51, (December 2002), pp.50062-50068.

Zingales, B.; Andrade, S. G.; Briones, M. R. S.; Campbell, D. A.; Chiari, E.; Fernandes, O.; Guhl, F.; Lages-Silva, E.; Macedo, A. M.; Machado, C. R.; Miles, M. A.; Romanha, A. J.; Sturm, N. R.; Tibayrenc, M. & Schijman, A. G. (2009), A new consensus for

Trypanosoma cruzi intraspecific nomenclature: second revision meeting recommends TcI to TcVI, Memórias Do Instituto Oswaldo Cruz, Vol.104, No.7, (November 2009), pp.1051-1054.

9

Expression of Estrogen Receptors in Placentas Originating from Premature Deliveries Induced by Arterial Hypertension

Andrzej Plewka[1], Danuta Plewka[2] and Grażyna Nowaczyk[3]
[1]Department of Proteomics, Medical University of Silesia in Sosnowiec
[2]Department of Histology, Medical University of Silesia in Katowice
[3] Department of Physiology, School of Health Care, Medical University of Silesia, Katowice,
Poland

1. Introduction

The role of sex steroids and their activity involve complex intracellular reactions and depend upon presence of a specific steroid receptor. Estrogens influence several processes in the human body, including tissues distant from genital organs. In the estrogen-dependent tissues the hormones control cell proliferation and influence cell differentiation.

Studies indicate that estrogens and estrogen receptors play important physiological roles in cardiovascular disease [1].

Estrogens act by controlling expression of specific genes in target cells [2,3]. Their transcriptional activity is mediated by two estrogen receptors, ER-α and ER-β, similar in structure and function.

Till the end of 1980s transmission of the message carried by the hormone was thought to be mediated by a single estrogen receptor only. In the mid 1990s studies were published which described the discovery of a new estrogen receptor in both animals and humans [4-7].

The new estrogen receptor, ER-β, proved to be highly homologous to the classical estrogen receptor, ER-α.

Functional differences at the molecular level between ER-α and ER-β are of principal importance for the body. Just as importantly, in the case of estrogen receptors the same ligand may play role of either an agonist or antagonist, depending on whether it binds to ER-α or ER-β. Therefore, following binding of the ligand ER-α and ER-β may induce distinct biological effects, linked to conformational changes of the receptor [8].

The transmission of estrogen-carried signal plays a significant role not only in normal but also in neoplastically altered tissues. The mediator in transmission of estrogen-carried message involves estrogen receptors, acting as transcription factors, activated by ligands [8-11] and by alternative pathways of growth factor intracellular signalling [12,13]. Their activity is subjected to intracellular control and is regulated by several tissue-dependent co-modulators. Tissue distribution of the latter determines the final effect, i.e., activation or repression of the estrogen-dependent genes. Co-modulators are significant for activity of estrogen receptors and represent the functional link between the receptor and transcriptional apparatus [14,15].

Gestosis represents a disease developing with an elevated arterial blood pressure. It may be accompanied by proteinuria and/or oedemas. The disease poses a high risk both to the mother and the fetus. There are several subtypes of the disease and it seems that the pregnancy-induced hypertension is of a key significance. Gestosis develops in as many as 8-10% pregnancies after their 20th week [16-20].

Pregnancy is associated with vascular adaptations. These adaptations are critical in pregnancy because their dysfunctions are implicated in pathological pregnancies, such as preeclampsia and other disorders [21-23]. The vascular adaptations are mediated by estrogens.

Development of a normally functioning placenta requires an extreme coordination between various cellular structures, depending on specific growth factors and highly related to reciprocal signalling between the cells.

We evaluated the two estrogen receptors, which participate in control of several functions [8,24,25]. We hoped that the investigations might prove helpful in evaluation of pathology developing in placentas obtained from mothers with pre-term delivery. In order to achieve the goal we evaluated differences in expression of selected receptors in placentas originating from normal pregnancies as compared to those from pre-term deliveries, burdened in addition by arterial hypertension in the mother.

Thus, the principal aim of the studies involved characterization of changes in ER-α and ER-β expression in placentas obtained from healthy women and from women who demonstrated pregnancy-induced hypertension and who developed pre-term delivery. It was also planned to examine changes in quantitative distribution of the two receptors in central portions of the placentas as compared to their peripheral fragments.

2. Material and methods

2.1 Material

The control group included placentas obtained from 20 women, aging 21 to 34 years, originating from deliveries at term, in 37th week of pregnancy, with a normal blood pressure during the entire pregnancy.

The experimental group I included placentas from 20 patients aging 22 to 34 years, originating from pre-term deliveries between 26th and 32nd week of pregnancy, induced by hypertension, which developed between 20th and 25th week of pregnancy.

The experimental group II consisted of placentas obtained from 20 mothers, aging 24 to 34 years, following pre-term deliveries between 33rd and 37th week of pregnancy, induced by hypertension, which developed between 20th and 25th week of pregnancy.

The placentas were macroscopically examined, their weight, width and thickness were recorded and then, their samples were taken, comprising full cross-section of placenta with all its components, including amnion epithelium and basal decidua.

Before isolation of placenta samples the patients were informed on the aim of the studies. The planned investigative procedures were approved by the Medical Bioethical Commission.

2.2 Sampling of the material

Placenta samples, 0.5-1.0 cm in width, were isolated from the central zone, around the umbilical cord, and from the peripheral zone.

Samples targeted for immunohistochemical and morphological investigations were immersed in a buffered solution of paraformaldehyde. The tissue samples were fixed in 4% (w/v) paraformaldehyde solution buffered with phosphates of physiological saline (PBS) for 24 hours, at the temperature of 4^0 C, and dehydrated in a row of alcohols of increasing concentration (50%, 70%, 95% and 100% - 3 times of 20 min each), clear in xylene (3x10 min), and left in 1:1 mixture of xylene and paraffin at room temperature overnight. Subsequently, the samples were transferred to paraffin of the temperature not higher than 60^0 C for three hours, exchanging paraffin every full hour, and were embedded in paraffin blocks.

The paraffin blocks were sectioned at 5 μm using a rotary microtome and the sections were placed on silanized microscope glasses. Before immunohistochemical tests the preparations were deparaffinized in an incubator (15 min, 56^0 C), and xylene (3 x 10 min) and rehydrated in a row of alcohols of a decreasing concentration, starting at the absolute alcohol and terminating at 30% alcohol, three minutes at every stem. Finally, the preparations were washed in distilled water and, then, in 10 mM PBS, pH 7.5.

In order to unmask antigens the preparations were boiled in a microwave oven (750 W) for 20 minutes in 10 mM citrate buffer, pH 6.0.

After cooling, they were washed in a buffer and activity of endogenous peroxidase was blocked by incubation with 1.5% (v/v) H_2O_2 in methanol for 10 minutes. Sites of non-specific binding were blocked using non-immunised, normal animal serum obtained from the animal in which later on secondary antibody was obtained, for 30 min at room temperature.

2.3 Antibodies

Monoclonal mouse anti-ER-α, directed against human estrogen receptor α, were purchased from Zymed Laboratories Inc., and used at the concentration of 1 μg/ml. Polyclonal rabbit anti-ER-β, directed to human estrogen receptor β, were obtained from Affinity Bioreagents Inc., and used at the concentration of 5 μg/ml.

2.4 Immunohistochemistry

After removal of serum, sections were overlaid with an appropriate primary antibody and left overnight at the temperature of 4^0 C. Sites of primary antibody binding were visualized using ABC technique. The sections were overlaid with appropriate secondary antibodies and, then, with avidin-biotinylated peroxidase complex (Vectastain ABC Kit, Vector Laboratories). The ABC complex was made visible using peroxidase substrate containing 3,3 diaminobenzidine (DAB) and hydrogen peroxide, in accordance with manufacturer's protocol (Vector Laboratories). The preparations were counterstained with Gill's hematoxylin, dehydrated and mounted. The negative control consisted of sections in which primary antibody was substituted by non-immunized serum of the animal in which subsequently primary antibody was obtained. In order to eliminate non-specific reactions the negative control was run in parallel on every slide.

An intra-organ and intra-cellular localization was evaluated under a light microscope (Nikon) at the magnification of 200x.

A quantitative analysis was conducted of ER-α and ER-β estrogen receptor contents. Using the KS100 computer software, optical density of microscope preparations was estimated in sites in which the colour immunohistochemical reaction developed. Absorption of the light wavelength pointed to optical density of cells in the cytoplasm, nucleus of which complexes of antibody with ER-α or ER-β were detected, reflecting the content of the reaction product.

The image analysis software of KS SA series was produced by Carl Zeiss Vision, Germany. The KS100/IBAS-C software was designed for measurements of interactively indicated geometric and densitometric parameters. At the stage of quantitative analysis autocalibration of the IBAS-C system takes place permitting calculations of surface area, mean lucidity, mean integrated lucidity, saturation coefficient, saturation coefficient in the scale of 1 to 255 and in % scale.

2.5 Statistical analysis

The results were collected in an Excel spread sheet (Microsoft, USA), and subsequently it was exported to STATISTICA software (Stat Soft, USA) to conduct statistical calculations.

For results of densitometric studies, estimation of significance of differences between placenta centre and periphery Student's t test for linked variables was used. On the other hand, Student's t test for unlinked variables was employed for inter-group differences. The differences were regarded significant at $p \leq 0.05$ level.

3. Results

3.1 Estrogen receptor ER-α

In the studies the placentas which were obtained from pre-term deliveries, were used in two groups: placentas from deliveries between 26th and 32nd week and those from deliveries between 33rd and 37th week. The control group consisted of placentas from at term deliveries.

Optical density of cells with expression of estrogen receptor reflects concentration of immunocytochemical reaction product in examined cells. Two types of the receptor, i.e., ER-α and ER-β were evaluated.

Appraisal of ER-α level in cytotrophoblast cells demonstrated a clearly decreasing optical density level of the product beginning at placentas from deliveries in the 26th-32nd week and ending at placentas from at term deliveries (Figures 1 and 2). The same analysis of peripheral parts of placentas showed that ER-α level was similar in the two experimental groups and in at term placentas (Figure 3).

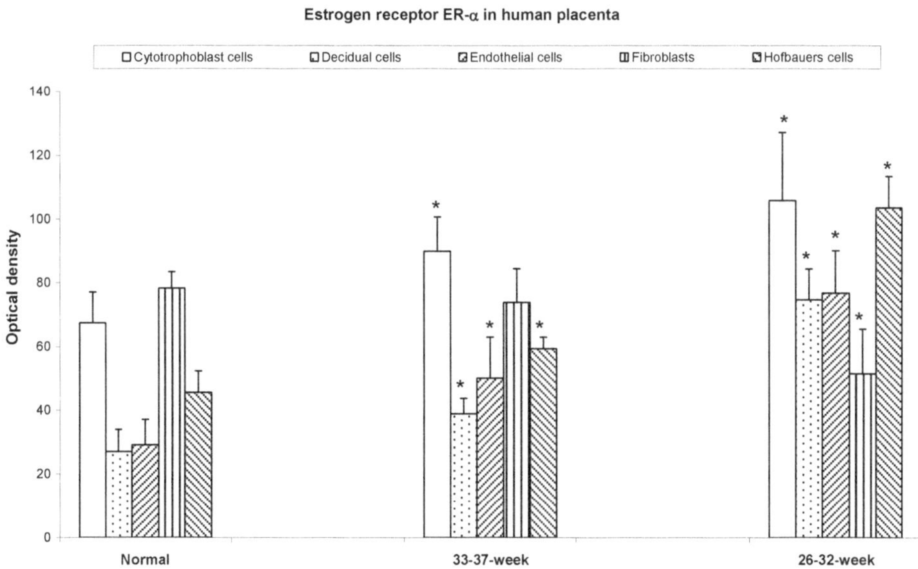

Fig. 1. Optical density of estrogen receptor ER-α in some cells originating from central part of human placentas originating from various periods of delivery. The data represent mean values ± SD. * - statistically significant ($p<0.05$) in comparison with normal group

No significant differences were detected between placenta centre and placenta periphery in cytotrophoblast cell optical density tested for expression of estrogen receptor ER-α.

Analysis of ER-α distribution in decidua cells documented an abrupt, almost 100% decrease in concentration of the receptor between the group of placentas from 26th-32nd week and the group from 33rd-37th week in the central portion of placenta (Figures 1 and 2). Even lower expression of the receptor was detected the control group, in which ER-α level was three fold lower than in the experimental group I. Peripheral portions of the placentas manifested no more pronounced differences in ER-α concentrations in decidua cells between the studied groups (Figure 3).

Comparisons of product content in decidua cells following reaction for estrogen receptor ER-α manifested significant differences between central and peripheral part of placentas from pre-term deliveries (33rd and 37th week) and placentas originating from at term deliveries.

In the central portion of placentas originating from pre-term deliveries in 26th-32nd week optical density of endothelial cells with expression of estrogen receptor ER-α reached the highest value. In the subsequent group of placentas, originating from deliveries between 33rd and 37th week, the documented value amounted to around 70% of the level typical for

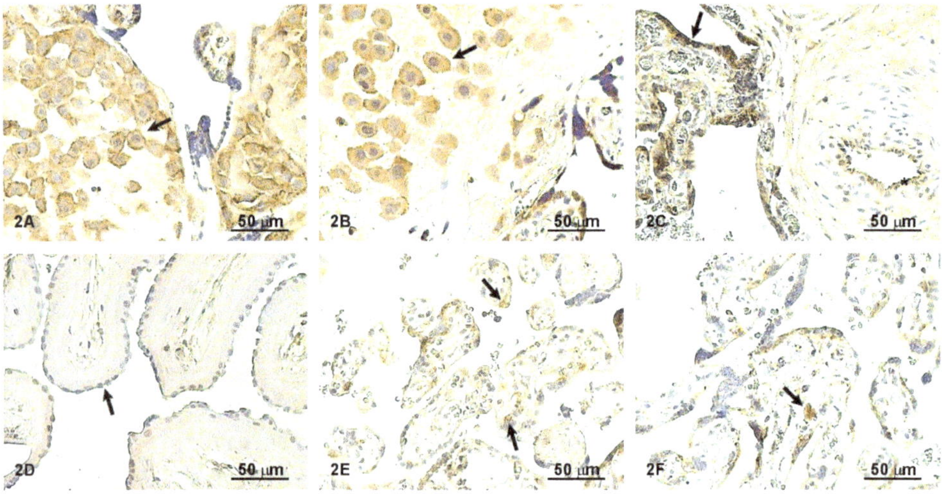

Fig. 2. Expression of estrogen receptor ER-α in decidual cells indicated by arrow (A,B), syncytiotrophoblasts (arrow) and endothelial cells (asterix) (C), cytotrophoblast cells (arrows) (E), Hofbauer's cells (arrow) (F), and no expression in amnion epithelium (arrow) (D) originating from peripheral parts of normal-term placentas (E,F) and central parts of placentas delivered between 26th and 32nd week of pregnancy (A,C) and 33rd and 37th week of pregnance (B,D).

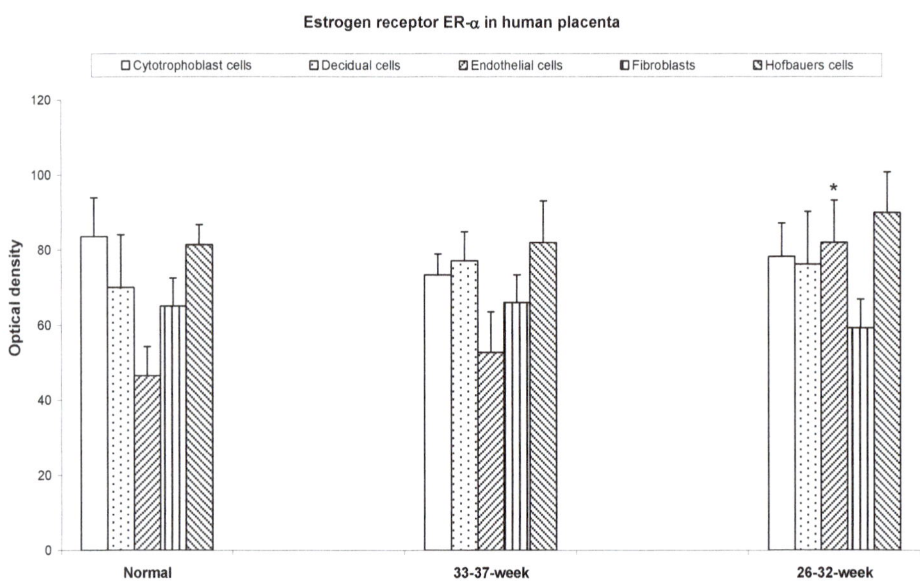

Fig. 3. Optical density of estrogen receptor ER-α in some cells originating from peripheral part of human placentas originating from various periods of delivery. The data represent mean values ± SD. * - statistically significant ($p<0.05$) in comparison with normal group

group I and in the control group it was even lower (Figure 1). All the detected differences between reaction product content following the reaction detecting estrogen receptor ER-α in endothelial cells of studied groups proved significant.

A similar tendency was disclosed in peripheral portions of placentas. Also in this case the highest optical density in endothelial cells with expression of estrogen receptor ER-α was detected in placentas from the pre-term deliveries between 26th and 32nd week of pregnancy. In the experimental group II, the content of reaction product following the reaction detecting estrogen receptor ER-α clearly decreased (Figure 3) and resembled the values noted in placentas from at term deliveries.

In the analyzed time periods of pregnancy no significant differences were disclosed in the content of reaction product following reaction for estrogen receptor ER-α between the centre and the periphery of placenta.

In fibroblasts of central placenta portions, originating from group I of pre-term deliveries optical density of cells with expression of estrogen receptor ER-α reached the lowest value (Figures 1 and 2). In the subsequent group a rising tendency was noted and in the placentas at term the detected level corresponded to 150% of the values observed in group I.

In peripheral portions of placentas originating from pre-term deliveries between 26th and 32nd week of pregnancy optical density of fibroblasts with expression of estrogen receptor ER-α was comparable to values obtained in the remaining two groups.

No significant differences were disclosed in the product content following the reaction for estrogen receptor ER-α between fibroblasts situated in the centre as compared to those at the periphery of placentas.

In central portions of placentas originating from pre-term deliveries between 26th and 32nd week of pregnancy optical density of Hofbauer's cells with expression of estrogen receptor ER-α reached the highest value. In the subsequent analyzed experimental groups a rapid decrease was noted in the content of reaction product following the test for estrogen receptor ER-α, and in the group of placentas originating from deliveries between 33rd and 37th week of pregnancy the level amounted to 60% of the group I level and in placentas from at term deliveries it was even lower (Figure 1).

In cases of peripheral placenta portions the content of reaction product in Hofbauer's cells following the test for estrogen receptor ER-α was comparable in all the three investigated groups of placentas (Figure 3).

Upon comparison of the reaction product content in Hofbauer's cells following the test for estrogen receptor ER-α between central and peripheral portions of the placentas significant inter-zone differences were disclosed in placentas originating from at term deliveries and pre-term deliveries of group II.

3.2 Estrogen receptor ER-β

Following evaluation of ER-β levels in decidua cells the central portions of placentas originating from deliveries from 26th - 32nd week and 33rd - 37th week contained a similar optical density of the reaction product and an evidently higher optical density than that noted in placenta following at term deliveries (Figures 4 and 5). The same analysis

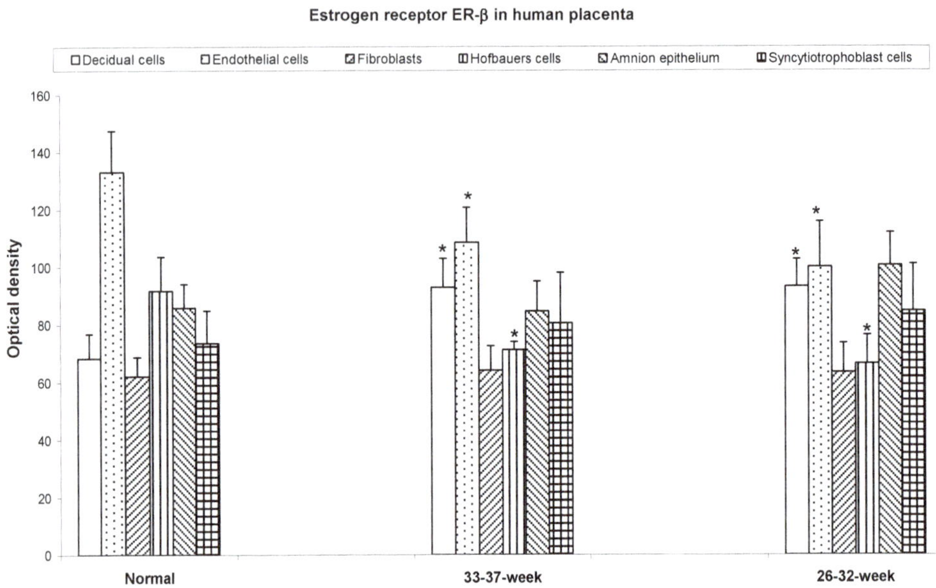

Fig. 4. Optical density of estrogen receptor ER-β in some cells originating from central part of human placentas originating from various periods of delivery. The data represent mean values ± SD. * - statistically significant ($p<0.05$) in comparison with normal group

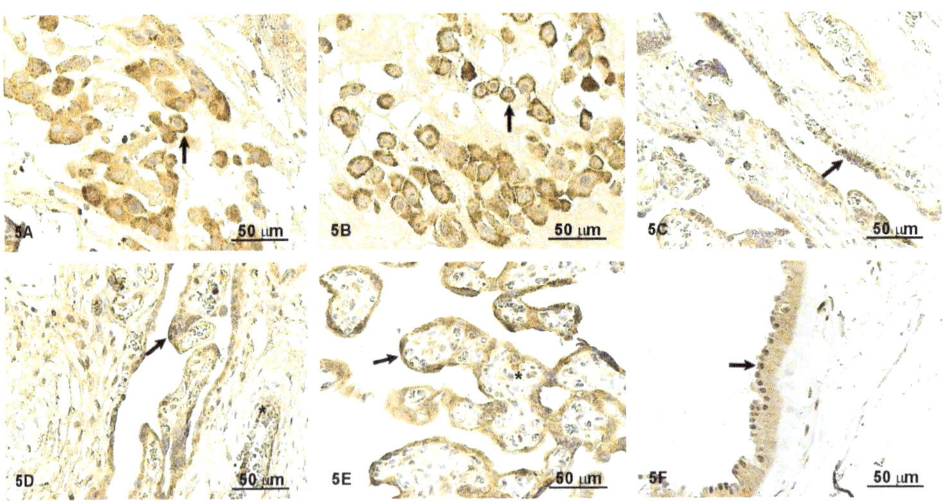

Fig. 5. Expression of estrogen receptor ER-β in decidual cells indicated by arrow (A,B), syncytiotrophoblasts (arrow) (C,D,E), endothelial cells (asterix) (C,D), and Hofbauer's cells (asterix) (E) and amnion epithelium (arrow) (F) originating from peripheral parts of normal-term placentas (B,D), central parts of placentas delivered between 26th and 32nd week of pregnancy (A,C) and 33rd and 37th week of pregnance (E,F).

performed in peripheral portions of the placentas detected in all cases the same levels of ER-β expression (Figure 6).

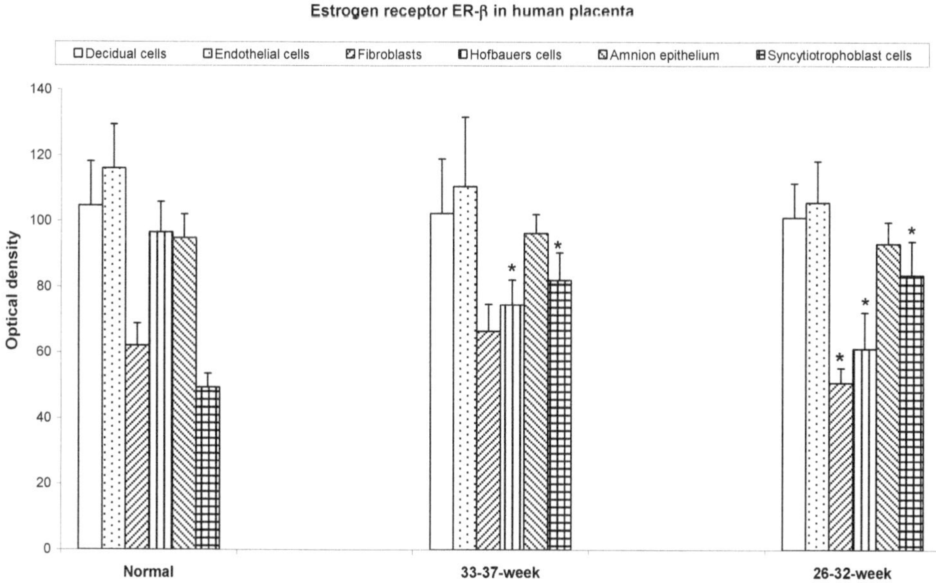

Fig. 6. Optical density of estrogen receptor ER-β in some cells originating from peripheral part of human placentas originating from various periods of delivery. The data represent mean values ± SD. * - statistically significant ($p<0.05$) in comparison with normal group

Upon comparison of the reaction product content following the test for estrogen receptor ER-β in decidua cells originating from either central or peripheral placenta portions significant differences were detected exclusively in the placenta originating from at term deliveries.

Analysis of ER-β distribution in endothelial cells of the central portion of placenta manifested a slight tendency for rising concentration of the receptor beginning at placentas from deliveries in 26th-32nd week and ending at placentas following at term deliveries (Figures 4 and 5). Comparable changes in concentrations of the receptor were noted in peripheral portions of placentas (Figure 6).

In the analyzed time periods of pregnancies no significant differences were observed between the centre and periphery of placentas in the content of reaction product in endothelial cells following the test for estrogen receptor ER-β.

The levels of ER-β receptor in fibroblasts were comparable in all studied groups, both in the central and the peripheral portions (Figures 4 and 6).

Analysis of the content of reaction product in fibroblasts following the test for estrogen receptor ER-β disclosed no significant differences between placental central and peripheral portions.

In contrast, levels of ER-β in Hofbauer's cells in the experimental groups proved to be significantly lower than in the control, both in the central and in the peripheral portions (Figures 4 and 6).

Upon comparison of reaction product content in Hofbauer's cells following the test for estrogen receptor ER-β in the central vs the peripheral portions of placenta no significant inter-zone differences were noted in the studied groups of placentas.

In central portions of placentas originating from deliveries between 26th and 32nd week of pregnancy amnion epithelial cells with expression of estrogen receptor ER-β demonstrated the highest optical density. In the subsequent experimental group a decrease was noted in the content in the product of a reaction for estrogen receptor ER-β, to the level comparable to that noted in placentas following at term deliveries.

Cells of amnion epithelium in peripheral portions of placentas originating from deliveries between 26th to 32nd week of pregnancy demonstrated optical density observed in the remaining two investigated groups of placentas.

Analysis of optical density in amnion epithelial cells with expression of estrogen receptor ER-β demonstrated no significant differences between centre and periphery of placenta.

In central portions of placentas optical density of the reaction product in syncytiotrophoblast cells following the test for estrogen receptor ER-β was analogous in all the investigated groups (Figure 4).

In peripheral portions of placentas optical density in syncytiotrophoblast cells with expression of estrogen receptor ER-β demonstrated a similar level in the experimental groups and a clearly lower level in the control group (Figure 6).

Comparison of optical densities in syncytiotrophoblast cells with expression of estrogen receptor ER-β disclosed no significant differences between experimental groups but they differed significantly in this respect from the control group.

4. Discussion

The presence of estrogens receptors in human tissues used to be evaluated by several investigators using various techniques, including RT-PCR, *in situ* hybridization and immunohistochemistry. The studies demonstrated their presence both in estrogen-dependent tissues and in tissues not recognized as estrogen-dependent, situated beyond the genital organs. Detailed recognition of estrogen receptor significance in organs and tissues functionally distant from generative functions is important for diagnosis and therapy of several diseases in men and women.

Expression of ER-α and ER-β has been examined in normal placentas and pre-term delivered placentas of women with diabetes mellitus and arterial hypertension. Pre-term placentas have demonstrated a clearly higher than normal level of ER-α, in line with the report of Schiessl et al. [26]. However, our observation pertained the central portion of placenta. Akram et al. [27] suggest the possible roles of ER and PR expression in the pathogenesis of both fetal growth restriction and preeclampsia, with lower levels contributing to higher likelihoods of disease outcome. ER-α is known to play a significant role in proliferation processes. High levels of the receptor may point to elevated requirements of estrogens. This may be linked to reconstruction of this portion of placenta. It should be kept in mind that in the third trimester of pregnancy and following the 32nd week of pregnancy in particular placenta may develop various abnormalities, frequently defined as senescence of placenta [28,29]. In general, the abnormalities are linked to degeneration of villi although they involve also interstitial fibrosis and swelling of sinusoids in the villi [30,31]. The more pronounced proliferation in this portion of placenta (unpublished data) may point to such alterations. However, we should remember that involvement of ER-β receptor is indispensable in terminal maturation of estrogen-dependent cells. In our studies expression of the receptor in placentas of experimental groups has been evidently higher than in normal placentas. Earlier a similar observation was published by Bukovsky et al. [32,33], who in addition documented the unique role of ER-β in the control of placental function. Since trophoblast represents the principal source of placental hormones, high expression of ER-α and ER-β in trophoblast cells may be linked to estrogen stimulation of placental hormone production.

The wide range of ER-β manifestation and its presence in organs which lack ER-α and in organs which till now have been thought to be untypical for effects of estrogens, such as lungs, intestines, urinary bladder, proves that ER-β does not just reproduce the classical receptor but that it carries its specific functions. A detailed recognition of significance of estrogen receptors in organs and tissues functionally distant from progenitor functions is important for diagnosis and therapy of multiple diseases both in women and men.

The observed augmented immunoreactivity of ER-β in our studies, e.g., decidual cells or in amnion epithelium should not be surprising. Taylor and Al-Azzawi [6] observed different distribution and expression of the receptor in resting and proliferating mammary gland. The same team demonstrated that in uterus ER-β was detected in cell nuclei of all stromal cells. This proves that ER-β may be of high significance in development of some organs.

According to our knowledge individual reports only pertained localization of estrogen receptors in human placenta and no data are available as to the cellular distribution of the receptors in vicinity of umbilical cord and, independently, at the periphery of placenta.

Both in central and peripheral placenta portions on its fetal side a nuclear and cytoplasmic localization of the receptors has been observed in variable intensities in various cells. Estrogen receptor ER-α has been noted in fibroblasts of amnion, in cell nuclei of cytotrophoblast cells of the chorionic plate. The cytoplasmic reaction has been detected in some stromal cells of chorionic trunks while nuclear and cytoplasmic reaction has been noted in endothelial cells of some large vessels. Within the villi a nuclear reaction has been documented in cytotrophoblast cells, nuclear and cytoplasmic reaction in vascular endothelium cells and a cytoplasmic reaction has been noted in Hofbauer's cells. Both nuclear and cytoplasmic reaction has been detected in decidua cells and fibroblasts while the nuclear reaction has characterized cytotrophoblast cells in basal membrane of the placenta. The observation has confirmed the earlier reports on the matter [6]. The data confirm that in certain tissues cells exhibit an exclusive expression of the nuclear receptor only while in other cells both the nuclear and the cytoplasmic forms of the receptor are produced.

In the analysed time periods of pregnancy no changes in localization of estrogen receptor ER-α have been disclosed in either central or peripheral portions of placenta but differences have been detected in the content of reaction product following the test for estrogen receptor

ER-α (Figures 1 and 3). Differences have also been noted in optical density of cells manifesting expression of estrogen receptor ER-α between centre and periphery of placentas in the analyzed groups.

On the fetal side, both in the central and peripheral portions of placenta, a nuclear reaction for estrogen receptor ER-β has been observed in epithelial cells of the amnion while both nuclear and cytoplasmic reaction has characterized fibroblasts of the amnion. In syncytiotrophoblast cells of chorionic plate a cytoplasmic reaction has been detected. In chorionic trunks and in villi nuclear reaction has been documented in endothelial cells and a cytoplasmic reaction in syncytiotrophoblast cells.

Within villi a cytoplasmic reaction has been seen also in Hofbauer's cells. Both nuclear and cytoplasmic reaction has been detected in decidua cells and in fibroblasts and a cytoplasmic reaction in syncytiotrophoblast cells in basal membrane of the placenta.

In analogy to the estrogen receptor ER-α, localization of estrogen receptor ER-β has shown no alterations in the studied periods on pregnancy. Even if in most tissues distribution of ER-β seems to be linked to expression of ER-α, expression of ER-β does not seem to be related to expression of ER-α. On the other hand, differences in optical density have been detected between cells with expression of estrogen receptor ER-β located in placenta centre as compared to placenta periphery and between groups of various duration of pregnancy (Figures 4 and 6). Moreover, differences have been documented in intensity of the reaction product following the test for estrogen receptor ER-β between central and peripheral portions of placentas in the analyzed groups.

Similarly to suggestions of Bukovsky et al. [32], our studies manifest that ER-α is sufficient for basic differentiation of estrogen-sensitive tissues. Lack of ER-β results in defects in morphology of terminally differentiated tissues and our results show that expression of ER-β is required for final differentiation of estrogen-dependent tissues. This applies to cytotrophoblast cells, decidua cells and Hofbauer's cells. If the placentas originating from pre-term deliveries contained degenerative lesions, the high level of ER-β expression in the above mentioned cells may indicate that highly advanced reparative processes develop in the placentas. Su et al. [33] hypothesize that endothelial ER-β appears to be a master regulator of prostanoid biosynthesis and contributes to high-resistance fetoplacental blood flow.

We were studied expression of estrogen receptors in term and pre-term delivered (induced by hypertension) placentas. Higher expression ER-α was observed in central zone of pre-term placentas than in term placentas. In peripheral there were no significant differences in ER-α content. ER-β expression was in pre-term placentas higher only in decidual cells and syncytiotrophoblast.

Its known that estrogen receptors play role in proliferation cells angiogenesis. Differences in ER contents in placentas from normal and pathological pregnancies may indicate on changes in estrogen synthesis or theirs placental transport, what may be reason of hypertension development.

5. References

[1] Tamura M, Nakayama T, Sato I, Sato N, Izawa N, Hishiki M, Mizutani Y, Furuya K, Yamamoto T. Haplotype-based case-control study of estrogen receptor alpha

(ESR1) gene and pregnancy-induced hypertension. Hypertens Res 2008;31:221-8.

[2] Rao BR. Isolation and characterization of an estrogen binding protein which may integrate the plethora of estrogenic actions in non-reproductive organs. J Steroid Biochem Mol Biol 1998;65:3-41.

[3] Zhu BT, Conney AH. Functional role of estrogen metabolism in target cells: review and perspectives. Carcinogenesis 1998;19:1-27.

[4] Mosselman S, Polman J, Dijkema R. ER beta: identification and characterization of a novel human estrogen receptor. FEBS Lett 1996;392:49-53.

[5] Pelletier G, Labrie C, Labrie F. Localization of oestrogen receptor alpha, oestrogen receptor beta and androgen receptors in the rat reproductive organs. J Endocrinol 2000;165:359-70.

[6] Taylor AH, Al-Azzawi F. Immunolocalisation of oestrogen receptor beta in human tissues. J Mol Endocrinol 2000;24:145-55.

[7] Tremblay GB, Tremblay A, Copeland NG, Gilbert DJ, Jenkins NA, Labrie F, Giguere V. Cloning, chromosomal localization, and functional analysis of the murine estrogen receptor beta. Mol Endocrinol 1997;11:353-65.

[8] Speroff L. A clinical understanding of the estrogen receptor. Ann NY Acad Sci 2000;900:26-39.

[9] Cheung E, Schwabish MA, Kraus WL. Chromatin exposes intrinsic differences in the transcriptional activities of estrogen receptors alpha and beta. EMBO J 2003;22:600-11.

[10] Matthews J, Gustafsson JA. Estrogen signaling: a subtle balance between ER alpha and ER beta. Mol Interv 2003;3:281-92.

[11] Moggs JG, Orphanides G. Estrogen receptors: orchestrators of pleiotropic cellular responses. EMBO Rep 2001;9:775-81.

[12] Ciana P, Raviscioni M, Mussi P, Vegeto E, Que I, Parker MG, Lowik C, Maggi A. In vivo imaging of transcriptionally active estrogen receptors. Nat Med 2003;9:82-6.

[13] Lemmen JG, Arends RJ, van Boxtel AL, van der Saag PT, van der Burg B. Tissue- and time-dependent estrogen receptor activation in estrogen reporter mice. J Mol Endocrinol 2004;32:689-701.

[14] Auboeuf D, Honig A, Berget SM, O'Malley BW. Coordinate regulation of transcription and splicing by steroid receptor coregulators. Science 2002;298:416-9.

[15] Klinge CM, Jernigan SC, Mattingly KA, Risinger KE, Zhang J. Estrogen response element-dependent regulation of transcriptional activation of estrogen receptors alpha and beta by coactivators and corepressors. J Mol Endocrinol 2004;33:387-410.

[16] Helske S, Vuorela P, Carpen O, Hornig C, Weich H, Halmesmaki E. Expression of vascular endothelial growth factor receptors 1, 2 and 3 in placentas from normal and complicated pregnancies. Mol Hum Reprod 2001;7:205–10.

[17] Kramer BW, Kaemmerer U, Kapp M, Herbst D, Marx A, Berg D, Groneck PA, Speer CP. Decreased expression of angiogenic factors in placentas with chorioamnionitis after preterm birth. Pediatr Res 2005;58:607-12.

[18] Kumazaki K, Nakayama M, Suehara N, Wada Y. Expression of vascular endothelial growth factor, placental growth factor, and their receptors Flt-1 and KDR in human placenta under pathologic conditions. Hum Pathol 2002;33:1069–77.

[19] Meher S, Duley L. Progesterone for preventing pre-eclampsia and its complications. Cochrane Database Syst Rev Oct 18 2006;(4):CD006175.

[20] Vuorela P, Carpen O, Tulppala M, Halmesmaki E. VEGF, its receptors and the tie receptors in recurrent miscarriage. Mol Hum Reprod 2000;6:276–82.
[21] Jobe SO, Ramadoss J, Koch JM, Jiang Y, Zheng J, Magness RR. Estradiol-17beta and its cytochrome P450- and catechol-O-methyltransferase-derived metabolites stimulate proliferation in uterine artery endothelial cells: role of estrogen receptor-alpha versus estrogen receptor-beta. Hypertension 2010;55:1005-11.
[22] Burton GJ, Charnock-Jones DS, Jauniaux E. Regulation of vascular growth and function in the human placenta. Reproduction 2009;138:895-902.
[23] Schiessl B, Innes BA, Bulmer JN, Otun HA, Chadwick TJ, Robson SC, Lash GE. Localization of angiogenic growth factors and their receptors in the human placental bed throughout normal human pregnancy. Placenta 200;30:79-87.
[24] Hall JM, McDonnell DP. The estrogen receptor beta-isoform (ERbeta) of the human estrogen receptor modulates ERalpha transcriptional activity and is a key regulator of the cellular response to estrogens and antiestrogens. Endocrinology 1999;140:5566-78.
[25] Knowlden JM, Gee JM, Robertson JF, Ellis IO, Nicholson RI. A possible divergent role for the oestrogen receptor alpha and beta subtypes in clinical breast cancer. Int J Cancer 2000;89:209-12.
[26] Schiessl B, Mylonas I, Hantschmann P, Kuhn C, Schulze S, Kunze S, Friese K, Jeschke U. Expression of endothelial NO synthase, inducible NO synthase, and estrogen receptors alpha and beta in placental tissue of normal, preeclamptic, and intrauterine growth-restricted pregnancies. J Histochem Cytochem 2005;53:1441–9.
[27] Akram SK, Sahlin L, Ostlund E, Hagenäs L, Fried G, Söder O. Placental IGF-I, estrogen receptor, and progesterone receptor expression, and maternal anthropometry in growth-restricted pregnancies in the Swedish population. Horm Res Paediatr 2011;75:131-7.
[28] Schneider H. Ontogenic changes in the nutritive function of the placenta. Placenta 1996;17:15-26.
[29] Smith SC, Baker PN, Symonds EM. Placental apoptosis in normal human pregnancy. Am J Obstet Gynecol 1997;177:57-65.
[30] Burton GJ, Reshetnikova OS, Milovanov AP, Teleshova OV. Stereological evaluation of vascular adaptations in human placental villi to differing forms of hypoxic stress. Placenta 1996;17:49-55.
[31] Iwahashi M, Ooshima A, Nakano R. Increase in the relative level of type V collagen during development and ageing of the placenta. J Clin Pathol 1996;49:916-9.
[32] Bukovsky A, Caudle MR, Cekanova M, Fernando RI, Wimalasena J, Foster JS, Henley DC, Elder RF. Placental expression of estrogen receptor beta and its hormone binding variant-comparison with estrogen receptor alpha and a role for estrogen receptors in asymmetric division and differentiation of estrogen-dependent cells. Reprod Biol Endocrinol Apr 15 2003;1:36.
[33] Bukovsky A, Cekanova M, Caudle MR, Wimalasena J, Foster JS, Henley DC, Elder RF. Expression and localization of estrogen receptor-alpha protein in normal and abnormal term placentae and stimulation of trophoblast differentiation by estradiol. Reprod Biol Endocrinol Feb 6 2003;1:13.
[34] Su EJ, Ernst L, Abdallah N, Chatterton R, Xin H, Monsivais D, Coon J, Bulun SE. Estrogen Receptor-β and Fetoplacental Endothelial Prostanoid Biosynthesis: A Link to Clinically Demonstrated Fetal Growth Restriction. J Clin Endocrinol Metab [First published ahead of print August 10, 2011 as doi:10.1210/lc.2011-1084.

Part 3

Immunology of Pregnancy

10

Placenta-Derived Exosomes and Their Role in the Immune Protection of the Fetus

Lucia Mincheva-Nilsson and Vladimir Baranov
Umeå University, Medical Faculty, Department of Clinical Microbiology Division of Clinical Immunology, Umeå, Sweden

1. Introduction

The mammalian pregnancy is an immunologic challenge to the maternal immune system. Considering the fact that transplant rejection is a well-defined immunologic phenomenon, the peaceful feto-maternal coexistence during mammalian pregnancy has been defined as "a paradox of nature" and puzzled immunologists for ages. In 1953, the immunologist and Nobel Prize laureate Sir Peter Medawar proposed that the maternal immune system is ignoring the fetus and defined his three well-known mechanisms for achievement of this: anatomical separation of the fetus and the mother, fetal antigenic immaturity and maternal inertness or indolence to the fetus (1). Although Medawar's proposal is still recognized and cited, it is only partly true and has been rightly revised in recent years. Today, it is well-proven that instead of being ignored, pregnancy is indeed recognized but tolerated by the maternal immune system, however, the responsible mechanisms for that remain unknown. The maternal-fetal interactions are highly complex and cannot be explained by, or subordinated to a single uniting theory of maternal tolerance to the fetus. In stead, multiple mechanisms, operating in concert at the systemic- as well as the local level are moulding the framework of successful pregnancy (reviewed in 2). Several of these mechanisms are mediated by the placenta, the key organ for successful mammalian reproduction (2).

Apart of its function as a hormonal, nutritional and oxygen provider of the fetus, placenta stands out as an important immunomodulatory organ actively secreting signal substances and factors that alter the maternal immune responses during pregnancy. Recently, several reports have shown that the human placenta participates in the feto-maternal cross-talk by secretion of nanometer-sized endosomally produced membrane-bound microvesicles (MV) called exosomes that act as fetal messengers and transfer packages of information to the maternal organism for adaptation to the ongoing pregnancy (3-8). The main focus of this chapter is on placenta-derived exosomes and their role in reproduction. A comparison to the placenta-released exosomes, larger placental microvesicles/microparticles, which are shed from the apical cell membrane of syncytiotrophoblast, will be presented and discussed. Initially, as a background, a short description of cell-cell communication and various microvesicles and their generation and roles is given.

2. Cell-cell communication – A basic necessity for all living organisms

Communication between individual cells is imperative for all living organisms. For a long time, cell communication was considered to be effectuated by three different ways: 1) by direct adhesion contacts between cells, such as receptor-ligand signalling and trogocytosis; 2) by soluble mediators, such as hormones, cytokines, chemokines and other signalling substances, bioactive ions and lipids, released in an autocrine and paracrine manner; and 3) by shuttling of information through intercellular channels called nanotubules (9, 10).

Recently, however, attention was focused on the fourth way of intercellular communication built on release and uptake of membrane-bound MVs. Communication by MV combines secretion of molecules with preservation of their membrane attachment and three-dimensional structure thus preserving the biologic activity of these molecules. Secreted or shed MVs execute cell-cell contact "by proxy", delivering information from a donor to a recipient/target cell in the near vicinity or at a distance. The exosomes are the smallest members of the MV family and the only ones that are produced in the endosomal compartment in multivesicular bodies (MVB) and secreted by exocytosis in the intercellular space, blood and various bodily fluids. The function of exosomes is highly diverse and dependent on the cells from which they originate. One very prominent feature is their immunomodulatory potency (reviewed in 9, 10). The rest of the MVs are larger in size and are produced and released from the plasma membrane by shedding or blebbing.

2.1 Microvesicles are everywhere

The existence of various membrane-bound MV in the intercellular space is easily observed by electron microscopy but for a long time was considered to be inert debris from cellular damage and of no importance. Thus, the first descriptions of exosome-like microvesicles during the 1980s by Heine et al. and Jonstone et al., who also named them exosomes and pointed out a biological role for these vesicles, were completely ignored (11-13). Only recently, less than 10 years ago were they rediscovered and identified as tools for intercellular communication. The realization that there are MVs produced by various cells and found in the blood and all bodily effusions in both health and disease has opened new perspectives in biology, understanding cell-cell communication and various biological mechanisms and their regulation. The MVs are a heterogeneous group, released both in health and disease. Their composition depends on and reflects the state of the cells that produce them and their physiological and/or pathogenetic roles are diverse depending on the donor cells, the recipient cells and in what environmental context they act. MVs are divided by size, morphology and mode of generation into (i) large MV, produced by budding of the cellular membrane, 0.1-2 μm in size with various roundish, oval or elongated shapes and (ii) small, nanosized (30-100 nm) MVs of endosomal origin called exosomes that will be separately discussed. The large MVs comprise two main types: those, produced by budding from the plasma membrane of living cells, including shed microvilli, called microvesicles or sometimes microparticles (14, 15); and those, produced by blebbing/fragmentation of the plasma membrane during the programmed dying of the cells, called apoptotic bodies/apoptotic blebs/apoptotic vesicles (16).

MVs, including exosomes, are produced by a vast variety of cells. Their "rediscovery" and upgrading in importance have caused a huge, exponential interest among scientists and literally an explosion of reports in the literature describing the MVs under different names, which can create confusion. In Table 1 a glossary with the names and definitions of various MV, described in the literature are given. The physical and morphological characteristics of the main MV types are presented in Table 2.

Microvesicle designation	**Definition**
Apoptotic bodies/blebs/ microvesicles/ microparticles	Microvesicles produced by fragmentation of the plasma membrane and the soma of dying cells. Carry membranal and cytosolic proteins and nucleic components like DNA.
Cardiosomes	Term used to designate exosomes produced by cardiomyocytes
Ectosomes	Vesicles shed from the plasma membrane of neutrophils and fibroblasts.
Endosomes	Nanovesicles (<100 nm in size) present in the multivesicular bodies (MVB), produced by inward budding of MVB's limiting membrane and secreted by exocytosis; called exosomes in secreted form.
Exovesicles	Microvesicles shed from the plasma membrane of dendritic cells.
Exosomes	30-100 nm-sized vesicles of endosomal origin secreted by fusion of MVB with the plasma membrane. Produced by a great variety of healthy and tumor cells and by the syncytiotrophoblast of the placenta.
Microparticles	Microvesicles shed by platelets, monocytes, and by the apical part of the syncytiotrophoblast plasma membrane, should not be confused with the syncytiotrophoblast-derived exosomes that are secreted through the exosomal compartment.
Microvesicles	The term is used in two ways: to designate all types of membrane-bound microvesicles, including exosomes and/or to designate larger microvesicles (>100 nm) produced and shed by the plasma membrane of normal and abnormal cells.
Prostasomes	Microvesicles of around 600 nm to 1μm in size, produced by shedding from the plasma membrane of normal prostate gland epithelium. Presence of prostasomes in prostate secretion is associated with fertility. However, the term has been used in a substantial amount of publications to designate exosomes.
Prominosomes	Microvesicles produced from the plasma membrane of the stem cells in the neural tube and the brain
STBM	Syncytiotrophoblast microvesicles or microparticles produced by the apical part of the plasma membrane, see microparticle definition above.
Tolerosomes	Exosomes, produced by the epithelial cells in the gastro-intestinal tract, involved in oral tolerance
Vexosomes	Microvesicles/exosomes engineered in vitro to carry viral vectors for gene therapy

Table 1. Glossary for terms and definitions used in scientific publication for description of microvesicles

Characteristics	Exosomes	Microvesicles/ Microparticles	Shed microvilli	Apoptotic bodies/vesicles
Size	30-100 nm	0.1-2 μm	> 400 nm	100–600to700 nm
Density in sucrose	1.13 - 1.19 g/ml	Undetermined	Undetermined	1.16-1.28 g/ml
Sedimentation (g)	100,000 -110,000	10,000 -100,000	10,000	1,500 - 100,000
Morphological shape	Cup shaped, electron translucent	Various shapes, electron-dense and/or electron translucent	Various shapes, round, elongated and cylinder-like	Irregular and heterogeneous in shape
Lipid membrane composition	Cholesterol-, sphingomyelin-, and ceramide-rich lipid rafts, expose phosphatidylserine	Expose phosphatidylserine, some enriched in cholesterol and diacylglycerol, some undetermined	Undetermined	Undetermined
Specific marker(s) for identification	Tetraspanins (CD63, CD9, CD83), ESCRT complex members (Alix, TSG101)	Integrins, selectins, CD40 and others, depending on the cell type	Various, depending on the cell type	Histones, DNA
Origin in the cell	Endosomal compartment - multivesicular bodies (MVB)	Plasma membrane	Plasma membrane	Fragments of dying cells, undetermined
Mechanism of sorting	Ceramide and ubiquitin dependent	Unknown	Unknown	Fragments of dying cells, undetermined
Intracellular storage	Yes	No	No	No
Mode of release/secretion	Exocytosis by fusion of MVB with the plasma membrane	Plasma membrane blebbing	Plasma membrane blebbing	Plasma membrane blebbing and cellular fragmentation

Adapted from ref. 10 with permission of Expert Reviews Ltd

Table 2. Some of the main characteristics of different types of microvesicles.*

2.2 Exosomes: definition and biogenesis

The exosomes are the smallest MVs that are produced in the multivesicular bodies (MVB) in the endosomal compartments of individual cells and secreted into the extracellular space by exocytosis. The exosomes are membrane bound nanometer-sized vesicles that carry a variety of proteins on their surface as well as inside, mRNA and microRNA and can be compared to parcels sent as "mail" between cells. The late endosomal compartment, where they are generated, can be viewed as "the post office". Each exosome carry proteins on its surface that serve as addresses of the sender and the recipient cell. Recent accumulating evidence shows that this "mail" can be powerful and transforming, determining the fate of the recipient cell.

The current definition of exosomes is: secreted membrane-bound nanovesicles that carry the following characteristics: 1) cup-shaped form, 2) 30-100 nm size, 3) tetraspanin presence in their lipid rich membrane, 4) buoyant density of 1.13-1,19 g/ml on sucrose gradient and 5) endosomal origin (9, 10).

The suggested pathway of biogenesis of exosomes separates them from all other known MVs. The exosomes are produced in the late endosomal compartment by inward budding of the limiting tetraspanin- and lipid-rich membrane of MVB and contain surface-bound and cytosolic proteins and RNA molecules. They are released when the MVB membrane fuses with the cellular plasma membrane and the MVB content of exosomes is emptied into the extracellular space. A detail schematic presentation of exosome biogenesis is shown in Figure 1B. There are two major pathways by which proteins are sorted to the MVB membrane that by inward budding becomes exosomal membrane: (i) protein recycling by endocytosis and transport of plasma membrane-expressed proteins to the early recycling endosomal compartment and from there to the late endosomal compartment and eventually to the MVB ending up on exosomes and (ii) direct transportation of proteins from the Golgi complex to the MVB where they are inserted into the MVB limiting membrane and further become expressed on the exosomal membrane as exosomes are produced in the MVB by inward budding. Previously, MVB were solely considered as an intermediate stage in the maturation of endosomes to lysosomes and were ascribed to be a "garbage station" of the cell - a dustbin for proteins aimed for destruction. Today it is known that instead of the lysosomal protein-destruction route, MVB can take an alternative route, moving to the plasma membrane and by fusion with it releasing their nanovesicle cargo as exosomes in the extracellular space. Thus, MVB are endosomal cellular organelles situated at a cross road in the cell where the fate of the proteins sorted to the MVB is decided - secretion by exosomes or degradation in lysosomes. Accordingly, two types of MVB have been suggested - degradative MVB taking the lysosomal pathway and exocytotic MVB involved in the secretion of exosomes. The process of sorting proteins to degradative MVB involves a multiprotein network called endosomal-sorting complexes required for transport (ESCRT) and ubiquitinylation process that tags with ubiquitin both cell surface and cytosolic proteins targeted for lysosomal degradation (17, 18). At present, the mechanism underlying the exocytotic MVB trafficking to the plasma membrane is less clear. The transmembrane protein TSAP6 is suggested to regulate exosome formation and Rab11, a member of the small GTPase family and calcium are considered to participate in the docking and fusion of exocytotic MVB with the plasma membrane (19, 20). Two pathways for protein sorting for exosome secretion have been suggested - the ESCRT multiprotein complex and an alternative ubiquitin-independent pathway based on sphingomyelin metabolites such as ceramide (18, 21). More studies are needed to establish the link between ubiquitin, phospholipids and ESCRT proteins and their role in the biogenesis of exosomes.

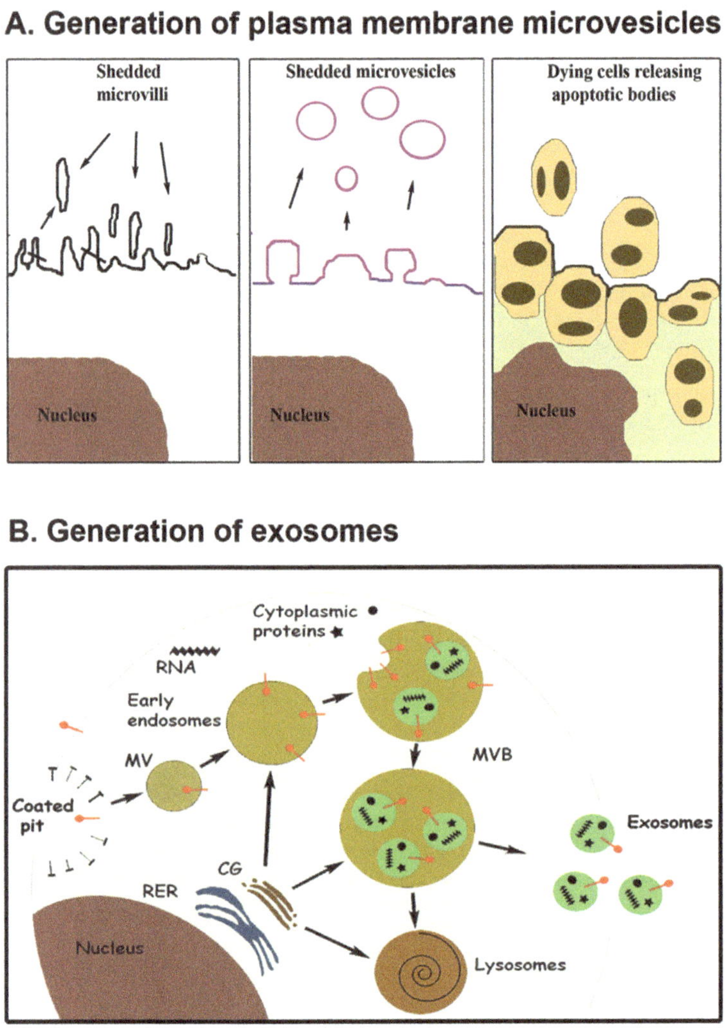

Adapted from reference #10 with permission of Expert Reviews Ltd.

Fig. 1. Generation of different microvesicles and their main characteristics. A) Shed microvilli, microvesicles and apoptotic bodies are all generated by the plasma membrane. B) Exosomes are generated in the endosomal compartment and carry both recycled proteins and proteins produced in the rough endoplasmic reticulum (RER) and directly sorted to the multivesicular bodies (MVB) from the Complex Golgi (CG). Note how the proteins are internalised in coated pits or inserted in the limiting membrane of the MVB and how exosomes are produced by inward budding of the limiting membrane - a way that ensures the same orientation of the membrane bound proteins on the exosomal membrane as that on the plasma membrane of the cell. The exosome-filled MVB are either fused with the plasma membrane to release exosomes or sent to lysosomes for degradation. The mechanisms deciding excretion or degradation of MVB are at present not known.

2.3 Exosomes: morphology, general biochemical composition and suggested roles

Electron microscopy is the method of choice for studies of exosomes biogenesis and morphology. Visualized *in situ* the exosomes are uniform spherical vesicles of 50-90 nm in size situated within the lumen of MVB. The electron microscopy image of isolated exosomes is different- the size varies between 30 to 100 nm, which is the upper size limit of exosomes and they have a typical cup-shaped form that is their hallmark. An illustration of isolated exosomes showing the typical heterogeneity in size and the cup shape is given in Figure 2A. The reason for the cap shape appearance is not known, but might be a consequence of the isolation procedure. The exosomal membrane is detergent and low temperature resistant and consists of lipid-rich bilayer of cholesterol, sphingolipids and tetraspanins where proteins with transmembrane or glycosylphosphinositol linkage are inserted.

Exosomes consist of proteins and RNA. The composition of the exosomes depends on the cells that have produced them and can vary even within the same cells, depending on their current differentiation and activation status. Thus exosomes reflect their donors and can influence their recipients. There is a conserved set of proteins common to all exosomes - cytosolic proteins such as tubulin, actin, actin-binding proteins, annexins, Rab proteins, heat shock proteins, signal transduction kinases, heterodimeric G proteins and the ESCRT members ALIX and TSG101. Common proteins expressed on the exosomal surface are adhesion molecules such as integrins and ICAM-1, MHC class I, and the tetraspanins like CD9, CD63, CD81 and CD82 (22).

There are many advantages of exosome-mediated cell-cell communication that can be listed as follows: (i) preservation of the 3D structure of the transported proteins and thus their biological activity; (ii) independence of cell-cell contact for signal delivery; (iii) independence of de novo synthesis; (iv) packages of carried molecules with a lower mobility and a higher concentration of the carried molecules; (v) biological effect at a distance.

Exosomes have been ascribed a variety of biological functions such as intracellular signalling, antigen presentation, immune regulation, receptor-ligand interactions, pro- and anti-apoptotic effects, delivery of proteins to plasma membrane of recipient cells thus changing their adhesive properties, transport of bioactive mRNA and microRNA, thus regulating gene expression and reprogramming recipient cells.

Exosomes can be divided into two major groups in relation to the immune defence system - exosomes with immunoactivating properties and those that are tolerogenic or immunosuppressive. In general, exosomes produced by immune cells such as antigen presenting cells (macrophages, dendritic cells and B cells) are immunoactivating. They can activate in various ways such as (i) directly by functioning as antigen presenters by proxy or indirectly by initiating immune response via dendritic cells that take up the exosomes and process the antigens carried by them; (ii) by activation T helper cells to cytokine production; (iii) by boostering cytotoxicity, antibody and cytokine production or priming of T cells (reviewed in 9, 10, 23). Interestingly, the cytolytic molecules perforin, granzyme and granulysin as well as FasL that are components of the cytotoxic machinery of cytotoxic T- and NK cells, are carried by exosome-like specialised vesicles in secretory lysosomes (24). The exosomes produced by epithelial cells and by the great majority of tumors are immune inhibitory. Normal epithelium secretes low amounts of exosomes that exert a mild immunosuppressive effect promoting homeostasis and immune tolerance. In contrast,

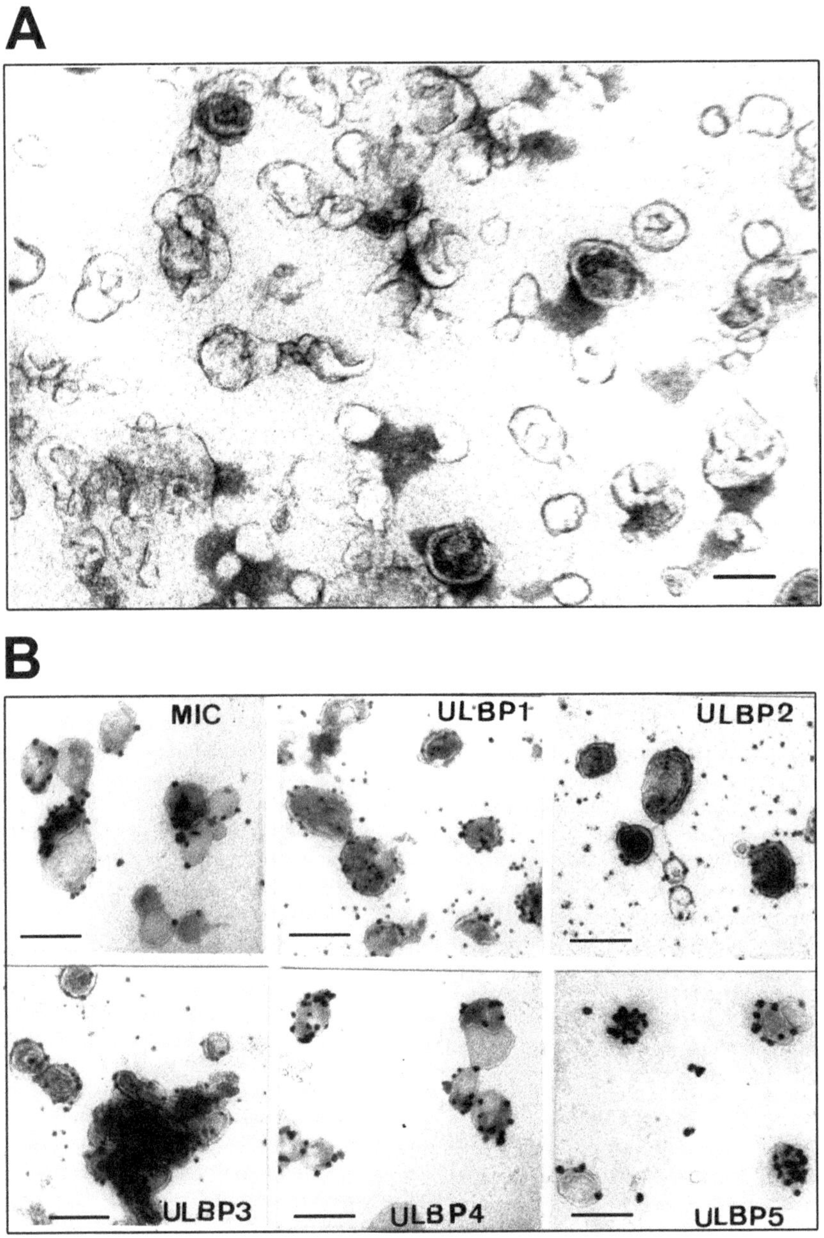

Bars represent 100 nm.
Reproduced from reference #10 with permission of Expert Reviews Ltd.

Fig. 2. Isolated exosomes from supernatants of placental explant cultures. A) Negative contrast staining showing their size and the typical cup-shaped form. B) Isolated exosomes stained with antibodies against the NKG2D ligands MIC and ULBP1-2 and immunogold.

epithelialy derived tumors such as various carcinomas secrete high amounts of immunosuppressive exosomes that carry immunoinhibitory molecules, proapoptotic molecules and receptor ligands that serve as decoys, dysregulating normal immune responses and impairing the immune system of the host. Thus the net effect of tumor exosomes originating from mammary, lung, colon, prostate and ovarian cancers is a powerful immune inhibition promoting the primary tumor to establish itself and spread metastases (25). Similar to tumors, placenta-derived exosomes, produced by the syncytiotrophoblast are suppressive and able to modulate the maternal immune system.

3. Human syncytiotrophoblast-a source of plasma membrane-derived shed microvesicles and endosomally secreted exosomes

The human syncytiotrophoblast, covering the placental villi, is the most important cell type of the human placenta with several functions such as being (i) the chief regulator of oxygen and nutritional and waste transport between the fetus and the mother necessary for fetal survival and growth; (ii) the site of synthesis of a variety of proteins - such as steroid and placental protein hormones, adhesion molecules and matrix metalloproteases, signal substances, and immunomodulatory molecules of crucial importance for the pregnancy success (26, 27). The syncytiotrophoblast is responsible for and carries out the "cross talk" between the mother and the fetus during pregnancy.

The human syncytiotrophoblast comprise a continuous layer of multinucleated finally differentiated trophoblast that makes a syncytium covering completely the multitudinous chorionic villi. The free apical part of the syncytium that is in direct contact with the maternal blood, is richly covered with numerous highly pleomorphic microvilli and branched surface projections suggesting a high mobility of the apical part of the syncytioplasm (27, 28). Comprehensive electron microscopic studies have shown that there is a constitutive shedding activity of plasma membrane-bound microvesicles and even whole microvilli from the apical syncytiotrophoblast surface membrane to the maternal blood. This normal shedding activity becomes forcefully enhanced by stress enforced by various pathologic pregnancy conditions, the most well-known and studied being preeclampsia (29). Besides the intensive shedding activity from the apical membrane surface the syncytiotrophoblast has an elaborate endosomal compartment and a high protein turnover activity. Scattered between the villi are numerous bristle-coated pits or caveolae, lipid-rich spots on the plasma membrane, associated with membrane molecule uptake and recycling. The syncytioplasm is very rich in free ribosomes and rough endoplasmic reticulum with dilated cisterns, Golgi complexes distributed at intervals in the syncytium and numerous mitochondria and tubular and numerous endosomal membranes and multivesicular bodies, all characteristic of vigorous protein synthesis and a well-developed endosomal compartment. The features of active protein synthesis, protein uptake and recycling and the elaborate MVB-rich endosomal compartment warrant for biogenesis and release of exosomes. Numerous nanometer-sized vesicles are seen in the MVB that reach the apical plasma membrane and open up to release their content. Thus, in addition to MV shedding from the plasma membrane, the syncytiotrophoblast of the human placenta simultaneously and constitutively releases exosomes.

The first provided ultrastructural evidence of biogenesis of exosomes in human placenta was shown for FasL and reported by Frängsmyr et al. (4). Using immunoelectron microscopy (IEM), it was shown that expression of FasL was completely devoid from the syncytioplasm and in stead directed to the MVB in the syncytiotrophoblast and secreted by exosomes of 60-100 nm in size (4). Furthermore, the NKG2D receptor ligands MHC class I chain related antigens A and B (MICA/B) and the human retinoic acid early transcript 1 (RAET1) proteins, also known as UL-16 binding protein (ULBP) 1-5, were used as marker molecules of the endosomal compartment in studies of the biogenesis of exosomes in the human syncytiotrophoblast (7, 8). Representative micrographs shown in Figure 3, illustrate MICA/B molecule expression in human syncytiotrophoblast. As can be seen in Figure 3A, besides surface expression these molecules are sorted to numerous MVB at different levels in the cytoplasm. Frequently, fusion of MVB with the apical microvillous membrane of the syncytiotrophoblast and release of microvesicles was seen (Figure 3B).

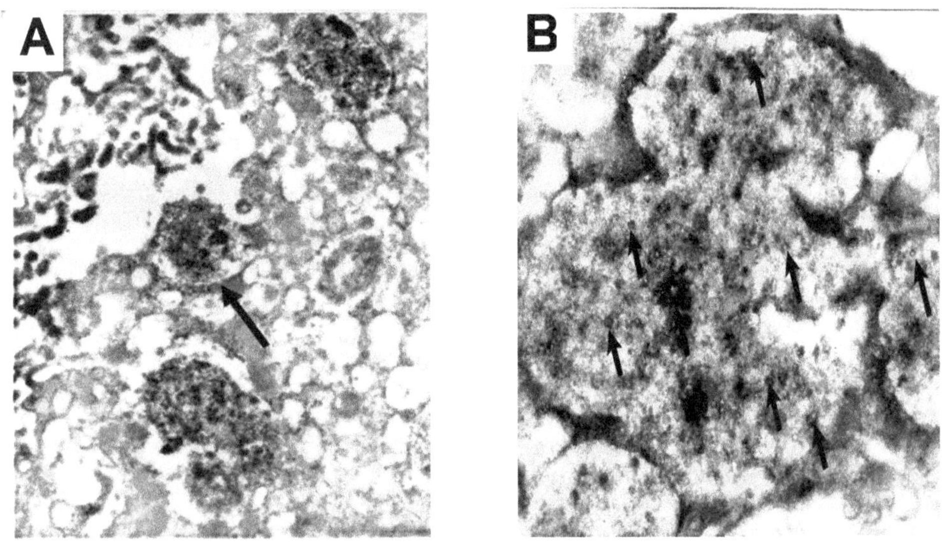

MICA/B: MHC class.I chain-related molecules A and B; MVB: multivesicular body.
Magnification: A) X 18,000; B) X 25,000.

Fig. 3. Biogenesis of MICA/B-expressing exosomes in the syncytiotrophoblast of human early normal placenta. A) Electron micrograph showing the apical microvillous surface and MVB stained with anti-MICA/B-antibodies. One of the MVB (arrow) is opening and releasing exosomes in the intervillous space. B) A magnification of MVB filled with exosomes and stained for MICA/B. Note also the staining of the limiting membrane. Arrows point at exosomes.

A logical question is how is it decided if a protein will be sorted to the endosomal compartment for exosome secretion? From our studies of exosome biogenesis in the syncytiotrophoblast (4, 7, 8) we propose two possible ways: (i) Proteins with lysine residues in their cytoplasmic tail such as MICB, FasL, ULBP4 and 5 are controlled by ubiquitinylation and will be sorted preferentially to MVB (30, 31). In support of this suggestion, we have reported that members of the ESCRT complex localize in the syncytiotrophoblastic MVB (8). (ii)By contrast, glycosylphosphoinositol (GPI)-linked proteins, such as ULBP1-3 and the transmembrane MICA are preferentially expressed in lipid rafts at the cell surface and by recycling can be sorted to the MVB. Such lipid raft domains have been proposed to support sorting of proteins to MVB and formation of exosomes (32, 33). In our studies (4, 7, 8) we found frequently lipid rafts and caveolae in the apical surface of the syncytiotrophoblast. In summary, we can conclude that both plasma membranal and exosomal expression of proteins is occurring in the human syncytiotrophoblast. The rich endosomal compartment with numerous MVB and the frequent signs of exosome release from the apical surface suggests that exosomal secretion is a constitutive feature of the villous syncytiotrophoblast.

The next question is if there is an advantage of exosomal secretion in pregnancy? Our studies of apoptosis-inducing molecules and the stress-inducible NKG2D ligands in human placenta clearly show that exosomal secretion is chosen over plasma membranal expression of these molecules and this choice is of crucial importance for the protection of the fetal allograft. If the apoptosis-inducing FasL was expressed on the cell surface, it would be immediately cleaved by the richly expressed placental matrix metalloproteases. The resulting soluble FasL would be easily involved in induction and promotion of unwanted inflammatory responses at the fetomaternal interface in a similar way as it promotes autoimmune inflammation and hypergammaglobulinemia in a systemic lupus erythematosus-like syndrome (34). In stead, exosomal FasL expression provides a membrane-bound form of the molecule that induced apoptosis of activated immune cells and thus promotes immunotolerance (4-6, 34). Furthermore, a strategy of releasing NKG2D ligands by placental exosomes would be a decoy mechanism downregulating the activating NK cell receptor NKG2D; by contrast a membranal expression of these molecules would make the villous syncytiotrophoblast a target for attack by NKG2D receptor-bearing maternal cytotoxic T and NK cells (7, 8). In conclusion, (i) the syncytiotrophoblast of the human placenta is a site of exosomal biogenesis and release; (ii) the exosomal secretion of important immunomodulatory molecules promotes the survival of the fetal allograft and is thus preferentially used by the human placenta as a fetal immune escape mechanism. In addition, the human syncytiotrophoblast is a vigorous protein produced with a MVB-rich endosomal compartment and thus an excellent model for studies of exosome biogenesis *per se*.

4. Placenta-derived exosomes: composition, structure and function

4.1 Methodological considerations in experimental work with exosomes

The difficulties in characterizing placental exosomes so far lie in the fact that the villous syncytiotrophoblast, which is the main exosome producer, simultaneously sheds microvesicles, sometimes called STBM or microparticles, from the apical plasma membrane. In several studies, a crude bulk of ultracentrifuged pellets are analysed as exosomes. It is important to realize that such pellets contain all kinds of large MVs, apoptotic bodies, other particles and protein precipitates together with exosomes. Thus, it is of extreme importance to pay attention to the isolation procedure when separating placental exosomes for characterization of their biochemical composition and functions. Firstly, it is absolutely necessary to apply a continuous sucrose gradient (floating density 1.13-1.19) or a sucrose cushion to ensure enrichment and collection of "maximally pure" exosomes. Secondly, when immunoflow cytometry is used for phenotypic characterization of molecules on the exosomal surface, an indirect approach by loading of the exosomes on beads should be applied, since most of the fluorescence-activated cell sorters have a discriminative capacity of around 300 nm and thus will exclude free unbound exosomes run directly in the cell sorter. Thirdly, the isolated fraction that is believed to be exosomes must be confirmed by analysing exosome specific markers, such as CD63, CD81, TSG101 and Alix.

4.2 Exosomal structure and composition

So far, studies of isolated placental exosomes have been performed on populations separated from placental explant cultures (7, 8) and peripheral blood of pregnant women (4, 5). Figure 2 illustrates syncytiotrophoblast-derived placental exosomes visualized by negative contrast staining and immunoelectron microscopy. The morphology is the typical cup shape and the size varies between 40 and 90 nm (Figure 2A). IEM reveals that they express the tetraspanins marker CD63 and the placenta-specific marker placental alkaline phosphatase, indicating their placental origin. In contrast to other exosomes, the placental exosomes are devoid of classical MHC molecules. Instead, they carry on their surface the stress inducible non-classical MHC class I chain-related molecules MICA/B and RAET1/ULBP1-5, ligands of the major cytotoxic receptor NKG2D (7, 8 Figure 2B). Besides the NKG2D ligands, placental exosomes express proapoptotic molecules such as FasL, TRAIL, and PD-L1 (3-6). In addition, they display a membranal expression of the regulatory cytokine TGFβ1. Recently, we performed proteomic analysis on placental explant culture-derived exosomes. An illustration of the major protein components are presented in Figure 4. In principal, the protein content can be divided into two compartments: proteins present on the exosomal membrane and those, entrapped in the exosomal lumen. The proteomic analysis revealed cytosolic proteins involved in biosynthesis and degradation, intracellular transport, fusion and signal transduction, heat-shock proteins and chaperons, and enzymes and ESCRT-associated proteins associated with exosome formation such as TSG101, Alix, vascular sorting protein 29 and charged MVB protein 1B and 4B (9, 10).

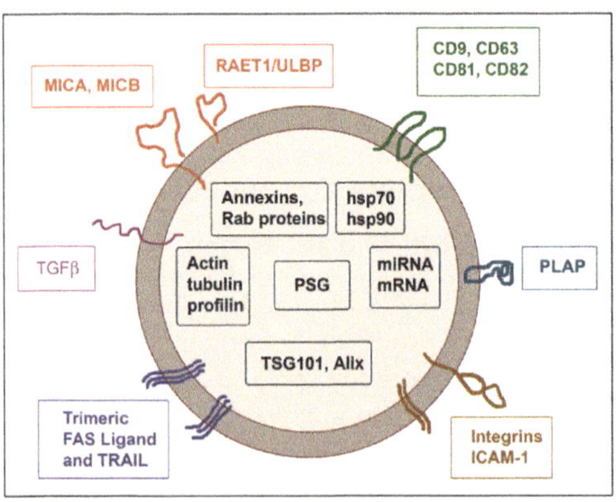

Human placental exosome-associated proteins

- Fas Ligand
- TRAIL
- MHC class I chain related proteins A and B
- Retinoic acid early transcript 1 (RAET1) proteins/ULBP1-5
- TGFβ1
- Placental alkaline phosphatase
- Placental leucine aminopeptidase
- Pregnancy specific glycoprotein 3
- Trophoblast glycoprotein 5T4

Fig. 4. Schematic presentation of a placental exosome and a list of some proteins, specific for placental exosomes.

Exosomes can transport selected mRNA and miRNA molecules from donor to recipient cells and thus influence and genetically reprogram recipient cells and regulate their intracellular metabolic pathways. So far, there are few studies of RNA content in placenta and placental exosomes. The first detailed miRNA study of placenta revealed that most placenta specific miRNAs were localized at a miRNA cluster on chromosome 19 (35) and were up- regulated during placental development. Six novel miRNA were identified and 4 of them were placenta-specific. Placenta-specific miRNA was also identified in plasma from pregnant women (36). Urged by these reports, exploration of miRNA content in placenta exosomes was undertaken. The trophoblast-derived cell line BeWo was used as a source of exosomes. Two placenta-specific miRNAs, MIR517A and MIR21 were found in the exosome-enriched supernatant fraction from BeWo cultures. A possible involvement of MIR17A in the regulation of TNF signal transduction has been suggested. This is the first and so far only mi RNA investigation of trophoblast-derived exosomes. Thus, these results need to be repeated, confirmed and extended to exosomes from placental cultures and normal and pathologic pregnancies at different times of gestation and of placenta differentiation. Thus, placental exosome-derived mRNAs and miRNAs and their capacity to enter and reprogram maternal cells awaits to be elucidated in future studies.

4.3 What do placental exosomes do?

As mentioned previously, the importance of enriching maximally pure exosome fractions for functional studies cannot be overemphasized. In numerous studies a mixture of several microvesicle subpopulations is phenotypically and functionally analysed. Such studies are difficult to interpret and reproduce and thus must be left out when discussing the function of placental exosomes. Thus, the information, reviewed here is taken from a limited number of investigations with "maximally pure" exosome fractions isolated from peripheral blood of pregnant women (4-8) and placental explant cultures. These studies can be summarized as follows: (i) Placental exosomes are able to impair T-cell immune responses by downregulation of the intracellular signalling through the CD3-z chain of the accessory molecule CD3 and the enzyme Janus kinase 3 (JAK3). (ii) NKG2D ligand-bearing placental exosomes act as decoy and downregulate the major activating NK cell receptor NKG2D on cytotoxic T-, NK- and γδT cells with a consequent impairment of the maternal cytotoxicity and protection of the fetal allograft against maternal cytotoxic immune attack. (iii) Placental exosomes carry the apoptosis-inducing molecules FasL, TRAIL and PD-L1 in active functional form that is able to induce apoptosis in activated immune cells. Thus it is clear that placental exosomes are involved in the control of critical immune mechanisms such as cytotoxicity, T cell response and apoptosis in the local vicinity and /or at a distance from the feto-maternal interface. These functions define the placental exosomes as immunosuppressive, using in a redundant way a number of mechanisms that inhibit the function of the maternal immune system during pregnancy and promote the survival of the fetal allograft. In other words, placental exosomes are important players in the establishment of the maternal tolerance towards the fetus.

5. Exosomes in amniotic fluid

Often, when discussing placental exosomes in pregnancy, exosomes in amniotic fluid are mentioned and discussed in the same terms as placental exosomes. However, placental exosomes and amniotic exosomes differ in origin and function and are thus different entities. The placenta specific exosomes are syncytiotrophoblast-derived and are secreted in the intervillous space of the chorionic villi directly into the maternal blood and influence the physiological adjustment of the maternal body to the ongoing pregnancy. The amniotic fluid stays in the amniotic cavity enveloped in the amniotic membranes and thus does not enter the maternal circulation. The fetus constantly produces amniotic fluid, most of which is fetal urine, and constantly swallows amniotic fluid throughout the pregnancy. At any developmental stage of pregnancy the amount of amniotic fluid is determined by the balance between these two processes. Convincing evidence has shown that the main source of amniotic fluid exosomes is the fetal kidney and the fetal urinary system. These exosomes carry on their surface CD24 as their specific address marker, annexin-1 and kidney markers such as aguaprin-2 and have a similar composition to exosomes from the urine of newborn infants (37, 39). It is logical to assume that their presence in the amniotic fluid is because of the fetal urine production rather than a special role in the immunomodulation of the maternal immune system. Amniotic exosomes have their niche and importance in monitoring the prenatal development of the renal system and in developing of prenatal diagnosis of kidney diseases and genetic malformations in the fetal kidney and urinary tract.

6. On the role of placental exosomes in human pregnancy: synthesis of facts and a proposed exosomal protective mechanism of action

Summarizing the current scientific data, there is no doubt that the syncytiotrophoblast of the human placenta continuously and constitutively produces and secretes exosomes. The placental exosomes are: (i) endosomally produced in the multivesicular bodies of the syncytiotrophoblast and released directly into the blood and systemic circulation of the pregnant women; (ii) pluripotent and immunosuppressive, carrying important bioactive molecules such as stress-inducible ligands, proapoptotic molecules, cytokines, other signaling molecules, mRNA and miRNA, thus being able to operate through different mechanisms and transform/reprogram recipient cells; (iii) acting by proxy to modulate the immune response of the mother locally or at a distance thus promoting maternal immune tolerance to the fetal allograft. A schematic drawing, suggesting two mechanisms that might be used by placental exosomes to alter the maternal immune response at the feto-maternal interface are presented in Figure 5. As can be seen, exosomes carrying NKG2D ligands can act as a decoy selectively downregulating cytotoxicity by internalization of the NKG2D receptor on cytotoxic T and NK cells without affecting the cytolytic machinery of the effector cells. Exosomes, bearing FasL, and/or TRAIL can induce apoptosis directed only towards activated Fas-expressing immune cells that might comprise a threat to the ongoing pregnancy. Furthermore, the exosomes, secreted by the syncytiotrophoblast to the maternal blood are most abundant in the intervillous space at the immediate vicinity of the chorion villi, where the highest risk for maternal attack and consequently the highest protection against the maternal immune cells is needed. The concentration of placental exosomes decreases with increasing distance from the placenta. Thus, the continuous secretion of exosomes by the syncytiotrophoblast creates an exosomal concentration gradient where the maternal immunosuppression and therefore immune protection of the fetus is strongest at the border between the syncytiotrophoblast and the maternal blood preventing a direct attack by the maternal immune cells. Moreover, the exosome turnover is very short, therefore the immunosuppressive influence of the placental exosomes would be "fading away" as the maternal blood leaves the placenta and enters the systemic maternal circulation. This could be one of the explanations why, although the maternal immune system during pregnancy is downregulated, it is not completely blunted. Pregnant women are more sensitive to infections during pregnancy; however, they are still able to mount a modified immune response. The temporarily "semi- immunocompromized" maternal defence during pregnancy is the price humans have to pay for the elaborate hemochorial mode of reproduction, required to provide the huge amount of oxygen and nourishment necessary for the fetal development of the highly complicated and sophisticated human brain. Several mechanisms work in concert to meet this challenge and modify the maternal immune system during pregnancy with a minimized loss of ability to fight infections and convincing evidence suggests that secretion of placental exosomes is one of them. The syncytiotrophoblast, producing and releasing exosomes puts up a shield around the hemochorial placenta to protect it against the risk of maternal immune attack that ultimately will damage the fetus. One can imagine that the fetus, together with the placenta, is "embedded" in a cloud of exosomes that creates a beneficial and protective milieu for the fetus to grow and develop.

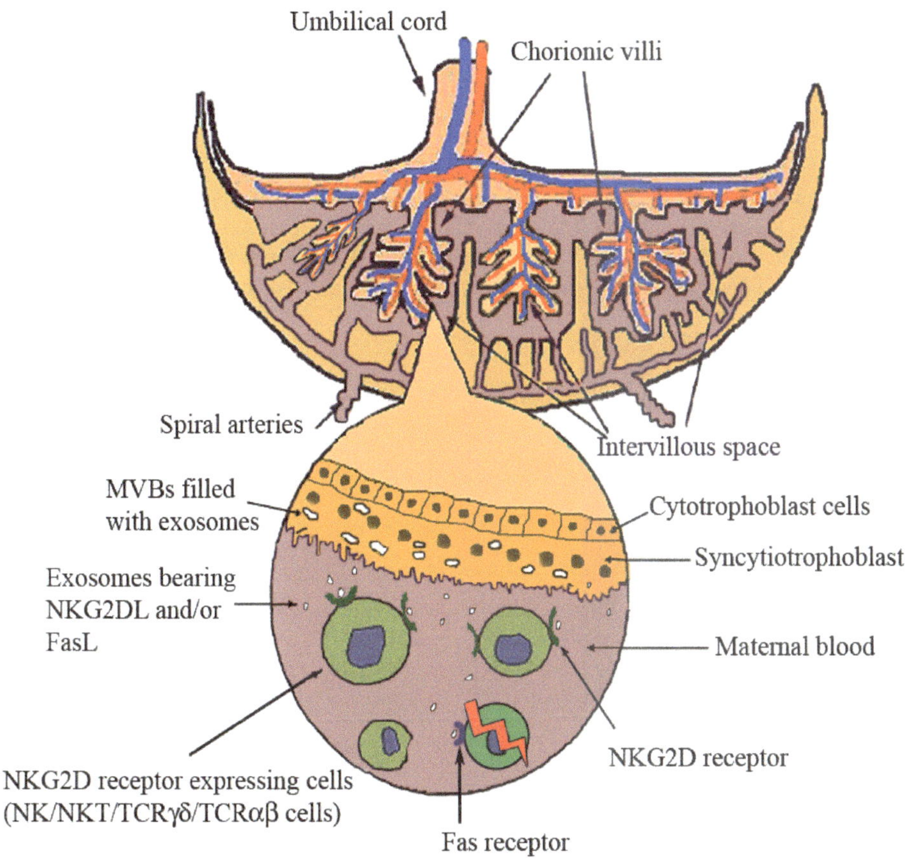

Adapted from reference #10 with permission of Expert Reviews Ltd.

Fig. 5. Schematic drawing of the human hemochorial placenta and a scenario suggesting how the pluripotent syncytiotrophoblast-released exosomes function at the feto-maternal border by down regulating the NKG2D receptor on cytotoxic lymphocytes and/or inducing apoptosis of activated Fas-expressing lymphocytes.

7. Future perspectives

The exosome research in reproduction is just at its beginning and it is logical to expect that more exosome-carried molecules and mechanisms of action will be revealed in the near future. Closing this chapter I would like to outline some issues that await elucidation. The first one is a detailed differential characterization of the placental exosomes, nanovesicles secreted through the endosomal compartment of the syncytiotrophoblast, in contrast to MV/STBM, larger vesicles shed by blebbing from the apical surface of the syncytiotrophoblast. Today, many investigations are done on mixture of exosomes and MV/STBM giving results difficult to interpret, reproduce or compare. The importance of adequate techniques for isolation of these two separate vesicle entities cannot be overestimated. Another issue is to identify and understand the exact mechanisms that govern exosome biogenesis *per se* both in general and in the placenta. Why and how do some MVB become degradative and sort to lysosomes for destruction whilst others are transported to the plasma membrane to release exosomes by exocytosis? The mRNA and miRNA content in placental exosomes has just started to shape up and needs confirmation and additional analyses to find a consensus. Finally, the role of exosomes in pathological pregnancies and related diseases, recurrent abortions, infertility and IVF failure awaits evaluation. Gaining knowledge in these areas will open possibilities for novel, exosome-based treatments of pregnancy failure and infertility. As for now, there is enough convincing evidence that the constitutively secreted immunosuppressive placental exosomes during normal pregnancy mount a protective exosomal shield around the feto-placental unit and comprise one of the keys for pregnancy success in human reproduction.

8. References

[1] Billingham RE, Medawar PD. "Actively required tolerance" of foreign cells. Nature 172, 603-606 (1953).

[2] Mincheva-Nilsson L. Immune cells and molecules in pregnancy: friends or foes to the fetus? *Expert Rev. Clin. Immunol.* 2(3), 447-460 (2006).

[3] Abrahams VM, Straszewski-Chavez SL, Guller S, *et al.* First trimester trophoblast cells secrete Fas ligand which induces immune cell apoptosis. *Mol. Hum. Reprod.* 10, 55-63 (2004).

[4] Frängsmyr L, Baranov V, Nagaeva O, *et al.* Cytoplasmic microvesicular form of Fas ligand in human early placenta: switching the tissue immune privilege hypothesis from cellular to vesicular level. *Mol. Hum. Reprod.* 11, 35-41 (2005).

[5] Taylor DD, Akyol S, Gercel-Taylor C. Pregnancy-associated exosomes and their modulation of T cell signaling. *J. Immunol.* 176, 1534-1542 (2006).

[6] Sabapatha A, Gercel-Taylor C, Taylor DD. Specific isolation of placenta-derived exosomes from the circulation of pregnant women and their immunoregulatory consequences. *Am. J. Reprod. Immunol.* 56, 345-355 (2006).

[7] Mincheva-Nilsson L, Nagaeva O, Chen T, *et al.* Placenta-derived soluble MHC class I chain-related molecules down-regulate NKG2D receptor on peripheral blood mononuclear cells during human pregnancy: a possible novel immune escape mechanism for fetal survival. *J. Immunol.* 176, 3585-3592 (2006).

[8] Hedlund M, Stenqvist A-C, Nagaeva O, *et al.* Human placenta expresses and secretes NKG2D ligands via exosomes that down-modulate the cognate receptor

expression: evidence for immunosuppressive function. *J. Immunol.* 183, 340-351, (2009).
[9] Mincheva-Nilsson L, Baranov V. The role of placental exosomes in reproduction. *Am. J. Reprod. Immunol.* 63 (6), 520-533 (2010).
[10] Mincheva-Nilsson L. Placental exosome-mediated immune protection of the fetus: feeling groovy in a cloud of exosomes. Exp. Rev. Obstet. Gynecol. 5(5), 619-634 (2010).
[11] Trams EG, Lauter CJ, Salem N Jr, *et al.* Exfoliation of membrane ecto-enzymes in form of microvesicles. *Biochim. Biophys. Acta* 645:63-70 (1981).
[12] Johnstone RM, Adam M, Hammond JR, *et al.* Vesicle formation during reticulocyte maturation. Association of plasma membrane activities with released vesicles (exosomes). *J. Biol. Chem.* 262, 9412-9420 (1987).
[13] Johnstone RM Revisiting the road to the discovery of exosomes. *Blood Cells Mol Dis* 34, 214-219 (2005).
[14] Beaudoin AR, Grondin G. Shedding of vesicular material from the cell surface of eukaryotic cells: different cellular phenomena. *Biochim. Biophys. Acta* 1071, 203-219 (1991).
[15] Cocucci E, Racchetti G, Meldolesi J: Shedding microvesicles: artefacts no more. *Trends Cell. Biol.* 19, 43-51 (2009).
[16] Ratajczak J, Wysoczynski M, Hayek F, *et al.* Membrane-derived microvesicles: important and underappreciated mediators of cell-cell communication. *Leukemia* 20, 1487-1495 (2006).
[17] Babst M. A protein's final ESCRT. *Traffic* 6, 2-9 (2005)
[18] Hurley JH. ESCRT complexes and the biogenesis of multivesicular bodies. *Curr. Opin. Cell. Biol.* 20, 4-11 (2008).
[19] Amzallag N, Passer BJ, Allanic D, *et al.* TSAP6 facilitates the secretion of translationally controlled tumor protein/histamine-releasing factor via a non-classical pathway. *J. Biol. Chem.* 279, 46104-46112 (2004).
[20] Savina A, Fader CM, Vidal M, *et al.* Rab 11 promotes docking and fusion of multivesicular bodies in a calcium-dependent manner. *Traffic* 6, 131-143 (2005).
[21] Trajkovic K, Hsu C, Chiantia S, *et al.* Ceramide triggers budding of exosome vesicles into multivesicular endosomes. *Science* 319, 1244-1247 (2008).
[22] Simpson RG, Lim GWE, Moritz RL, *et al.* Exosomes: proteomic insides and diagnostic potential. *Expert Rev. Proteomics* 6, 267-283 (2009).
[23] Thery C, Ostrowski M, Segura E: Membrane vesicles as conveyors of immune responses. *Nat. Rev. Immunol.* 9, 581-593 (2009).
[24] Mincheva-Nilsson L, Nagaeva O, Sundqvist KG, *et al.* γδT cells of human early pregnancy decidua: evidence for cytotoxic potency. *Int. Immunol.* 12, 585-596 (2000).
[25] Valenti R, Huber V, Iero M, *et al.* Tumor-released microvesicles as vehicles of immunosuppression. *Cancer Res.* 67, 2912-2915 (2007).
[26] Blackburn DG, Taylor JM, Padykula HA. Trophoblast concept as applied to therian mammals. *J. Morphol.* 196, 127-136 (1988).
[27] Fuchs R, Ellinger I. Endocytic and transcytic processes in villous syncytiotrophoblast: role in nutrient transport to the human fetus. *Traffic* 5, 725-738 (2004).
[28] Enders AC. Formation of syncytium from cytotrophoblast in the human placenta. *Obstet. Gynecol.* 25, 378-386 (1965).

[29] Redman CWG, Sargent IL. Microparticles and immunomodulation in pregnancy and pre-eclampsia. *J. Reprod. Immunol.* 76, 61-67 (2007).
[30] Cerwenka A. New twist on the regulation of NKG2D ligand expression. *J. Exp. Med.* 206, 265-268 (2009).
[31] Zuccato E, Blott EJ, Holt O, *et al.* Sorting of Fas ligand to secretory lysosomes is regulated by mono-ubiquitinylation and phosphorylation. *J. Cell. Sci.*120, 191-199 (2007).
[32] Eleme K, Taner ST, Önfelt B, Collinson LM, *et al.* Cell surface organization of stress-inducible proteins ULBP and MICA that stimulate human NK cells and T cells via NKG2D. *J. Exp. Med.* 199, 1005-1010 (2004).
[33] Ashiru O, Boutet P, Fernandez-Messina L, Aguiera-Gonzales S, *et al.* Natural killer cell cytotoxicity is suppressed by exposure to the human NKG2D ligand MICA*008 that is shed by tumor cells in exosomes *Cancer Res.* 70, 481-489 (2010).
[34] O'Reilly LA, Tai L, Lee, L, *et al.* Membrane-bound Fas ligand only is essential for Fas-induced apoptosis. *Nature* 461, 659-663 (2009).
[35] Luo SS, Ishibashi O, Ishikawa G, *et al.* Human villous trophoblast express and secrete placenta-specific microRNAs into maternal circulation via exosomes. *Biol. Reprod.* 81, 717-729 (2009).
[36] Chim SS, Shing TK, Hung EC, *et al.* Detection and characterization of placental micro RNAs in maternal plasma. *Clin. Chem.* 54, 482-490 (2008).
[37] Pisitkun T, Shen RF, Knepper MA. Identification and proteomic analysis of exosomes in human urine. *Proc. Natl. Acad. Sci. USA*, 101, 13368-13373 (2004).
[38] Keller S, Rupp C, Stoek A, *et al.* CD24 is a marker of exosomes secreted into urine and amniotic fluid. *Kidney International*, 72, 1095-1102 (2007).

11

Cytokines and the Innate Immune Response at the Materno-Fetal Interface

Aled H. Bryant and Catherine A. Thornton
Institute of Life Science, Swansea University, UK

1. Introduction

Labour is the climax of pregnancy resulting in the expulsion of the fetus from the uterus. It is a complex process and the mechanisms involved in the initiation of labour are poorly understood despite decades of investigation. Generally, labour is not a sudden occurrence but one for which the body prepares: numerous physiological, biochemical and immunological events take place at the materno-fetal interface, and in both mother and fetus in the lead up to parturition (Hendricks, Brenner et al. 1970). These same processes might be accelerated or other pathways brought into play when labour occurs prematurely. The bulk of perinatal morbidity and mortality is associated with premature labour and delivery of a preterm infant (Tucker and McGuire 2004; Steer 2005). Understanding the mechanisms of labour in health and in adverse obstetric outcomes should provide insight into the pathogenesis of preterm birth.

2. Labour, inflammation and cytokines

Human labour and delivery have been compared to an inflammatory response (Aboussahoud, Bruce et al. 2010; Liggins, Fairclough et al. 1973) of at least three physiologically interdependent processes: remodelling of the cervix to allow it to stretch open to the width of the reproductive tract, weakening and rupture of the membranes in the region that overlies the cervix, and the initiation of rhythmic contractions of increasing amplitude and frequency that ultimately force the fetus and placenta from the uterus. Pro-inflammatory cytokines have a role in most of these processes, suggesting that the immune privileges that the fetal-placental unit has enjoyed during pregnancy might be revoked at the time of labour (Aboussahoud, Bruce et al. 2010; Bayraktar, Peltier et al. 2009). Other beneficial effects of strong pro-inflammatory activity during labour could include removal of placental fragments and a heightened innate immune response in the postpartum uterus to combat the pathogens undoubtedly encountered at this time.

2.1 Cervical ripening

Re-modelling of the extracellular matrix, including decreased collagen concentration and the dispersion of collagen fibrils, is a feature of cervical ripening (Leppert 1995; Winkler and Rath 1999). This is facilitated by increased local production of many pro-inflammatory cytokines and chemokines, such as interleukin-1β (IL-1β), IL-6, IL-8, monocyte chemotactic protein-1 (MCP-1; CCL2) and tumour necrosis factor α (TNFα) (Osman, Young et al. 2003; Tornblom, Klimaviciute et al. 2005), and an influx of neutrophils and macrophages that also secrete cytokine and chemokines and amplify the inflammatory response via the recruitment of other inflammatory cells to the cervix (Rodney W; Sennstrom, Brauner et al. 1997; Sakamoto, Moran et al. 2005). Cytokines such as TNFα and IL-1β activate the nuclear factor (NF)κB pathway, leading to increased production of proteases, cathepsins and matrix metalloproteinases (MMPs), that allow for the digestion of collagen (Watari, Watari et al. 1999). Inhibitors of MMP are down-regulated by IL-1β, and IL-1β also increases production of cyclooxygenase (COX)-2 and prostaglandin E_2 (PGE_2) which further increases production of proteinases and modulates leukocyte trafficking (Sato, Michizu et al. 2001). Murine models show that mechanisms regulating cervical ripening might differ in preterm and term birth, and with underlying cause of labour: preterm birth subsequent to progesterone withdrawal in the absence of infection was comparable to term cervical ripening but preterm ripening in response to infection (using lipopolysaccharide (LPS)) was associated with a robust pro-inflammatory response including neutrophil influx and activation of the prostaglandin synthesis cascade (Holt, Timmons et al. 2011).

2.2 Membrane rupture

Membrane rupture is also characterised by extracellular matrix remodeling: fibronectin is degraded by MMPs and other proteases (Lockwood, Senyei et al. 1991; Vadillo-Ortega, Hernandez et al. 1996) facilitating separation of the previously fused chorioamniontic membranes and deciduas. Similar to the cervix, production of MMPs is increased in response to the augmented production of pro-inflammatory cytokines such as IL-8, IL-6, TNFα and IL-1β (Laham, Brennecke et al. 1996a, 1996b, 1999.). Inflammatory cytokines decrease rupture strength of fetal membranes. This is achieved by induction of prostaglandin and reactive oxygen species production, and collagen remodelling via the release of proteases such as MMP9 (Moore, Novak et al. 2009).

2.3 Myometrial contractions

A similar pattern of cytokine activity is observed in the myometrium: increased levels of IL-6, IL-1β, TNFα and IL-8 result in increased production of COX-2 and PGE_2 (Pollard and Mitchell 1996; Young, Thomson et al. 2002). IL-6 in particular promotes increased production of oxytocin and expression of the oxytocin receptor by myometrial cells (Friebe-Hoffmann, Chiao et al. 2001). PGE_2 and oxytocin in combination are responsible for intracellular calcium increase which are essential for contractions (Thornton, Gillespie et al. 1992).

3. Preterm birth

Birth prior to 37 weeks of gestation is the leading cause of perinatal morbidity and mortality in the Western world; 75% of perinatal mortality and nearly 50% of long-term neurological morbidity are associated with preterm birth (PTB) (Goldenberg, Culhane et al. 2008). Preterm infants are prone to higher rates of complications of the gastrointestinal, renal and respiratory systems (Saigal and Doyle 2008). Increasing PTB rates over the past 30 years in industrialised countries reflects increased indicated preterm births for reasons such as preeclampsia and intrauterine growth restriction (IUGR), and the fallout of multiple gestations associated with assisted reproductive technologies (ART). Other risk factors for preterm birth include ethnicity, previous preterm birth, low maternal body mass index (BMI), genetic variation, infection including periodontal disease, and adverse behaviours. Annual estimates currently suggest that 12.9 million (about 10%) infants worldwide are born prematurely (Beck, Wojdyla et al. 2010). The prevention and management of PTB is one of the major challenges of contemporary obstetrics and gynaecology. PTB also has a large economic impact. The cost of preterm birth to the public sector in England and Wales is approximately £3 billion; the average preterm baby is one and a half times more costly than a full term neonate with the estimated incremental cost per PTB infant at around £30,000 in England and Wales (Mangham, Petrou et al. 2009). Recent decades have seen improvements in the survival rates of preterm infants due to advances in neonatal care and the increased use of antenatal steroids but little change in the ability to prevent preterm birth (Elovitz and Mrinalini 2004).

Preterm delivery for maternal and/or fetal indications accounts for around 30% of preterm births (Hamilton, Martin et al. 2006). Other obstetric precursors of preterm birth are spontaneous preterm labour (sPTL) with intact membranes and preterm premature rupture of the membranes (PPROM). Spontaneous preterm labour, defined as regular uterine contractions with accompanying cervical changes before 37 weeks gestation accounts for 45%, while PPROM, defined as spontaneous membrane rupture accounts for 15% (Goldenberg, Culhane et al. 2008). Both sPTL and PPROM are the outcome of maternal and/or fetal inflammatory responses that can have a systemic component or remain localised to the reproductive tract.

Intrauterine infection is a common mechanism of preterm labour accounting for 25 - 40% of all sPTL cases, although limitations in microbiological culture techniques might make this a conservative estimate (Goldenberg, Hauth et al. 2000). Several routes have been suggested for microbial invasion into the intrauterine cavity. The most common route is the ascension of microorganisms from the vagina through the cervix and into the uterus. The infection can ultimately gain access to the amniotic fluid thereby exposing the fetus to infection (Kim, Romero et al. 2009). Other routes of infection include hematogenous spread through the placenta of non-genital tract infections such as those from the oral cavity (Bearfield, Davenport et al. 2002). Irrespective of the route, microbial invasion results in infection at various sites including the placenta, the fetal membranes, the amniotic fluid, the umbilical cord, and the fetus itself. Many microorganisms have been associated with PPROM, sPTL and PTB. Common microorganisms resulting in intrauterine infection include *Escherichia coli* (Naeye 1979), *Ureaplasma urealyticum* (Yoon, Romero et al. 1998), *Streptococcus agalactiae* (Gibbs, Romero et al. 1992) and *Chlamydia trachomatis* (Gibbs, Romero et al. 1992) among many others. For example, genital mycoplasmas have been associated with a higher maternal white blood count and C-reactive protein (CRP), and more leukocytes in the amniotic fluid (Oh, Lee et al. 2010).

4. Inflammation and cytokines in healthy and adverse pregnancy outcomes

A wealth of evidence indicates that labour is an inflammatory process (Bowen, Chamley et al. 2002). Inflammation is a primary response mechanism resulting from the biological activity of cytokines and other mediators produced in response to harmful stimuli of both infectious and non-infectious origins. Cytokines are small proteins secreted by various cells that function as extracellular signalling molecules to facilitate communication between various cells of the body, a response induced by binding to specific receptors expressed by target cells. Cytokines including IL-6, IL-8 and TNFα are key immunological and inflammatory mediators which can act in an autocrine, paracrine or endocrine manner.

The pathophysiological mechanisms underlying preterm birth are largely unknown but might relate to premature activation of the normal labour process or the response to an insult. Proposed triggers of preterm birth include: uterine over-distension, stress, infection and inflammation, and other immunologically-mediated processes. Irrespective of the triggering event, local and systemic inflammation tends to be a feature of preterm labour and delivery. Understanding the inflammatory pathways that contribute to the initiation and maintenance of preterm (and term) labour could be used to develop strategies to: (i) identify those women most at risk of preterm labour and birth, and (ii) prevent preterm birth. Whilst infection-associated PTB is the focus of this chapter, clinical studies have revealed an association between infection and other pregnancy complications such as preeclampsia and IUGR (Hsu and Witter 1995; Arechavaleta-Velasco, Koi et al. 2002).

A burgeoning body of literature implicates numerous cytokines in the normal physiological processes of pregnancy (e.g. implantation, placental function, parturition) and in the inflammatory response during infection associated preterm labour. The analysis of changes in candidate cytokines has proved worthwhile in identifying potential underlying mechanisms of PTB. IL-1, the first cytokine implicated, is up-regulated in response to microbial products in the human decidua, resulting in the production of prostaglandins by the amnion and deciduas (Romero, Brody et al. 1989a; Romero, Durum et al. 1989b; Romero, Wu et al. 1989c). Mid-trimester amniotic fluid levels of IL-1β levels are associated positively with preterm delivery (Puchner, Iavazzo et al. 2011), and IL-6 concentrations in amniotic fluid are considered a marker for infection (Romero, Avila et al. 1990; Yoon, Romero et al. 1995). Other cytokines including IL-10 (Gotsch, Romero et al. 2008), TNFα (Romero, Manogue et al. 1989d), colony stimulating factor (CSF) (Saito, Kato et al. 1992) and IL-18 (Pacora, Romero et al. 2000) among others have been linked to infection associated preterm labour. There are now a number of groups developing strategies to identify cytokine and other protein signatures that might rapidly identify those women most at risk of delivering prematurely especially in the setting of intrauterine infection. Mass spectrometry-based proteomic profiling of amniotic fluid from women with PTL or PPROM found an inverse relationship between time to delivery and severity of intra-amniotic inflammation as determined by measurement of 4 biomarkers. While minimal inflammation was also associated with preterm birth, the extent of intra-amniotic inflammation correlated with negative outcomes for the neonate (Buhimschi, Bhandari et al. 2007). The potential of proteomic profiling of cervico-vaginal fluid also has been evaluated in a non-human primate model of intra-amniotic infection. Differential expression of proteins was observed in control versus infected samples and this might offer a relatively non-invasive strategy for detection of infection via signatures created by specific biomarkers (Gravett, Thomas et al. 2007).

The cytokines of interest are made by cells normally present in the gestation-associated tissues such as trophoblast cells and macrophages, and by leukocytes that infiltrate these tissues in response to inflammatory stimuli. An accumulation of leukocytes evident upon histological analysis of the placental membranes, so-called chorioamnionitis, occurs in around one-third of preterm deliveries. Chorioamnionitis was once considered a hallmark of infection but it was soon recognised to occur in the absence of any detectable signs of infection. Now, two types of chorioamnionitis have been classified: acute chorioamnionitis (ACA) associated with infection, and chronic chorioamnionitis (CCA) of immunologic origin related to maternal anti-fetal allograft rejection and graft-versus-host disease in the placenta (Lee, Romero et al. 2011). The local cytokine profile differs with the type of chorioamnionitis: IL-6 is the prototypic cytokine elevated in amniotic fluid in ACA whereas for CCA amniotic fluid levels of CXCL10 (IP-10 - interferon-inducible protein-10) are increased and there is elevated gene expression of CXCL9 (MIG - monokine induced by interferon gamma), CXCL10 and CXCL11 (I-TAC - interferon-inducible T-cell alpha chemoattractant) (Kim, Romero et al. 2010).

While chorioamnionitis generally is associated with adverse pregnancy outcomes, around 9 - 20% of term deliveries have evidence of histologic chorioamnionitis and the duration of labour might impact on the occurrence of this (Lee 2011, Romero et al.; Park, Romero et al. 2010). Notably chorioamnionitis is also increased in spontaneous versus induced preterm birth (Kim, Romero et al. 2010). Preterm chorioamnionitis is accompanied by villitis in around 40% of cases (Kim, Romero et al. 2010). Placental villous macrophages (Hofbauer cells) in particular increase when there is evidence of chorioamnionitis. It has been suggested that fibroblast production of MCP-1 in response to bacterial products such as LPS or inflammatory cytokines such as IL-1β or TNFα might drive the accumulation of macrophages within placental villi in this setting (Toti, Arcuri et al. 2011).

5. The innate immune response and inflammation: pattern recognition receptors and cytokine production

Changes in cytokine production at the maternal-fetal interface are a feature of both term and preterm labour. This has generated much interest in the mechanisms of cytokine production in the placenta and attached membranes, and whether such changes precede labour or are simply a consequence of it. Signalling pathways of the innate immune system which produce a defined cytokine output in response to microbial stimuli have been postulated as central to this. Several studies have found a link between the treatment of various gestation-associated tissues with microbial stimuli and cytokine outputs (Holmlund, Cebers et al. 2002; Wang and Hirsch 2003; Elovitz and Mrinalini 2004; Kim, Romero et al. 2004; Kumazaki, Nakayama et al. 2004). These studies have shown that microbial products such as LPS can trigger key molecular events ultimately leading to the production of relevant cytokines.

The innate immune system uses evolutionary conserved germline encoded receptors, termed pattern recognition receptors (PRRs), to recognise and respond to a variety of pathogenic and non-pathogenic microorganisms. Identification of PRRs was initially demonstrated by work on the *Drosophila* protein Toll, a protein involved in development of dorsoventral polarity during embryonic development. However, Hoffman and colleagues demonstrated that Toll was also required for an effective immune response to *Aspergillus fumigates* in the fly (Lemaitre, Nicolas et al. 1996). This realisation inspired a search for mammalian homologues of Toll, which lead to the discovery initially of Toll-like receptor 4

(TLR4), and consequently the remainder of the Toll-like receptor family (TLRs) (Medzhitov, Preston-Hurlburt et al. 1997). As increasing research attention has been placed on the mechanisms of innate immune recognition and signalling, other pattern recognition families have been discovered. These include; RIG-I (retinoic acid-inducible gene I)-like receptors (RLRs) (Yoneyama and Fujita 2007), NOD (nucleotide oligomerisation domain)-like receptors (NLRs) (Mathews, Sprakes et al. 2008), C-type lectin receptors (CLRs) (Netea, Ferwerda et al. 2005) and DAI (DNA dependent activator of IFN regulatory factors)-like receptors (DLRs) (Takaoka, Wang et al. 2007). Each family of PRRs has numerous members.

PRRs detect conserved molecular patterns called pathogen associated molecular patterns (PAMPs) on a wide range of pathogens. Detection of a PAMP by its specific PRR, activates intracellular signalling, leading to cytokine gene expression and eventual activation of inflammatory and antimicrobial responses (Ishii, Koyama et al. 2008). Examples of PAMPs include lipopolysaccharide (LPS), a cell wall component of Gram-negative bacteria, and peptidoglycan (PGN), a component of Gram-positive bacteria cell walls (Janeway and Medzhitov 2002). PRRs have also been shown to recognise damage associated molecular pattern patterns (DAMPs) released by the host (Bianchi 2007).

Below is an overview of each PRR family including some detail about cellular expression, signalling pathways, and the exogenous and endogenous ligands that might initiate activity via each pathway. This will be too much detail for some readers but for others will provide some insight into the constantly growing complexity of the innate immune response. Following this we review the current knowledge of expression and activity of components of each of these pathways/families in gestation-associated tissues.

5.1 Toll-like Receptors

The first characterised mammalian TLR was TLR4, and a further 12 mammalian TLRs have since been identified (Akira 2004). Only TLRs 1 - 10 are expressed and functional in humans. TLRs 1-9 are functional in both human and mice, however TLR10 is likely non-functional in mice due to substitution of the C-terminal half of the mouse TLR10 gene with a non-productive sequence. In contrast, a stop codon in the human TLR11 gene, results in the gene not being expressed, while mouse TLR11 is functional and has a role in urogenital tract infections in particular (Zhang, Zhang et al. 2004). Stimulation of TLRs by their specific PAMPs initiates an intracellular signalling cascade involving numerous proteins, most notably MyD88. Activation of these signalling molecules ultimately leads to the activation of NFκB and other transcription factors to induce the production of inflammatory cytokines.

TLRs are type I transmembrane glycoproteins. The extracellular N-terminal end of all TLRs is composed of leucine-rich repeats (LRRs), which mediate PAMP binding and receptor dimerisation (Akira 2004). The LRR domain is composed of 19-25 tandem LRR motifs, of 24-29 amino acids in length (Matsushima, Tanaka et al. 2007). The mechanisms by which TLRs can differentiate between PAMPs or how any one TLR can respond to multiple PAMPs are only now being revealed. It has been suggested that specific ligand binding sites are created in each TLR by specific insertions of the PAMP into the LRR (Bell, Mullen et al. 2003). The conserved cytoplasmic region of each TLR is termed the Toll/IL-1 receptor (TIR) domain due its similarity to the cytoplasmic domains of the interleukin-1 receptor family. The TIR domain varies between 135 and 160 amino acids in length and functions as a binding site for downstream adaptor molecules (Akira and Takeda 2004).

TLRs can be characterised into two groups based on their cellular location and ligand specificity: plasma membrane localised TLRs - 1, 2, 4, 5 and 6 – that generally recognise lipid based PAMPs; TLRs localised to intracellular endosomes - 3, 7, 8 and 9 – that recognise nucleic acid based PAMPs. While the ligand(s) for TLR10 are unknown its localisation to the plasma membrane suggests these would be lipid based.

The most extensively studied member of the TLR family is TLR4. TLR4 is expressed on various haematopoietic cells including monocytes, macrophages, polymorphonuclear (PMN) cells, dendritic cells, and B cells. It is also expressed by non-haematopoietic cells including epithelial cells and fibroblasts (Ospelt and Gay 2010). TLR4 predominantly recognises lipopolysaccaride (LPS), a cell wall component of Gram-negative bacteria, composed of O-antigen, lipid A (endotoxin) and an oligosaccharide core (Hoshino, Takeuchi et al. 1999). TLR4 recognition of LPS requires formation of a complex with CD14 and MD2 (Shimazu, Akashi et al. 1999). MD2 binds to the extracellular region of TLR4, enabling it to bind to the lipid A component of LPS. CD14, a glycosyl phosphatidylinositol (GPI)-anchored, high affinity membrane protein, binds LPS in the presence of LPS-binding protein (LBP). LBP exchanges monomers of LPS for other lipids bound in its lipid binding site prior to transferring the LPS monomers to CD14. This enables CD14 to concentrate the LPS which is released from the bacterium in small amounts prior to presenting the LPS to the TLR4-MD2 complex (Lu, Yeh et al. 2008). TLR4 also has been implicated in the detection of fungal PAMPs including glucuronoxylomannan of *Cryptococcus neoformans,* and mannan derived from *Saccharomyces cerevisiae* and *Candida albicans* (Netea, Van Der Graaf et al. 2002).

TLR2, which has a similar expression profile to TLR4, recognises a variety of PAMPs from both Gram-positive and Gram-negative bacteria including lipoproteins/lipopeptides and peptidoglycan, glycolipids, lipoteichoic acid and non-endobacterial LPS (Takeuchi, Hoshino et al. 1999). TLR2 also recognises fungal PAMPs including cell surface phospholipomannan of *C. albicans,* and *S. cerevisiae* derived zymosan (Netea, Van Der Graaf et al. 2002; Netea, Van der Graaf et al. 2004). TLR2 forms a heterodimer with its structural relatives, TLR1 or TLR6 (Takeuchi and Akira; Takeuchi, Kawai et al. 1999). These heterodimers - TLR2/TLR1 and TLR2/TLR6 - can detect subtle variations in the lipid component of lipoproteins: tri-acetylated lipopeptides by TLR2/TLR1 and di-acetylated lipopeptides by TLR2/TLR6 (Takeuchi and Akira). Recognition of di-acetylated lipopeptides by TLR2/TLR6, is facilitated by the co-receptor CD36, a class II scavenger protein (Hoebe, Georgel et al. 2005). Expression patterns of TLR1 and TLR6 are similar to that of TLR2, although it has been shown that they are both highly expressed on B cells, while TLR2 is not (Ospelt and Gay 2010). However the regulation of TLR2 expression differs between various cell types depending on their specific function, which is not the case for TLR1 and TLR6 (Ospelt and Gay 2010).

TLR5 recognises bacterial flagellin, a structural protein which is the major component of flagella of Gram-negative bacteria (Hayashi, Smith et al. 2001). Recognition of flagellin by TLR5 is possibly via highly conserved regions in the flagellin protein (Hawn, Verbon et al. 2003). A common stop codon in TLR5 is associated with loss of signalling to flagellin and increased susceptibility to pneumonia caused by *Legionella pneumophila* (Hawn, Verbon et al. 2003). In addition to the conventional expression of TLR5 by haematopoietic cells, TLR5 is expressed on the basolateral surface of healthy human intestinal epithelium, suggesting that bacterial recognition by TLR5 only occurs as the bacteria invade across the epithelium (Gewirtz, Navas et al. 2001).

TLR3 is involved in the recognition of double-stranded RNA (dsRNA) from double-stranded viruses, such as reovirus, or that are generated during viral replication of single stranded viruses (Alexopoulou, Holt et al. 2001; Wang, Town et al. 2004). Multiple haematopoietic cells, such as dendritic cells, and non-haematopoietic cells, such as epithelial cells, express TLR3 which is located within endosomes. Recognition of dsRNA by TLR3 was first demonstrated using TLR3 deficient mice, which showed susceptibility to mouse cytomegalovirus (Tabeta, Georgel et al. 2004). The type I interferon (IFN) inducing dsRNA synthetic analog, polyinosine-deoxycytidylic acid (poly I:C) is often used *in vitro* to induce TLR3 activity (Alexopoulou, Holt et al. 2001).

TLR7 and TLR8 are structurally highly conserved and recognise uridine or guanosine-rich single stranded RNAs from a variety of viruses, including the influenza virus and human immunodeficienty virus (HIV) (Heil, Ahmad-Nejad et al. 2003; Heil, Hemmi et al. 2004; Lund, Alexopoulou et al. 2004). Additionally, they can recognise several synthetic imidazoquinoline-like molecules, such as resiquimod, which have potent antiviral activities due to their structural similarity to ribonucleic acids. While TLR7 and TLR8 recognise viral nucleic acid structures (Diebold, Kaisho et al. 2004; Heil, Hemmi et al. 2004) their expression within endosomes prohibits, under normal circumstances, interaction with host derived ssRNA.

TLR9 recognises the commonly found unmethylated CpG motifs of single-stranded DNA present in the genomes of many viruses and bacteria (Lund, Sato et al. 2003; Hochrein, Schlatter et al. 2004; Krug, Luker et al. 2004). DNA viruses shown to induce inflammatory cytokine and type 1 IFN production via TLR9, include Herpes simplex virus-1 (HSV-1), HSV-2 and murine cytomegalovirus (MCM). Two structurally different forms of CpG exist: A-type CpG oligodeoxynucleotides (ODNs) which stimulate plasmacytoid DCs (pDCs) to produce IL-12 and IFNα, and B-type CpG ODNs, which induce IL-6, IL-12 and TNFα production by pDCs. In addition B-type CpG ODNs also up-regulate expression of MHC Class II and the costimulatory molecules CD80 and CD86 on B cells and pDCs (Verthelyi, Ishii et al. 2001; Krug, Luker et al. 2004). TLR9 might also recognise host derived CpGs but these are weak inducers of activation due to the presence of highly methylated cytosine bases.

5.1.1 TLRs: recognition and response

Binding of PAMPs leads to the dimerisation of TLRs, which triggers the activation of the TLR mediated signalling pathways and the expression of various genes involved in the immune response. As previously described TLR2 forms a heterodimer with either TLR1 or TLR6, the remaining TLRs form homodimers (Saitoh, Akashi et al. 2004). TLR signalling originates from the TIR domain of the receptor, which associates with an adaptor containing a TIR domain. Various adaptors have been characterised including MyD88, TRIF, TRAM and TIRAP; each are involved in slightly different signalling pathways, dependent on which TLR is activated (Watters, Kenny et al. 2007). Two principle TLR signalling pathways have been described: the MyD88-dependent pathway and the MyD88-independent pathway also known as the TRIF-dependent pathway.

The adaptor MyD88, which has a C-terminal TIR domain in addition to an N-terminal death domain, associates with the TIR domain of the TLR. Upon activation of a TLR, MyD88 recruits IRAK-4, a member of the IL-1 receptor associated kinase (IRAK) family, via interactions between the death domains of both molecules. This enables activation of IRAK-1 by IRAK-4 mediated phosphorylation. IRAK-1 then associates with TRAF6 (TNF receptor associated factor 6), resulting in the eventual activation of the IκB kinase (IKK) complex, which consists of IKKα, IKKβ and NEMO/IKKγ. The IKK complex induces the phosphorylation of IκB, resulting in translocation of the nuclear transcription factor NF-κB, from the cytosol to the nucleus. Once in the nucleus NF-κB can induce expression of multiple inflammatory cytokines (Chen, Bhatia et al. 2006; Adhikari, Xu et al. 2007; Kawagoe, Sato et al. 2008). Alternatively, activation of TRAF6 can lead to the activation of MAP kinases, resulting in AP-1 transcription factor activation. As shown in MyD88-deficient mice, MyD88 is vital for signalling via this pathway. A second adaptor, TIRAP (TIR domain-containing adaptor protein)/Mal (MyD88-adaptor-like) has been shown to be associated with the MyD88-dependent pathway for signalling via TLR2 and TLR4 (Yamamoto, Sato et al. 2002).

Evidence for a My88-independent pathway was first shown in MyD88-deficient macrophages, in which NFκB activation was not observed but production of inflammatory cytokines was (Kawai, Adachi et al. 1999). Further investigation noted that TLR4 stimulation results in IRF3 activation, a transcription factor involved in the production of IFNα (Kawai, Takeuchi et al. 2001). Additionally IRF3 was activated in response to dsRNA or viral infection, via TLR3, suggesting that both TLR3 and TLR4 can utilise a common MyD88-independent pathway (Yoneyama, Suhara et al. 1998).

In addition to TIRAP/Mal, two other main adaptors have been identified as involved in the MyD88-independent pathway: TRIF (TIR domain containing adaptor inducing IFNα) also known as TICAM-1 (TIR domain containing molecule), and TRAM (TRIF-related adaptor molecule) or TICAM-2. TRIF has been associated with MyD88-independent signalling via TLR3, while TRIF and TRAM are associated with MyD88-independent signalling via TLR4 (Oshiumi, Matsumoto et al. 2003; Oshiumi, Sasai et al. 2003; Yamamoto, Sato et al. 2003). The TIR domain of TRIF is located in the centre of the molecule and the flanking N-terminal and C-terminal regions can both mediate the activation of NFκB but by two different actions: the N-terminal region associates with TRAF6, while the C-terminal region associates with RIP1 (receptor interacting protein) (Sato, Sugiyama et al. 2003; Meylan, Burns et al. 2004). Activation of the IFNα promoter is exclusively via the N-terminal region in association with the non-canonical IKKs, TBK1 and IKKi/IKKε, which mediate the phosphorylation and nuclear translocation of IRF3, resulting in the induction of IRF3 dependent IFNβ production.

5.1.2 TLRs: negative regulation

Excessive production of inflammatory cytokines in response to PAMPs by TLRs can lead to detrimental outcomes including sepsis and autoimmune disease. Thus negative regulatory mechanisms have developed in response to TLR-mediated signalling. Once such mechanism is the phenomenon known as tolerance, in which a subsequent challenge by a PAMP results in a reduced response. This was first documented in relation to LPS, however the exact mechanisms are not yet fully understood. A number of inhibitors of TLR signalling have also been described. One such molecule is IRAK-M. IRAK-M lacks kinase activity and prevents the dissociation of IRAK-1/IRAK4 from MyD88 which in turn prevents the IRAK-1/TRAF6 complex forming (Wesche, Gao et al. 1999; Kobayashi, Inohara et al. 2002).

Another inhibitor SOCS1 (suppressor of cytokine synthesis) has been shown to directly modulate TLR signalling (Yasukawa, Sasaki et al. 2000).

5.2 C-type Lectin Receptors (CLRs)

CLRs are a family of receptors that recognise and bind carbohydrates in a calcium-dependent manner. Binding is mediated via a conserved carbohydrate recognition domain (CRD) first identified on circulating mannose binding lectin (MBL). Other than MBL, CLRs are primarily expressed on antigen presenting cells (APCs) such as macrophages and dendritic cells, and are involved particularly in fungal recognition and modulation of the anti-fungal innate immune response. CLR intracellular signalling is activated via immunoreceptor tyrosine-based activation (ITAM)-like motifs present in the cytoplasmic tail of the receptor or on ITAM containing adaptors. Examples of such CLRs include; Dectin-1, Dectin-2, macrophage-inducible C-type lectin (MINCLE), DC-SIGN and the mannose receptor (Netea, Ferwerda et al. 2005).

Mannose binding lectin has two to six clusters of CRDs which facilitate the identification of and attachment to repetitive mannose and fucose residues found on various microorganisms. The fixed orientation of the CRDs requires not only the presence of these residues but their specific spatial arrangement to initiate interaction between MBL and the target micro-organism. Recognition of mannose and fucose by MBL leads to the activation of the lectin complement pathway and enhanced polymorphonuclear cell uptake (Ji, Gewurz et al. 2005; Ji, Olinger et al. 2005; van Asbeck, Hoepelman et al. 2008).

The mannose receptor (MR) has similar recognition strategies to MBL. Primarily expressed by macrophages and dendritic cells, the mannose receptor is a type-1 membrane protein with eight tandemly arranged CRD domains. These allow the recognition of various carbohydrates terminating in L-fucose, D-mannose and N-acetyl glucosamine (Taylor, Gordon et al. 2005). In addition to CRDs at the extracellular region, MR has two additional domains, an N-terminal cysteine-rich domain and a fibronectin II domain, these are involved in calcium-independent binding to sulphated sugars and collagen, respectively. Unlike the CRDs, these additional domains are only involved in the recognition of endogenous ligands and not those of microbial origin (Taylor, Gordon et al. 2005; Napper, Drickamer et al. 2006). The role of the MR in host defence remains a mystery: animal knockout models do not demonstrate an increased susceptibility to pathogens such as *Candida albicans* and mycobacteria which are known to contain MR ligands (Wojcikiewicz, Zhang et al. 2003; Appelmelk, den Dunnen et al. 2008).

The most widely studied CLR is Dectin-1. Dectin-1, also known as C-type lectin domain family 7 member A (CLEC7A), is a small (33kDa) type II glycosylated transmembrane receptor with an extracellular CRD connected to a cytoplasmic ITAM-like motif by a stalk domain. Two functional isoforms exist - Dectin-1A, and Dectin-1B which lacks the stalk domain, due to alternative splicing (Herre, Gordon et al. 2004). Dectin-1 expression in humans can be found on myeloid cells, including neutrophils, monocytes/macrophages and dendritic cells, however limited expression has been noted on other cell types (Herre, Gordon et al. 2004). Dectin-1 recognises specifically the glucose polymers β-1-3 and/or β-1-6-glucans primarily found in the cell walls of fungi, including *Candida albicans* and *Saccharomyces cerevisiae*, but which can also be found in the cell walls of some plants (Brown and Gordon 2001). Upon binding of the appropriate PAMP, phosphorylation of Dectin-1 occurs by a non-receptor tyrosine kinase, Src, via interaction with its ITAM motif. This leads to the activation of another kinase, Syk, which induces the activation of the CARD9-Bc110-Malt1 adaptor complex leading ultimately to the activation of NFκB and the production of pro-inflammatory cytokines (Gross, Gewies et al. 2006). In addition, activation of Dectin-1 mediates the production of reactive oxygen species (ROS) and further modulation of cytokine expression via the NFAT pathway (Underhill, Rossnagle et al. 2005; Goodridge, Simmons et al. 2007). Attenuation of the Dectin-1 mediated pro-inflammatory response has been linked to internalisation of the receptor (Hernanz-Falcon, Joffre et al. 2009). It has been shown that signalling via Dectin-1 and TLR2/TLR6 combined enhances the response triggered by each receptor alone (Gantner, Simmons et al. 2003).

Similarly to Dectin-1, ITAM-dependent signalling via MINCLE leads to the activation of NFκB and the NFAT pathway, via recognition of numerous exogenous PAMPs and endogenous DAMPS, including mycobacteria, *C. albicans* and necrotic cells (Yamasaki, Ishikawa et al. 2008). The identification of necrotic and damaged cells is mediated via recognition of splicesome-associated protein 130 (SAP130), secreted by these cells. MINCLE was the first known example of a CLR that can interact with PAMPs and DAMPs (Yamasaki, Ishikawa et al. 2008). MINCLE and another CLR, Galectin-3, have a role in anti-*Candida* defence, by recognition of β-mannose, resulting in MINCLE interacting with the Fc receptor common γ-chain (FcRγ), leading to Syk and CARD9-depedent activation of NFκB (Jouault, El Abed-El Behi et al. 2006; Yamasaki, Ishikawa et al. 2008). MINCLE also recognises the immunostimulatroy component of *Mycobacterium tuberculosis* - trehalose-6′6′-dimycolate better known as cord factor (Ishikawa, Ishikawa et al. 2009).

Other CLRs, such as DC-SIGN and Dectin-2, are involved in the recognition and uptake of *Candida albicans* by detecting highly mannose structures (McGreal, Rosas et al. 2006). DC-SIGN, expressed primarily on monocyte-derived dendritic cells, is a type II transmembrane receptor with only one C-type lectin domain. DC-SIGN also interacts with *Leishmania* but has gained increasing interest because of its involvement in the recognition of several viruses including human immunodeficiency virus (HIV)(Geijtenbeek, van Vliet et al. 2001; Cambi, Gijzen et al. 2003; Koppel, van Gisbergen et al. 2005). Dectin-2 which can be found on myeloid cells, has been suggested to have a role in hyphal recognition (Netea, Ferwerda et al. 2005). In response to *Candida albicans*, Dectin-2 induces the production of TNF, via interaction with FcγR (Nakahara, Nakagawa et al. 2006). Additionally, Dectin-2 has been implicated in Th17 inducing activity in response to *Candida* (Robinson, Osorio et al. 2009).

5.3 Nod-like Receptors (NLRs)

NLRs (also known as CATERPILLERs) consist of a large family of 23 human intracellular (cytosolic) PRRs, which recognise both PAMPs and/or DAMPs. Acitvation via NLRs leads to cytokine production via NFκB, or the inflammasome (see section 5.3.1) (Ting and Davis 2005; Kanneganti, Lamkanfi et al. 2007; Shaw, Reimer et al. 2008). NLRs have also been implicated in autophagy, a lysosomal degradation and cell death pathway that follows infection (Ting, Willingham et al. 2008). Structurally, NLRs are characterised by the presence of a trimodular structure: a central nucleotide binding domain (NBD) flanked by leucine rich repeats (LRRs) at the C-terminal and a protein binding domain - caspase activation and recruitment domain (CARD), baculovirus inhibitor of apoptosis protein repeat (BIR), death effector domain (DED) or pyrin domain (PYD) - at the N-terminal. These N-terminal domains, also termed the effector region, are responsible for the protein-protein interactions needed to activate downstream signal transduction. NLRs can be categorised into subfamilies based on this effector domain including: NLRC (Nod-like receptor containing a CARD domain) and CIITA or NLRA (class II, major histocompatibility complex, transactivator) all contain CARD effector domains, while NLRPs contain a pyrin effector domain, and NAIPs or NLRBs contain three BIR domains (Kanneganti, Lamkanfi et al. 2007; Kumar, Kawai et al. 2009).

The first identified and most widely studied NLRs are NOD1 and NOD2. These belong to the NLRC subfamily and are highly expressed in monocytes, macrophages and dendritic cells, in addition to other hematopoietic cells and epithelial cells (Fritz, Ferrero et al. 2006). Both NOD1 and NOD2 recognise peptidoglycan (PGN) an essential building block of Gram-positive bacterial cell walls and to a lesser extent Gram-negative bacteria. PGN consists of glycan chains cross-linked via short peptides (Girardin, Travassos et al. 2003), NOD1 and NOD2 recognise different motifs in this structure: NOD2 recognises the conserved muramyl dipeptide (MDP) motif found in all PGNs (McDonald, Inohara et al. 2005), whereas NOD1 recognises D-γ-glutamyl-meso-DAP dipeptide (iE-DAP), which is present in all Gram-negative, but only some Gram-positive PGNs (Chamaillard, Hashimoto et al. 2003; Benko, Philpott et al. 2008). NOD2 can also recognise viral ssRNA and mycobacterial N-glycolylmuramyl dipeptides (Coulombe, Divangahi et al. 2009; Sabbah, Chang et al. 2009). Thus both NOD1 and NOD2 are involved in the recognition of a variety of pathogenic bacteria including: *E. coli*, *Chlamydia spp*, *Haemophilus influenza* by NOD1, and *M. tuberculosis* and *Streptococcus pneumonia* by NOD2 (Kumar, Kawai et al. 2009). Since the majority of these bacteria replicate outside of the cytoplasm where NOD1 and NOD2 are located, a mechanism by which PGN can cross the cell membrane to activate them is required. Although numerous transport proteins including PepT1, PepT2, and pannexin have been identified to facilitate MDP passage into the cytoplasm, an exact mechanism is not fully understood (Vavricka, Musch et al. 2004; Lee, Tattoli et al. 2009; Marina-Garcia, Franchi et al. 2009).

In general, activation of NOD1 and NOD2 by their respective ligands results in a conformational change allowing interaction with CARD domain containing receptor–interacting serine-threonine kinase 2 (RIP2) in a homophilic CARD-CARD manner. Cellular inhibitors of apoptosis 1 and 2 (cIAP1 and 2) are also involved (Kobayashi, Inohara et al. 2002). RIP2 can then mediate the ubiquitination of NFκB essential modulator (NEMO)/IKKγ, subsequently leading to the activation of NFκB and the production of pro-inflammatory cytokines and antimicrobial peptides (Inohara, Koseki et al. 2000). Activation of NOD2 by MDP also can result in the activation of the mitogen activated protein kinase (MAPK) pathways via the adapter CARD9 (Kobayashi, Chamaillard et al. 2005).

5.3.1 The inflammasome

Certain members of the NLR family detect microbial components in the cytosol and trigger the assembly of a large caspase 1 activating complex termed the inflammasome. This complex supports the autocatalytic cleavage of caspase-1 which enables the processing and secretion of IL-1β and IL-18. NLRP1, NLRP3, NLRC4 and the adapter apoptosis-associated speck-like protein containing a CARD (ASC) are critical components of the inflammasome but emerging components include NLRP6 (Bauernfeind 2011, Ablasser et al.; Kersse 2011,

Bertrand et al.; Franchi, Eigenbrod et al. 2009). While much of the focus has been on the caspase-1 inflammasome, other caspases are also associated with an inflammasome-triggered response in a caspase-1-independent manner (Kayagaki, Warming et al. 2011).

The NLRP3 inflammasome is the most extensively studied: it comprises NLRP3, ASC, and caspase-1 (Martinon and Tschopp 2004). Like other NLRP family members, NLRP3 is composed of a C-terminal LRR domain, a central NOD domain and an N-terminal PYD domain. NLRP3 is expressed in many types of hematopoietic cells, in addition to osteoblasts, skin keratinocytes and transitional epithelium of the urinary tract (Elinav, Strowig et al. 2011). A wide variety of pathogens of bacterial, fungal and viral origin can initiate NLRP3 inflammasome formation: *Listeria monocytogenes, Staphylococcus aureus, C. albicans, Saccharomyces cerevisiae*, and adenovirus and influenza viruses. A number of host-derived DAMPs indicative of cellular injury, including extracellular ATP and uric acid among others, have been shown to activate the inflammasome (Mariathasan, Weiss et al. 2006; Gasse, Riteau et al. 2009). The mechanisms involved in the recognition of these stimuli by NLRP3 are currently not fully understood. Interaction of cellular mediators with a variety of PAMPs and DAMPs, ultimately relaying signals to NLRP3 has been postulated but physical interaction between NLRP3 and the PAMPs/DAMPs has not been ruled out (Marina-Garcia, Franchi et al. 2008). Following activation, NLRP3 oligomerisation leads to the clustering of PYD domains which can then recruit the CARD containing adaptor ASC which by a CARD-CARD interaction can then recruit pro-caspase-1. The clustering of pro-capase-1 results in its autocleavage to the active caspase-1 p10/p20 tetramer enabling the processing of cytokine proforms to yield mature molecules for secretion. Production of these proforms depends on NFκB driven transcriptional activity resulting from signalling from other PRRs such as NOD2 and TLRs (Schroder and Tschopp 2010).

Less is known about the NLRP1 inflammasome, which is comprised of ASC, caspase-1, caspase-5, and NLRP1 (Martinon and Tschopp 2004). NLRP1 is expressed in various haematopoietic cells including: T and B cells, monocytes, dendritic cells and granulocytes, on non-haematopoietic cells within the testes, and neurons (Elinav, Strowig et al. 2011). The structure of NLRP1 is different to that of NLRP3, as NLRP1 contains a C-terminal CARD domain, allowing NLRP1 to interact directly with pro-caspase-1. However ASC forms part of the inflammasome complex, allowing for the recruitment of caspase-5 providing additional inflammasome activity (Martinon and Tschopp 2004).

NLRC4 (also known as IPAF) is expressed primarily in lymphoid tissue. Like NOD1 and NOD2 it has a C-terminal LRR domain, a central NOD domain, and an N-terminal CARD domain (Hu, Elinav et al. 2010). Activation of the NLRC4 by microbial flagellin leads to the activation of caspase-1, IL-1β secretion and pyroptosis, a rapid form of cell death (Lightfield, Persson et al. 2008; Miao, Ernst et al. 2008). Similar to NLRP1, NLRC4 can interact directly with pro-caspase-1 via its CARD domain. The role of ASC in the NLRC4 inflammasome remains inconclusive: ASC cannot interact with NLRC4 which lacks a PYD domain but a role for ASC in regulation of this inflammasome has been suggested (Schroder and Tschopp 2010).

5.4 RIG-I like Receptors (RLRs)

The cytoplasmic RNA helicases that comprise the RIG-I like family of receptors play a major role in host anti-viral defence. RLRs include the highly characterised RIG-1 (retinoic acid-inducible gene I), MDA5 (melanoma differentiation associated factor 5) and LGP2 (laboratory of genetics and physiology 2). These are able to detect a variety of viral RNA ligands present in the cytoplasm and triggering the activation of transcription factors resulting in the production of type 1 interferons (IFN) in addition to expression of other anti-viral genes (Yoneyama and Fujita 2007). Viral recognition also occurs via TLR3. It seems that RIG-1 and MDA5 play a greater role in viral recognition by fibroblasts, macrophages and myeloid dendritic cells whereas TLR3 plays a more important role in viral recognition by plasmacytoid dendritic cells (Kato, Sato et al. 2005).

Both RIG-1 and MDA5 share a number of structural similarities. They contain a central DExD/H box RNA helicase domain flanked by an N-terminal of tandem CARD domains and a C-terminal domain (CTD). In the case of RIG-1 the CTD also contains a repressor domain (RD), involved in autoregulation, which is not present in the CTD of MDA5. Despite their similar structures, RIG-1 and MDA5 are able to detect distinct viral species: RIG-1 is involved in the recognition of Paramyxoviridae, Filoviridae and Rhabdoviridae among others, whereas MDA5 is important in the recognition of Picornaviruses (Loo and Gale 2011). More is known about RLR signalling in regard to RIG-1, however its believed that both RIG-1 and MDA5 share a common signalling pathway, involving the adaptor ISP-1 (Kawai, Takahashi et al. 2005). Prior to recognition of RNA by the RD or CTD region, RIG-1 is inactive in a "closed" conformation, where the CARD domain is bound to the RD. Activation of RIG-1 results in a conformational change whereby CARD is released from the RD, allowing the CARD domain to interact with the adaptor ISP-1 (Loo and Gale 2011). ISP-1 can then initiate two distinct signalling routes resulting in the activation of various transcription factors including NFκB which induces the production of pro-inflammatory cytokines, and IRF3 and IRF7 which are responsible for the expression of type 1 IFNs (Kawai, Takahashi et al. 2005). Unlike RIG-1, MDA5 does not contain a RD to regulate its activation and when expressed ectopically signalling occurs in the absence of RNA recognition (Terness, Kallikourdis et al. 2007). Unlike RIG-I and MDA5, LGP2 lacks the N-terminal CARD domain, consisting only of the RNA helicase domain and the C-terminal domain containing an RD. It has been suggested that LGP2 is involved in the negative regulation of RIG-1 and possibly MDA5 (Loo and Gale 2011). This negative feedback is thought to take place on many levels including acting as a competitor for dsRNA, interaction with ISP-1, and maybe direct binding to RIG-1 via RD interactions (Terness, Kallikourdis et al. 2007).

5.5 Other pattern recognition receptors

Other less well characterised groups of pattern recognition receptors have also been described, including DAI (DNA dependent activator of IFN regulatory factors)-like receptors (DLRs) and scavenger receptors (SR). DAI (also known as DLM-1 and ZBP1) is the only DLR receptor to be described to date. It was first identified in mouse macrophages and mouse tumour stromal cells. DAI was up-regulated by exposure to cytosolic DNA or interferon gamma (IFNγ) suggesting that DAI functions as a DNA sensor (Fu, Comella et al. 1999; Ishii, Coban et al. 2006). A human homologue containing two N-terminal Zα domains and a C-terminal domain has since been described but it is of unknown function (Rothenburg, Schwartz et al. 2002). Activation of DAI by either microbial or host derived DNA, results in the activation of both the NFκB pathway and the IRF pathway (Takaoka and Taniguchi 2008).

Scavenger receptors (SRs) are a group of cell surface transmembrane receptors that are important in the clearance of several pathogens, host modified molecules, and apoptotic cells by endocytotic internalisation. These receptors also play a role in lipid metabolism. Expressed primarily on myeloid cells and some endothelial cells, both their expression and structure are regulated by various cytokines. Numerous SRs have been shown to play a role in innate immunity, including SR-A I, SR-A II, CD36, LOX-1, MARCO, SR-CL I, SR-CL II, SCARF1 and DSR-C1 (Peiser, Mukhopadhyay et al. 2002; Means, Mylonakis et al. 2009).

6. Pattern recognition receptors at the maternal-fetal interface

The discovery of an association between intrauterine infection, inflammation and certain adverse pregnancy outcomes has lead to increased interest in the innate immune response at the maternal-fetal interface (Goncalves, Chaiworapongsa et al. 2002). The production by gestation-associated tissues of cytokines in response to microbial products has been well documented. Since pattern recognition receptors are a key component of the innate immune response, linking infection by various microorganisms to the production of inflammatory mediators, a role for PRRs at the maternal–fetal interface has been postulated. To date studies have principally focused on the role of TLRs and most recently NLRs, primarily in the placenta and the trophoblast.

6.1 Placenta

Expression of transcripts for TLR 1-10 in the term placenta has been demonstrated with all but TLR9 shown to be functional (note that TLR10 function has not been studied due to the lack of an identified ligand). Changes were observed in both mRNA expression and functional cytokine outputs in response to labour at term (Patni, Wynen et al. 2009). TLR2 and TLR4 protein has been localised to term syncytiotrophoblast and intermediate trophoblast cells and both receptors are highly expressed in first trimester placental tissue (Holmlund, Cebers et al. 2002; Abrahams and Mor 2005). First trimester trophoblast cells also express TLR6. TLR6 blocks apoptosis induced by PGN via TLR1 and TLR2 and mediates NFκB activation and secretion of IL-6 and IL-8 leading to the postulate that TLR6 might regulate the balance of apoptosis and inflammation in response to Gram-positive infection (Abrahams, Aldo et al. 2008).

The NLRs, NOD1 and NOD2 are both expressed in the first trimester placenta where they are localised to the syncytiotrophoblast and cytotrophoblast. In contrast only NOD1 is expressed in term trophoblast cells. This corresponds to the functional outputs of first versus third trimester trophoblast cells; first trimester cells respond to both MDP and iE-DAP, and third trimester cells only respond to iE-DAP (Abrahams 2011; Cardenas, Mulla et al. 2011). The NOD1 ligand, iEDAP, can induce preterm delivery in a murine model. When lower doses that did not induce preterm delivery were used there was heightened inflammation at the materno-fetal interface and in the fetus itself (Cardenas, Mulla et al. 2011). Immunohistochemical studies have shown that the CLR DC-SIGN is expressed by fetal macrophages (Hofbauer cells) within the chorionic villi of the term placenta (Geijtenbeek, van Vliet et al. 2001). Viral ssRNA also activates cytokine, chemokine, and type I interferon production by primary first trimester trophoblast cells. This ligand also induces apoptosis in trophoblast cells in an IFNβ-dependent fashion (Aldo, Mulla et al. 2010).

6.2 Amnion

Amniotic epithelial cells represent the first line of defence against intra-amniotic infection. Earlier studies were restricted to TLR2 and TLR4 and found that both of these receptors are up-regulated in the amnion from women with chorioamnionitis compared to those without (Kim, Romero et al. 2004) although not all studies support this finding (Choi, Jung et al. 2011). Transcripts for TLRs 1-10 have been detected in human amniotic epithelial cells. However only TLR2/6, TLR4 and TLR5 have been reported to be functional: activation of TLR2/6 and TLR5 resulted in increased production of IL-6 and IL-8, while activation of TLR4 reduced cell viability via apoptosis (Gillaux, Mehats et al. 2011). Immunohistochemical studies of human fetal membranes have shown that the expression of TLR4 is greater in the chorion than the amnion, that expression decreases with gestational age but that expression does not differ by anatomic location within the uterus (Choi, Jung et al. 2011).

6.3 Decidua

Despite its juxtaposition to the myometrium the expression and function of PRRs within the maternally derived decidua is not studied extensively. Transcripts for TLRs 1-6 have been detected in term decidual cells but only TLR1, TLR2, TLR4 and TLR6 where shown to be functional via production of IL-8 in response to stimulation with LPS or PGN (Canavan and Simhan 2007). Immunohistochemical studies have demonstrated the expression of NOD1 and NOD2 in first trimester decidualised stroma (King, Horne et al. 2009). DC-SIGN has also been detected on decidual macrophages (Repnik, Tilburgs et al. 2008).

7. PRRs and adverse pregnancy outcomes

PRRs expressed at the maternal-fetal interface could play an important role in the pathogenesis of infection-associated preterm birth and other adverse pregnancy outcomes (Abrahams 2005a). This possibility has been studied mostly with regards to TLRs, especially TLR4. LPS from Gram-negative bacteria has been implicated in infection associated preterm birth and there have been a number of studies exploring the possible role of TLR4 in preterm labour. Functional TLR4 has been implicated in preterm labour triggered by administration of heat killed *E.coli* in mice (Wang and Hirsch 2003) . Evidence for a role for TLRs in infection-associated preterm birth also comes from genetic studies. A polymorphism (Asp299Gly) known to be associated with impaired TLR4 function and an increased likelihood of Gram-negative sepsis (Agnese DM 2002) was carried more often by preterm infants than term infants or by mothers delivering preterm than at term (Vacca, Cantoni et al. 2010). Genetic variation in TLRs is also associated with other adverse obstetric outcomes: *TLR4*, *TLR9* and *TLR1* but not *TLR2* variants are associated with placental malaria (low birth weight and maternal anaemia; no difference in parasite densities) (Hamann, Bedu-Addo et al. 2010). Other genetic variants are also associated with risk of PTB: maternal genetic variants in extracellular matrix metabolism with risk of PPROM and fetal genetic variation (e.g. IL-6R1) are associated with risk of PTB (Romero, Friel et al. 2010).

While LPS has been used as the model for many years it is worth noting that LPS from different species of bacteria might differentially regulate inflammatory responses from gestation-associated tissues such as the amniochorion (Chang, Jain et al. 2010). Also tissue processing for ex vivo investigations can impact on cytokine measurements. For example, in a comparison of punch biopsies of amnion or choriodecidua versus dual compartment transwells, the punch biopsies typically made greater amounts of cytokines (Miller 2010. and Loch-Caruso). Such observations highlight the need to take these factors into account when designing studies and when comparing data from different studies.

In addition to the direct pro-inflammatory effects initiated by exposure to infection, disturbances in the regulation of apoptosis might also be associated with sub-optimal pregnancy outcome (Jerzak and Bischof 2002). Increased trophoblast apoptosis is seen during the first trimester of pregnancies complicated with IUGR or preeclampsia (Saito, Kato et al. 1992; Smith, Baker et al. 1997), and elevated trophoblast apoptosis has been observed in preterm births (Kakinuma, Kuwayama et al. 1997; Balkundi, Ziegler et al. 2003). It has been suggested that the direct or indirect effects of infectious microorganisms upon trophoblast cell survival might depend upon which TLRs are activated with TLR2-mediated events presumably favouring apoptosis.

Recently there has been growing interest in how a viral infection might itself cause preterm birth and also how it might increase the risk of pregnancy failure during subsequent or concurrent bacterial infection. In a murine model, intraperitoneal injection of a synthetic TLR3 ligand, poly I:C, caused preterm delivery within 24 hours. This was associated with inflammation in multiple gestation-associated tissues (polymorphonuclear cell infiltrate, necrosis and haemorrhage), infiltration of NK cells and macrophages into the placenta, and placental cytokine (e.g. IL-6) and chemokine (e.g. MCP-1) production that could also be detected systemically. This did not occur in TLR3 knock out animals. The cytokine response could be replicated *in vitro* by polyI:C treatment of primary murine trophoblast and a human trophoblast cell line and involved activation of NFκB (Koga, Cardenas et al. 2009). In contrast, intra-peritoneal injection of murine herpes virus was associated with evidence of inflammation in the placenta and spleen but no adverse pregnancy outcomes. Evidence of viral infection in the placenta and decidua but not the fetus led the investigators to postulate that these tissues act as a barrier to capture virus and prevent infection of the fetus. However, this might not prevent developmental impacts on the fetus. Human primary first trimester trophoblast also can be infected with herpes virus *in vitro* but unlike the response to poly I:C treatment, cytokine and chemokine production tended to be down-regulated. Viral infection but not polyI:C induced increased expression of TLR2 and TLR4 in human trophoblast cells and in the accompanying mouse model, viral infection sensitised for a response - preterm delivery in less than 24hrs in all mice accompanied by 100% fetal death - to intraperitoneal infection of LPS (Cardenas 2010, 2011 respectively, Means et al.; Cardenas 2010, 2011 respectively, Mor et al.).

These observations have highlighted a need for better understanding of the expression and activity of viral detecting PRRs at the materno-fetal interface. Although the focus of this chapter is the placenta and attached membranes it is also worth noting that there is incredible interest in how anti-viral responses by women are affected by pregnancy.

Preeclampsia, a pregnancy specific hypertensive disorder, also is characterised by inflammation. Pathways related to stress, inflammation (including TLR signalling pathways), growth, tissue remodelling, and metabolism are all altered during preeclampsia (Sado, Naruse et al. 2011). The differences might reflect acute inflammation secondary to microbial infection versus chronic inflammation secondary to oxidative stress. Possible involvement of the inflammasome in preeclampsia has been suggested. Uric acid is known to activate the inflammasome: circulating uric acid levels increase prior to clinical manifestations of preeclampsia and levels relate to disease severity. Components of the inflammasome, including ASC, are expressed in first and third trimester trophoblasts and monosodium urate up-regulates IL-1β production in an inflammasome-dependent manner (Mulla, Myrtolli et al. 2011). There is also interest in the potential role of viral PAMPs or related DAMPs from necrotic cells in preeclampsia. Activation via TLR3 or the RLRs RIG-1 and MDA-5 leading to downstream inflammation, anti-angiogenesis and oxidative stress converging on endothelial dysfunction has been postulated (Chatterjee, Weaver et al. 2011).

8. Regulating the inflammatory response at the materno-fetal interface

The resolution of inflammation is essential for immune homeostasis. It has become apparent that there are intracellular stress proteins that have extracellular properties related to the regulation of the innate immune response and inflammation. These so-called RAMPs (resolution-associated molecular patterns) (Shields, Panayi et al. 2011) have anti-inflammatory activity or the ability to resolve inflammation and counterbalance the activity of PAMPs and DAMPs. There is keen interest in the potential therapeutic use of these.

There are also a number of cytokines well recognised for their anti-inflammatory activity. These include IL-4, IL-10 and IL-13. IL-10 can down-regulate LPS- and LTA-induced cytokine/chemokine responses by the healthy term placenta (Bayraktar, Peltier et al. 2009). Paradoxically, IL-10 is increased in amniotic fluid from women in term labour and women with intra-amniotic infection at term and preterm, and is also increased in those without infection who delivered preterm rather than term (Gotsch, Romero et al. 2008). Elevated IL-10 in these circumstances might represent a compensatory mechanism that has failed. Similarly, an anti-inflammatory cytokine (IL-4, IL-10 and IL-13) bias within the cervix prior to 16 weeks of gestation might identify those women most likely to suffer microbial invasion of the utero-placental unit and then spontaneous preterm labour and delivery (Simhan, Bodnar et al. 2011). Whether the greater anti-inflammatory milieu permits ascending infection or is a compensatory response to a pro-inflammatory response to existing infection that when no longer controlled tips in favour of the pro-inflammatory response and the initiation of labour remains to be determined.

There is also a need to better understand the bioactivity of key cytokines at the materno-fetal interface. The biological effect of any cytokine depends on the expression of cognate receptors on target cells and this can be modified by the presence of soluble receptors, macromolecules that bind the cytokine, and the relative abundance of other cytokines. IL-6 provides a relevant example. IL-6 is a multi-functional cytokine: while its pro- and anti-inflammatory properties are of particular interest in the context of this review it is also involved in the acute phase reaction and regulates haematopoiesis. Classic signaling by IL-6 is mediated via interaction with the non-signaling transmembrane IL-6 receptor followed by homodimerisation of signalling gp130. IL-6R-negative cells can utilize IL-6 *trans*-signaling via IL-6 binding to soluble IL-6R (sIL-6R) for interaction with membrane expressed gp130. The presence of soluble gp130 (sgp130) inhibits *trans*-signaling by offering an alternative binding site for IL-6/sIL-6R thereby prohibiting interaction with the membrane bound form of gp130 and downstream intracellular signalling. Although sgp130 cannot bind directly to IL-6 it has been shown recently to also inhibit classic signaling depending on the ratio of IL-

6 and sIL-6R (Garbers, Thaiss et al. 2011). Human amniotic fluid contains IL-6, sIL-6R and sgp130 with levels of sgp130 declining with increasing gestational age. Amniotic fluid IL-6 and sIL-6R are increased when there is evidence of intraamniotic infection: the fetal membranes are a key source of these mediators. Increased IL-6R, either membrane or soluble, combined with decreased sgp130 in intraamniotic infection would favour IL-6 pro-inflammatory signalling. Indeed, sgp130 but not sIL-6R modulates LPS-mediated MMP9 production by fetal membranes (Lee, Buhimschi et al. 2011). Reduced IL-6 *trans*-signalling mainly due to reduced circulating soluble gp130 also has been implicated in recurrent spontaneous abortion via a postulated role in modulating activity of regulatory T ell at materno-fetal interface (Arruvito, Billordo et al. 2009).

9. Conclusion

The study of PRR-mediated inflammation at the maternal-fetal interface has only just begun. A better understanding of these receptors and the signal transduction cascades they initiate might explain why some pregnancies are complicated by PTL and PPROM whereas others are only affected by PPROM. Moreover, investigations into the endogenous activators of PRRs might explain how PTL and PPROM can occur in the absence of infection (e.g. preeclampsia, multiple gestation, teenage pregnancy, or excessive tobacco and alcohol consumption). These molecules (either the receptors or their signalling molecules) might therefore be excellent targets for therapeutic strategies because they are upstream effectors of the pro-inflammatory cascade that ultimately results in premature labour and preterm birth.

10. References

Aboussahoud, W., C. Bruce, et al. (2010). "Activation of Toll-like receptor 5 decreases the attachment of human trophoblast cells to endometrial cells in vitro." *Hum Reprod* 25(9): 2217-2228.

Abrahams, V. M. (2005a). "Toll-like receptors in the cycling female reproductive tract and during pregnancy." *Current Women's Health Review* 1: 35-42.

Abrahams, V. M. (2011). "The role of the Nod-like receptor family in trophoblast innate immune responses." *J Reprod Immunol* 88(2): 112-7.

Abrahams, V. M., P. B. Aldo, et al. (2008). "TLR6 Modulates First Trimester Trophoblast Responses to Peptidoglycan." *J Immunol* 180(9): 6035-6043.

Abrahams, V. M. and G. Mor (2005). "Toll-like receptors and their role in the trophoblast." *Placenta* 26(7): 540-7.

Adhikari, A., M. Xu, et al. (2007). "Ubiquitin-mediated activation of TAK1 and IKK." *Oncogene* 26(22): 3214-26.

Agnese DM, C. J., Hahm SJ, Coyle SM, Corbett SA, Calvano SE, Lowry SF. (2002). "Human toll-like receptor 4 mutations but not CD14 polymorphisms are associated with an increased risk of gram-negative infections." *J Infect Dis.* Nov 15;186(10):1522-5.

Akira, S. (2004). "Toll receptor families: structure and function." *Semin Immunol* 16(1): 1-2.

Akira, S. and K. Takeda (2004). "Toll-like receptor signalling." *Nat Rev Immunol* 4(7): 499-511.

Aldo, P. B., M. J. Mulla, et al. (2010). "Viral ssRNA Induces First Trimester Trophoblast Apoptosis through an Inflammatory Mechanism." *Am J Reprod Immunol* 64(1): 27-37.

Alexopoulou, L., A. C. Holt, et al. (2001). "Recognition of double-stranded RNA and activation of NF-kappaB by Toll-like receptor 3." *Nature* 413(6857): 732-8.

Appelmelk, B. J., J. den Dunnen, et al. (2008). "The mannose cap of mycobacterial lipoarabinomannan does not dominate the Mycobacterium-host interaction." *Cell Microbiol* 10(4): 930-44.

Arechavaleta-Velasco, F., H. Koi, et al. (2002). "Viral infection of the trophoblast: time to take a serious look at its role in abnormal implantation and placentation?" *J Reprod Immunol* 55(1-2): 113-21.

Arruvito, L., A. Billordo, et al. (2009). "IL-6 trans-signaling and the frequency of CD4+FOXP3+ cells in women with reproductive failure." *J Reprod Immunol* 82(2): 158-165.

Balkundi, D. R., J. A. Ziegler, et al. (2003). "Regulation of FasL/Fas in human trophoblasts: possible implications for chorioamnionitis." *Biol Reprod* 69(2): 718-24.

Bauernfeind, F., A. Ablasser, et al. (2011). "Inflammasomes: current understanding and open questions." *Cell Mol Life Sci* 68(5): 765-783.

Bayraktar, M., M. Peltier, et al. (2009). "IL-10 Modulates Placental Responses to TLR Ligands." *Am J Reprod Immunol* 62(6): 390-399.

Bearfield, C., E. S. Davenport, et al. (2002). "Possible association between amniotic fluid micro-organism infection and microflora in the mouth." *BJOG* 109(5): 527-33.

Beck, S., D. Wojdyla, et al. (2010). "The worldwide incidence of preterm birth: a systematic review of maternal mortality and morbidity." *Bull World Health Organ* 88(1): 31-8.

Bell, J. K., G. E. Mullen, et al. (2003). "Leucine-rich repeats and pathogen recognition in Toll-like receptors." *Trends Immunol* 24(10): 528-33.

Benko, S., D. J. Philpott, et al. (2008). "The microbial and danger signals that activate Nod-like receptors." *Cytokine* 43(3): 368-73.

Bianchi, M. E. (2007). "DAMPs, PAMPs and alarmins: all we need to know about danger." *J Leukoc Biol* 81(1): 1-5.

Bowen, J. M., L. Chamley, et al. (2002). "Cytokines of the placenta and extra-placental membranes: roles and regulation during human pregnancy and parturition." *Placenta* 23(4): 257-73.

Brown, G. D. and S. Gordon (2001). "Immune recognition. A new receptor for beta-glucans." *Nature* 413(6851): 36-7.

Buhimschi, C. S., V. Bhandari, et al. (2007). "Proteomic Profiling of the Amniotic Fluid to Detect Inflammation, Infection, and Neonatal Sepsis." *PLoS Med* 4(1): e18.

Cambi, A., K. Gijzen, et al. (2003). "The C-type lectin DC-SIGN (CD209) is an antigen-uptake receptor for Candida albicans on dendritic cells." *Eur J Immunol* 33(2): 532-8.

Canavan, T. P. and H. N. Simhan (2007). "Innate immune function of the human decidual cell at the maternal-fetal interface." *J Reprod Immunol* 74(1-2): 46-52.

Cardenas, I., R. E. Means, et al. (2010). "Viral Infection of the Placenta Leads to Fetal Inflammation and Sensitization to Bacterial Products Predisposing to Preterm Labor." *J Immunol* 185(2): 1248-1257.

Cardenas, I., G. Mor, et al. (2011). "Placental Viral Infection Sensitizes to Endotoxin-Induced Pre-Term Labor: A Double Hit Hypothesis." *Am J Reprod Immunol* 65(2): 110-117.

Cardenas, I., M. J. Mulla, et al. (2011). "Nod1 activation by bacterial iE-DAP induces maternal-fetal inflammation and preterm labor." *J Immunol* 187(2): 980-6.

Chamaillard, M., M. Hashimoto, et al. (2003). "An essential role for NOD1 in host recognition of bacterial peptidoglycan containing diaminopimelic acid." *Nat Immunol* 4(7): 702-7.

Chang, J., S. Jain, et al. (2010). "Differential host response to LPS variants in amniochorion and the TLR4/MD-2 system in Macaca nemestrina." *Placenta* 31(9): 811-817.

Chatterjee, P., L. E. Weaver, et al. (2011). "Do double-stranded RNA receptors play a role in preeclampsia?" *Placenta* 32(3): 201-205.

Chen, F., D. Bhatia, et al. (2006). "Finding NEMO by K63-linked polyubiquitin chain." *Cell Death Differ* 13(11): 1835-8.

Choi, S. J., S. H. Jung, et al. (2011). "Immunohistochemical distribution of toll-like receptor 4 in preterm human fetal membrane." *J Obstet Gynaecol Res*.

Coulombe, F., M. Divangahi, et al. (2009). "Increased NOD2-mediated recognition of N-glycolyl muramyl dipeptide." *J Exp Med* 206(8): 1709-16.

Diebold, S. S., T. Kaisho, et al. (2004). "Innate antiviral responses by means of TLR7-mediated recognition of single-stranded RNA." *Science* 303(5663): 1529-31.

Elinav, E., T. Strowig, et al. (2011). "Regulation of the antimicrobial response by NLR proteins." *Immunity* 34(5): 665-79.

Elovitz, M. A. and C. Mrinalini (2004). "Animal models of preterm birth." *Trends Endocrinol Metab* 15(10): 479-87.

Franchi, L., T. Eigenbrod, et al. (2009). "The inflammasome: a caspase-1-activation platform that regulates immune responses and disease pathogenesis." *Nat Immunol* 10(3): 241-247.

Friebe-Hoffmann, U., J. P. Chiao, et al. (2001). "Effect of IL-1beta and IL-6 on oxytocin secretion in human uterine smooth muscle cells." *Am J Reprod Immunol* 46(3): 226-31.

Fritz, J. H., R. L. Ferrero, et al. (2006). "Nod-like proteins in immunity, inflammation and disease." *Nat Immunol* 7(12): 1250-7.

Fu, Y., N. Comella, et al. (1999). "Cloning of DLM-1, a novel gene that is up-regulated in activated macrophages, using RNA differential display." *Gene* 240(1): 157-63.

Gantner, B. N., R. M. Simmons, et al. (2003). "Collaborative induction of inflammatory responses by dectin-1 and Toll-like receptor 2." *J Exp Med* 197(9): 1107-17.

Garbers, C., W. Thaiss, et al. (2011). "Inhibition of classic signaling is a novel function of soluble GP130 which is controlled by the ratio of interleukin 6 and soluble interleukin 6 receptor." *J Biol Chem* 286(50):42959-70.

Gasse, P., N. Riteau, et al. (2009). "Uric acid is a danger signal activating NALP3 inflammasome in lung injury inflammation and fibrosis." *Am J Respir Crit Care Med* 179(10): 903-13.

Geijtenbeek, T. B., S. J. van Vliet, et al. (2001). "DC-SIGN, a dentritic cell-specific HIV-1 receptor present in placenta that infects T cells in trans-a review." *Placenta* 22 Suppl A: S19-23.

Gewirtz, A. T., T. A. Navas, et al. (2001). "Cutting edge: bacterial flagellin activates basolaterally expressed TLR5 to induce epithelial proinflammatory gene expression." *J Immunol* 167(4): 1882-5.

Gibbs, R. S., R. Romero, et al. (1992). "A review of premature birth and subclinical infection." *Am J Obstet Gynecol* 166(5): 1515-28.

Gillaux, C., C. Mehats, et al. (2011). "Functional screening of TLRs in human amniotic epithelial cells." *J Immunol* 187(5): 2766-74.
Girardin, S. E., L. H. Travassos, et al. (2003). "Peptidoglycan molecular requirements allowing detection by Nod1 and Nod2." *J Biol Chem* 278(43): 41702-8.
Goldenberg, R. L., J. F. Culhane, et al. (2008). "Epidemiology and causes of preterm birth." *Lancet* 371(9606): 75-84.
Goldenberg, R. L., J. C. Hauth, et al. (2000). "Intrauterine infection and preterm delivery." *N Engl J Med* 342(20): 1500-7.
Goncalves, L. F., T. Chaiworapongsa, et al. (2002). "Intrauterine infection and prematurity." *Ment Retard Dev Disabil Res Rev* 8(1): 3-13.
Goodridge, H. S., R. M. Simmons, et al. (2007). "Dectin-1 stimulation by Candida albicans yeast or zymosan triggers NFAT activation in macrophages and dendritic cells." *J Immunol* 178(5): 3107-15.
Gotsch, F., R. Romero, et al. (2008). "The anti-inflammatory limb of the immune response in preterm labor, intra-amniotic infection/inflammation, and spontaneous parturition at term: A role for interleukin-10." *J Matern Fetal Neonatal Med* 21(8): 529-547.
Gotsch, F., R. Romero, et al. (2008). "The anti-inflammatory limb of the immune response in preterm labor, intra-amniotic infection/inflammation, and spontaneous parturition at term: a role for interleukin-10." *J Matern Fetal Neonatal Med* 21(8): 529-47.
Gravett, M. G., A. Thomas, et al. (2007). "Proteomic analysis of cervical-vaginal fluid: identification of novel biomarkers for detection of intra-amniotic infection." *J Proteome Res* 6(1): 89-96.
Gross, O., A. Gewies, et al. (2006). "Card9 controls a non-TLR signalling pathway for innate anti-fungal immunity." *Nature* 442(7103): 651-6.
Hamann, L., G. Bedu-Addo, et al. (2010). "The toll-like receptor 1 variant S248N influences placental malaria." *Infection, Genetics and Evolution* 10(6): 785-789.
Hamilton, B. E., J. A. Martin, et al. (2006). "Births: preliminary data for 2005." *Natl Vital Stat Rep* 55(11): 1-18.
Hawn, T. R., A. Verbon, et al. (2003). "A Common Dominant TLR5 Stop Codon Polymorphism Abolishes Flagellin Signaling and Is Associated with Susceptibility to Legionnaires' Disease." *J Exp Med* 198(10): 1563-1572.
Hayashi, F., K. D. Smith, et al. (2001). "The innate immune response to bacterial flagellin is mediated by Toll-like receptor 5." *Nature* 410(6832): 1099-103.
Heil, F., P. Ahmad-Nejad, et al. (2003). "The Toll-like receptor 7 (TLR7)-specific stimulus loxoribine uncovers a strong relationship within the TLR7, 8 and 9 subfamily." *Eur J Immunol* 33(11): 2987-97.
Heil, F., H. Hemmi, et al. (2004). "Species-specific recognition of single-stranded RNA via toll-like receptor 7 and 8." *Science* 303(5663): 1526-9.
Hendricks, C. H., W. E. Brenner, et al. (1970). "Normal cervical dilatation pattern in late pregnancy and labor." *Am J Obstet Gynecol* 106(7): 1065-82.
Hernanz-Falcon, P., O. Joffre, et al. (2009). "Internalization of Dectin-1 terminates induction of inflammatory responses." *Eur J Immunol* 39(2): 507-13.
Herre, J., S. Gordon, et al. (2004). "Dectin-1 and its role in the recognition of beta-glucans by macrophages." *Mol Immunol* 40(12): 869-76.

Hochrein, H., B. Schlatter, et al. (2004). "Herpes simplex virus type-1 induces IFN-alpha production via Toll-like receptor 9-dependent and -independent pathways." *Proc Natl Acad Sci U S A* 101(31): 11416-21.

Hoebe, K., P. Georgel, et al. (2005). "CD36 is a sensor of diacylglycerides." *Nature* 433(7025): 523-7.

Holmlund, U., G. Cebers, et al. (2002). "Expression and regulation of the pattern recognition receptors Toll-like receptor-2 and Toll-like receptor-4 in the human placenta." *Immunology* 107(1): 145-51.

Holt, R., B. C. Timmons, et al. (2011). "The Molecular Mechanisms of Cervical Ripening Differ between Term and Preterm Birth." *Endocrinology* 152(3): 1036-1046.

Hoshino, K., O. Takeuchi, et al. (1999). "Cutting edge: Toll-like receptor 4 (TLR4)-deficient mice are hyporesponsive to lipopolysaccharide: evidence for TLR4 as the Lps gene product." *J Immunol* 162(7): 3749-52.

Hsu, C. D. and F. R. Witter (1995). "Urogenital infection in preeclampsia." *Int J Gynaecol Obstet* 49(3): 271-5.

Hu, B., E. Elinav, et al. (2010). "Inflammation-induced tumorigenesis in the colon is regulated by caspase-1 and NLRC4." *Proc Natl Acad Sci U S A* 107(50): 21635-40.

Inohara, N., T. Koseki, et al. (2000). "An induced proximity model for NF-kappa B activation in the Nod1/RICK and RIP signaling pathways." *J Biol Chem* 275(36): 27823-31.

Ishii, K. J., C. Coban, et al. (2006). "A Toll-like receptor-independent antiviral response induced by double-stranded B-form DNA." *Nat Immunol* 7(1): 40-8.

Ishii, K. J., S. Koyama, et al. (2008). "Host innate immune receptors and beyond: making sense of microbial infections." *Cell Host Microbe* 3(6): 352-63.

Ishikawa, E., T. Ishikawa, et al. (2009). "Direct recognition of the mycobacterial glycolipid, trehalose dimycolate, by C-type lectin Mincle." *J Exp Med* 206(13): 2879-88.

Janeway, C. A., Jr. and R. Medzhitov (2002). "Innate immune recognition." *Annu Rev Immunol* 20: 197-216.

Jerzak, M. and P. Bischof (2002). "Apoptosis in the first trimester human placenta: the role in maintaining immune privilege at the maternal-foetal interface and in the trophoblast remodelling." *Eur J Obstet Gynecol Reprod Biol* 100(2): 138-42.

Ji, X., H. Gewurz, et al. (2005). "Mannose binding lectin (MBL) and HIV." *Mol Immunol* 42(2): 145-52.

Ji, X., G. G. Olinger, et al. (2005). "Mannose-binding lectin binds to Ebola and Marburg envelope glycoproteins, resulting in blocking of virus interaction with DC-SIGN and complement-mediated virus neutralization." *J Gen Virol* 86(Pt 9): 2535-42.

Jouault, T., M. El Abed-El Behi, et al. (2006). "Specific recognition of Candida albicans by macrophages requires galectin-3 to discriminate Saccharomyces cerevisiae and needs association with TLR2 for signaling." *J Immunol* 177(7): 4679-87.

Kakinuma, C., C. Kuwayama, et al. (1997). "Trophoblastic apoptosis in mice with preterm delivery and its suppression by urinary trypsin inhibitor." *Obstet Gynecol* 90(1): 117-24.

Kanneganti, T. D., M. Lamkanfi, et al. (2007). "Intracellular NOD-like receptors in host defense and disease." *Immunity* 27(4): 549-59.

Kato, H., S. Sato, et al. (2005). "Cell type-specific involvement of RIG-I in antiviral response." *Immunity* 23(1): 19-28.

Kawagoe, T., S. Sato, et al. (2008). "Sequential control of Toll-like receptor-dependent responses by IRAK1 and IRAK2." *Nat Immunol* 9(6): 684-91.
Kawai, T., O. Adachi, et al. (1999). "Unresponsiveness of MyD88-deficient mice to endotoxin." *Immunity* 11(1): 115-22.
Kawai, T., K. Takahashi, et al. (2005). "IPS-1, an adaptor triggering RIG-I- and Mda5-mediated type I interferon induction." *Nat Immunol* 6(10): 981-8.
Kawai, T., O. Takeuchi, et al. (2001). "Lipopolysaccharide stimulates the MyD88-independent pathway and results in activation of IFN-regulatory factor 3 and the expression of a subset of lipopolysaccharide-inducible genes." *J Immunol* 167(10): 5887-94.
Kayagaki, N., S. Warming, et al. (2011). "Non-canonical inflammasome activation targets caspase-11." *Nature* 479(7371): 117-121.
Kersse, K., M. J. M. Bertrand, et al. (2011). "NOD-like receptors and the innate immune system: Coping with danger, damage and death." *Cytokine Growth Factor Rev 22(5-6):257-76.*
Kim, C. J., R. Romero, et al. (2010). "The frequency, clinical significance, and pathological features of chronic chorioamnionitis: a lesion associated with spontaneous preterm birth." *Mod Pathol* 23(7): 1000-1011.
Kim, M. J., R. Romero, et al. (2009). "Widespread microbial invasion of the chorioamniotic membranes is a consequence and not a cause of intra-amniotic infection." *Lab Invest* 89(8): 924-36.
Kim, Y. M., R. Romero, et al. (2004). "Toll-like receptor-2 and -4 in the chorioamniotic membranes in spontaneous labor at term and in preterm parturition that are associated with chorioamnionitis." *Am J Obstet Gynecol* 191(4): 1346-55.
King, A. E., A. W. Horne, et al. (2009). "Differential expression and regulation of nuclear oligomerization domain proteins NOD1 and NOD2 in human endometrium: a potential role in innate immune protection and menstruation." *Mol Hum Reprod* 15(5): 311-9.
Kobayashi, K., N. Inohara, et al. (2002). "RICK/Rip2/CARDIAK mediates signalling for receptors of the innate and adaptive immune systems." *Nature* 416(6877): 194-9.
Kobayashi, K. S., M. Chamaillard, et al. (2005). "Nod2-dependent regulation of innate and adaptive immunity in the intestinal tract." *Science* 307(5710): 731-4.
Koga, K., I. Cardenas, et al. (2009). "Activation of TLR3 in the Trophoblast is Associated with Preterm Delivery." *Am J Reprod Immunol* 61(3): 196-212.
Koppel, E. A., K. P. van Gisbergen, et al. (2005). "Distinct functions of DC-SIGN and its homologues L-SIGN (DC-SIGNR) and mSIGNR1 in pathogen recognition and immune regulation." *Cell Microbiol* 7(2): 157-65.
Krug, A., G. D. Luker, et al. (2004). "Herpes simplex virus type 1 activates murine natural interferon-producing cells through toll-like receptor 9." *Blood* 103(4): 1433-7.
Kumar, H., T. Kawai, et al. (2009). "Pathogen recognition in the innate immune response." *Biochem J* 420(1): 1-16.
Kumazaki, K., M. Nakayama, et al. (2004). "Immunohistochemical distribution of Toll-like receptor 4 in term and preterm human placentas from normal and complicated pregnancy including chorioamnionitis." *Hum Pathol* 35(1): 47-54.

Laham, N., S. P. Brennecke, et al. (1996a). "Differential release of interleukin-6 from human gestational tissues in association with labour and in vitro endotoxin treatment." *J Endocrinol* 149(3): 431-9.

Laham, N., S. P. Brennecke, et al. (1996b). "Labour-associated increase in interleukin-1 alpha release in vitro by human gestational tissues." *J Endocrinol* 150(3): 515-22.

Laham, N., S. P. Brennecke, et al. (1999). "Interleukin-8 release from human gestational tissue explants: effects of gestation, labor, and chorioamnionitis." *Biol Reprod* 61(3): 823-7.

Lee, J., R. Romero, et al. (2011). "A Signature of Maternal Anti-Fetal Rejection in Spontaneous Preterm Birth: Chronic Chorioamnionitis, Anti-Human Leukocyte Antigen Antibodies, and C4d." *PLoS ONE* 6(2): e16806.

Lee, J., I. Tattoli, et al. (2009). "pH-dependent internalization of muramyl peptides from early endosomes enables Nod1 and Nod2 signaling." *J Biol Chem* 284(35): 23818-29.

Lee, S. Y., I. A. Buhimschi, et al. (2011) "IL-6 Trans-Signaling System in Intra-Amniotic Inflammation, Preterm Birth, and Preterm Premature Rupture of the Membranes." *J Immunol* 186(5): 3226-3236.

Lemaitre, B., E. Nicolas, et al. (1996). "The dorsoventral regulatory gene cassette spatzle/Toll/cactus controls the potent antifungal response in Drosophila adults." *Cell* 86(6): 973-83.

Leppert, P. C. (1995). "Anatomy and physiology of cervical ripening." *Clin Obstet Gynecol* 38(2): 267-79.

Liggins, G. C., R. J. Fairclough, et al. (1973). "The mechanism of initiation of parturition in the ewe." *Recent Prog Horm Res* 29: 111-59.

Lightfield, K. L., J. Persson, et al. (2008). "Critical function for Naip5 in inflammasome activation by a conserved carboxy-terminal domain of flagellin." *Nat Immunol* 9(10): 1171-8.

Lockwood, C. J., A. E. Senyei, et al. (1991). "Fetal fibronectin in cervical and vaginal secretions as a predictor of preterm delivery." *N Engl J Med* 325(10): 669-74.

Loo, Y. M. and M. Gale, Jr. (2011). "Immune signaling by RIG-I-like receptors." *Immunity* 34(5): 680-92.

Lu, Y.-C., W.-C. Yeh, et al. (2008). "LPS/TLR4 signal transduction pathway." *Cytokine* 42(2): 145-151.

Lund, J., A. Sato, et al. (2003). "Toll-like receptor 9-mediated recognition of Herpes simplex virus-2 by plasmacytoid dendritic cells." *J Exp Med* 198(3): 513-20.

Lund, J. M., L. Alexopoulou, et al. (2004). "Recognition of single-stranded RNA viruses by Toll-like receptor 7." *Proc Natl Acad Sci U S A* 101(15): 5598-603.

Mangham, L. J., S. Petrou, et al. (2009). "The cost of preterm birth throughout childhood in England and Wales." *Pediatrics* 123(2): e312-27.

Mariathasan, S., D. S. Weiss, et al. (2006). "Cryopyrin activates the inflammasome in response to toxins and ATP." *Nature* 440(7081): 228-32.

Marina-Garcia, N., L. Franchi, et al. (2009). "Clathrin- and dynamin-dependent endocytic pathway regulates muramyl dipeptide internalization and NOD2 activation." *J Immunol* 182(7): 4321-7.

Marina-Garcia, N., L. Franchi, et al. (2008). "Pannexin-1-mediated intracellular delivery of muramyl dipeptide induces caspase-1 activation via cryopyrin/NLRP3 independently of Nod2." *J Immunol* 180(6): 4050-7.

Martinon, F. and J. Tschopp (2004). "Inflammatory caspases: linking an intracellular innate immune system to autoinflammatory diseases." *Cell* 117(5): 561-74.
Mathews, R. J., M. B. Sprakes, et al. (2008). "NOD-like receptors and inflammation." *Arthritis Res Ther* 10(6): 228.
Matsushima, N., T. Tanaka, et al. (2007). "Comparative sequence analysis of leucine-rich repeats (LRRs) within vertebrate toll-like receptors." *BMC Genomics* 8: 124.
McDonald, C., N. Inohara, et al. (2005). "Peptidoglycan signaling in innate immunity and inflammatory disease." *J Biol Chem* 280(21): 20177-80.
McGreal, E. P., M. Rosas, et al. (2006). "The carbohydrate-recognition domain of Dectin-2 is a C-type lectin with specificity for high mannose." *Glycobiology* 16(5): 422-30.
Means, T. K., E. Mylonakis, et al. (2009). "Evolutionarily conserved recognition and innate immunity to fungal pathogens by the scavenger receptors SCARF1 and CD36." *J Exp Med* 206(3): 637-53.
Medzhitov, R., P. Preston-Hurlburt, et al. (1997). "A human homologue of the Drosophila Toll protein signals activation of adaptive immunity." *Nature* 388(6640): 394-7.
Meylan, E., K. Burns, et al. (2004). "RIP1 is an essential mediator of Toll-like receptor 3-induced NF-kappa B activation." *Nat Immunol* 5(5): 503-7.
Miao, E. A., R. K. Ernst, et al. (2008). "Pseudomonas aeruginosa activates caspase 1 through Ipaf." *Proc Natl Acad Sci U S A* 105(7): 2562-7.
Miller, M. F. and R. Loch-Caruso (2010) "Comparison of LPS-stimulated release of cytokines in punch versus transwell tissue culture systems of human gestational membranes." *Reprod Biol Endocrinol* 8: 121.
Moore, R. M., J. B. Novak, et al. (2009). "Alpha-Lipoic Acid Inhibits Tumor Necrosis Factor-Induced Remodeling and Weakening of Human Fetal Membranes." *Biology of Reproduction* 80(4): 781-787.
Mulla, M. J., K. Myrtolli, et al. (2011) "Uric Acid Induces Trophoblast IL-1β Production Via the Inflammasome: Implications for the Pathogenesis of Preeclampsia." *Am J Reprod Immunol* 65(6): 542-548.
Naeye, R. L. (1979). "Causes of the excessive rates of perinatal mortality and prematurity in pregnancies complicated by maternal urinary-tract infections." *N Engl J Med* 300(15): 819-23.
Nakahara, K., M. Nakagawa, et al. (2006). "Maternal ghrelin plays an important role in rat fetal development during pregnancy." *Endocrinology* 147(3): 1333-42.
Napper, C. E., K. Drickamer, et al. (2006). "Collagen binding by the mannose receptor mediated through the fibronectin type II domain." *Biochem J* 395(3): 579-86.
Netea, M. G., G. Ferwerda, et al. (2005). "The Frameshift Mutation in Nod2 Results in Unresponsiveness Not Only to Nod2- but Also Nod1-activating Peptidoglycan Agonists." *JJ Biol Chem* 280(43): 35859-35867.
Netea, M. G., C. Van der Graaf, et al. (2004). "Recognition of fungal pathogens by Toll-like receptors." *Eur J Clin Microbiol Infect Dis* 23(9): 672-6.
Netea, M. G., C. A. Van Der Graaf, et al. (2002). "The role of toll-like receptor (TLR) 2 and TLR4 in the host defense against disseminated candidiasis." *J Infect Dis* 185(10): 1483-9.
Oh, K. J., K. A. Lee, et al. (2010) "Intraamniotic infection with genital mycoplasmas exhibits a more intense inflammatory response than intraamniotic infection with other

microorganisms in patients with preterm premature rupture of membranes." *Am J Obstet Gynecol* 203(3): 211.e1-211.e8.

Oshiumi, H., M. Matsumoto, et al. (2003). "TICAM-1, an adaptor molecule that participates in Toll-like receptor 3-mediated interferon-beta induction." *Nat Immunol* 4(2): 161-7.

Oshiumi, H., M. Sasai, et al. (2003). "TIR-containing adapter molecule (TICAM)-2, a bridging adapter recruiting to toll-like receptor 4 TICAM-1 that induces interferon-beta." *J Biol Chem* 278(50): 49751-62.

Osman, I., A. Young, et al. (2003). "Leukocyte density and pro-inflammatory cytokine expression in human fetal membranes, decidua, cervix and myometrium before and during labour at term." *Mol Hum Reprod* 9(1): 41-5.

Ospelt, C. and S. Gay (2010) "TLRs and chronic inflammation." *Int J Biochem Cell Biol* 42(4): 495-505.

Pacora, P., R. Romero, et al. (2000). "Participation of the novel cytokine interleukin 18 in the host response to intra-amniotic infection." *Am J Obstet Gynecol* 183(5): 1138-43.

Park, H. S., R. Romero, et al. (2010) "Histologic Chorioamnionitis is More Common after Spontaneous Labor than after Induced Labor at Term." *Placenta* 31(9): 792-795.

Patni, S., L. P. Wynen, et al. (2009). "Expression and activity of Toll-like receptors 1-9 in the human term placenta and changes associated with labor at term." *Biol Reprod* 80(2): 243-8.

Peiser, L., S. Mukhopadhyay, et al. (2002). "Scavenger receptors in innate immunity." *Curr Opin Immunol* 14(1): 123-8.

Pollard, J. K. and M. D. Mitchell (1996). "Intrauterine infection and the effects of inflammatory mediators on prostaglandin production by myometrial cells from pregnant women." *Am J Obstet Gynecol* 174(2): 682-6.

Puchner, K., C. Iavazzo, et al. (2011) "Mid-trimester amniotic fluid interleukins (IL-1beta, IL-10 and IL-18) as possible predictors of preterm delivery." *In Vivo* 25(1): 141-8.

Repnik, U., T. Tilburgs, et al. (2008). "Comparison of macrophage phenotype between decidua basalis and decidua parietalis by flow cytometry." *Placenta* 29(5): 405-12.

Robinson, M. J., F. Osorio, et al. (2009). "Dectin-2 is a Syk-coupled pattern recognition receptor crucial for Th17 responses to fungal infection." *J Exp Med* 206(9): 2037-51.

Kelly, R.W. (2002) "Inflammatory mediators and cervical ripening." *J Reprod Immunol* 57(1-2): 217-224.

Romero, R., C. Avila, et al. (1990). "Amniotic fluid interleukin 6 in preterm labor. Association with infection." *J Clin Invest* 85(5): 1392-400.

Romero, R., D. T. Brody, et al. (1989a). "Infection and labor. III. Interleukin-1: a signal for the onset of parturition." *Am J Obstet Gynecol* 160(5 Pt 1): 1117-23.

Romero, R., S. Durum, et al. (1989b). "Interleukin-1 stimulates prostaglandin biosynthesis by human amnion." *Prostaglandins* 37(1): 13-22.

Romero, R., L. A. Friel, et al. (2010) "A genetic association study of maternal and fetal candidate genes that predispose to preterm prelabor rupture of membranes (PROM)." *Am J Obstet Gynecol* 203(4): 361.e1-361.e30.

Romero, R., K. R. Manogue, et al. (1989d). "Infection and labor. IV. Cachectin-tumor necrosis factor in the amniotic fluid of women with intraamniotic infection and preterm labor." *Am J Obstet Gynecol* 161(2): 336-41.

Romero, R., Y. K. Wu, et al. (1989c). "Human decidua: a source of interleukin-1." *Obstet Gynecol* 73(1): 31-4.

Rothenburg, S., T. Schwartz, et al. (2002). "Complex regulation of the human gene for the Z-DNA binding protein DLM-1." *Nucleic Acids Res* 30(4): 993-1000.

Sabbah, A., T. H. Chang, et al. (2009). "Activation of innate immune antiviral responses by Nod2." *Nat Immunol* 10(10): 1073-80.

Sado, T., K. Naruse, et al. (2011) "Inflammatory pattern recognition receptors and their ligands: factors contributing to the pathogenesis of preeclampsia." *Inflamm Res* 60(6): 509-520.

Saigal, S. and L. W. Doyle (2008). "An overview of mortality and sequelae of preterm birth from infancy to adulthood." *Lancet* 371(9608): 261-9.

Saito, S., Y. Kato, et al. (1992). "Amniotic fluid granulocyte colony-stimulating factor in preterm and term labor." *Clin Chim Acta* 208(1-2): 105-9.

Saitoh, S., S. Akashi, et al. (2004). "Lipid A antagonist, lipid IVa, is distinct from lipid A in interaction with Toll-like receptor 4 (TLR4)-MD-2 and ligand-induced TLR4 oligomerization." *Int Immunol* 16(7): 961-9.

Sakamoto, Y., P. Moran, et al. (2005). "Macrophages and not granulocytes are involved in cervical ripening." *J Reprod Immunol* 66(2): 161-73.

Sato, S., M. Sugiyama, et al. (2003). "Toll/IL-1 receptor domain-containing adaptor inducing IFN-beta (TRIF) associates with TNF receptor-associated factor 6 and TANK-binding kinase 1, and activates two distinct transcription factors, NF-kappa B and IFN-regulatory factor-3, in the Toll-like receptor signaling." *J Immunol* 171(8): 4304-10.

Sato, T., H. Michizu, et al. (2001). "Hormonal regulation of PGE2 and COX-2 production in rabbit uterine cervical fibroblasts." *J Appl Physiol* 90(4): 1227-1231.

Schroder, K. and J. Tschopp (2010). "The inflammasomes." *Cell* 140(6): 821-32.

Sennstrom, M. K., A. Brauner, et al. (1997). "Interleukin-8 is a mediator of the final cervical ripening in humans." *Eur J Obstet Gynecol Reprod Biol* 74(1): 89-92.

Shaw, M. H., T. Reimer, et al. (2008). "NOD-like receptors (NLRs): bona fide intracellular microbial sensors." *Curr Opin Immunol* 20(4): 377-82.

Shields, A. M., G. S. Panayi, et al. (2011) "Resolution-associated molecular patterns (RAMP): RAMParts defending immunological homeostasis?" *Clin Exp Immunol* 165(3): 292-300.

Shimazu, R., S. Akashi, et al. (1999). "MD-2, a molecule that confers lipopolysaccharide responsiveness on Toll-like receptor 4." *J Exp Med* 189(11): 1777-82.

Simhan, H. N., L. M. Bodnar, et al. (2011) "Lower genital tract inflammatory milieu and the risk of subsequent preterm birth: an exploratory factor analysis." *Paediatr Perinat Epidermiol* 25(3): 277-282.

Smith, S. C., P. N. Baker, et al. (1997). "Placental apoptosis in normal human pregnancy." *Am J Obstet Gynecol* 177(1): 57-65.

Steer, P. (2005). "The epidemiology of preterm labor--a global perspective." *J Perinat Med* 33(4): 273-6.

Tabeta, K., P. Georgel, et al. (2004). "Toll-like receptors 9 and 3 as essential components of innate immune defense against mouse cytomegalovirus infection." *Proc Natl Acad Sci U S A* 101(10): 3516-21.

Takaoka, A. and T. Taniguchi (2008). "Cytosolic DNA recognition for triggering innate immune responses." *Adv Drug Deliv Rev* 60(7): 847-57.

Takaoka, A., Z. Wang, et al. (2007). "DAI (DLM-1/ZBP1) is a cytosolic DNA sensor and an activator of innate immune response." *Nature* 448(7152): 501-5.

Takeuchi, O. and S. Akira "Pattern recognition receptors and inflammation." *Cell* 140(6): 805-20.

Takeuchi, O., K. Hoshino, et al. (1999). "Differential roles of TLR2 and TLR4 in recognition of gram-negative and gram-positive bacterial cell wall components." *Immunity* 11(4): 443-51.

Takeuchi, O., T. Kawai, et al. (1999). "TLR6: A novel member of an expanding toll-like receptor family." *Gene* 231(1-2): 59-65.

Taylor, P. R., S. Gordon, et al. (2005). "The mannose receptor: linking homeostasis and immunity through sugar recognition." *Trends Immunol* 26(2): 104-10.

Terness, P., M. Kallikourdis, et al. (2007). "Tolerance signaling molecules and pregnancy: IDO, galectins, and the renaissance of regulatory T cells." *Am J Reprod Immunol* 58(3): 238-54.

Thornton, S., J. I. Gillespie, et al. (1992). "Mobilization of calcium by the brief application of oxytocin and prostaglandin E2 in single cultured human myometrial cells." *Exp Physiol* 77(2): 293-305.

Ting, J. P. and B. K. Davis (2005). "CATERPILLER: a novel gene family important in immunity, cell death, and diseases." *Annu Rev Immunol* 23: 387-414.

Ting, J. P., S. B. Willingham, et al. (2008). "NLRs at the intersection of cell death and immunity." *Nat Rev Immunol* 8(5): 372-9.

Tornblom, S. A., A. Klimaviciute, et al. (2005). "Non-infected preterm parturition is related to increased concentrations of IL-6, IL-8 and MCP-1 in human cervix." *Reprod Biol Endocrinol* 3: 39.

Toti, P., F. Arcuri, et al. (2011) "Focal Increases of Fetal Macrophages in Placentas from Pregnancies with Histological Chorioamnionitis: Potential Role of Fibroblast Monocyte Chemotactic Protein-1." *Am J Reprod Immunol* 65(5): 470-479.

Tucker, J. and W. McGuire (2004). "Epidemiology of preterm birth." *Bmj* 329(7467): 675-8.

Underhill, D. M., E. Rossnagle, et al. (2005). "Dectin-1 activates Syk tyrosine kinase in a dynamic subset of macrophages for reactive oxygen production." *Blood* 106(7): 2543-50.

Vacca, P., C. Cantoni, et al. (2010) "Crosstalk between decidual NK and CD14+ myelomonocytic cells results in induction of Tregs and immunosuppression." *Proceedings of the Proc Natil Acad Sci USA* 107(26): 11918-11923.

Vadillo-Ortega, F., A. Hernandez, et al. (1996). "Increased matrix metalloproteinase activity and reduced tissue inhibitor of metalloproteinases-1 levels in amniotic fluids from pregnancies complicated by premature rupture of membranes." *Am J Obstet Gynecol* 174(4): 1371-6.

van Asbeck, E. C., A. I. Hoepelman, et al. (2008). "Mannose binding lectin plays a crucial role in innate immunity against yeast by enhanced complement activation and enhanced uptake of polymorphonuclear cells." *BMC Microbiol* 8: 229.

Vavricka, S. R., M. W. Musch, et al. (2004). "hPepT1 transports muramyl dipeptide, activating NF-kappaB and stimulating IL-8 secretion in human colonic Caco2/bbe cells." *Gastroenterology* 127(5): 1401-9.

Verthelyi, D., K. J. Ishii, et al. (2001). "Human peripheral blood cells differentially recognize and respond to two distinct CPG motifs." *J Immunol* 166(4): 2372-7.

Wang, H. and E. Hirsch (2003). "Bacterially-induced preterm labor and regulation of prostaglandin-metabolizing enzyme expression in mice: the role of toll-like receptor 4." *Biol Reprod* 69(6): 1957-63.

Wang, T., T. Town, et al. (2004). "Toll-like receptor 3 mediates West Nile virus entry into the brain causing lethal encephalitis." *Nat Med* 10(12): 1366-73.

Watari, M., H. Watari, et al. (1999). "Pro-inflammatory cytokines induce expression of matrix-metabolizing enzymes in human cervical smooth muscle cells." *Am J Pathol* 154(6): 1755-62.

Watters, T. M., E. F. Kenny, et al. (2007). "Structure, function and regulation of the Toll/IL-1 receptor adaptor proteins." *Immunol Cell Biol* 85(6): 411-9.

Wesche, H., X. Gao, et al. (1999). "IRAK-M is a novel member of the Pelle/interleukin-1 receptor-associated kinase (IRAK) family." *J Biol Chem* 274(27): 19403-10.

Winkler, M. and W. Rath (1999). "Changes in the cervical extracellular matrix during pregnancy and parturition." *J Perinat Med* 27(1): 45-60.

Wojcikiewicz, E. P., X. Zhang, et al. (2003). "Contributions of molecular binding events and cellular compliance to the modulation of leukocyte adhesion." *J Cell Sci* 116(12): 2531-2539.

Yamamoto, M., S. Sato, et al. (2003). "TRAM is specifically involved in the Toll-like receptor 4-mediated MyD88-independent signaling pathway." *Nat Immunol* 4(11): 1144-50.

Yamamoto, M., S. Sato, et al. (2002). "Cutting edge: a novel Toll/IL-1 receptor domain-containing adapter that preferentially activates the IFN-beta promoter in the Toll-like receptor signaling." *J Immunol* 169(12): 6668-72.

Yamasaki, S., E. Ishikawa, et al. (2008). "Mincle is an ITAM-coupled activating receptor that senses damaged cells." *Nat Immunol* 9(10): 1179-88.

Yasukawa, H., A. Sasaki, et al. (2000). "Negative Regulation of Cytokine Signaling Pathways." *Ann Rev Immunol* 18(1): 143-164.

Yoneyama, M. and T. Fujita (2007). "Function of RIG-I-like receptors in antiviral innate immunity." *J Biol Chem* 282(21): 15315-8.

Yoneyama, M. and T. Fujita (2007). "RIG-I family RNA helicases: cytoplasmic sensor for antiviral innate immunity." *Cytokine Growth Factor Rev* 18(5-6): 545-51.

Yoneyama, M., W. Suhara, et al. (1998). "Direct triggering of the type I interferon system by virus infection: activation of a transcription factor complex containing IRF-3 and CBP/p300." *Embo J* 17(4): 1087-95.

Yoon, B. H., R. Romero, et al. (1995). "Amniotic fluid interleukin-6: a sensitive test for antenatal diagnosis of acute inflammatory lesions of preterm placenta and prediction of perinatal morbidity." *Am J Obstet Gynecol* 172(3): 960-70.

Yoon, B. H., R. Romero, et al. (1998). "Microbial invasion of the amniotic cavity with Ureaplasma urealyticum is associated with a robust host response in fetal, amniotic, and maternal compartments." *Am J Obstet Gynecol* 179(5): 1254-60.

Young, A., A. J. Thomson, et al. (2002). "Immunolocalization of proinflammatory cytokines in myometrium, cervix, and fetal membranes during human parturition at term." *Biol Reprod* 66(2): 445-9.

Zhang, D., G. Zhang, et al. (2004). "A toll-like receptor that prevents infection by uropathogenic bacteria." *Science* 303(5663): 1522-6.

12

Mechanisms of Maternal Immune Tolerance During Pregnancy

John E. Schjenken[1], Jorge M. Tolosa[1,2],
Jonathan W. Paul[1], Vicki L. Clifton[3] and Roger Smith[1]
[1]*Mothers and Babies Research Centre, University of Newcastle, New Lambton Heights, NSW,*
[2]*Faculty of Medical Sciences, University of Santiago of Chile, Santiago,*
[3]*Robinson Institute, Lyell McEwin Hospital, Elizabeth Vale, SA*
[1,3]*Australia*
[2]*Chile*

1. Introduction

Throughout their evolution, animals have developed mechanisms which protect them against parasites or infections by detecting and destroying foreign biological material within their own bodies. These mechanisms for excluding "non-self" biological materials whilst at the same time maintaining the integrity of the "self" have evolved for hundreds of millions of years into a highly complex body system, the immune system (Bainbridge, 2000). Any disbalance or alteration of the mechanisms maintaining the dynamic equilibrium between the "self" and "non-self" recognition could translate into a pathological state (or condition) like autoimmune disease at one end of the scale or immunodeficiency at the other.

The immunological system in placental mammals has been particularly challenged throughout the course of evolution, not just because of the exposure to a wide range of pathogens ("non-self") but because the evolution of the placenta allowed females to maintain fetuses within the reproductive tract for prolonged periods. One of the most intriguing features of mammalian embryo development is the re-organization of the maternal uterine tissue (endometrium) by embryo derived cells (trophoblast cells) in order to establish an intimate association with the mother. This process starts with embryo implantation and is characterized by the invasion of uterine tissues by the embryonic cells (trophoblast cells), culminating with the formation of the placenta, which permits intrauterine nourishment of the fetus, removal of waste metabolites, and the exchange of respiratory gasses to and from the fetal circulation until the moment of birth.

The intimate association between mother and embryo in placental mammals creates the potential problem of two genetically distinct individuals having to coexist for the duration of the pregnancy. This means that during pregnancy, the mothers' immune system has to tolerate the presence of paternal alloantigens ("nonself") from the placenta and/or the fetus (Bainbridge, 2000). In this context, pregnancy is a unique immunological challenge and it has been compared to the transplantation of a tissue or organ from a donor that is tolerated by the recipient (mother) and not rejected.

The paradox of the fetal allograft (transplant), as this process has been called, has been the dominant hypothesis driving research and debate in the field of reproductive immunology and the question why the mother does not reject the feto-placental unit remains unanswered. No other tissue, when surgically transplanted between genetically different individuals, enjoys the impunity from lethal host immune responses that characterizes the maternal-fetal relationship.

More than 50 years have passed since Peter Medawar (Medawar, 1953) made one of the most influential contributions to the field of Reproductive Immunology with his essay entitled "Some Immunological and Endocrinological Problems Raised by the Evolution of Viviparity in Vertebrates". Based on his pioneering studies demonstrating the role of tissue antigens in the recognition and rejection of skin grafts between genetically different individuals, and the work of others (reviewed in (Billington, 2003)) on the genetic basis of tumor transplant rejection in mice, Medawar recognized the truly paradoxical nature of the immunological relationship between the mother and her fetus. In his words: "The immunological problem of pregnancy may be formulated thus: How does the pregnant mother contrive to nourish within itself, for many weeks or months, a fetus that is an antigenically foreign body?" (Medawar, 1953).

This immunological paradox exists because according to the laws of tissue transplantation, fetal alloantigens encoded by polymorphic genes inherited from the father should provoke maternal immune responses leading to fetal rejection soon after blastocyst implantation in the uterine wall (Billingham, 1964; Medawar, 1953). From a genetic perspective, mother and fetus are never identical in outbred populations because the fetus inherits a different set of polymorphic genes from each parent and multiple tissue antigens differ between fetus and mother. Even more extraordinary is the case of surrogate mothers, where the feto-placental unit represents a bigger alloantigen challenge for the mother and can be considered a perfect example of a successful allotransplantation (at least temporarily).

Originally, Medawar proposed three explanations to answer the question as to how the fetus does not usually provoke an immunological reaction from its mother: (1) the anatomical separation of fetus from mother; (2) the antigenic immaturity of the fetus; and (3) the immunological indolence or inertness of the mother" (Medawar, 1953).

Medawar himself was convinced that the anatomical separation of fetus from mother, by a barrier considered at that time to be impermeable to maternal cells, was by far the most important of these possible explanations. Very early on, Billingham (Billingham, 1964) drew attention to the growing evidence for bi-directional transfer of cellular elements between mother and fetus, indicating that the placenta cannot be regarded as an absolute barrier. It is now known that in species with hemochorial placentation, as in humans and rodents, the mother and the fetus are not separated by an intact layer of epithelial cells, and placental trophoblast cells are thus exposed to maternal immune cells. A bidirectional transfer of cells between mother and fetus is common during human and murine pregnancy, and can lead to microchimerism (Nelson et al., 2007).

The second hypothesis proposed by Medawar, that the conceptus lacked immunogenicity, has been shown in studies by Hoskin and others (Elbe-Burger et al., 2000; Hoskin and Murgita, 1989) not to occur as immune reactions against fetal cells have been described. Hoskin and Murgita (Hoskin and Murgita, 1989) showed an immune reaction against fetal cells in the mouse. In this study, splenic T cells with a helper phenotype obtained from primiparous CBA/J mice pregnant by syngeneic matings were found to proliferate in response to co-culture with fetal thymus cells. Maternal anti-fetal lymphoproliferative responses were also shown to be blocked by the addition of antibodies against major histocompatibility complex (MHC) molecules (Hoskin and Murgita, 1989). More recently, studies have shown that fetal tissue expresses MHC molecules which are required for immune recognition and activation (reviewed in (Bainbridge, 2000)). All together, these data showed that the conceptus had immunogenic properties.

In reference to Medawar's third hypothesis, there is ample evidence that pregnancy is recognized by the immune system. Antibodies against fetal antigens have been detected in the sera of pregnant women showing that maternal recognition of fetal antigens does occur (reviewed in (Billington, 1992)). Women undergoing normal pregnancy preferentially release type 2 helper T cell (Th2) cytokines, whereas women who have recurrent spontaneous abortions induce the production of type 1 helper T cell (Th1) cytokines (Raghupathy, 1997). Thus the maternal immune system not only recognizes pregnancy but responds in a way which can determine the success or failure of pregnancy.

The maternal immune system is clearly active, and under certain conditions may contribute to fetal damage/death. Well-defined pathological processes include destruction of fetal erythrocytes (Rh antigen, erythroblastosis) and platelets (HPA-1 and -2, alloimmune thrombocytopenia) by maternal antibodies and infections of pregnancy, where activated macrophages secreting high levels of Th1-type cytokines alter the delicate cytokine balance at the maternal-fetal interface (Hunt, 1989; Marzi et al., 1996). Yet even with a demonstrably active maternal immune system, mothers usually seem to tolerate rather than reject their genetically disparate fetuses (Hunt et al., 2005). Because of this, it has been necessary to reconsider the physiological interactions and physical contacts between fetal and maternal elements as a dynamic entity occurring at different levels during the course of pregnancy.

Following on from Medawar's original hypotheses, a fourth conceptual proposal was advanced by Billingham in 1964 (Billingham, 1964). Billingham proposed that the uterus may be an immune privileged site, where fetal tissue directs the maternal immune response towards a protective, tolerant one. The concept of immune-privileged sites has been recognized by immunologists for nearly 135 years, since the Dutch ophthalmologist Van Dooremaal observed prolonged survival of a mouse skin graft placed into the anterior chamber of a dog's eye (reviewed in (Stein-Streilein and Streilein, 2002)). Together with the anterior chamber of the eye, other tissues such brain, ovary, testis, pregnant uterus, and placenta, display many of the characteristics of immune-privileged sites where immune reactions are not initiated in response to tissues displaying histocompatibility differences either by setting up anatomical and/or physiological barriers, which prevent access to cells of the immune system (Trowsdale and Betz, 2006).

Experimental studies have since shown that transplant immunity can be both elicited and expressed in a normal manner in the uterus. This was shown initially by Poppa *et al.*, in 1964, who demonstrated the rejection of intrauterine parathyroid allografts in pseudopregnant parathyroidectomized rats (Poppa et al., 1964). Also, the possibility of ectopic pregnancies demonstrates that the uterus does not uniquely protect the conceptus as an immune privileged site (Billington, 2003).

So the question is how does the mother's immune system recognize and respond to feto-placental antigens in a way that promotes successful pregnancy and not immune rejection? It is known from extensive studies in transplantation that a semi-allogeneic graft will be promptly rejected without adequate pharmacological control of the recipient's immune system, whereas the semi-allogeneic fetus which expresses antigens derived from both the mother and the father can survive throughout normal pregnancy without immunological rejection (Billington, 2003). This suggests that the developing fetus has mechanisms which prevent a maternal immune response against paternal/fetal antigens. Indeed, studies have shown that during pregnancy, paternal alloantigens can avoid maternal immune rejection. Tafuri *et al.*, showed that female mice would accept an allogeneic tumor graft while pregnant with a conceptus from a father matching the allograft but if the tumor cells were transplanted from a third party allogeneic donor, they would be rejected. Further, after the delivery of the mice, paternal tumors would be rejected showing that this tolerance only occurred during pregnancy (Tafuri et al., 1995).

The immune regulatory processes operating at the level of the maternal-fetal interface are highly dynamic and invoke multiple and sometimes redundant mechanisms and/or factors to reduce the likelihood of maternal immune rejection. Together with this redundancy, it is widely accepted that fetal factors drive changes in maternal immune responses and that both the fetus and the mother actively contribute to the development and maintenance of the pregnant uterus as an immune privileged site.

To understand the physiological mechanisms of maternal immune tolerance of the semi-allogeneic fetus during pregnancy has relevant implications not just for the field of Reproductive Immunology but also is clinically relevant for immune-mediated diseases (e.g., autoimmunity and asthma/allergy), cancer and for cell and organ transplantation. While the precise cellular interactions and mechanisms involved in maternal tolerance to the semi-allograft feto-placental unit are not yet completely understood, the identity of some of the critical factors and mechanisms have been uncovered and some details follow.

2. Mechanisms of maternal immune tolerance

2.1 Complement system

The innate branch of the immune system comprises the cells and mechanisms that defend the host from foreign organisms in a non-specific manner. Central to innate immune responses is the complement system (Girardi, 2008). Over 30 proteins are involved in its activation and they act in concert to protect the host against invading organisms (Girardi, 2008; Girardi et al., 2006). Activation of the complement cascade promotes chemotaxis of inflammatory cells and osmotic lysis of mammalian and bacterial cells through the formation of membrane attack complexes and is commonly used by the immune system to kill foreign or cancerous cells (Danilova, 2006). The complement cascade is regulated by complement regulatory proteins (CRP) that are expressed on cells and are critical for protecting tissues from inflammation that occurs in response to complement activation.

The complement cascade can be activated by three different pathways: the classical, the mannose binding lectin, and the alternative pathway. These pathways are activated as a result of different stimuli. The classical pathway is triggered by the presence of antibody bound to a target antigen, the lectin pathway is initiated by carbohydrates on microbial surfaces and the alternative pathway is spontaneously and constantly activated on biological surfaces in plasma and in most other body fluids allowing for rapid complement activation in response to foreign antigens (Zipfel and Skerka, 2009). These three activation pathways lead to the cleavage of the C3 component and the generation of C3a and C3b fragments. C3a causes the activation and release of inflammatory mediators such as histamine while C3b activates additional members of the complement cascade until the binding of C5b initiates the recruitment of the membrane attack complex (MAC). The MAC is a pore forming lipophilic complex that activates cell lysis, which results in permeabilization of the cell membrane and ultimately, cell death (Girardi, 2008; Zipfel and Skerka, 2009).

In transplantation, the activation of complement has been shown to be involved in acute graft rejections. The use of monoclonal antibodies to complement proteins has demonstrated that complement is activated and deposited on the vascular endothelium of the transplanted tissue in a significant number of acute rejections (Wasowska et al., 2007). However, complement can be regulated and the process of regulation can be controlled by the stimulation or inhibition of complement activation. Due to the similarities between pregnancy and tissue or organ transplantation, it has been suggested that appropriate complement inhibition is a requirement for successful pregnancy (Girardi, 2008). Indeed, as complement may be one of the components in the maternal blood which may damage trophoblast cells after its activation by antibodies, trophoblast cells have protective mechanisms which allow them to avoid complement activation. The placenta expresses three CRP: decay-accelerating factor (DAF), membrane co-factor protein (MCP), and CD59 (Tedesco et al., 1993). These regulatory proteins inhibit complement at different stages of the activation sequence. DAF and MCP both act early in the complement cascade to control C3 activation whilst CD59 is an inhibitor of the MAC (Morgan and Holmes, 2000) . Thus, the expression of CRP at the maternal/fetal interface is a critical adaptation for protecting the fetus from injury inflicted by inflammation provoked by complement activation (Holmes et al., 1992).

The role of CRP in trophoblast complement inhibition is further supported in studies by Tedesco *et al.*, 1993 (Tedesco et al., 1993), who tested the role of CRP in the vulnerability of human trophoblast to complement activation. In these studies the inhibition of MCP and CD59 resulted in an increased susceptibility of trophoblast cells to complement mediated immunological activation suggesting the inhibition of complement by MCP and CD59 is required for pregnancy to proceed as normal. The protective function of DAF was unable to be tested due to its reduced expression on isolated trophoblasts compared to normal placental tissue.

In rare cases, individuals deficient in DAF or CD59 have been reported, but no MCP deficiencies have been found. Individuals lacking DAF or CD59 survive pregnancy apparently unscathed making it unlikely that either regulator is essential for fetal survival but it is tempting to speculate that since there are no reported cases of individuals deficient in MCP, this protein may have an essential role in complement inhibition in pregnancy. It is possible that the reason that this deficiency has not been identified is because it is without consequence (Morgan and Holmes, 2000). However, mutations in MCP have been identified in some patients predisposed to preeclampsia, leading to the suggestion that dysregulation of complement activation can be a risk factor for preeclampsia (Salmon et al., 2011).

The most convincing evidence of complement inhibition in pregnancy comes from studies in mice and rats. These species express the three complement regulators detailed above but they also carry another regulator not found in other species called Crry (Trowsdale and Betz, 2006). Xu *et al.*, 2000 generated mice that were deficient in Crry (Crry$^{(-/-)}$) and showed that survival of Crry$^{(-/-)}$ embryos was compromised due to complement deposition and placental inflammation. This study demonstrated that complement was responsible for the fetal loss as breeding to C3$^{(-/-)}$ rescued Crry$^{(-/-)}$ from lethality (Xu et al., 2000).

2.2 Phosphocholination

Phosphocholination is a post-translational modification which involves the addition of the small haptenic molecule phosphocholine to the polysaccharide moiety of certain secretory glycoproteins. This modification is characteristic of a wide variety of prokaryotic organisms (e.g. bacteria) as well as eukaryotic organisms (e.g. parasites). In parasites it has been suggested that phosphocholine containing proteins are secreted into host organisms and have an effect on immune cells leading to immunosuppression (Lovell et al., 2007). In particular, phosphocholinated proteins in filarial nematodes have been shown to inhibit normal proliferative responses of both T and B lymphocytes *in vitro*. These effects have been attributed to the phosphocholine moiety as phosphocholine coupled to bovine serum albumin has the same inhibitory effects on T and B lymphocytes as phosphocholinated filarial nematode proteins (Harnett and Harnett, 1993; Lal et al., 1990).

Recent studies have shown that phosphocholination can occur in mammalian species. Foulds *et al.*, (Foulds et al., 2008) identified lyso-glycerophosphocholine as an endogenous immunosuppressive agent in bovine and rat gonadal fluids. In these studies, the immunosuppressive fractions of rat testicular interstitial fluid and bovine ovarian follicular fluid were assayed by sequential reverse phase high performance liquid chromatography (HPLC) and sequenced using capillary electrophoresis electrospray ionization mass spectrometry. These molecules were shown to inhibit T cell proliferation and induce apoptosis of T cells in a time and dose dependent manner (Foulds et al., 2008).

In the placenta, Lovell et al., (Lovell et al., 2007) showed that a large number of placental polypeptides and proteins carry phosphocholine as a tissue specific post translational modification and suggested the presence of phosphocholine groups on placental secretory proteins and peptides may play a major role in maternal immune tolerance during pregnancy. In these studies, placental neurokinin B and the precursors of corticotropin releasing hormone (CRH), adrenocorticotropin, hemokinin, activin and follistatin were shown to be post-translationally modified by the addition of phosphocholine using a combination of HPLC and two site immunometric analyses. Lowry (Lowry, 2008) suggested that the addition of phosphocholine moieties in placental secreted peptides and proteins may be the rule rather than the exception and that this post translational modification may play an important role in maternal immune tolerance during pregnancy.

2.3 Programmed Death Ligand 1 (PDL1)

The activation of T lymphocytes requires two signals, one of which is delivered by the T cell receptor complex after antigen recognition and the other which requires the engagement of costimulatory receptors. The second signal can be either positive, which leads to full T cell activation, or negative, which can downregulate immune responses (Rothstein and Sayegh, 2003). In regards to negative T cell signaling, the inhibitory costimulatory receptor molecule programmed death 1 (PD1) and its ligands, PDL1 and PDL2 have been shown to play a role in regulating immune responses *in vivo* (Guleria et al., 2005).

PD1 is a 55kDa type 1 transmembrane receptor that was initially identified in a murine T-cell hybridoma undergoing activation induced cell death (Ishida et al., 1992) and is a member of the CD28 IgG superfamily (Rothstein and Sayegh, 2003). It has been shown to be constitutively expressed by double negative thymocytes (hematopoietic progenitor cells present in the thymus which are negative for CD4 and CD8) and natural killer (NK) cells, and its expression can be induced on activated CD4 and CD8 T cells, B cells and macrophages. The ligands for PD1, PDL1/2, are expressed on antigen presenting cells following cellular activation or exposure to interferon gamma (IFN-γ). PDL-1 has also been found on a subpopulation of activated T cells. In addition, the ligands can be constitutively expressed or induced by a variety of parenchymal or endothelial cells, including heart, kidney, pancreas and placenta (Blank et al., 2005).

Binding of either ligand to PD1 inhibits antigen stimulated T cell activation through several mechanisms including the control of proliferation, alteration of cytokine production, and the induction of apoptosis (Blank et al., 2005; Hori et al., 2006). *In vivo* studies have shown the critical importance of PD1 in maintaining immunological self tolerance. PD1 knockout mice have fatal autoimmune disease and in humans, polymorphisms in PD1 are associated with several autoimmune diseases (Nishimura and Honjo, 2001; Prokunina et al., 2002). Further, this inhibitory receptor and its ligand have also been shown to prevent allograft rejection suggesting an important role in negative T cell signaling (Wang et al., 2007).

As a result of their established role in negative T cell signaling, it was hypothesized that PD1/PDL(1/2) signaling may play an important role in maternal immune tolerance. During pregnancy, PDL2 is expressed on the syncytiotrophoblast in early pregnancy, while PDL1 is expressed on all trophoblast populations throughout pregnancy. Expression of PDL1 is low in first trimester placenta and increases throughout gestation whereas PDL2 is prominent in the syncytiotrophoblast of the early placenta and decreases throughout gestation (Petroff et al., 2003; Petroff et al., 2005). Interestingly, in the mouse the source of PDL1 is the maternal decidua and not the trophoblast suggesting that the decidua may participate in the suppression of alloantigen specific T cells.

Experimental studies on mice using blocking antibodies against PDL1 and PDL2 showed a dramatic loss of allogeneic fetuses in animals treated with the PDL1 but not PDL2 blocking antibody. No effect of the inhibition of PDL1 signaling was observed in syngeneic fetuses suggesting that PDL1 is participating in maternal immune tolerance (Guleria et al., 2005). However, in contrast to the above study, Taglauer *et al.* (Taglauer et al., 2009), showed that the absence of maternal PD1 and PDL1 had no detectable effects on gestation length, litter size, or pup weight at birth in both syngeneic or allogeneic pregnancies. The discrepancies between the two studies are hard to explain but the lack of rejection seen in Taglauer *et al.*, (Taglauer et al., 2009) may be explained by the existence of redundant or compensatory immunosuppressive mechanisms at the maternal fetal interface.

As detailed above, The PD1/PDL1 pathway can inhibit T lymphocytes through several mechanisms. In regards to maternal immune tolerance, it has been speculated that the role of PD1/PDL1 in maternal-fetal tolerance is to control the abundance of T cells by inducing apoptosis of paternal antigen specific T cells. Taglauer *et al.*, 2009 (Taglauer et al., 2009) showed that fetal antigen-specific lymphocytes upregulate PD1 following recognition of fetal antigen. In the absence of PD1, lymphocytes were seen to accumulate in the maternal uterine draining lymph nodes suggesting that PD-1 may be responsible for their deletion.

2.4 Major Histocompatibility Complex (MHC) and the non-classical Human Leukocyte Antigen (HLA) class 1bGenes (HLA-E, -G and –F) expressed on Trophoblast cells

All mammalian species studied to date possess a tightly linked cluster of genes, the Major Histocompatibility Complex (MHC) complex, which are involved in intercellular immune recognition and antigen presentation to T lymphocytes. Based on the observation that in most of the cases of transplant rejection the immune response is directed against a few proteins encoded by the MHC genetic region, the study of the immunological status of the mammalian fetus has been primarily directed towards determining which MHC are expressed on trophoblast cells (Bainbridge, 2000). The MHC, which is referred to as the Human Leukocyte Antigen (HLA) complex in humans, is organized into three regions based on the types of molecules that are produced. Class I molecules encode glycoproteins which are expressed on the surface of nearly all nucleated cells, class II molecules encode glycoproteins primarily expressed on antigen presenting cells and class III molecules encode secreted proteins associated with the immune process (e.g. soluble serum proteins) (Kuby, 1997).

In organ transplantation, allelic differences between MHC class II and class I molecules form the primary basis for transplant rejection. Therefore it is relevant to note that trophoblast cells of the placenta are unique because they are one of the few mammalian cell types that do not express classical MHC class II antigens, either constitutively or after exposure to IFN-γ (Murphy et al., 2004). This is arguably one of the most important immune evasion strategies during pregnancy.

Initially it was thought that trophoblast cells did not display HLA antigens and that this phenomenon could completely account for immunological protection of the fetus (Faulk and Temple, 1976; Goodfellow et al., 1976; Hunt et al., 1988). It was later discovered that placental cells express specific genes within the MHC loci. The expressed class I genes are subdivided into class Ia, which includes HLA-A, -B, and -C, and class Ib, which includes HLA-E, -F, and -G. Human trophoblast cells do not express the two main polymorphic classical class Ia antigens HLA-A and B (Redman et al., 1984) and only express one class Ia molecule (HLA-C) and all three class Ib molecules. These class Ib antigens are distinguished by low numbers of alleles that differ at the protein level.

HLA-G was the first trophoblast HLA molecule to be identified and is of great interest due to the strong evidence which suggests that this class Ib molecule may be important in preventing maternal immune attack against the fetus during pregnancy (Le Bouteiller, 1996). Interestingly, HLA-G like proteins have also been identified in the placentas of non-human primates supporting the concept that HLA-G like proteins may be important in maternal immune tolerance.

HLA-G can be expressed as seven isoforms, of which four are membrane bound (HLA-G1 to G4) and three are soluble (HLA-G5 to -G7) (Carosella et al., 2008). In contrast to classical

HLA alleles, HLA-G has a very low level of polymorphism with only 8 protein variants. Most of the polymorphisms that are encountered in the HLA-G gene are not predicted to alter the amino acid sequence, or, if they do, will not change the secondary structure of the molecule. Due to the low level of polymorphisms, paternal HLA-G expressed on the surface of trophoblast cells will be almost identical to maternal HLA-G. This minimizes the risk of immune rejection.

Early studies identified HLA class I antigen expression as being specific to extra-villous trophoblast (EVT) populations, with the proteins being prominent in cells adjacent to the decidua throughout gestation (Hunt and Langat, 2009). However, the antibody used to identify these antigens required MHC light chain and MHC heavy chain associations which are not present on all HLA-G isoforms. More recent studies using different antibodies which are capable of detecting previously undetectable HLA-G alleles showed that HLA-G isoforms are present throughout the placenta and within the chorion membrane, decidua and maternal blood (Hunt and Langat, 2009).

Since HLA-G is produced at high levels at the maternal interface it has been suggested to have a role in maternal tolerance induction. The effects of HLA-G in different tissues include impacts on NK cell killing activity, migration and cell viability, proliferation and IFN-γ production, regulation of cytokine production, suppression of cytotoxic T lymphocyte killing activity and viability, inhibition of proliferation and induction of a suppressive phenotype in T helper cells, and alteration of dendritic cell stimulatory capacity and maturation of this lineage (reviewed in (Hunt, 2006)).

There are currently no reported cases of pregnancy from women in which all the forms of the HLA-G are absent. However, mutations in HLA-G alleles have been identified. For example, Ober *et al.,* (Ober et al., 1998) identified a single base pair deletion at position 1597 of exon 3 of HLA-G which is present on 7.4% of African American and 2.9% Hispanic chromosomes. This deletion causes a frameshift mutation and results in amino acid substitutions in all of the residues of the second half of exon 3. Individuals with this mutation, have no detectable HLA-G1 protein but are still able to go through normal pregnancy suggesting that certain HLA-G alleles are not essential for pregnancy. Other studies have shown that certain polymorphisms such as a 14 base pair insertion in exon 8 of the 3′-UTR may be associated with pregnancy complications such as preeclampsia and recurrent spontaneous abortion (Larsen and Hviid, 2009). However, these data are not well supported in the literature and different studies show different effects of HLA-G polymorphisms.

Studies of MHC molecules in the trophoblast of the mouse have shown that mice predominantly express only one MHC class I antigen, H-2K, at the cell surface of trophoblast giant cells and appear to lack the expression of non-classical MHC molecules (Madeja et al., 2011). However, recent studies have hypothesized that mice may have a functional homolog of HLA-G, with both Qa-2 and Blastocyst MHC being postulated to play this role. The mouse Qa-2 gene has some of the structural characteristics of HLA-G and is expressed on pre-implantation embryos (Comiskey et al., 2003) while Blastocyst MHC is selectively expressed in the blastocyst and placenta (Tajima et al., 2003). Interestingly, both of these putative homologs have been implicated in immune regulation (Comiskey et al., 2003; Tajima et al., 2003) suggesting that they may play a similar role to HLA-G.

Altogether, these data suggest that non-classical MHC molecules may play an important role in the generation of maternal immune tolerance.

2.5 Tryptophan catabolism mediated by indoleamine 2,3,-dioxygenase (IDO)

Indoleamine 2,3-dioxygenase (IDO) is an enzyme that catabolizes the essential amino acid L-tryptophan that is required for the biosynthesis of proteins. IDO was initially described in 1967 by Yamamoto and Hayaishi in the rabbit intestine as an enzyme that could oxidize both L- and D-tryptophan (Yamamoto and Hayaishi, 1967) and was later shown to have an important role in microbial resistance by allowing cells to deplete tryptophan from intracellular pools or the local microenvironment (Mellor and Munn, 1999). When an infectious agent invades a tissue, leukocytes and lymphocytes accumulate at the site of infection and secrete IFNs into the inflammatory milieu. The presence of IFN triggers IDO production and subsequent tryptophan catabolism which inhibits the growth of the infectious agent (Grohmann et al., 2003).

As tryptophan is an indispensible requirement for cell growth, it was proposed that IDO may have other important roles. Indeed, there are intriguing associations between altered tryptophan metabolism and cell-mediated immune responses. For example, enhanced tryptophan catabolism by macrophages has been shown to inhibit T cell proliferation and it appears that the expression of IDO by cells allows them to suppress unwanted T cell responses (Munn et al., 1999). Further, emerging evidence is linking the IDO pathway with T-regulatory (Treg) cell biology. Firstly, studies have shown that IDO competent dendritic cells can drive the generation of Tregs through high levels of IDO. Secondly, IDO can prevent the reprogramming of Tregs into proinflammatory T-helper-like cells *in vivo* (Munn, 2011). In support of the above statements, studies have shown that patients receiving tryptophan for a variety of disorders experience a high frequency of autoimmune disease (Mellor and Munn, 1999). In addition, studies of the potential role of IDO in transplantation tolerance have shown that the presence of this enzyme in pancreatic islet, lung, heart and corneal allografts can significantly extend graft survival (reviewed in (Mulley and Nikolic-Paterson, 2008). Collectively, these data suggest that IDO can modulate immunity.

IDO expression is not detected in most tissues of healthy mammals but can be increased by infection and inflammation due to the production of IFNs and other factors (Baban et al., 2004). The only tissues where IDO is expressed at constitutively high levels is the proximal male epididymis and at the maternal-fetal interface during mammalian pregnancy (Baban et al., 2004). Munn *et al.,* (Munn et al., 1998) proposed that in the mouse the expression of IDO by the placenta is crucial in the prevention of T cell responses against the fetus. In this study Munn *et al.,* demonstrated that tryptophan is catabolized by the placenta during pregnancy and that this process suppresses T cell activity and defends the fetus against rejection. Rapid T cell-induced rejection of all allogeneic but no syngeneic fetuses occurred when pregnant mice were treated with the IDO inhibitor, 1-methyl-tryptophan (Munn et al., 1998).

In humans, Kudo *et al.,* showed that IDO activity and messenger RNA (mRNA) expression can be positively regulated by cytokines such as IFN-γ and that tryptophan transport into the trophoblast is the rate limiting step for IDO mediated tryptophan degradation (Kudo and Boyd, 2000; Kudo and Boyd, 2001). Knowing that IDO had similar actions in humans as in mice, Kudo *et al.,* examined the potential role of IDO in the human placenta. In these studies, Kudo *et al.*, showed that tryptophan degradation by IDO inhibited lymphocyte proliferation in placental tissues. Media conditioned by placental villi in the presence of IFN-γ (inducer of IDO) was more depleted of tryptophan than control media and the proliferation of mononuclear cells, specifically $CD4^+$ T lymphocytes was markedly inhibited by tryptophan degradation. This inhibition could be reversed by the addition of 1-methyl tryptophan (Kudo et al., 2001).

Despite all of these reports which support a role for IDO in maternal immune tolerance, a number of studies have shown that IDO is not essential for pregnancy. Baban *et al.*, developed an IDO knockout mouse and showed that in allogeneic matings, the mice were capable of producing litters of normal sizes and rates compared to control mice suggesting that redundant mechanisms may protect allogeneic fetuses in IDO knockout mice (Baban et al., 2004). Also, in humans it has been reported that IDO expression does not differ between proven fertile women and women with a history of miscarriages.

2.6 Progesterone

Since the 1970s, evidence detailing the production of various hormones and cytokines by the placenta has expanded our knowledge on mechanisms by which uterine tissue functions as well as the putative roles of these hormones and cytokines in pregnancy (Petraglia et al., 1996). The production and modulation of hormones during pregnancy is essential and many important processes, such as the transport of sperm and oocytes, implantation and labor are controlled by alterations in the hormonal environment (Szekeres-Bartho, 2002). Placental steroid hormones have also been considered as possible mediators of immunosuppression during pregnancy because of the immunosuppressive properties of natural and synthetic glucocorticoids (Siiteri et al., 1977).

Among the hormones present in maternal serum, progesterone, the hallmark of pregnancy, appears to play a major role in reducing the maternal response to the fetal allograft (Beagley and Gockel, 2003). Progesterone has been shown to be essential in the maintenance of pregnancy in a number of mammalian species. In humans, progesterone is produced autonomously by the placenta at high levels (up to 250 mg a day) (Szekeres-Bartho, 2002). Shortly after delivery the concentration of progesterone in maternal blood falls precipitously.

Early studies showed that high concentrations of progesterone can prolong the survival of xenogeneic and allogeneic grafts (reviewed in (Szekeres-Bartho, 2002)). For example, Hansen *et al.*, (Hansen et al., 1986) studied the effect of progesterone on skin transplants placed in the uterine lumen of ovariectomized ewes. Allografts placed in the uterine lumen of progesterone treated ewes were present 30 days after engraftment while allografts placed in control animals were completely resorbed. Other studies have shown that progesterone can affect various phases of the immune response *in vivo*. Siiteri et al (Siiteri *et al.*, 1977) showed in rats, using progesterone concentrations that mimic the high intrauterine concentration in pregnancy, that progesterone can effectively block cellular immune responses both *in vitro* and *in vivo*. Stites *et al.*, (Stites et al., 1983) using human blood cultures showed that progesterone was capable of inhibiting monocyte dependent T cell activation.

Progesterone can induce its immunological changes by a number of different cellular and molecular mechanisms. It has been shown to stimulate the activity of specific enzyme matrix metalloproteinases and adhesion molecules, inhibit antibody production and suppress T-cell activation and cytotoxicity, modify the activity of natural killer cells and induce the secretion of protective asymmetric antibodies (reviewed in (Kyurkchiev et al., 2010).

In pregnancy, the immunosuppressive effects of progesterone are determined on the one hand by its concentration and also by the progesterone-binding capacity of lymphocytes. Lymphocytes carried by the maternal blood during pregnancy are extremely sensitive to progesterone which suggests receptor mediated action of progesterone on the lymphocytes. Szekeres-Batho *et al.*, (Szekeres-Bartho et al., 1990) showed that $CD8^+$ lymphocytes produced peripherally during pregnancy were reactive to progesterone receptor monoclonal antibodies and that the level of progesterone receptor positive lymphocytes increased throughout gestation.

The biological effects of progesterone during pregnancy are manifested by a 34kDa protein, called the progesterone induced blocking factor (PIBF), which is released by lymphocytes of pregnant women following binding of progesterone to its receptors (Szekeres-Bartho, 2002). In pregnant women, the PIBF concentration gradually increases until the 37th week of gestation, followed by a slow decrease until term. PIBF signals through the JAK/STAT pathway and has been shown to: alter the cytokine balance resulting in a preferential production of Th2 type cytokines in mice, inhibit NK cell activity through mediation by cytokines, and regulate anti-abortive effects (Kozma et al., 2006; Szekeres-Bartho, 2002; Szekeres-Bartho and Wegmann, 1996; Szekeres-Bartho et al., 2008). In peripheral blood of healthy pregnant women, the percentage of PIBF positive lymphocytes is significantly higher in all trimesters of pregnancy than in women at risk for premature pregnancy termination (Szekeres-Bartho et al., 1995).

Interestingly, recent studies have suggested that progesterone may have a role in the generation of Treg cells in both mice and humans. In these studies, physiological doses of progesterone were shown to significantly increase the population of Treg cells (Lee et al., 2011; Mao et al., 2010). However, in contrast to these data, Mjosberg *et al.* showed using an *in vitro* model, that progesterone reduced the Treg cell population in PBMC from non-pregnant women (Mjosberg et al., 2009). While the potential role of progesterone in the stimulation of Treg cells is exciting, further studies are required.

2.7 Th1-Th2 cytokine balance in pregnancy

The best studied peripheral immune cells in pregnancy are T-lymphocytes. Within this population there are two main subsets which are defined as helper T lymphocytes and cytotoxic T lymphocytes. Helper T lymphocytes are particularly important in the context of pregnancy as they affect the function of other immune cells by producing cytokines (Veenstra van Nieuwenhoven et al., 2003). Helper T lymphocytes can be further separated into Th1 and Th2 based on their profile of cytokine production. Th1 produce tumor necrosis factor (TNF)-α, IFN-γ and interleukin (IL)-2 which promote cellular immune responses while Th2 produce IL-4, IL-5, IL-9, IL-10 and IL-13 which promote humoral responses (Mosmann et al., 1986; Veenstra van Nieuwenhoven et al., 2003).

It has been shown that T cells mediate many of their effects through the secretion of cytokines and in pregnancy it has been hypothesized that a correctly regulated cytokine environment determines the growth and survival of the feto-placental unit. Studies by Chaouat *et al.*, (Chaouat et al., 1995; Chaouat et al., 1990) examined fetal survival following the injection of various cytokines in mice and showed that granulocyte macrophage colony stimulating factor (GM-CSF), IL-3 and IL-10 enhanced fetal survival and promoted intrauterine growth while TNF-α, IFN-γ and IL-2 had deleterious effects which led to fetal death. These studies, and the studies of others led to the Th1/Th2 paradigm proposed by Wegmann *et al.*, in 1993 (Wegmann et al., 1993) which hypothesized that Th2 cytokines inhibit Th1 responses, improving fetal survival and impairing responses against some pathogens. It is important to note that this hypothesis was in reference to the post-implantation period till labor (Chaouat, 2007) and was never meant to be extended to implantation and conception where inflammatory cells and molecules play an important role in preparing the female reproductive tract for pregnancy (Robertson, 2010).

As detailed above, the Th1/Th2 paradigm stated that "successful pregnancy is a Th2 phenomenon " (Wegmann et al., 1993). Indeed, pregnancy is characterized by an increase in Th2 immune responses. Studies in humans and in mice have shown that the maternal immune response is biased toward a Th2 humoral response and away from cell-mediated immunity which could be harmful to the fetus (Raghupathy, 1997; Wegmann et al., 1993). In women who suffer from recurrent spontaneous abortions their peripheral blood mononuclear cells (PBMCs) respond *in vitro* to trophoblast antigens by producing high levels of the Th1 cytokine IFN-γ and TNF-α (Chaouat et al., 1990; Hill et al., 1995). Conversely, in PBMC from women who are not prone to recurrent spontaneous abortions a preferential production of the Th2 cytokine IL-10 is observed (Hill et al., 1995). It is also interesting to note that humoral associated autoimmune diseases such as lupus tend to flare up during pregnancy while cell-mediated ones such as rheumatoid polyarthritis, often enter remission (reviewed in (Chaouat, 2007)).

Several different cells and soluble factors have been proposed as potential regulators of the altered Th1/Th2 ratio characteristic of pregnancy. The syncytiotrophoblast and cytotrophoblast are known to produce cytokines and these cells can influence cytokine production by acting on the Th1/Th2 balance (de Moraes-Pinto et al., 1997). Decidual cells and cells of the uterine draining lymph node have also been shown to suppress immune responses *in vitro*. Factors such as progesterone, PIBF and IDO have been proposed to alter the Th1/Th2 balance and cytokines themselves may play extremely important roles in modifying the immune system to favor a Th2 environment. Both transforming growth factor (TGF)-β and IL-10 appear to assist in maintaining the Th1/Th2 balance. IL-10 plays an important role in preventing spontaneous pregnancy failure in mice. The injection of IL-10 alone into pregnant mice has been shown to lead to the prevention of fetal resorption. This effect can be reversed by the addition of anti-IL-10 antibodies (Chaouat et al., 1995). TGF-β has been correlated with the immunosuppressive activity of decidual supernatants, appears to be reduced or absent in mice undergoing fetal resorptions and also appears to have an essential role in priming the immune system to tolerate seminal antigens (Raghupathy, 1997; Robertson et al., 2002).

However, Th2 dominant immunity has also been observed in recurrent abortion cases and Th2 knockout mice can proceed normally through a pregnancy suggesting that in addition to the Th1/Th2 phenomena, there are other mechanisms which may contribute to maternal immune tolerance (Chaouat et al., 2003). With this in mind, the Th1/Th2 paradigm has been expanded into the Th1/Th2/Th17/Treg paradigm. In this paradigm, Th17 cells, which produce IL-17 and are reported to be expressed at high levels in spontaneous abortion, are mediators of inflammation along with Th1 cells, while Treg cells which are potent suppressors of inflammatory immune responses and are essential to prevent autoimmunity (Saito et al., 2010), may be important in the induction of antigen specific tolerance.

TGF-β super family members are pleiotropic cytokines with well-known roles in a wide range of developmental processes including tissue differentiation, morphogenesis, proliferation, and migration. TGF-β1, TGF-β2 and TGF-β3 are abundant in mammalian reproductive tissues. TGF-β fulfils a pivotal role in the peripheral immune system through mediating the acquisition of immune tolerance (Schmidt-Weber and Blaser, 2004). TGF-β can inhibit T helper type 1 (Th1) responses, which may be detrimental to pregnancy (Raghupathy, 2001), and is an important regulator of NK cell behavior, down-regulating IFN-γ induced activation and inflammatory cytokine production. Lymphocyte populations secreting TGF-β are causally linked with pregnancy success in mice (Arck et al., 1999) and are diminished in the event of miscarriage. Indeed, in mice prone to a high pregnancy failure rate, TGF-β mRNA is significantly decreased in both uterine epithelial and metrial gland (NK) cells (Gorivodsky et al., 1999).

It has been reported that the intravaginal administration of bioactive TGF-β3 can enhance success of pregnancy in vivo in an established mouse model of abortion (resorptions) (the CBA/J × DBA/2 mouse model) (Clark et al., 2008). This result could be explained by the independent ability of TGF-β to promote a Treg cell response.

Recent reports have suggested a role for TGF-β in the generation of Treg cells from CD4+CD25− precursors (Ayatollahi et al., 2007; Chen et al., 2003; Zheng et al., 2007). These data suggest that Treg cells maintain transplantation tolerance through a TGF-β-dependent FOXP3 induction (Horwitz et al., 2008; Zheng et al., 2008). Thus, TGF-β is a key regulator of the signaling pathways which initiate and maintain FOXP3 expression and suppressive function among CD4+CD25− precursors.

A reduction in TGF-β1 has been observed in samples from non-pregnant women, compared with those of pregnant women, which might confirm the effect of TGF-β1 in controlling the development and function of the immune system during pregnancy (Ayatollahi et al., 2007; Power et al., 2002).

In addition to the known individual effects of TGF-β and IL-10 on lymphocytes and antigen-presenting cells, there is evidence for both cytokines working together to determine an immune response in a synergic way (Nagaeva et al., 2002). It has been shown that suppressive effects of TGF-β and IL-10 added together is greater than each acting alone (Chen et al., 2003; Horwitz et al., 2003; Horwitz et al., 2008; Zheng et al., 2008).

In spite of TGF-β having a central role in the induction of Foxp3 and regulatory capacity in CD4+ T cells for transplantation tolerance, recently, however, the general anti-inflammatory role of TGF-β in CD4+ T cell polarization has been questioned by the discovery that, in the presence of inflammatory cytokines such as IL-6 or IL-1, TGF-β drives the differentiation of Th17 cells associated with transplant rejection (Regateiro et al., 2011).

2.8 Regulatory T cells

The term Tregs (regulatory T-cells) refers to a subpopulation of T-lymphocytes with pivotal suppressive/regulatory properties that are devoted to maintaining antigen-specific T-cell tolerance, diminishing destructive immune responses and preventing autoimmune disease. Three main subsets of CD4+ regulatory T-cells with distinctive suppressive mechanisms have been identified and can be distinguished by their phenotype, cytokine secretion and tissue origin. These are type 1 regulatory T-cells (Tr1), T-helper 3 cells and $CD4^+$ $CD25^+$ Treg cells. Each of these subsets has the capacity to inhibit the proliferation and effector function of other T cells. Treg cells have two main physiological roles: control T-cell reaction with self antigens that have escaped negative selection by the thymus, and limit the extent and duration of responses exerted by T-cells reactive with alloantigens and other exogenous antigens (Guerin et al., 2009).

Treg cells have fast become established as perhaps the most potent and widespread suppressive cell lineage in the immune system and they are involved in immune tolerance, autoimmunity, inflammation, transplantation and cancer (Guerin et al., 2009). Studies into the biological action of Treg cells have shown that they are potent suppressors of inflammatory immune responses and are an essential requirement to prevent autoimmunity and to promote the tolerance of allogeneic organ grafts (Groux et al., 1997; Kingsley et al., 2002). These unique properties of T cells have led to speculation that they may have an important role in reproduction (Guerin et al., 2009).

Studies in mice have indicated that Treg cells are essential during the first days of pregnancy, even prior to embryo implantation. In mice, the Treg cell population expands as early as 2 days after mating where it is required to control the maternal immune response during peri-conception. It has been postulated that factors which promote the expansion of Treg cells are contained in seminal fluid. Soluble factors in seminal fluid such as members of the TGF-β family and prostaglandins have previously been linked with the generation of Treg cells (Robertson et al., 2009). These early Treg cells play an important role in implantation as studies have shown that depletion of Treg cells prior to implantation leads to a reduction in the percentage of pregnant mice (Zenclussen et al., 2005).

Following implantation in the mouse, Treg cell number is seen to increase throughout gestation and these cells are able to suppress both autoimmune responses and allogeneic responses directed against the fetus. The physiological significance of $CD4^+CD25^+$ Treg cells in pregnancy was demonstrated in studies using an adoptive transfer model, where complete T-cell populations or populations depleted of $CD4^+CD25^+$ Treg cells were transferred into pregnant T-cell deficient mice. In these studies, Aluvihare *et al.,* (Aluvihare et al., 2004) observed that in the absence of $CD4^+CD25^+$ Treg cells, allogeneic fetuses were promptly rejected, whereas syngeneic fetuses were unaffected. In addition, Zenclussen *et al.,* (Zenclussen et al., 2005) showed that *in vivo* prevention of fetal rejection in abortion prone mice could only be achieved after adoptive transfer of Treg cells from normal pregnant mice.

A similar increase in Treg cell populations is evident in pregnant women. Studies have shown that circulating human $CD4^+CD25^+$ Treg cells increase throughout gestation with a peak during the second trimester and then a subsequent decline postpartum. Isolated human $CD4^+CD25^+$ Treg were further shown to suppress proliferative responses of autologous $CD4^+CD25^-$ T-cells to allogeneic dendritic cells (Somerset et al., 2004). The role of

Treg cells in maternal immune tolerance is further supported in studies which show that paternal antigen stimulation of Treg cells is required for optimal protection of fetuses from rejection. Mjosberg *et al.*, showed that Treg cells from peripheral blood of pregnant and non-pregnant women can suppress alloantigen responses *in vitro*, with increased capacity to suppress anti-paternal as opposed to irrelevant alloantigens (Mjosberg et al., 2007).

The importance of Treg cells in pregnancy is further supported by studies of individuals who had complications of pregnancy. In preeclampsia, $CD4^{+}CD25^{high}$ Treg cells are significantly reduced in both peripheral blood and decidual tissue compared to normal pregnant women (Sasaki et al., 2007). In spontaneous abortions, the levels of $CD4^{+}CD25^{+}$ Treg cells are significantly lower in patients who had a spontaneous abortion compared to samples from induced abortions (Sasaki et al., 2004). Unexplained infertility is also associated with a reduction in the expression of the Treg cell marker FOXP3 mRNA in endometrial tissue (Jasper et al., 2006). Furthermore, cells expressing the Treg cell activation marker CTLA-4 are more prevalent in peripheral blood and term deciduas of normal healthy pregnant women compared with non-pregnant women (Heikkinen et al., 2004). Therefore, impaired differentiation and recruitment of uterine Treg cells may increase the chance of pregnancy complications.

Collectively, these results suggest that Treg cells may have an important role in maternal immune tolerance.

2.9 Corticotropin Releasing Hormone (CRH) and its regulation of FasL expression

CRH is a 41 amino acid peptide hormone that acts as the main neurotransmitter orchestrating the stress response through the secretion of adrenocorticotropic hormone (ACTH) or corticotropin from corticotropes of the anterior pituitary (McLean and Smith, 2001; Vale et al., 1981). In addition to its function in the hypothalamic-pituitary-adrenal axis, expression of CRH has been recognized at several different sites, including the placenta (McLean and Smith, 2001).

Despite the knowledge of the role of CRH in the hypothalamic-pituitary-adrenal axis, the precise biological role/s for CRH in feto-maternal tissues are yet to be elucidated. In the placenta and fetal membranes CRH appears to have a wide variety of functions, including the regulation of trophoblast cell growth and invasion, tissue remodeling through the secretion of the matrix degrading protease matrix metalloproteinase 9, control of placental vascular tone through the activation of the nitric oxide pathway, direct modulation of endocrine function, especially prostaglandin generation and bioavailability, gestation length and the onset of labor (reviewed in (Grammatopoulos, 2008)). In addition to these roles, CRH is also known to have immunological effects.

Traditionally hypothalamic CRH has been considered to act indirectly in an anti-inflammatory fashion as the end product of the hypothalamic-pituitary-adrenal axis is cortisol which is a well known anti-inflammatory compound. However CRH produced at peripheral inflammatory sites has been shown to possess potent proinflammatory properties that can influence both innate and acquired immune responses (Kalantaridou et al., 2007). In the reproductive system, intrauterine and ovarian CRH can have proinflammatory properties. For intrauterine CRH, various studies have shown that it may participate in the acute aseptic inflammatory response that is characteristic of embryo implantation (Makrigiannakis et al.,

2001). Ovarian CRH can also participate in the inflammatory processes of ovulation and luteolysis (Kalantaridou et al., 2007). However, following implantation, the embryo suppresses the inflammatory response and prevents immune rejection. It has been hypothesized that the anti-inflammatory role of CRH may play a role in this process through interactions with the proapoptotic cytokine, Fas Ligand (FasL) (Makrigiannakis et al., 2001).

FasL is a type II membrane protein of approximately 280 amino acids that belongs to the TNF superfamily. FasL has a high level of conservation amongst species and is highly expressed on several immune cells including activated T and B lymphocytes, NK cells, monocytes and macrophages. The major function of FasL is to induce apoptosis in cells which express its receptor, Fas (Lee and Ferguson, 2003). Fas, a membrane protein that belongs to the TNF and nerve growth factor receptor family, is also expressed at high levels in several immune cells, including activated B and T lymphocytes, NK cells, monocytes, and macrophages (reviewed in (Houston and O'Connell, 2004)). Due to the expression of Fas at high levels in several immune cells, it has been hypothesized that Fas/FasL interactions may be important in immune tolerance.

FasL expression has also been reported in nonhemopoietic cells, mainly from immune-privileged tissues, including testis, cornea, trophoblast (Makrigiannakis et al., 2001), and cancer cells (Houston and O'Connell, 2004), suggesting that the Fas-FasL system may play an important role in the mechanism underlying this immune-privileged status (Griffith et al., 1995).

The Fas-FasL system is involved in apoptosis and is extensively used by the immune system during lymphopoiesis and immunopoiesis. It is also a major mechanism during clonal deletion of autoimmune cells inside the central and peripheral lymphoid organs and is involved in the cytolytic pathways of NK cells, Th1 cells and cytotoxic T cells. The Fas/FasL system is also implicated in the regulation of cellular turnover, tumor cell elimination, antiviral responses and protection of particular tissues against potential danger represented mainly by activated lymphocytes (reviewed in (Houston and O'Connell, 2004; Thellin et al., 2000)).

During human pregnancy, FasL is expressed on the trophoblast and decidualized endometrial cells. (Makrigiannakis et al., 2004; Taylor et al., 2006). Studies on placental exosomes have also shown the presence of cytoplasmic microvesicular forms of FasL in syncytiotrophoblast (Frangsmyr et al., 2005) and its secretion into maternal blood (Taylor et al., 2006). As a result of this expression profile, FasL has been speculated to have a role in embryo implantation and maternal immune tolerance. Makrigiannakis *et al.*, (Makrigiannakis et al., 2001) examined the role of FasL in implantation and early pregnancy and showed that CRH increased FasL expression in human EVT cells which in turn increased the levels of activated T cell apoptosis in PBMC isolated from newborn children. Neutralizing antibodies to FasL were shown to inhibit CRH-induced apoptosis suggesting that this effect was mediated by Fas/FasL interactions.

To determine the relevance of these *in vitro* findings, Makrigiannakis used an *in vivo* rat model to study embryo implantation. These studies showed that administration of the CRH-R1 antagonist, antalarmin, to female rats resulted in a marked decrease in FasL expression, implantation sites and live embryos. As with the *in vitro* studies, these studies showed that this was a T cell dependent process as T cell deficient rats treated with antalarmin had no difference in the number of implantation sites compared to control animals (Makrigiannakis et al., 2001).

However, as with IDO and PDL-1, studies have shown that Fas/FasL interactions are not obligatory for successful pregnancy. Hunt *et al.,* (Hunt et al., 1997) examined whether the absence of FasL affected pregnancy using *gld* mice (mice unable to express a functional FasL). In these mice, extensive leukocytic infiltrates and necrosis at the decidual-placental interface were observed which resulted in increased embryo resorption and a decrease in litter size. Interestingly, the lack of FasL in this mutant strain did not abrogate fertility suggesting that there may be other mechanisms which can control the maternal immune response in the absence of FasL.

2.10 Placental endogenous retroviral envelope proteins

Retroviruses can be defined as a class of enveloped viruses that have their genetic material in the form of RNA and use the enzyme reverse transcriptase to translate their RNA into DNA in a host cell (Ryan, 2004). All retroviruses contain information coding for three defined sets of regions of genes: *gag* (group specific antigen), *pol* (polymerase) and *env* (envelope). *Gag* directs the synthesis of internal virion proteins that form the capsid and nucleoprotein structure; *pol* contains the information for the reverse transcriptase and integrase enzymes and *env* contains the surface and transmembrane subunits of the virion envelope protein, which are involved in cell fusion, immunosuppression and receptor recognition (Sandrin et al., 2004).

Human endogenous retroviruses (HERVs) are evolutionary fossils inherited in a Mendelian fashion and are derived from retroviruses which, at some ancient time-point, have infected germline cells (Urnovitz and Murphy, 1996) and because of that, they are present in all human cells. HERVs represent about 8% of the human genome (Ryan, 2004). The analysis by Tristem (Tristem, 2000) confirms previous reports that the vast majority of HERV elements are defective by virtue of deletions or stop codons in *gag, pol* or *env* genes. Although many HERVs are defective, some still have open reading frames that are free from deletions and mutations. From these sequences, several types of expression are seen, from subgenomic and full length RNA transcripts, to complete retroviral particles with polymerase and protease activity.

The most abundant expression of different HERVs is seen in the placenta and embryonic tissues, and other reproductive tissues or cells, such as the testis and oocyte. From as early as the 1970s repeated electron microscope observations have been made of the presence of C-type ERVs within both human and animal placental tissue (Harris, 1991). The presence of ERV particles and proteins in these tissues suggests a normal function for these proteins in this environment (Mwenda, 1994).

In 1999, Blond et al. (Blond et al., 1999) described a HERV *env* gene belonging to the HERV-W family encoding a protein expressed in the syncytiotrophoblast which was called syncytin by Mi et al. (Mi et al., 2000). Syncytin (syncytin-1) was shown to fuse human trophoblasts cells and it has been proposed that syncytin-1 may be a key factor in regulating syncytialization during placenta formation (Blond et al., 2000; Mi et al., 2000). Later on, a second fusogenic envelope protein belonging to the HERV-FRD family was identified in the placenta and named syncytin-2 (env-FRD) (Blaise et al., 2003). We now know that human (Blaise et al., 2003; Mi et al., 2000), mouse, rat, gerbil, vole, hamster (Dupressoir et al., 2005), rabbit (Heidmann et al., 2009) and most recently bovine (Koshi et al., 2011) all express in their placenta, endogenous retroviral envelope proteins which appear to play an important biological role.

In addition to their role in cell-cell fusion, it has been hypothesized that placental ERV envelope proteins may have a role in maternal immune tolerance (Mangeney et al., 2007). Retroviral infections are commonly associated with immunosuppression in many species which can result in susceptibility to other infections (Haraguchi et al., 1997). The majority of studies on the immunosuppressive effects of retroviruses have focused on exogenous retroviruses (Blaise et al., 2001; Mangeney and Heidmann, 1998; Peterson et al., 1963) however there is growing evidence that ERVs may play an immunosuppressive role at the maternal-fetal interface (Mangeney et al., 2001; Villarreal, 1997). The source of this immunosuppression is a highly conserved amino acid sequence called the immunosuppressive domain (ISD) present in the transmembrane subunit of the envelope protein of most retroviruses (Cianciolo et al., 1985). Both syncytin-1 and syncytin-2 carry a sequence with a degree of homology to the ISD.

A synthetic peptide with the 17 amino acid consensus sequence of the ISD called CKS-17, was originally produced by Cianciolo *et al.,* (Cianciolo et al., 1985) and has been extensively studied (reviewed in (Haraguchi et al., 2008)). Initially, CKS-17 was shown to inhibit the proliferation of an IL-2 dependent murine cytotoxic T cell line as well as alloantigen stimulated proliferation of murine and human lymphocytes (Cianciolo et al., 1985). Since these initial studies by Cianciolo, CKS-17 has been shown to have important immunological effects ultimately resulting in an inhibition of cell-mediated immunity (Th1 type responses) and a shift towards humoral immunity (Th2 type responses) (Haraguchi et al., 2008). The maintenance of pregnancy has also been correlated with a shift from Th1 to Th2 type immune responses (Wegmann et al., 1993).

The immunosuppressive properties of the retroviral ISD have been further explored *in vivo.* Exogenous retroviral envelope proteins from MMuLV (Mangeney and Heidmann, 1998) and Mason Pfizer Monkey Virus (MPMV) (Blaise et al., 2001) as well as the endogenous HERV-H (Mangeney et al., 2001) have been shown to have immunosuppressive properties using an *in vivo* mouse tumor model. Allogeneic tumor cells that would normally be rejected by the mice were transfected with the envelope protein of the retroviruses and tumor cell growth and proliferation was examined. Retroviral envelope expression was able to block immune-mediated elimination of the tumor cells (Blaise et al., 2001; Mangeney et al., 2001; Mangeney and Heidmann, 1998). Interestingly, in studies on MPMV, this immunosuppression was shown to be specific to tumor cells expressing the envelope protein, as tumor cells not expressing the envelope protein injected simultaneously into the same mouse were rejected (Mangeney and Heidmann, 1998).

Mangeney *et al.,* 2007 (Mangeney et al., 2007) provided the first evidence for an immunosuppressive function for placental syncytins. Human syncytin-1 and -2, and mouse syncytin-A and –B were transfected into an allogeneic tumor cell line and transplanted subcutaneously into mice. Tumor cell growth was used as a measure of immunosuppression. This study showed that in both humans and mice, one of the two syncytin proteins (syncytin-2 in humans, syncytin-B in mice) was immunosuppressive, while the other is not (syncytin-1 in humans, syncytin-A in mice).

To further characterize placental syncytins immunosuppressive properties, Mangeney analyzed the humoral immune response of syncytin-1 and -2 using recombinant syncytin ectodomains, which are 63- or 64-residue-long fragments respectively and which include the ISD. These ectodomains are large enough to adopt the proper physiological conformation (Kobe et al., 1999; Mangeney et al., 2007; Renard et al., 2005). An assay was designed based on the production of antibodies by mice injected with the purified ectodomain. The human syncytin ectodomain proteins were injected twice at a 1 week interval and sera were collected 4 days after the last injection for analysis of IgG titers. The results showed that a humoral response was only mounted against the "non-immunosuppressive" syncytin-1 suggesting that syncytin-2 had no stimulatory effect on the production of antibodies (Mangeney et al., 2007).

The findings of Mangeney *et al.,* (Mangeney et al., 2007) are rather puzzling as the localization of the immunosuppressive syncytin-2 is within the villous cytotrophoblast cells where it is not directly exposed to the maternal circulation while syncytin-1 is localized in the maternal blood bathed syncytiotrophoblast (Kudaka et al., 2007; Malassine et al., 2008). Also, while syncytin-1 levels have been shown to increase throughout pregnancy, syncytin-2 has a decreasing pattern of expression (Okahara et al., 2004). Transcriptional levels of syncytin-2 are also about 10-fold lower than syncytin-1 in the first trimester and 40-fold lower at term.

To our knowledge, no further studies have been completed on the immunosuppressive properties of syncytin-2, -A and –B so further analysis of these proteins are required. In regards to syncytin-1, it is clear that the current knowledge on the involvement of this protein in maternal immune tolerance requires further characterization. However, it is clear from these studies that placental retroviral envelope proteins may contribute to the altered maternal immune environment during pregnancy.

2.11 Placental exosomes

Recently it has become apparent that placental exosomes also may play an important role in maternal immune tolerance (reviewed in (Mincheva-Nilsson and Baranov, 2010)). The authors would like to point the reader's attention to Chapter: 12. by Lucia Mincheva-Nilsson and Vladimir Baranov for a detailed review on the role of placental exosomes in immune modulation.

3. Conclusion

Despite over half of a century of systematic research and the advance of new and more precise research methods on the mechanisms behind maternal immune tolerance, there is still no answer to the question originally formulated by Medawar: "*How does the pregnant mother contrive to nourish within itself, for many weeks or months, a foetus that is an antigenically foreign body?*" (Medawar, 1953). Undoubtedly more research needs to be done in this field to allow a better understanding of the critical mechanisms involved in maternal immune tolerance. The mechanisms that are detailed above (for overview of the mechanisms discussed, please refer to Figure 1) are all capable of inducing immune tolerance, but not all of them are necessarily required for pregnancy to be successful (Baban et al., 2004; Chaouat et al., 2003). There appear to be many redundant mechanisms that exist to provide robustness to the system that is essential for mammalian pregnancy.

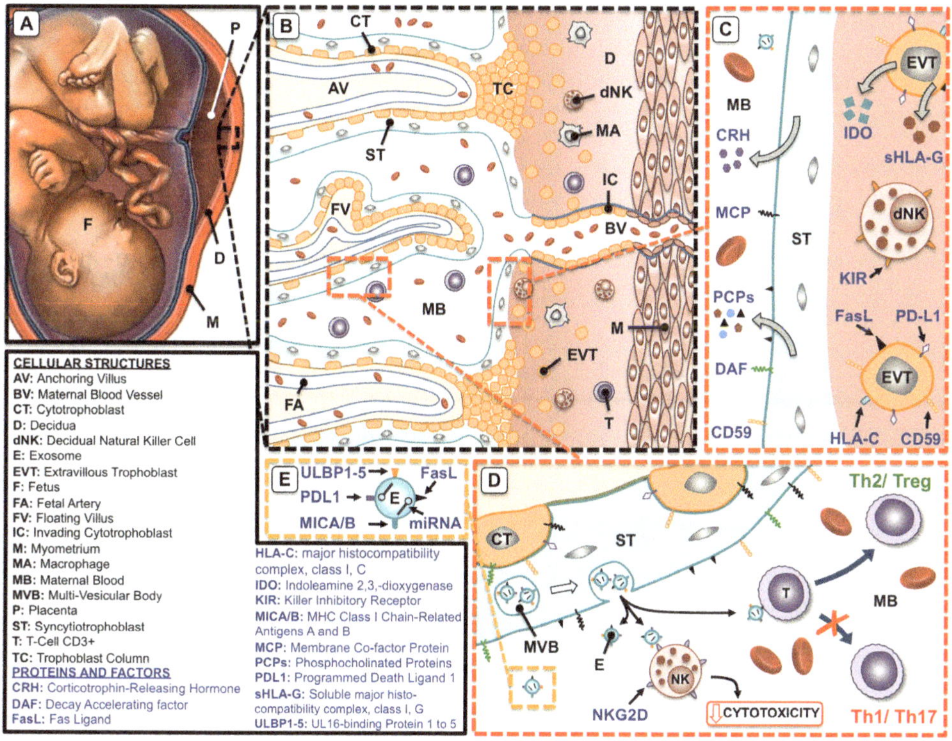

Fig. 1. **Some of the mechanisms operating at the feto maternal interface that contribute to the immune tolerance towards fetal antigens.** The immune regulatory processes operating at the level of the maternal fetal interface are highly dynamic and invoke multiple and sometimes redundant mechanisms and/or factors to reduce the likelihood of maternal immune rejection. Together with this redundancy, it is widely accepted that fetal factors drive changes in maternal immune responses and that both the fetus and the mother actively contribute to the successful pregnancy. **A)** General overview of the anatomical relationship between the feto placental unit within the uterus. **B)** Humans have a haemochorial placenta characterized by a high level of infiltration of maternal tissues by extravillous trophoblast cells and the release of maternal blood into the intervillous space. In this form of placentation the mother and the fetus are separated by a villous trophoblast layer which consists of an outer syncytiotrophoblast layer and an inner cytotrophoblast layer. The syncytiotrophoblast is formed by the fusion of the underlying mononuclear cytotrophoblast layer to form a multinucleated syncytium. **C)** Numerous factors are expressed at the maternal fetal interface which can regulate the maternal immune system to tolerate the presence of fetal antigens. These factors can be carried by either syncytiotrophoblast or extravillous trophoblast or may even be produced by maternal immune cell subtypes present in the decidua. Multiple strategies are used by trophoblast cells to avoid maternal immune cells and antibody-mediated cell destruction, including altered HLA expression (HLA-G, HLA-C), synthesis of immunosuppressive molecules such as FasL, PDL1, IDO, and expression of high levels of complement regulatory proteins (DAF, MCP, CD59) that protect the extraembryonic tissues from maternal anti-paternal cytotoxic

antibodies. Uterine changes during pregnancy also help contribute to maternal immune adaptation, including alterations in the relative proportions, phenotype, and functions of leukocyte subpopulations, induction of immunosuppressive molecules (progesterone, prostaglandins), and changes in cytokine profiles across gestation. **D)** More recently, studies detailing the secretion of immunosuppressive exosomes by trophoblast cells have led to the hypothesis that placental derived exosomes may play an important role in the shift from a Th1/Th17 immune response, which promotes rejection, toward a Th2/Treg cell response that promotes tolerance as it inhibits Natural Cell Killer cytotoxicity against trophoblast cells. **E)** A number of immunosuppressive molecules have been documented as being carried by placental exosomes, including FasL, PDL1, MHC molecules, NKG2D ligands as well as miRNAs that may modulate the immune response.

The knowledge gained from research into the mechanisms of maternal immune tolerance can lead to a greater understanding of the processes vital to the establishment and maintenance of tolerance. These findings can not only contribute to developing therapeutic strategies to treat pregnancy immune related disorders such as preeclampsia or some infertilities but also to develop interventions to address malignancies in cancer and also to improve transplantation success rates.

4. References

Aluvihare, V. R., Kallikourdis, M. and Betz, A. G. (2004). Regulatory T cells mediate maternal tolerance to the fetus. *Nat Immunol*, Vol. 5, No. 3, pp. 266-71.

Arck, P. C., Ferrick, D. A., Steele-Norwood, D., Egan, P. J., Croitoru, K., Carding, S. R., Dietl, J. and Clark, D. A. (1999). Murine T cell determination of pregnancy outcome. *Cell Immunol*, Vol. 196, No. 2, pp. 71-9.

Ayatollahi, M., Geramizadeh, B., Yazdani, M. and Azarpira, N. (2007). Effect of the immunoregulatory cytokines on successful pregnancy depends upon the control of graft rejection mechanisms. *Transplant Proc*, Vol. 39, No. 1, pp. 244-5.

Baban, B., Chandler, P., McCool, D., Marshall, B., Munn, D. H. and Mellor, A. L. (2004). Indoleamine 2,3-dioxygenase expression is restricted to fetal trophoblast giant cells during murine gestation and is maternal genome specific. *J Reprod Immunol*, Vol. 61, No. 2, pp. 67-77.

Bainbridge, D. R. (2000). Evolution of mammalian pregnancy in the presence of the maternal immune system. *Rev Reprod*, Vol. 5, No. 2, pp. 67-74.

Beagley, K. W. and Gockel, C. M. (2003). Regulation of innate and adaptive immunity by the female sex hormones oestradiol and progesterone. *FEMS Immunol Med Microbiol*, Vol. 38, No. 1, pp. 13-22.

Billingham, R. E. (1964). Transplantation Immunity and the Maternal-Fetal Relationship. *N Engl J Med*, Vol. 270, No. pp. 667-72.

Billington, W. D. (1992). Transfer of antigens and antibodies between mother and fetus. In *Immunological Obstetrics* eds. C. B. Coulam W. P. Faulk and J. McIntyre), pp. 290-304. New York: W.W. Norton and Co.

Billington, W. D. (2003). The immunological problem of pregnancy: 50 years with the hope of progress. A tribute to Peter Medawar. *J Reprod Immunol*, Vol. 60, No. 1, pp. 1-11.

Blaise, S., de Parseval, N., Benit, L. and Heidmann, T. (2003). Genomewide screening for fusogenic human endogenous retrovirus envelopes identifies syncytin 2, a gene conserved on primate evolution. *Proc Natl Acad Sci U S A*, Vol. 100, No. 22, pp. 13013-8.

Blaise, S., Mangeney, M. and Heidmann, T. (2001). The envelope of Mason-Pfizer monkey virus has immunosuppressive properties. *J Gen Virol*, Vol. 82, No. Pt 7, pp. 1597-600.

Blank, C., Gajewski, T. F. and Mackensen, A. (2005). Interaction of PD-L1 on tumor cells with PD-1 on tumor-specific T cells as a mechanism of immune evasion: implications for tumor immunotherapy. *Cancer Immunol Immunother*, Vol. 54, No. 4, pp. 307-14.

Blond, J. L., Beseme, F., Duret, L., Bouton, O., Bedin, F., Perron, H., Mandrand, B. and Mallet, F. (1999). Molecular characterization and placental expression of HERV-W, a new human endogenous retrovirus family. *J Virol*, Vol. 73, No. 2, pp. 1175-85.

Blond, J. L., Lavillette, D., Cheynet, V., Bouton, O., Oriol, G., Chapel-Fernandes, S., Mandrand, B., Mallet, F. and Cosset, F. L. (2000). An envelope glycoprotein of the human endogenous retrovirus HERV-W is expressed in the human placenta and fuses cells expressing the type D mammalian retrovirus receptor. *J Virol*, Vol. 74, No. 7, pp. 3321-9.

Carosella, E. D., Moreau, P., Lemaoult, J. and Rouas-Freiss, N. (2008). HLA-G: from biology to clinical benefits. *Trends Immunol*, Vol. 29, No. 3, pp. 125-32.

Chaouat, G. (2007). The Th1/Th2 paradigm: still important in pregnancy? *Semin Immunopathol*, Vol. 29, No. 2, pp. 95-113.

Chaouat, G., Assal Meliani, A., Martal, J., Raghupathy, R., Elliott, J. F., Mosmann, T. and Wegmann, T. G. (1995). IL-10 prevents naturally occurring fetal loss in the CBA x DBA/2 mating combination, and local defect in IL-10 production in this abortion-prone combination is corrected by in vivo injection of IFN-tau. *J Immunol*, Vol. 154, No. 9, pp. 4261-8.

Chaouat, G., Ledee-Bataille, N., Zourbas, S., Ostojic, S., Dubanchet, S., Martal, J. and Frydman, R. (2003). Cytokines, implantation and early abortion: re-examining the Th1/Th2 paradigm leads to question the single pathway, single therapy concept. *Am J Reprod Immunol*, Vol. 50, No. 3, pp. 177-86.

Chaouat, G., Menu, E., Clark, D. A., Dy, M., Minkowski, M. and Wegmann, T. G. (1990). Control of fetal survival in CBA x DBA/2 mice by lymphokine therapy. *J Reprod Fertil*, Vol. 89, No. 2, pp. 447-58.

Chen, Z. M., O'Shaughnessy, M. J., Gramaglia, I., Panoskaltsis-Mortari, A., Murphy, W. J., Narula, S., Roncarolo, M. G. and Blazar, B. R. (2003). IL-10 and TGF-beta induce alloreactive CD4+CD25- T cells to acquire regulatory cell function. *Blood*, Vol. 101, No. 12, pp. 5076-83.

Cianciolo, G. J., Bogerd, H. P., Kipnis, R. J., Copeland, T. D., Oroszlan, S. and Snyderman, R. (1985). Inhibition of lymphocyte proliferation by a synthetic peptide homologous to envelope proteins of human and animal retroviruses. *Trans Assoc Am Physicians*, Vol. 98, No. pp. 30-41.

Clark, D. A., Fernandes, J. and Banwatt, D. (2008). Prevention of spontaneous abortion in the CBA x DBA/2 mouse model by intravaginal TGF-beta and local recruitment of CD4+8+ FOXP3+ cells. *Am J Reprod Immunol*, Vol. 59, No. 6, pp. 525-34.

Comiskey, M., Goldstein, C. Y., De Fazio, S. R., Mammolenti, M., Newmark, J. A. and Warner, C. M. (2003). Evidence that HLA-G is the functional homolog of mouse Qa-2, the Ped gene product. *Hum Immunol*, Vol. 64, No. 11, pp. 999-1004.

Danilova, N. (2006). The evolution of immune mechanisms. *J Exp Zool B Mol Dev Evol*, Vol. 306, No. 6, pp. 496-520.

de Moraes-Pinto, M. I., Vince, G. S., Flanagan, B. F., Hart, C. A. and Johnson, P. M. (1997). Localization of IL-4 and IL-4 receptors in the human term placenta, decidua and amniochorionic membranes. *Immunology*, Vol. 90, No. 1, pp. 87-94.

Dupressoir, A., Marceau, G., Vernochet, C., Benit, L., Kanellopoulos, C., Sapin, V. and Heidmann, T. (2005). Syncytin-A and syncytin-B, two fusogenic placenta-specific murine envelope genes of retroviral origin conserved in Muridae. *Proc Natl Acad Sci U S A*, Vol. 102, No. 3, pp. 725-30.

Elbe-Burger, A., Mommaas, A. M., Prieschl, E. E., Fiebiger, E., Baumruker, T. and Stingl, G. (2000). Major histocompatibility complex class II- fetal skin dendritic cells are potent accessory cells of polyclonal T-cell responses. *Immunology*, Vol. 101, No. 2, pp. 242-53.

Faulk, W. P. and Temple, A. (1976). Distribution of beta2 microglobulin and HLA in chorionic villi of human placentae. *Nature*, Vol. 262, No. 5571, pp. 799-802.

Foulds, L. M., Boysen, R. I., Crane, M., Yang, Y., Muir, J. A., Smith, A. I., de Kretser, D. M., Hearn, M. T. and Hedger, M. P. (2008). Molecular identification of lyso-glycerophosphocholines as endogenous immunosuppressives in bovine and rat gonadal fluids. *Biol Reprod*, Vol. 79, No. 3, pp. 525-36.

Frangsmyr, L., Baranov, V., Nagaeva, O., Stendahl, U., Kjellberg, L. and Mincheva-Nilsson, L. (2005). Cytoplasmic microvesicular form of Fas ligand in human early placenta: switching the tissue immune privilege hypothesis from cellular to vesicular level. *Mol Hum Reprod*, Vol. 11, No. 1, pp. 35-41.

Girardi, G. (2008). Complement inhibition keeps mothers calm and avoids fetal rejection. *Immunol Invest*, Vol. 37, No. 5, pp. 645-59.

Girardi, G., Bulla, R., Salmon, J. E. and Tedesco, F. (2006). The complement system in the pathophysiology of pregnancy. *Mol Immunol*, Vol. 43, No. 1-2, pp. 68-77.

Goodfellow, P. N., Barnstable, C. J., Bodmer, W. F., Snary, D. and Crumpton, M. J. (1976). Expression of HLA system antigens on placenta. *Transplantation*, Vol. 22, No. 6, pp. 595-603.

Gorivodsky, M., Torchinsky, A., Zemliak, I., Savion, S., Fein, A. and Toder, V. (1999). TGF beta 2 mRNA expression and pregnancy failure in mice. *Am J Reprod Immunol*, Vol. 42, No. 2, pp. 124-33.

Grammatopoulos, D. K. (2008). Placental corticotrophin-releasing hormone and its receptors in human pregnancy and labour: still a scientific enigma. *J Neuroendocrinol*, Vol. 20, No. 4, pp. 432-8.

Griffith, T. S., Brunner, T., Fletcher, S. M., Green, D. R. and Ferguson, T. A. (1995). Fas ligand-induced apoptosis as a mechanism of immune privilege. *Science*, Vol. 270, No. 5239, pp. 1189-92.

Grohmann, U., Fallarino, F. and Puccetti, P. (2003). Tolerance, DCs and tryptophan: much ado about IDO. *Trends Immunol*, Vol. 24, No. 5, pp. 242-8.

Groux, H., O'Garra, A., Bigler, M., Rouleau, M., Antonenko, S., de Vries, J. E. and Roncarolo, M. G. (1997). A CD4+ T-cell subset inhibits antigen-specific T-cell responses and prevents colitis. *Nature*, Vol. 389, No. 6652, pp. 737-42.

Guerin, L. R., Prins, J. R. and Robertson, S. A. (2009). Regulatory T-cells and immune tolerance in pregnancy: a new target for infertility treatment? *Hum Reprod Update*, Vol. 15, No. 5, pp. 517-35.

Guleria, I., Khosroshahi, A., Ansari, M. J., Habicht, A., Azuma, M., Yagita, H., Noelle, R. J., Coyle, A., Mellor, A. L., Khoury, S. J. et al. (2005). A critical role for the programmed death ligand 1 in fetomaternal tolerance. *J Exp Med*, Vol. 202, No. 2, pp. 231-7.

Hansen, P. J., Bazer, F. W. and Segerson, E. C., Jr. (1986). Skin graft survival in the uterine lumen of ewes treated with progesterone. *Am J Reprod Immunol Microbiol*, Vol. 12, No. 2, pp. 48-54.

Haraguchi, S., Good, R. A., Cianciolo, G. J., Engelman, R. W. and Day, N. K. (1997). Immunosuppressive retroviral peptides: immunopathological implications for immunosuppressive influences of retroviral infections. *J Leukoc Biol*, Vol. 61, No. 6, pp. 654-66.

Haraguchi, S., Good, R. A. and Day-Good, N. K. (2008). A potent immunosuppressive retroviral peptide: cytokine patterns and signaling pathways. *Immunol Res*, Vol. 41, No. 1, pp. 46-55.

Harnett, W. and Harnett, M. M. (1993). Inhibition of murine B cell proliferation and down-regulation of protein kinase C levels by a phosphorylcholine-containing filarial excretory-secretory product. *J Immunol*, Vol. 151, No. 9, pp. 4829-37.

Harris, J. R. (1991). The evolution of placental mammals. *FEBS Lett*, Vol. 295, No. 1-3, pp. 3-4.

Heidmann, O., Vernochet, C., Dupressoir, A. and Heidmann, T. (2009). Identification of an endogenous retroviral envelope gene with fusogenic activity and placenta-specific expression in the rabbit : a new "syncytin" in a third order of mammals. *Retrovirology*, Vol. 6, No. 1, pp. 107.

Heikkinen, J., Mottonen, M., Alanen, A. and Lassila, O. (2004). Phenotypic characterization of regulatory T cells in the human decidua. *Clin Exp Immunol*, Vol. 136, No. 2, pp. 373-8.

Hill, J. A., Polgar, K. and Anderson, D. J. (1995). T-helper 1-type immunity to trophoblast in women with recurrent spontaneous abortion. *Jama*, Vol. 273, No. 24, pp. 1933-6.

Holmes, C. H., Simpson, K. L., Okada, H., Okada, N., Wainwright, S. D., Purcell, D. F. and Houlihan, J. M. (1992). Complement regulatory proteins at the feto-maternal interface during human placental development: distribution of CD59 by comparison with membrane cofactor protein (CD46) and decay accelerating factor (CD55). *Eur J Immunol*, Vol. 22, No. 6, pp. 1579-85.

Hori, J., Wang, M., Miyashita, M., Tanemoto, K., Takahashi, H., Takemori, T., Okumura, K., Yagita, H. and Azuma, M. (2006). B7-H1-induced apoptosis as a mechanism of immune privilege of corneal allografts. *J Immunol*, Vol. 177, No. 9, pp. 5928-35.

Horwitz, D. A., Zheng, S. G. and Gray, J. D. (2003). The role of the combination of IL-2 and TGF-beta or IL-10 in the generation and function of CD4+ CD25+ and CD8+ regulatory T cell subsets. *J Leukoc Biol*, Vol. 74, No. 4, pp. 471-8.

Horwitz, D. A., Zheng, S. G. and Gray, J. D. (2008). Natural and TGF-beta-induced Foxp3(+)CD4(+) CD25(+) regulatory T cells are not mirror images of each other. *Trends Immunol*, Vol. 29, No. 9, pp. 429-35.

Hoskin, D. W. and Murgita, R. A. (1989). Specific maternal anti-fetal lymphoproliferative responses and their regulation by natural immunosuppressive factors. *Clin Exp Immunol*, Vol. 76, No. 2, pp. 262-7.

Houston, A. and O'Connell, J. (2004). The Fas signalling pathway and its role in the pathogenesis of cancer. *Curr Opin Pharmacol*, Vol. 4, No. 4, pp. 321-6.

Hsi, B. L., Hunt, J. S. and Atkinson, J. P. (1991). Differential expression of complement regulatory proteins on subpopulations of human trophoblast cells. *J Reprod Immunol*, Vol. 19, No. 3, pp. 209-23.

Hunt, J. S. (1989). Cytokine networks in the uteroplacental unit: macrophages as pivotal regulatory cells. *J Reprod Immunol*, Vol. 16, No. 1, pp. 1-17.

Hunt, J. S. (2006). Stranger in a strange land. *Immunol Rev*, Vol. 213, No. pp. 36-47.

Hunt, J. S., Fishback, J. L., Andrews, G. K. and Wood, G. W. (1988). Expression of class I HLA genes by trophoblast cells. Analysis by in situ hybridization. *J Immunol*, Vol. 140, No. 4, pp. 1293-9.

Hunt, J. S. and Langat, D. L. (2009). HLA-G: a human pregnancy-related immunomodulator. *Curr Opin Pharmacol*, Vol. 9, No. 4, pp. 462-9.

Hunt, J. S., Petroff, M. G., McIntire, R. H. and Ober, C. (2005). HLA-G and immune tolerance in pregnancy. *Faseb J*, Vol. 19, No. 7, pp. 681-93.

Hunt, J. S., Vassmer, D., Ferguson, T. A. and Miller, L. (1997). Fas ligand is positioned in mouse uterus and placenta to prevent trafficking of activated leukocytes between the mother and the conceptus. *J Immunol*, Vol. 158, No. 9, pp. 4122-8.

Ishida, Y., Agata, Y., Shibahara, K. and Honjo, T. (1992). Induced expression of PD-1, a novel member of the immunoglobulin gene superfamily, upon programmed cell death. *Embo J*, Vol. 11, No. 11, pp. 3887-95.

Jasper, M. J., Tremellen, K. P. and Robertson, S. A. (2006). Primary unexplained infertility is associated with reduced expression of the T-regulatory cell transcription factor Foxp3 in endometrial tissue. *Mol Hum Reprod*, Vol. 12, No. 5, pp. 301-8.

Kalantaridou, S. N., Zoumakis, E., Makrigiannakis, A., Godoy, H. and Chrousos, G. P. (2007). The role of corticotropin-releasing hormone in blastocyst implantation and early fetal immunotolerance. *Horm Metab Res*, Vol. 39, No. 6, pp. 474-7.

Kingsley, C. I., Karim, M., Bushell, A. R. and Wood, K. J. (2002). CD25+CD4+ regulatory T cells prevent graft rejection: CTLA-4- and IL-10-dependent immunoregulation of alloresponses. *J Immunol*, Vol. 168, No. 3, pp. 1080-6.

Kobe, B., Center, R. J., Kemp, B. E. and Poumbourios, P. (1999). Crystal structure of human T cell leukemia virus type 1 gp21 ectodomain crystallized as a maltose-binding protein chimera reveals structural evolution of retroviral transmembrane proteins. *Proc Natl Acad Sci U S A*, Vol. 96, No. 8, pp. 4319-24.

Koshi, K., Ushizawa, K., Kizaki, K., Takahashi, T. and Hashizume, K. (2011). Expression of endogenous retrovirus-like transcripts in bovine trophoblastic cells. *Placenta*, Vol. 32, No. 7, pp. 493-9.

Kozma, N., Halasz, M., Palkovics, T. and Szekeres-Bartho, J. (2006). The progesterone-induced blocking factor modulates the balance of PKC and intracellular Ca. *Am J Reprod Immunol*, Vol. 55, No. 2, pp. 122-9.

Kuby, J. (1997). Major Histocompatibility Complex. In *Immunology* (ed. D. Allen), pp. 223-248: W.H. Freeman and Company.

Kudaka, W., Oda, T., Jinno, Y., Yoshimi, N. and Aoki, Y. (2007). Cellular Localization of Placenta-Specific Human Endogenous Retrovirus (HERV) Transcripts and their Possible Implication in Pregnancy-Induced Hypertension. *Placenta*, Vol. 29, No. 3, pp. 282-289.

Kudo, Y. and Boyd, C. A. (2000). Human placental indoleamine 2,3-dioxygenase: cellular localization and characterization of an enzyme preventing fetal rejection. *Biochim Biophys Acta*, Vol. 1500, No. 1, pp. 119-24.

Kudo, Y. and Boyd, C. A. (2001). The role of L-tryptophan transport in L-tryptophan degradation by indoleamine 2,3-dioxygenase in human placental explants. *J Physiol*, Vol. 531, No. Pt 2, pp. 417-23.

Kudo, Y., Boyd, C. A., Sargent, I. L. and Redman, C. W. (2001). Tryptophan degradation by human placental indoleamine 2,3-dioxygenase regulates lymphocyte proliferation. *J Physiol*, Vol. 535, No. Pt 1, pp. 207-15.

Kyurkchiev, D., Ivanova-Todorova, E. and Kyurkchiev, S. D. (2010). New target cells of the immunomodulatory effects of progesterone. *Reprod Biomed Online*, Vol. 21, No. 3, pp. 304-11.

Lal, R. B., Kumaraswami, V., Steel, C. and Nutman, T. B. (1990). Phosphocholine-containing antigens of Brugia malayi nonspecifically suppress lymphocyte function. *Am J Trop Med Hyg*, Vol. 42, No. 1, pp. 56-64.

Larsen, M. H. and Hviid, T. V. (2009). Human leukocyte antigen-G polymorphism in relation to expression, function, and disease. *Hum Immunol*, Vol. 70, No. 12, pp. 1026-34.

Le Bouteiller, P. (1996). HLA Class I Genes and Products. In *HLA and the maternal-fetal relationship* (ed. J. S. Hunt), pp. 51-85. Heidelberg: R.G. Landes company.

Lee, H. O. and Ferguson, T. A. (2003). Biology of FasL. *Cytokine Growth Factor Rev*, Vol. 14, No. 3-4, pp. 325-35.

Lee, J. H., Ulrich, B., Cho, J., Park, J. and Kim, C. H. (2011). Progesterone promotes differentiation of human cord blood fetal T cells into T regulatory cells but suppresses their differentiation into th17 cells. *J Immunol*, Vol. 187, No. 4, pp. 1778-87.

Lovell, T. M., Woods, R. J., Butlin, D. J., Brayley, K. J., Manyonda, I. T., Jarvis, J., Howell, S. and Lowry, P. J. (2007). Identification of a novel mammalian post-translational modification, phosphocholine, on placental secretory polypeptides. *J Mol Endocrinol*, Vol. 39, No. 3, pp. 189-98.

Lowry, P. J. (2008). The placenta is simply a neuroendocrine parasite. *J Neuroendocrinol*, Vol. 20, No. 6, pp. 700-4.

Madeja, Z., Yadi, H., Apps, R., Boulenouar, S., Roper, S. J., Gardner, L., Moffett, A., Colucci, F. and Hemberger, M. (2011). Paternal MHC expression on mouse trophoblast affects uterine vascularization and fetal growth. *Proc Natl Acad Sci U S A*, Vol. 108, No. 10, pp. 4012-7.

Makrigiannakis, A., Zoumakis, E., Kalantaridou, S. and Chrousos, G. (2004). Endometrial and placental CRH as regulators of human embryo implantation. *J Reprod Immunol*, Vol. 62, No. 1-2, pp. 53-9.

Makrigiannakis, A., Zoumakis, E., Kalantaridou, S., Coutifaris, C., Margioris, A. N., Coukos, G., Rice, K. C., Gravanis, A. and Chrousos, G. P. (2001). Corticotropin-releasing hormone promotes blastocyst implantation and early maternal tolerance. *Nat Immunol*, Vol. 2, No. 11, pp. 1018-24.

Malassine, A., Frendo, J. L., Blaise, S., Handschuh, K., Gerbaud, P., Tsatsaris, V., Heidmann, T. and Evain-Brion, D. (2008). Human endogenous retrovirus-FRD envelope protein (syncytin 2) expression in normal and trisomy 21-affected placenta. *Retrovirology*, Vol. 5, No. 1, pp. 6.

Mangeney, M., de Parseval, N., Thomas, G. and Heidmann, T. (2001). The full-length envelope of an HERV-H human endogenous retrovirus has immunosuppressive properties. *J Gen Virol*, Vol. 82, No. Pt 10, pp. 2515-8.

Mangeney, M. and Heidmann, T. (1998). Tumor cells expressing a retroviral envelope escape immune rejection in vivo. *Proc Natl Acad Sci U S A*, Vol. 95, No. 25, pp. 14920-5.

Mangeney, M., Renard, M., Schlecht-Louf, G., Bouallaga, I., Heidmann, O., Letzelter, C., Richaud, A., Ducos, B. and Heidmann, T. (2007). Placental syncytins: Genetic disjunction between the fusogenic and immunosuppressive activity of retroviral envelope proteins. *Proc Natl Acad Sci U S A*, Vol. 104, No. 51, pp. 20534-9.

Mao, G., Wang, J., Kang, Y., Tai, P., Wen, J., Zou, Q., Li, G., Ouyang, H., Xia, G. and Wang, B. (2010). Progesterone increases systemic and local uterine proportions of CD4+CD25+ Treg cells during midterm pregnancy in mice. *Endocrinology*, Vol. 151, No. 11, pp. 5477-88.

Marzi, M., Vigano, A., Trabattoni, D., Villa, M. L., Salvaggio, A., Clerici, E. and Clerici, M. (1996). Characterization of type 1 and type 2 cytokine production profile in physiologic and pathologic human pregnancy. *Clin Exp Immunol*, Vol. 106, No. 1, pp. 127-33.

McLean, M. and Smith, R. (2001). Corticotrophin-releasing hormone and human parturition. *Reproduction*, Vol. 121, No. 4, pp. 493-501.

Medawar, P. B. (1953). Some immunological and endocrinological problems raised by the evolution of viviparity in vertebrates. *Symp. Soc. Exp. Biol.*, Vol. 44, No. pp. 320-338.

Mellor, A. L. and Munn, D. H. (1999). Tryptophan catabolism and T-cell tolerance: immunosuppression by starvation? *Immunol Today*, Vol. 20, No. 10, pp. 469-73.

Mi, S., Lee, X., Li, X., Veldman, G. M., Finnerty, H., Racie, L., LaVallie, E., Tang, X. Y., Edouard, P., Howes, S. et al. (2000). Syncytin is a captive retroviral envelope protein involved in human placental morphogenesis. *Nature*, Vol. 403, No. 6771, pp. 785-9.

Mincheva-Nilsson, L. and Baranov, V. (2010). The role of placental exosomes in reproduction. *Am J Reprod Immunol*, Vol. 63, No. 6, pp. 520-33.

Mjosberg, J., Berg, G., Ernerudh, J. and Ekerfelt, C. (2007). CD4+ CD25+ regulatory T cells in human pregnancy: development of a Treg-MLC-ELISPOT suppression assay and indications of paternal specific Tregs. *Immunology*, Vol. 120, No. 4, pp. 456-66.

Mjosberg, J., Svensson, J., Johansson, E., Hellstrom, L., Casas, R., Jenmalm, M. C., Boij, R., Matthiesen, L., Jonsson, J. I., Berg, G. et al. (2009). Systemic reduction of functionally suppressive CD4dimCD25highFoxp3+ Tregs in human second trimester pregnancy is induced by progesterone and 17beta-estradiol. *J Immunol*, Vol. 183, No. 1, pp. 759-69.

Morgan, B. P. and Holmes, C. H. (2000). Immunology of reproduction: protecting the placenta. *Curr Biol*, Vol. 10, No. 10, pp. R381-3.

Mosmann, T. R., Cherwinski, H., Bond, M. W., Giedlin, M. A. and Coffman, R. L. (1986). Two types of murine helper T cell clone. I. Definition according to profiles of lymphokine activities and secreted proteins. *J Immunol*, Vol. 136, No. 7, pp. 2348-57.

Mulley, W. R. and Nikolic-Paterson, D. J. (2008). Indoleamine 2,3-dioxygenase in transplantation. *Nephrology (Carlton)*, Vol. 13, No. 3, pp. 204-11.

Munn, D. H. (2011). Indoleamine 2,3-dioxygenase, Tregs and Cancer. *Curr Med Chem*, Vol. 18, No. 15, pp. 2240-6.

Munn, D. H., Shafizadeh, E., Attwood, J. T., Bondarev, I., Pashine, A. and Mellor, A. L. (1999). Inhibition of T cell proliferation by macrophage tryptophan catabolism. *J Exp Med*, Vol. 189, No. 9, pp. 1363-72.

Munn, D. H., Zhou, M., Attwood, J. T., Bondarev, I., Conway, S. J., Marshall, B., Brown, C. and Mellor, A. L. (1998). Prevention of allogeneic fetal rejection by tryptophan catabolism. *Science*, Vol. 281, No. 5380, pp. 1191-3.

Murphy, S. P., Choi, J. C. and Holtz, R. (2004). Regulation of major histocompatibility complex class II gene expression in trophoblast cells. *Reprod Biol Endocrinol*, Vol. 2, No. pp. 52.

Mwenda, J. M. (1994). Possible biological functions for the expression of endogenous retroviral gene products in human placental tissues. *Cell Mol Biol (Noisy-le-grand)*, Vol. 40, No. 2, pp. 105-9.

Nagaeva, O., Jonsson, L. and Mincheva-Nilsson, L. (2002). Dominant IL-10 and TGF-beta mRNA expression in gammadeltaT cells of human early pregnancy decidua suggests immunoregulatory potential. *Am J Reprod Immunol*, Vol. 48, No. 1, pp. 9-17.

Nelson, J. L., Gillespie, K. M., Lambert, N. C., Stevens, A. M., Loubiere, L. S., Rutledge, J. C., Leisenring, W. M., Erickson, T. D., Yan, Z., Mullarkey, M. E. et al. (2007). Maternal microchimerism in peripheral blood in type 1 diabetes and pancreatic islet beta cell microchimerism. *Proc Natl Acad Sci U S A*, Vol. 104, No. 5, pp. 1637-42.

Nishimura, H. and Honjo, T. (2001). PD-1: an inhibitory immunoreceptor involved in peripheral tolerance. *Trends Immunol*, Vol. 22, No. 5, pp. 265-8.

Ober, C., Aldrich, C., Rosinsky, B., Robertson, A., Walker, M. A., Willadsen, S., Verp, M. S., Geraghty, D. E. and Hunt, J. S. (1998). HLA-G1 protein expression is not essential for fetal survival. *Placenta*, Vol. 19, No. 2-3, pp. 127-32.

Okahara, G., Matsubara, S., Oda, T., Sugimoto, J., Jinno, Y. and Kanaya, F. (2004). Expression analyses of human endogenous retroviruses (HERVs): tissue-specific and developmental stage-dependent expression of HERVs. *Genomics*, Vol. 84, No. 6, pp. 982-90.

Peterson, R. D., Hendrickson, R. and Good, R. A. (1963). Reduced Antibody Forming Capacity During the Incubation Period of Passage a Leukemia in C3h Mice. *Proc Soc Exp Biol Med*, Vol. 114, No. pp. 517-20.

Petraglia, F., Florio, P., Nappi, C. and Genazzani, A. R. (1996). Peptide signaling in human placenta and membranes: autocrine, paracrine, and endocrine mechanisms. *Endocr Rev*, Vol. 17, No. 2, pp. 156-86.

Petroff, M. G., Chen, L., Phillips, T. A., Azzola, D., Sedlmayr, P. and Hunt, J. S. (2003). B7 family molecules are favorably positioned at the human maternal-fetal interface. *Biol Reprod*, Vol. 68, No. 5, pp. 1496-504.

Petroff, M. G., Kharatyan, E., Torry, D. S. and Holets, L. (2005). The immunomodulatory proteins B7-DC, B7-H2, and B7-H3 are differentially expressed across gestation in the human placenta. *Am J Pathol*, Vol. 167, No. 2, pp. 465-73.

Poppa, G., Simmons, R. L., David, D. S. and Russell, P. S. (1964). The Uterus as a Recipient Site for Parathyroid Homotransplantation. *Transplantation*, Vol. 2, No. pp. 496-502.

Power, L. L., Popplewell, E. J., Holloway, J. A., Diaper, N. D., Warner, J. O. and Jones, C. A. (2002). Immunoregulatory molecules during pregnancy and at birth. *J Reprod Immunol*, Vol. 56, No. 1-2, pp. 19-28.

Prokunina, L., Castillejo-Lopez, C., Oberg, F., Gunnarsson, I., Berg, L., Magnusson, V., Brookes, A. J., Tentler, D., Kristjansdottir, H., Grondal, G. et al. (2002). A regulatory polymorphism in PDCD1 is associated with susceptibility to systemic lupus erythematosus in humans. *Nat Genet*, Vol. 32, No. 4, pp. 666-9.

Raghupathy, R. (1997). Th1-type immunity is incompatible with successful pregnancy. *Immunol Today*, Vol. 18, No. 10, pp. 478-82.
Raghupathy, R. (2001). Pregnancy: success and failure within the Th1/Th2/Th3 paradigm. *Semin Immunol*, Vol. 13, No. 4, pp. 219-27.
Redman, C. W., McMichael, A. J., Stirrat, G. M., Sunderland, C. A. and Ting, A. (1984). Class 1 major histocompatibility complex antigens on human extra-villous trophoblast. *Immunology*, Vol. 52, No. 3, pp. 457-68.
Regateiro, F. S., Howie, D., Cobbold, S. P. and Waldmann, H. (2011). TGF-beta in transplantation tolerance. *Curr Opin Immunol*, Vol. No. pp.
Renard, M., Varela, P. F., Letzelter, C., Duquerroy, S., Rey, F. A. and Heidmann, T. (2005). Crystal structure of a pivotal domain of human syncytin-2, a 40 million years old endogenous retrovirus fusogenic envelope gene captured by primates. *J Mol Biol*, Vol. 352, No. 5, pp. 1029-34.
Robertson, S. A. (2010). Immune regulation of conception and embryo implantation-all about quality control? *J Reprod Immunol*, Vol. 85, No. 1, pp. 51-7.
Robertson, S. A., Guerin, L. R., Moldenhauer, L. M. and Hayball, J. D. (2009). Activating T regulatory cells for tolerance in early pregnancy - the contribution of seminal fluid. *J Reprod Immunol*, Vol. 83, No. 1-2, pp. 109-16.
Robertson, S. A., Ingman, W. V., O'Leary, S., Sharkey, D. J. and Tremellen, K. P. (2002). Transforming growth factor beta--a mediator of immune deviation in seminal plasma. *J Reprod Immunol*, Vol. 57, No. 1-2, pp. 109-28.
Rothstein, D. M. and Sayegh, M. H. (2003). T-cell costimulatory pathways in allograft rejection and tolerance. *Immunol Rev*, Vol. 196, No. pp. 85-108.
Ryan, F. P. (2004). Human endogenous retroviruses in health and disease: a symbiotic perspective. *J R Soc Med*, Vol. 97, No. 12, pp. 560-5.
Saito, S., Nakashima, A., Shima, T. and Ito, M. (2010). Th1/Th2/Th17 and regulatory T-cell paradigm in pregnancy. *Am J Reprod Immunol*, Vol. 63, No. 6, pp. 601-10.
Salmon, J. E., Heuser, C., Triebwasser, M., Liszewski, M. K., Kavanagh, D., Roumenina, L., Branch, D. W., Goodship, T., Fremeaux-Bacchi, V. and Atkinson, J. P. (2011). Mutations in complement regulatory proteins predispose to preeclampsia: a genetic analysis of the PROMISSE cohort. *PLoS Med*, Vol. 8, No. 3, pp. e1001013.
Sandrin, V., Muriaux, D., Darlix, J. L. and Cosset, F. L. (2004). Intracellular trafficking of Gag and Env proteins and their interactions modulate pseudotyping of retroviruses. *J Virol*, Vol. 78, No. 13, pp. 7153-64.
Sasaki, Y., Darmochwal-Kolarz, D., Suzuki, D., Sakai, M., Ito, M., Shima, T., Shiozaki, A., Rolinski, J. and Saito, S. (2007). Proportion of peripheral blood and decidual CD4(+) CD25(bright) regulatory T cells in pre-eclampsia. *Clin Exp Immunol*, Vol. 149, No. 1, pp. 139-45.
Sasaki, Y., Sakai, M., Miyazaki, S., Higuma, S., Shiozaki, A. and Saito, S. (2004). Decidual and peripheral blood CD4+CD25+ regulatory T cells in early pregnancy subjects and spontaneous abortion cases. *Mol Hum Reprod*, Vol. 10, No. 5, pp. 347-53.
Schmidt-Weber, C. B. and Blaser, K. (2004). Regulation and role of transforming growth factor-beta in immune tolerance induction and inflammation. *Curr Opin Immunol*, Vol. 16, No. 6, pp. 709-16.
Siiteri, P. K., Febres, F., Clemens, L. E., Chang, R. J., Gondos, B. and Stites, D. (1977). Progesterone and maintenance of pregnancy: is progesterone nature's immunosuppressant? *Ann N Y Acad Sci*, Vol. 286, No. pp. 384-97.

Somerset, D. A., Zheng, Y., Kilby, M. D., Sansom, D. M. and Drayson, M. T. (2004). Normal human pregnancy is associated with an elevation in the immune suppressive CD25+ CD4+ regulatory T-cell subset. *Immunology*, Vol. 112, No. 1, pp. 38-43.

Stein-Streilein, J. and Streilein, J. W. (2002). Anterior chamber associated immune deviation (ACAID): regulation, biological relevance, and implications for therapy. *Int Rev Immunol*, Vol. 21, No. 2-3, pp. 123-52.

Stites, D. P., Bugbee, S. and Siiteri, P. K. (1983). Differential actions of progesterone and cortisol on lymphocyte and monocyte interaction during lymphocyte activation--relevance to immunosuppression in pregnancy. *J Reprod Immunol*, Vol. 5, No. 4, pp. 215-28.

Szekeres-Bartho, J. (2002). Immunological relationship between the mother and the fetus. *Int Rev Immunol*, Vol. 21, No. 6, pp. 471-95.

Szekeres-Bartho, J., Faust, Z. and Varga, P. (1995). The expression of a progesterone-induced immunomodulatory protein in pregnancy lymphocytes. *Am J Reprod Immunol*, Vol. 34, No. 6, pp. 342-8.

Szekeres-Bartho, J., Szekeres, G., Debre, P., Autran, B. and Chaouat, G. (1990). Reactivity of lymphocytes to a progesterone receptor-specific monoclonal antibody. *Cell Immunol*, Vol. 125, No. 2, pp. 273-83.

Szekeres-Bartho, J. and Wegmann, T. G. (1996). A progesterone-dependent immunomodulatory protein alters the Th1/Th2 balance. *J Reprod Immunol*, Vol. 31, No. 1-2, pp. 81-95.

Szekeres-Bartho, J., Wilczynski, J. R., Basta, P. and Kalinka, J. (2008). Role of progesterone and progestin therapy in threatened abortion and preterm labour. *Front Biosci*, Vol. 13, No. pp. 1981-90.

Tafuri, A., Alferink, J., Moller, P., Hammerling, G. J. and Arnold, B. (1995). T cell awareness of paternal alloantigens during pregnancy. *Science*, Vol. 270, No. 5236, pp. 630-3.

Taglauer, E. S., Yankee, T. M. and Petroff, M. G. (2009). Maternal PD-1 regulates accumulation of fetal antigen-specific CD8+ T cells in pregnancy. *J Reprod Immunol*, Vol. 80, No. 1-2, pp. 12-21.

Tajima, A., Tanaka, T., Ebata, T., Takeda, K., Kawasaki, A., Kelly, J. M., Darcy, P. K., Vance, R. E., Raulet, D. H., Kinoshita, K. et al. (2003). Blastocyst MHC, a putative murine homologue of HLA-G, protects TAP-deficient tumor cells from natural killer cell-mediated rejection in vivo. *J Immunol*, Vol. 171, No. 4, pp. 1715-21.

Taylor, D. D., Akyol, S. and Gercel-Taylor, C. (2006). Pregnancy-associated exosomes and their modulation of T cell signaling. *J Immunol*, Vol. 176, No. 3, pp. 1534-42.

Tedesco, F., Narchi, G., Radillo, O., Meri, S., Ferrone, S. and Betterle, C. (1993). Susceptibility of human trophoblast to killing by human complement and the role of the complement regulatory proteins. *J Immunol*, Vol. 151, No. 3, pp. 1562-70.

Thellin, O., Coumans, B., Zorzi, W., Igout, A. and Heinen, E. (2000). Tolerance to the foeto-placental 'graft': ten ways to support a child for nine months. *Curr Opin Immunol*, Vol. 12, No. 6, pp. 731-7.

Tristem, M. (2000). Identification and characterization of novel human endogenous retrovirus families by phylogenetic screening of the human genome mapping project database. *J Virol*, Vol. 74, No. 8, pp. 3715-30.

Trowsdale, J. and Betz, A. G. (2006). Mother's little helpers: mechanisms of maternal-fetal tolerance. *Nat Immunol*, Vol. 7, No. 3, pp. 241-6.

Urnovitz, H. B. and Murphy, W. H. (1996). Human endogenous retroviruses: nature, occurrence, and clinical implications in human disease. *Clin Microbiol Rev*, Vol. 9, No. 1, pp. 72-99.

Vale, W., Spiess, J., Rivier, C. and Rivier, J. (1981). Characterization of a 41-residue ovine hypothalamic peptide that stimulates secretion of corticotropin and beta-endorphin. *Science*, Vol. 213, No. 4514, pp. 1394-7.

Veenstra van Nieuwenhoven, A. L., Heineman, M. J. and Faas, M. M. (2003). The immunology of successful pregnancy. *Hum Reprod Update*, Vol. 9, No. 4, pp. 347-57.

Villarreal, L. P. (1997). On viruses, sex, and motherhood. *J Virol*, Vol. 71, No. 2, pp. 859-65.

Wang, L., Han, R. and Hancock, W. W. (2007). Programmed cell death 1 (PD-1) and its ligand PD-L1 are required for allograft tolerance. *Eur J Immunol*, Vol. 37, No. 10, pp. 2983-90.

Wasowska, B. A., Lee, C. Y., Halushka, M. K. and Baldwin, W. M., 3rd. (2007). New concepts of complement in allorecognition and graft rejection. *Cell Immunol*, Vol. 248, No. 1, pp. 18-30.

Wegmann, T. G., Lin, H., Guilbert, L. and Mosmann, T. R. (1993). Bidirectional cytokine interactions in the maternal-fetal relationship: is successful pregnancy a TH2 phenomenon? *Immunol Today*, Vol. 14, No. 7, pp. 353-6.

Xu, C., Mao, D., Holers, V. M., Palanca, B., Cheng, A. M. and Molina, H. (2000). A critical role for murine complement regulator crry in fetomaternal tolerance. *Science*, Vol. 287, No. 5452, pp. 498-501.

Yamamoto, S. and Hayaishi, O. (1967). Tryptophan pyrrolase of rabbit intestine. D- and L-tryptophan-cleaving enzyme or enzymes. *J Biol Chem*, Vol. 242, No. 22, pp. 5260-6.

Zenclussen, A. C., Gerlof, K., Zenclussen, M. L., Sollwedel, A., Bertoja, A. Z., Ritter, T., Kotsch, K., Leber, J. and Volk, H. D. (2005). Abnormal T-cell reactivity against paternal antigens in spontaneous abortion: adoptive transfer of pregnancy-induced CD4+CD25+ T regulatory cells prevents fetal rejection in a murine abortion model. *Am J Pathol*, Vol. 166, No. 3, pp. 811-22.

Zheng, S. G., Wang, J. and Horwitz, D. A. (2008). Cutting edge: Foxp3+CD4+CD25+ regulatory T cells induced by IL-2 and TGF-beta are resistant to Th17 conversion by IL-6. *J Immunol*, Vol. 180, No. 11, pp. 7112-6.

Zheng, S. G., Wang, J., Wang, P., Gray, J. D. and Horwitz, D. A. (2007). IL-2 is essential for TGF-beta to convert naive CD4+CD25- cells to CD25+Foxp3+ regulatory T cells and for expansion of these cells. *J Immunol*, Vol. 178, No. 4, pp. 2018-27.

Zipfel, P. F. and Skerka, C. (2009). Complement regulators and inhibitory proteins. *Nat Rev Immunol*, Vol. 9, No. 10, pp. 729-40.

Part 4

Placental Vasculature

13

Role of EG-VEGF in Human Placentation: Physiological and Pathological Implications

P. Hoffmann, S. Brouillet, M. Benharouga, J.J. Feige and N. Alfaidy
University Joseph Fourier, INSERM U1036, CEA - Grenoble, France

1. Introduction

Pre-eclampsia (PE, also called gravidic toxemia) is a hypertensive disorder that affects 5% of all pregnancies. It occurs during the second half of pregnancy (Carty et al, 2010). Affected women experience high blood pressure, fluid retention, nausea, and headaches. If not treated, PE leads to convulsions (eclampsia), kidney failure, liver failure and death. Screening tests for PE are poorly predictive and the "gold standard marker" is still to be discovered in order to assist the clinician in the prognosis of the pathology. The underlying causes of the development of the pathology are often unknown and the late diagnosis of the disease results in premature delivery of the fetus, which is considered to be the most definitive method to minimize PE complications. PE is still a major problem in Obstetrics and Gynecology and is the cause of several maternal deaths.

PE is a multifactorial disease whose pathogenesis is not solely vascular, genetic, immunologic, or environmental, but is a complex combination of factors (Ilekis et al., 2007). The heterogeneity of the disease is suggested by diverse clinical manifestations such as mild or severe PE, early onset (<34 weeks) or late onset (>34 weeks) of the disease and presence or absence of associated IUGR (intrauterine growth restriction) (Dekker, 1999). Also women with asthma, obesity, maternal infections, insulin resistance or adverse lipid metabolic profile have an increased incidence of PE. (Carty et al., 2010) Moreover, a population-based cohort study suggests that women with early-onset PE are at greater risk of cardiovascular disease later in life (Irgens, 2007). Although its aetiology remains unclear, there have been significant advances in the understanding of the pathophysiology of the disorder. The primary lesion is thought to be due to deficient trophoblast invasion of the maternal spiral arteries by the end of first trimester of pregnancy and the beginning of the second trimester, leading to underperfusion of the uteroplacental unit. It is well documented today that the cause of the development of PE is a shallow invasion of maternal decidua and spiral arteries by extravillous trophoblasts (EVTs) (Fisher, 2004, McMaster et al., 2004). Successful human placentation depends on adequate transformation of the uteroplacental vasculature by EVT following proliferation, migration, and invasion of these cells into the maternal decidua (Cross et al., 1994, Strickland & Richards, 1992), this process of vascular remodeling rises to a peak by the end of the first trimester and declines rapidly thereafter (Aplin, 1991). At around 10-12 weeks of gestation (wg), cytotrophoblasts (CT) that are present in anchoring villi generate multilayered columns of EVTs that colonize the interstitium of the maternal decidua, the inner third of the myometrium and the uterine blood vessels. This invasion results in the formation of a low resistance vascular system that is essential for fetal growth (Charnock-Jones et al., 2004). This developmental period is characterized by an important physiological switch in oxygen tension during the opening of the intervillous space. Before 9 wg, placental oxygen tension is low (~20 mm Hg) and after the first trimester, it increases to ~55 mm Hg (Jauniaux et al., 2000). During pregnancy, the depth of invasion by EVT into the uterine wall is critical and finely controlled. Poor invasion causes a lack of remodeling of the spiral arterioles and leads to a sustained hypoxic environment over the first trimester of pregnancy. This abnormal condition potentially leads to pathological conditions such as PE, IUGR, spontaneous abortion and stillbirth (Carty et al., 2010, Myatt & Miodovnik, 1999, Redman & Sargent, 2005). For instance, a limited trophoblast invasion of maternal vessels has been correlated to both PE (Sibai et al., 2005) and fetal growth restriction, whereas an excessive trophoblast invasion is associated with invasive mole, placenta accreta and choriocarcinoma (Wells, 2007).

In PE, several aspects have been reported to contribute to the poor remodeling of the spiral arteries, including defective EVT differentiation toward the invasive phenotype, increased apoptosis, an imbalanced control of migratory and invasive EVT functions (Huppertz & Peeters, 2005, Kingdom et al., 2000). However, despite many years of extensive research on the disorders that are associated with abnormal placentation, the mechanisms leading to a successful pregnancy are far from being fully understood. It is likely that a fine balance between the expression of pro- and anti-invasive factors might regulate the depth and rate of placental invasion. Various growth factors and cytokines, such as EGF, HGF, TGF-α, amphiregulin, IGF-II, and IL-1β, stimulate trophoblast differentiation toward an invasive phenotype (Cartwright et al., 1999,Lysiak et al., 1993); by contrast, limited data exist regarding possible negative regulators of trophoblast differentiation. Graham and Lala, (Graham & Lala, 1991) first demonstrated that TGF-β produced primarily by the decidua inhibits trophoblast invasion. Subsequent studies revealed that TGF-β3 inhibits trophoblast invasion following an interaction with endoglin, a component of the TGF-β receptor complex (Caniggia et al., 1997, Irving & Lala, 1995). Recently, improved understanding of the pathogenesis of PE has raised the possibility that blood levels of antiangiogenic proteins might eventually be used to predict this devastating condition. Investigations on the cause of PE development have also pointed out the potential importance of angiogenic factors and their receptors. For instance, low VEGF (vascular endothelial growth factor) levels or increased production of VEGF antagonists such as the soluble fms-like tyrosine kinase-1 (sFlt-1, also referred to as sVEGFR-1) have been proposed as possible mediators of PE (Levine et al., 2004). A key discovery in the field was the understanding that PE major phenotypes, such as hypertension and proteinuria are due to an excess of sFlt-1 that is made by the placenta and acts by neutralizing the pro-angiogenic proteins (VEGF) and placental growth factor (PlGF). More recently, soluble endoglin, another circulating anti-angiogenic protein was found to synergize with sFlt-1 and to contribute to the pathogenesis of PE. Abnormalities in these circulating angiogenic proteins are not only present during clinical PE, but seem also to antedate clinical symptoms by several weeks. Altogether these findings suggest that sequential angiogenic factor changes could have predictive value in PE. Therefore, current research in this field aims to discover more specific markers of the disease.

Although VEGF is selectively acting on any type of endothelial cell including placental endothelial cells, it is ubiquitously expressed. The existence of organ-specific angiogenic and/or anti-angiogenic factors has been postulated for many years (Dellian et al., 1996, Stewart & Wiley, 1981), but only recently received confirmation when a new factor named endocrine gland-derived vascular endothelial growth factor (EG-VEGF), was characterized and sequenced (LeCouter et al., 2001). This factor was found to be expressed in testis, adrenal gland, ovary and placenta (LeCouter et al., 2001), in addition, its angiogenic action appeared to be restricted to endothelial cells derived from endocrine tissues (LeCouter et al., 2001). In endothelial cells isolated from steroidogenic tissues, EG-VEGF was shown to promote proliferation, survival and chemotaxis (LeCouter et al., 2001). *In vivo* delivery of adenoviruses encoding EG-VEGF resulted in endocrine tissue-specific angiogenesis (LeCouter et al., 2003).

EG-VEGF also called prokineticin 1 (PROK1) is a member of a class of proteins named prokineticins (PROK) family that also includes Bv8, a frog peptide purified from the skin secretion of the yellow-bellied toad *Bombina variegata* (LeCouter et al., 2001), also known as prokineticin-2 (PROK2). Human EG-VEGF and Bv8 share the same G protein-coupled receptors, termed PROKR1 and PROKR2 (Masuda et al., 2002).

2. Prokineticins

The Prokineticin family comprises EG-VEGF/PROK1 and Bv8/PROK2, which were identified in frog, fish, reptiles and mammals. The names PROK1 and PROK2 were assigned to these proteins by Li et al. (M. Li et al., 2001) to reflect their functions in inducing specific and potent contractions of the smooth muscle of the gastrointestinal tract. Subsequently, LeCouter et al. (LeCouter et al., 2001) described a growth factor which induced a strong and specific mitogenic response in endocrine gland-derived endothelial cells. The similar effects induced by this protein and by VEGF led it to be named, EG-VEGF. Although there are several similarities in the functions of VEGF and EG-VEGF, the two factors are structurally unrelated. EG-VEGF and Bv8 share 44% amino acid identity and share a common protein structure motif. They have a conserved N-terminal sequence (AVITGA), which is essential for the activity of these proteins. Mutations to this sequence, by insertion of a methionine preceding the Nterminal alanine, substitution of the N-terminal alanine with a methionine or deletion of the first two amino acids (Negri et al., 2005), produce PROK receptor (PROKR) antagonists. Another feature of the PROKs is the presence of ten conserved cysteines, which are predicted to form five disulfide bonds (Boisbouvier et al., 1998, M. Li et al., 2001). The PROKs are the cognate ligands for two closely related G-protein-coupled receptors (GPCRs), termed PROKR1 and PROKR2, which share 85% amino acid identity and exhibit the greatest differences in their N-terminal sequences (D.C. Lin et al., 2002, Masuda et al., 2002). Their sequences are almost identical in the transmembrane domains (Soga et al., 2002), suggesting that their activation mechanisms are identical and that small molecule analogues will not discriminate between the receptors, as is the case for EG-VEGF and Bv8. The affinity of these factors for their receptors is similar, with Bv8 showing a moderately higher affinity for both receptors. PROKRs have been reported to couple either to Gs, Gi or to Gq proteins (D.C. Lin et al., 2002, Soga et al., 2002). In adrenal cortex capillary endothelial (ACE) cells, activation of the receptors has been shown to be inhibited by pertussis toxin, suggesting Gi coupling. By contrast, in transfected CHO cells activation of the receptors has been shown to induce calcium mobilization and phosphoinositide hydrolysis (D.C. Lin et al., 2002, Soga et al.,

2002), suggesting Gq coupling. Signalling through these receptors is linked to phospholipase C activation and generation of diacylglycerol and inositol phosphate, with potential downstream activation of protein kinase C, extracellular-signal regulated kinases (ERK) 1 and 2, Akt and nitric oxide synthase (Hoogerwerf, 2006,D.C. Lin et al., 2002,R. Lin et al., 2002).

3. Prokineticins in reproduction

Prokineticins were originally identified as regulators of intestinal contraction but subsequently shown to affect vascular function, neuronal survival, nociception, immune responses, and gonadotropin releasing hormone systems (Battersby et al., 2004, Dorsch et al., 2005, LeCouter et al., 2003, Maldonado-Perez et al., 2007). Quickly after their discovery, the members of this family showed differential specificities of expression and preferential sites of actions. While Bv8/PROK2 was associated to the neuronal system, EG-VEGF was more associated to the reproductive tract. EG-VEGF has been well studied in the ovary, uterus, testis, prostate and placenta (Battersby et al., 2004, Brouillet et al., 2010, Dorsch et al., 2005, Fraser et al., 2005,Hoffmann et al., 2007,2006, Hoffmann et al., 2009, LeCouter et al., 2001, LeCouter et al., 2003, Maldonado-Perez et al., 2007, Pasquali et al., 2006).

3.1 Prokineticin expression in human reproductive systems

Since its discovery, EG-VEGF has been reported to be highly expressed in the reproductive system, and it is now believed to play important roles in diverse facets of reproduction processes. While our group has been interested in the study of EG-VEGF and its receptors in the placenta, other groups have studied this factor in endometrium, ovary, prostate, uterus and testis.

In the testis, EG-VEGF is predominantly expressed in testosterone-producing Leydig cells, and its receptors are expressed in vascular endothelial cells (LeCouter et al., 2001). The exact role of each type of receptor remains however to be elucidated.

In the normal ovary, EG-VEGF is expressed in a dynamic way in elements of the sex cord–stroma lineage. Maturing secondary follicles maintain strong EG-VEGF expression. However, in the antral follicle, EG-VEGF is expressed at low levels in theca cells. In the corpus luteum, the mRNA expression of EG-VEGF increases as the corpus luteum matures. The actions of EG-VEGF in the ovary are likely to be mediated by both PROKR1 and PROKR2.

In the endometrium, EG-VEGF, PROKR1 and PROKR2 expression peak during the window of implantation, a period that corresponds to the maximum of receptivity, and there is no temporal variation in the expression of PROK2, PROKR1, or PROKR2 during the same period. EG-VEGF and its receptors were localized to multiple cellular compartments, including glandular epithelial, stromal, endothelial cells in the endometrium and endothelial and smooth muscle cells in the myometrium. The elevation in EG-VEGF expression in the secretory phase of the menstrual cycle indicated a potential regulation of EG-VEGF by progesterone (Fraser et al., 2005, Kisliouk et al., 2003).

Further support for a role of PROKs in reproductive functions can be gleaned from PROKR2 and PROK2 knockout mice, which show hypoplasia of the reproductive tract (Dode et al., 2006, Martin et al.). This phenotype has been explained by the lack of GnRH neurons in the hypothalamus of these animals. Interestingly, mutations in PROK2 and PROKR2 have been identified in patients with Kallmann syndrome, a pathology that is defined by the association of hypogonadotropic hypogonadism (HH) with olfactory abnormalities (anosmia or hyposmia). Recently, homozygous loss-of-function mutations of PROK2 were described in families with HH, suggesting an autosomal recessive inheritance disorder. Hence PROKs seem to be directly involved in a major pathology of the reproductive system that is due to failure in sexual maturation. However, it is possible that the loss of PROKs might also have a direct local impact on to the observed atrophy of these tissues.

3.2 Prokineticins in human placenta and decidua

In the placenta, the expression of EG-VEGF was briefly reported by the group of Ferrara in 2001. However, insightful work on EG-VEGF throughout pregnancy came from our group with a focus on early pregnancy and from the group of Dr Jabbour with more focus on the decidual unit, at the term of human gestation (Catalano et al., 2010 , Maldonado-Perez et al., 2007).

3.2.1 Prokineticins at term of the pregnancy

The group of Jabbour (Cook et al., 2010,Evans et al., 2008, Maldonado-Perez et al., 2007) has reported the localization of EG-VEGF and that of its receptors in term placenta and decidua; studied its signaling pathways, and demonstrated the effect of EG-VEGF on the expression of two inflammatory and vascular mediators, the cyclooxygenase (COX)-2 and IL-8 in third-trimester placentas. IL-8 is a potent neutrophil chemoattractant and angiogenic factor, promoting endothelial cell chemotaxis (Winkler, 2003), whereas COX-2 is the inducible isoform of the enzyme involved in the synthesis of prostaglandins from arachidonic acid. Their results showed that EG-VEGF and PROKR1 were highly expressed in term placenta and were immunolocalized to syncytiotrophoblasts, cytotrophoblasts, fetal endothelium, and macrophages. EG-VEGF induced a time-dependent increase in the expression of IL-8 and COX-2. These data suggest that EG-VEGF may have a novel role as a mediator of the inflammatory response in the placenta at the time of parturition.

3.2.2 Prokineticins in early pregnancy: focus on the placenta

As mentioned above, among the prokineticin members, EG-VEGF appeared to be an important actor for reproductive functions with indications of its potential involvement in human pregnancy, and particularly in placentation processes. The next paragraphs will summarize our main findings in this field.

3.2.2.1 Hypothesis

EG-VEGF was shown to be specific of the reproductive system and to be highly expressed in the placenta. Since its levels of expression were up-regulated by hypoxia, a strong attribute of placentation processes; and since a predictive marker for the launch of PE is still to be discovered; we performed a series of investigations to determine whether EG-VEGF could be a such marker.

3.2.2.2 Methods

To investigate the role of EG-VEGF in normal and pathological pregnancies, we used both human and mouse material. This consisted of placental tissues and sera collected at different gestational ages. First-trimester human placentas were obtained from elective terminations of pregnancies. Shortly after collection, tissues were snap-frozen in dry ice and stored at -80°C (for protein and mRNA extraction), fixed in paraformaldehyde at room temperature (for immunohistochemistry), or used for *in vitro* primary culture. Collection and processing of human placentas was approved by the University Hospital Ethics Committee, and informed consent was obtained from each patient (Brouillet et al., 2010, Hoffmann et al., 2007, 2006, Hoffmann et al., 2009). Mouse placentas were also collected at different gestational ages. Animal surgery was conducted following both institutional and European Community guidelines for the use of experimental animals.

To test our hypotheses, different methods were used. The main ones will be emphasized in each paragraph.

4. Main results

4.1 Expression of prokineticins in human and mouse placenta

Our first study on prokineticins in the placenta has reported the pattern of expression of EG-VEGF and its analog, Bv8 (PROK2). This set of experiment has been performed using immunohistochemistry and western blot analysis. Whereas no expression of Bv8 was observed in the placenta, EG-VEGF was highly present in this tissue during the first trimester of pregnancy, with a strong expression in the syncytiotrophoblast. A comparison of EG-VEGF localization to that of VEGF showed that these factors are not localized to the same cell types, but rather show complementary localizations (Figure 1).

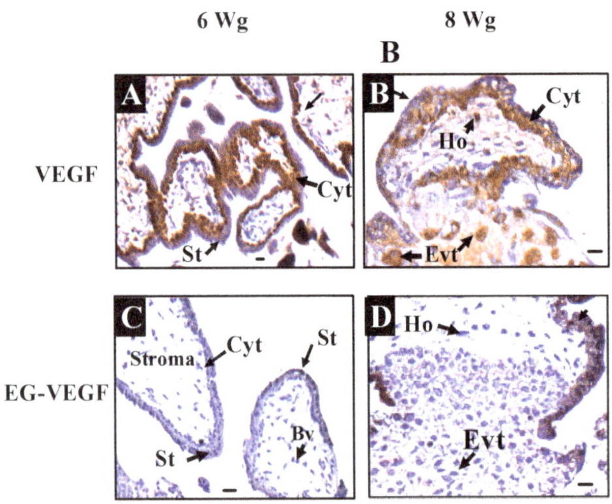

Fig. 1. **Comparison of VEGF and EG-VEGF Immunoreactivity (Ir) in placental villous tissues. A, B** show representative VEGF Ir, (brown color) at 6 and 8 weeks of gestation (wg), respectively. **C, D** show EG-VEGF Ir (brown color) at the same wg. Note that VEGF staining is present from 6 wg and EG-VEGF staining is only present at 8 wg. EG-VEGF and VEGF exhibit complementary sites of Ir in chorionic villi and EVT. Cytotrophoblast (Ct), Hobfauer cells (Ho), Extravillous trophoblast (EVT), syncytiotrophoblast (St). Scale bar = 20 μm

EG-VEGF receptors were found in trophoblast cells, endothelial cells and EVT, suggesting potential roles of this factor in the control of placental development (Hoffmann et al., 2007, 2006). Using quantitative RT-PCR we determined the pattern of expression of EG-VEGF and its receptors during the first trimester of human pregnancy. PROKR1 expression exhibited the same profile of expression as EG-VEGF, and PROKR2 was stably expressed during the first trimester with a slight increase by the end of this period (Figure.2).

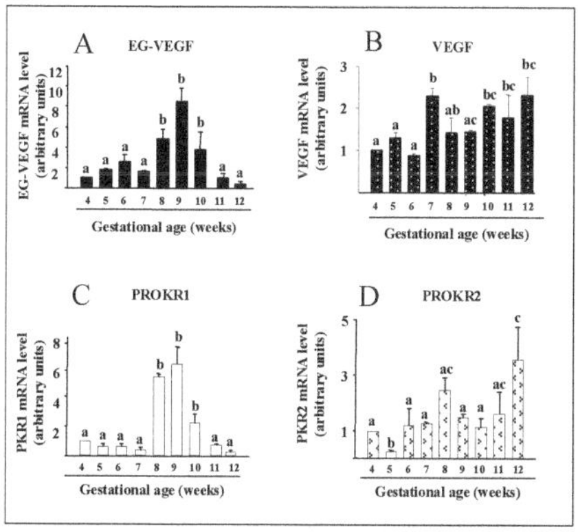

Fig. 2. **EG-VEGF (A), VEGF (B), PROKR1 (C) and PROKR2 (D) mRNA expression during the first trimester of pregnancy**. Values overwritten with different letters are significantly different from each other ($P < 0.05$).

The same results were found in mouse placenta during the first 10.5 days post coitum (dpc), corresponding to the first trimester of human pregnancy (Figure.3). We showed that EG-VEGF and VEGF exhibit different patterns of expression and different localizations in the mouse placenta. EG-VEGF was mainly localized in the labyrinth whereas VEGF was present in glycogen and giant cells. EG-VEGF mRNA and protein levels were the highest before 10.5 dpc whereas those of VEGF showed stable expression throughout gestation. PROKR1 protein was localized to the labyrinth layer and showed the same pattern of expression as EG-VEGF, whereas PROKR2 expression was maintained over 10.5 dpc with both trophoblastic and endothelial cell localizations. Altogether these findings suggest that EG-VEGF may have a direct effect on both endothelial and trophoblast cells and is likely to play an important role in placentation (Hoffmann et al., 2007, 2006).

4.2 Role of EG-VEGF in the trophoblast invasion

In the light of the data obtained in our first publications on the expression of this factor and its receptors, we decided to investigate the potential role of EG-VEGF in the control of trophoblast invasion into the maternal decidua, a requisite process for successful pregnancy. Human placental explants and EVT were used to determine EG-VEGF effect on migration, invasion and tube-like organization of EVT. We used the HTR-8/SVneo cells as a model for EVT cells (Graham et al., 1993). A wound healing assay was performed to examine the effect of EG-VEGF on HTR motility. Cells were seeded in equal number into six-well plates. At confluence, cells were scratched and allowed to heal for 24 h. Our results showed that EG-VEGF is a potent inhibitor of EVT and migration. Measurement of EVT tube-like formation was performed

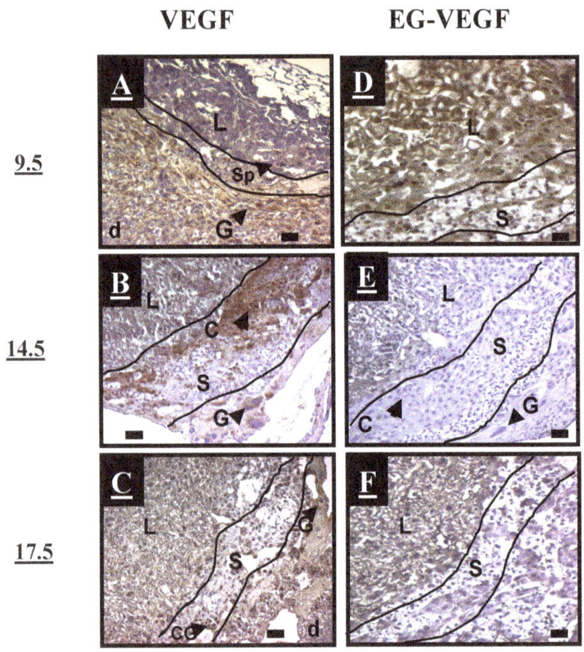

Fig. 3. **Immunolocalizations of VEGF and EG-VEGF in mouse placenta.** at 9.5, 14.5 and 17.5 dpc. Labyrinth (L), Glycogen cells (GC), Giant cells (Gi), spongiotrophoblast (Sp). Scale bar = 50 μm

using time lapse microscopy. Our results showed that EG-VEGF inhibited the tube-like organization of EVT cells. The control of EVT invasion by EG-VEGF was confirmed in a set of experiments that employed placental explants. Villous explant cultures were established from first trimester human placentas (10–12 wg) as described previously (Caniggia et al., 1999, Genbacev et al., 1993). It was particularly relevant to study EG-VEGF effects on trophoblast differentiation towards an invasive phenotype in a system in which the placental villous tissue architecture is maintained. Placental villous explants in culture preserve the topology of intact villi and closely mimic the formation of anchoring villi occurring *in vivo* by the end of first trimester of pregnancy (Caniggia et al., 1999, Genbacev et al., 1993). Figure. 4 shows representative photographs of placental villous tips at day 3 of culture in the absence or presence of EG-VEGF (50 ng/ml). In the control condition there was an obvious outgrowth of EVT from the distal end of the villous tip and migration into Matrigel. In contrast, in the presence of EG-VEGF, there was almost no outgrowth or migration of EVT into Matrigel. In additional experiments we demonstrated that these effects were mediated by the type 2 receptor of EG-VEGF, PROKR2 and involved MMP2 and 9 activities, (Hoffmann et al., 2009).

4.3 Role of EG-VEGF in placental angiogenesis.

Pro-angiogenic effects of EG-VEGF were reported in many reproductive systems, confirming its direct involvement in angiogenesis. Using appropriate angiogenesis assays

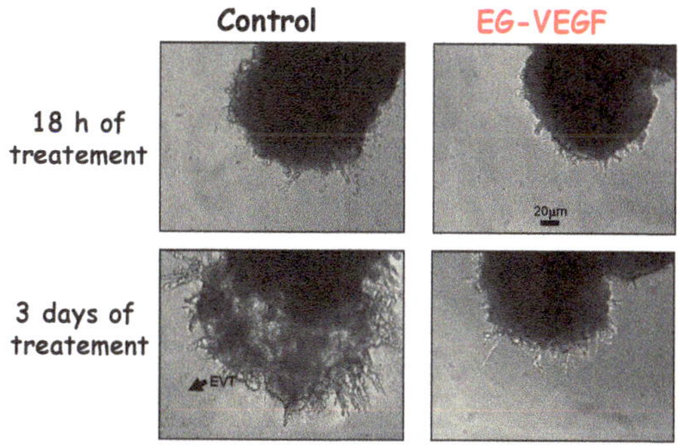

Fig. 4. **Effect of EG-VEGF on the invasion of EVT.** Villous explants from 10 to 12 wg were maintained in culture for 6 days. EG-VEGF (50 ng/ml) treatment started 24 h after the launch of the culture and was assessed for 24h. Control experiments were run in parallel using explants from the same placenta.

(Proliferation, migration, pseudo-vascular organization, spheroid sprouting) and functional studies (microvascular permeability and paracellular transport) we were able to answer an important biological question related to the role of EG-VEGF in placental development. EG-VEGF effects were analyzed in placental microvascular endothelial cells "HPEC" and in macrovascular umbilical vein endothelial cells "HUVEC". First, we showed that HPEC and HUVEC express both types of receptors, with a much higher level of expression in HPEC, (Brouillet et al., 2010). Furthermore, we showed that EG-VEGF increased HPEC but not HUVEC proliferation and migration (Brouillet et al., 2010).

To determine EG-VEGF effect on the sprout formation, a three-dimensional *in vitro* angiogenesis system was used. Whereas no effect of EG-VEGF was observed on HUVEC sprouting, this factor increases HPEC sprouting. Figure. 5 shows representative photographs of HPEC spheroids at the time of their incubation and 12h later. To control the response of the cells, we examined the effect of the potent angiogenic factors, FGF-2. As expected, FGF-2 induced significant sprouting of the spheroids as compared to the control conditions. EG-VEGF induced the same level of sprouting in HPEC spheroids compared to that obtained with FGF2.

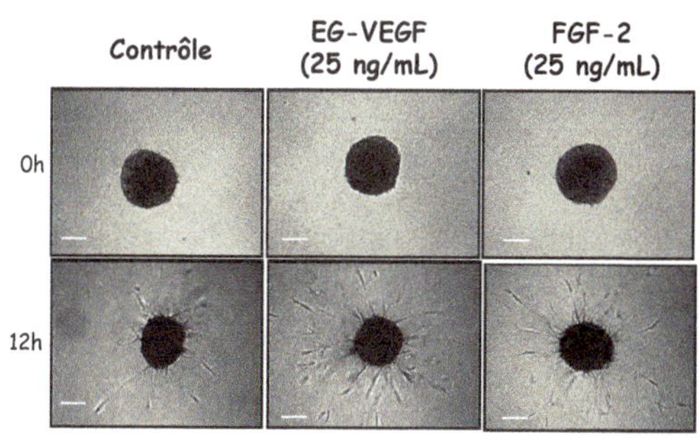

Fig. 5. **EG-VEGF, effect on the sprouting of HPEC spheroids.** Representative photographs of spheroids formed from HPEC cells and cultured in collagen gel for 0 or 12h in the absence or presence of EG-VEGF (25ng/ml), FGF-2 (25 ng/ml).

In the placenta, the microvascular endothelium is known to participate in angiogenesis, maintenance of blood fluidity and is also a discriminating barrier in materno-fetal transports of solutes and nutrients (Murray, 2003, Rodgers, 1988), therefore a maintenance of a semi-permeable barrier by the endothelium is critically important in endothelial cell function. Both permeability and paracellular transport of HPEC monolayers were assessed. HPEC permeability was measured in response to EG-VEGF and thrombin, an enhancer of electrolyte transport. The endothelial barrier was evaluated by trans-endothelial electrical resistance (TEER). Figure. 6A shows the percentage of increase in permeability of a monolayer of HPEC in response to thrombin (70 U/ml), EG-VEGF (25 ng/ml), or VEGF (25 ng/ml). TEER was recorded every 5 min for 35 min. As expected, thrombin significantly increased HPEC permeability. Under EG-VEGF treatment, HPEC permeability increased as early as 5 min after treatment and was maintained for up to 20 minutes. The effect of EG-VEGF on the paracellular transport was measured using [^{3}H]-mannitol. The data summarizing the permeability coefficients for [^{3}H]-mannitol transport in response to thrombin and EG-VEGF are presented in Figure. 6B. The basal permeability Coefficient (Papp) in HPEC was 1.7 x10^{-5}cm/s. Thrombin almost doubled [^{3}H]-mannitol transport through HPEC, and EG-VEGF increased this transport to almost the same levels achieved by

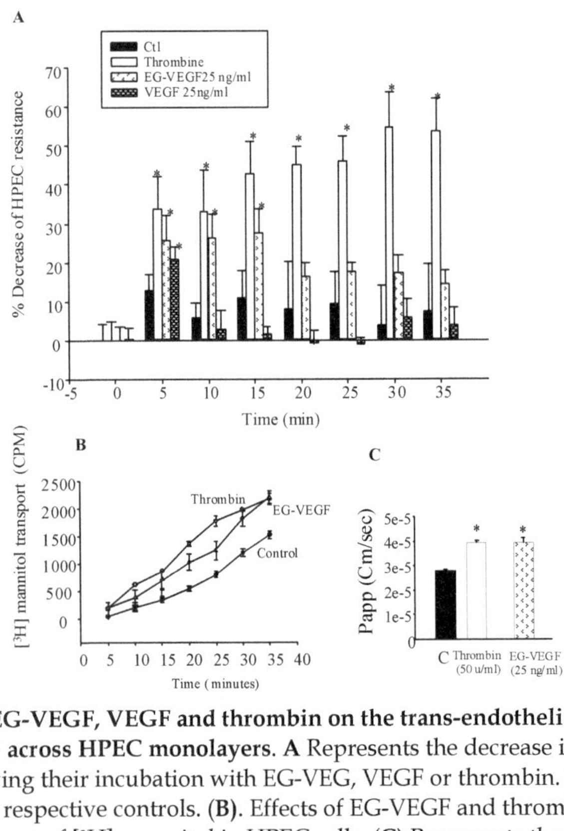

Fig. 6. **Effects of EG-VEGF, VEGF and thrombin on the trans-endothelial electrical resistance (TEER) across HPEC monolayers. A** Represents the decrease in the TEER of HPEC cells following their incubation with EG-VEG, VEGF or thrombin. The results were normalized to the respective controls. **(B)**. Effects of EG-VEGF and thrombin on the paracellular transport of [^{3}H]-mannitol in HPEC cells. **(C)** Represents the permeability coefficient of EG-VEGF and thrombin.

thrombin, Figure. 6C. More importantly, using siRNA and antibody blocking techniques, we demonstrated that PROKR1 mediates EG-VEGF angiogenic effects, whereas PROKR2 is rather involved in its effects on cellular permeability (Brouillet et al, 2010). Altogether, our results showed, for the first time, that EG-VEGF is a potent new angiogenic and survival factor for microvascular endothelial cells, and characterized the EG-VEGF mediated angiogenic processes. These finding propose a novel view of the regulation of angiogenesis normal placentation, (Brouillet et al, 2010).

4.4 EG-VEGF regulation in human placenta

4.4.1 Regulation by oxygen tension

Low oxygen tension is a key parameter that controls gene expression during the first trimester of pregnancy. Moreover, the highest level of expression level of EG-VEGF and its receptor PROKR1 is observed during the hypoxic period of human placentation (Hoffmann et al., 2007, 2006). This observation prompted us to hypothesize that EG-VEGF and PROKR1 mRNA might be regulated by oxygen tension in human trophoblast cells. To test this hypothesis, we incubated trophoblast cells isolated from first trimester placentas under either 20% O2 or 3% O2 and measured EG-VEGF and PROKR1 mRNA abundance using quantitative RT-PCR. As shown in Figure. 7A, a significant increase in both EG-VEGF (160% of normoxic control) and PROKR1 (200% of normoxic control) mRNA levels was observed under hypoxic conditions (3% O2). We then examined the effects of transcription and translation inhibitors on the hypoxic regulation of EG-VEGF expression. In the presence of the RNA polymerase inhibitor DRB, the hypoxic induction of EG-VEGF was completely abolished, whereas it was preserved in the presence of cycloheximide, a potent inhibitor of translation, Figure. 7B. These data suggest that hypoxia regulates EG-VEGF gene expression at the transcriptional level.

EG-VEGF levels appeared to greatly vary during early pregnancy, progressively increasing until the 10th wg and rapidly dropping afterward. These dramatic changes appear to be correlated with the hypoxic developmental period of the placenta. This correlation is supported by the transcriptionally controlled up-regulation of EG-VEGF mRNA and concomitant increase of its protein levels that were observed in primary cultures of trophoblasts after 24 h of culture under reduced oxygen tension. This regulation was not unexpected as a functional hypoxia-response element (TACGTGCGGC) able to bind the hypoxia-inducible factor-1 has been identified in the human EG-VEGF promoter (LeCouter et al., 2001). Regulation of placental growth factors expression by oxygen tension is well established and has been described for several angiogenic factors, including VEGF, TGFβ3 (Schaffer et al., 2003), and the soluble form of VEGF receptor-1 (s-flt) (H. Li et al., 2005, Nagamatsu et al., 2004). We also observed up-regulation of PROKR1 receptor expression under hypoxic conditions. A GenBank screen of the human PROKR1 promoter revealed the presence of one putative HIF-1α binding site, suggesting that the oxygen effect on PROKR1 expression might occur through a pathway that involves HIF-1α. However, we cannot totally exclude that other factors presenting peaks in their expression during the first trimester of pregnancy may also participate in the regulation of EG-VEGF expression. Human chorionic gonadotropin (hCG) and progesterone are two such candidates because they have been recently shown to stimulate EG-VEGF mRNA expression in human luteinized granulosa cells (Fraser et al., 2005) and human endometrial tissue (Battersby et al., 2004), respectively.

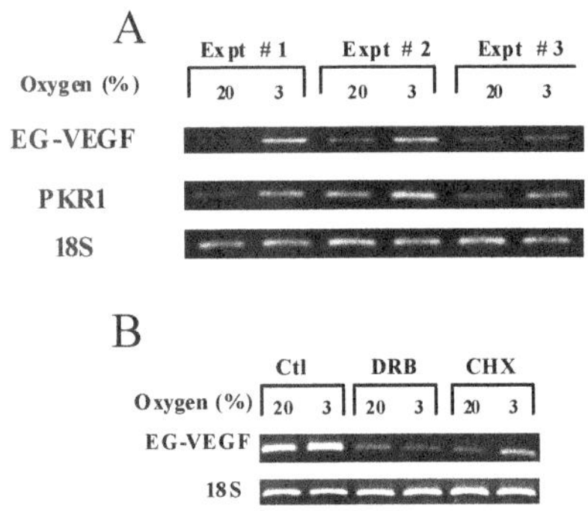

Fig. 7. **Effect of hypoxia on EG-VEGF and PROKR1 mRNA expression in human trophoblast cells.** Cytrophoblasts were isolated from 10 different placentas collected at 7-10 weeks of gestation and cultured under either normoxic or hypoxic conditions. Panel **A** shows the RT-PCR amplification products for EG-VEGF and PROKR1 under either 20% or 3% O_2. **B.** shows the effect of DRB and CHX on basal and hypoxia-induced EG-VEGF mRNA expression in trophoblast cells.

4.4.2 Regulation by human chorionic gonadotropin (hCG)

During placental development, the hypoxic environment occurs from the beginning of implantation to the end of the first trimester. However, the strongest expression of EG-VEGF is between the 8th and 11th wg, suggesting that other factors than hypoxia might regulate the EG-VEGF/ PROKR1/PROKR2 system. To date, little is known about the regulation of EG-VEGF and its receptors, and there is no enlightenment for the peak of expression of EG-VEGF by the end of the first trimester of pregnancy. During the first trimester of pregnancy, one dominant hormone, hCG exhibits the same pattern of expression as of EG-VEGF and displays similar effects on placental development (Licht et al., 2001, Malassine & Cronier, 2002). One of the earliest endocrine roles of hCG is to stimulate the corpus luteum to produce enough progesterone in order to establish pregnancy at the outset. In the placenta, hCG is well known to facilitate trophoblastic differentiation (Licht et al., 2001, Malassine & Cronier, 2002), and was reported to induce the expression of specific genes such as VEGF, leukemia inhibitory factor, and MMP-9, all central to the establishment of the feto-maternal interface (Licht et al., 2007, Zygmunt et al., 2002). In human placenta, hCG is primarily produced by the syncytiotrophoblast and to a certain extent by the cytotrophoblast (Kirkegaard et al., 2011, Krantz et al., 2004, Rao & Lei, 2007, Shi et al., 1993). In normal pregnancies, detectable levels of hCG begin to appear in the maternal circulation about 2-3 weeks after conception and the peak is observed at ~8-9 wg before declining significantly in the later stages of pregnancy. High serum hCG levels at mid-late pregnancy have been associated with PE, IUGR and Down's syndrome (DS).

We investigated the regulation of EG-VEGF expression, and its receptors by hCG. Both placental explants (PEX) and primary cultures of trophoblast from the first trimester of pregnancy were used to investigate this hypothesis. Our results show that **i**) LH/CGR, the hCG receptor, is expressed both in cyto- and syncytiotrophoblasts **ii**) hCG increases EG-VEGF, PROKR1 and PROKR2 mRNA and protein expression in a dose and time-dependent manners **iii**) hCG increases the release of EG-VEGF from PEX conditioned media **iv**) hCG effects are transcriptional and post- transcriptional and **v**) the hCG effects are mediated by cAMP via cAMP response elements present in the EG-VEGF promoter region. Altogether, these results demonstrate a new role for hCG in the regulation of an emerging regulatory system of trophoblast invasion, EG-VEGF and its receptors (Figure 8).

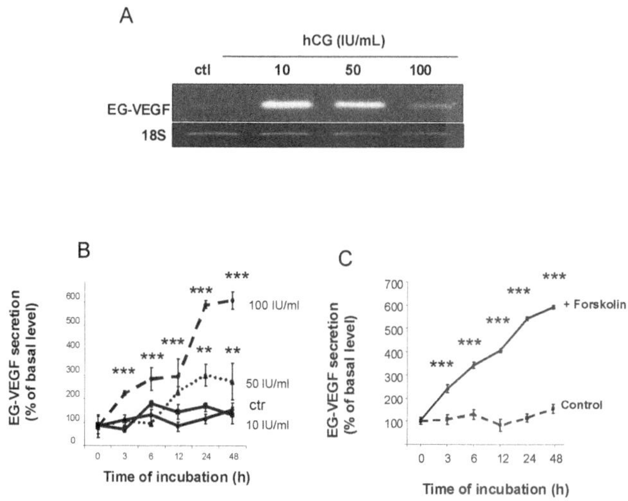

Fig. 8. **hCG effect on EG-VEGF expression and secretion. A** shows a representative analysis of hCG (10, 50 and 100 IU/ml) effect on EG-VEGF mRNA expression in syncytiotrophoblast cells. **B** shows a temporal (0 to 48 h) and a dose dependence analysis of hCG effect on EG-VEGF secretion in placental conditioned media. **C** shows a time course (0h- 48h) effect of Forskolin on EG-VEGF secretion.

5. EG-VEGF and pregnancy pathologies

5.1 Prematurity

Compelling recent findings suggest that PROKs and their receptors might play a crucial role in premature onset of labor. The labor onset is known to be associated with inflammatory cascades in the uteroplacental unit, and EG-VEGF has been shown to regulate the production of proinflammatory cytokines and to be involved in the inflammatory response in the placenta (Catalano et al., 2010 , Denison et al., 2008, Evans et al., 2008). Therefore, antagonism of prokineticin action may provide a therapy for preterm labor caused by early inflammation and contractile pathways. Further investigations are however required to demonstrate a direct involvement of EG-VEGF in the mechanisms of term and preterm labor. A particular interest should be given to EG-VEGF potential actions on the expression of factors that trigger parturition, particularly in the fetal membranes, major sites of prostaglandins synthesis and metabolism.

5.2 Preeclampsia and IUGR.

5.2.1 EG-VEGF and Preeclampsia

Since the discovery of EG-VEGF, our group has been interested in its study in PE. In fact, the combination of our previous data showing that EG-VEGF was abundantly expressed in human placenta during the first trimester of pregnancy; that its expression was up regulated by hypoxia; and that EG-VEGF regulates EVT invasion, suggested to us that EG-VEGF circulating levels might be altered in PE. We were first to report EG-VEGF circulating levels throughout human pregnancy and to show that they were significantly higher during the third trimester of pregnancy in PE patients compared to controls (Figure 9). These data raise the possibility that inappropriate expression or function of EG-VEGF or that of its receptors might contribute to major complications of pregnancy, such as PE, which is associated with abnormal trophoblast invasion and placental development. We now know that the origin of PE takes place during the first trimester of pregnancy and that any changes in protein expression after the establishment of the disease are considered to be consequences of the disease rather than causes of its development. Our data show that EG-VEGF expression is at its lowest levels by the end of the first trimester, suggesting that its greatest role should occur within that trimester. Moreover, given the correlation between the pattern of EG-VEGF and PROKR1 expression with the hypoxic period of placental development and knowing that failure in placental angiogenesis is thought to contribute to PE development, one can speculate on the potential implication of this factor and/or its receptors in the development of PE. However, only a prospective study examining the expression of EG-VEGF and/or PROKR1 during the first trimester of pregnancy in women who go on to develop PE will allow to provide an answer to this question. Clinical studies are ongoing to examine these hypotheses. Future studies are also required to determine the biological activities triggered by EG-VEGF in the human placenta and identify whether dysregulation of EG-VEGF expression may result in placental pathologies.

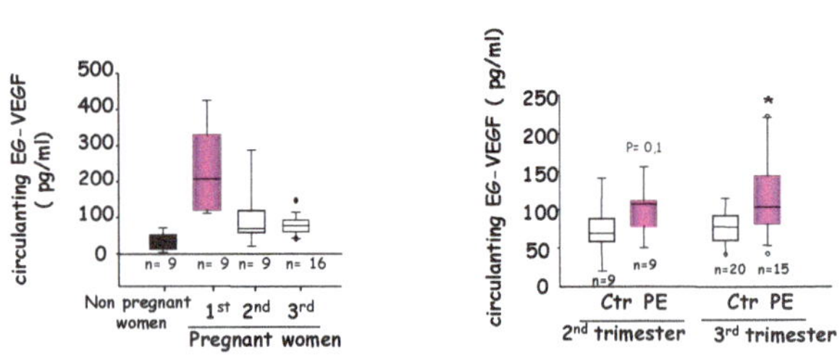

Fig. 9. **EG-VEGF serum levels in non-pregnant and in pregnant women at the first, second and third trimesters.** (graph on the left) and in PE women at second and third trimesters. Box plot demonstrates 10th, 25th, 50th, 75th, and 90th percentiles. (* $P < 0.05$, by ANOVA followed by Dunn's Method).

5.2.2 EG-VEGF and IUGR

Nowadays, our group has been interested in the study of the direct effects of EG-VEGF on placental development and particularly on its direct actions on the villi growth and survival, under stressful conditions. These studies were performed in the perspective to investigate the role of EG-VEGF in the second most important pathology of human pregnancy, IUGR.

Hence, we investigated EG-VEGF effects on i) trophoblast proliferation, both in primary cytotrophoblast (CT) and in placental explants culture, and on trophoblast survival, ii) cytotrophoblast syncytialisation (measurement of syncytin 1 and 2 and β-hCG mRNA expression). To further investigate the role of EG-VEGF and its receptors in placental development, we determined their levels of expression, both at the mRNA and protein levels, in normal and IUGR placentas. We also determined the circulating levels of EG-VEGF in sera collected from normal and IUGR pregnant women. Our results show that EG-VEGF i) increased CT proliferation; both in primary and explant cultures ii) did not affect syncytin 1, syncytin 2 and β-hCG mRNA expression iii) EG-VEGF, PROKR1 and PROKR2 mRNA and proteins levels are significantly increased in IUGR placentas, and iv) EG-VEGF circulating levels are significantly higher in IUGR patients. Altogether, these results identify a new placental growth factor during the first trimester of pregnancy, and provide evidence for its dysregulation in IUGR placentas. Changes in EG-VEGF, PROKR1 and PROKR2 in IUGR placentas, may well occur as a compensatory mechanism for this pathological condition. Further clinical investigations are required to demonstrate whether dysregulations in EG-VEGF and receptors in IUGR pregnancies are causes or consequences of the occurrence of this pathology.

6. Future directions for research on EG-VEGF in human placentation

6.1 EG-VEGF and implantation

It has been demonstrated that EG-VEGF, but not PROK2, expression peaks during the midluteal window of implantation, with immunolocalization to endometrial glandular epithelium, stromal and endothelial cells, and myometrial vascular endothelium as well as smooth muscle (Evans et al., 2009,Ngan et al., 2006,Salker et al.). In addition, it has been suggested that EG-VEGF could have a role in mediating the dysregulated vascular permeability that occur in ovarian hyperstimulation syndrome. The expression of PROKs and their receptors has also been reported in the fallopian tube from women with ectopic pregnancy (Tiberi et al.,2010). A dysregulation of these factors and their receptors has been demonstrated, suggesting a potential role for PROKs in fallopian tube function (Shaw et al.,2010). It has been postulated that these dysregulations could affect smooth muscle contractility in fallopian tube and embryo-tubal transport, providing a potential cause for ectopic pregnancy. More studies are required to evaluate whether PROKs are involved in these processes.

We have shown that EG-VEGF acts as a permeability factor during the first trimester of pregnancy, one can therefore speculate that EG-VEGF might also act on the endometrium to facilitate implantation by increasing endothelial leakage at the implantation site, one of the earliest signs of implantation. More studies are also required to evaluate whether PROKs are involved in perimplantation, spiral arteriole formation and recruitment of immune cells, including uterine natural killer cells, which have been shown to increase in number during the implantation window and in early pregnancy (King et al., 1996a, King et al., 1996b).

6.2 EG-VEGF and preeclampsia

Although there is abundant evidence for the role of circulating anti-angiogenic factors as mediators of the clinical signs and symptoms of PE (Ahmed et al., 2000), there are no definitive data linking early abnormalities in angiogenic factors with the impaired placentation in PE. Nowadays, our team is conducting a clinical study that aims to answer this question for EG-VEGF. This work relies on using blood samples collected from 500 pregnant women during early pregnancy with a follow up of their pregnancies outcome. A positive correlation between high EG-VEGF levels and PE occurrence will suggest that this factor is directly involved in alterations that lead to PE development. Moreover, it will suggest that sequential measurement of anti-angiogenic factors may be useful as a screening test for premature PE, possibly when combined with other early predictive tests such as Doppler ultrasound (Grill et al., 2009). This will be important for timely referral of patients at high risk of developing early PE and for indicating the need for therapeutic measures when they become available. Large prospective studies with longitudinal specimen collection from early pregnancy are required to definitely assess whether sequential changes in angiogenic proteins can be used to predict preterm PE.

7. Conclusion

During the last six years, we were able to assemble interesting data in regards to the expression, role and regulation of EG-VEGF in normal and pathological human pregnancies. The combination between our fundamental research and clinical approaches allowed us to strongly propose EG-VEGF as a potential marker for PE. Our ongoing clinical study will allow us to undeniably determine the role of this factor in normal placentation and to conclude on its potential relevance as a marker of PE. Furthermore we plan to develop an animal model to test whether dysregulations in EG-VEGF levels are a cause or consequence of the development of this pathology.

8. Acknowledgments

We thank the staff of the Department of Gynecology/Obstetrics, Grenoble Hospital (Pr. F. Sergent). We acknowledge the following sources of funding: INSERM (U1036), University Joseph Fourier, CEA, Région Rhône-Alpes (CIBLE-2008) and the Fondation pour la Recherche Médicale.

9. References

Ahmed, A.; Dunk, C.; Ahmad, S. et al. (2000). Regulation of placental vascular endothelial growth factor (VEGF) and placenta growth factor (PIGF) and soluble Flt-1 by oxygen--a review, *Placenta,* Vol.21 Suppl A, pp. S16-24

Aplin, J.D. (1991). Implantation, trophoblast differentiation and haemochorial placentation: mechanistic evidence in vivo and in vitro, *J Cell Sci,* Vol.99 (Pt 4), pp. 681-692

Battersby, S.; Critchley, H.O.; Morgan, K. et al. (2004). Expression and regulation of the prokineticins (endocrine gland-derived vascular endothelial growth factor and Bv8) and their receptors in the human endometrium across the menstrual cycle, *J Clin Endocrinol Metab,* Vol.89, No.5, pp. 2463-2469

Boisbouvier, J.; Albrand, J.P.; Blackledge, M. et al. (1998). A structural homologue of colipase in black mamba venom revealed by NMR floating disulphide bridge analysis, *J Mol Biol,* Vol.283, No.1, pp. 205-219

Brouillet, S.; Hoffmann, P.; Benharouga, M. et al. Molecular characterization of EG-VEGF-mediated angiogenesis: differential effects on microvascular and macrovascular endothelial cells, *Mol Biol Cell,* Vol.21, No.16, pp. 2832-2843

Caniggia, I.; Grisaru-Gravnosky, S.; Kuliszewsky, M. et al. (1999). Inhibition of TGF-beta 3 restores the invasive capability of extravillous trophoblasts in preeclamptic pregnancies, *J Clin Invest*, Vol.103, No.12, pp. 1641-1650

Caniggia, I.; Taylor, C.V.; Ritchie, J.W. et al. (1997). Endoglin regulates trophoblast differentiation along the invasive pathway in human placental villous explants, *Endocrinology*, Vol.138, No.11, pp. 4977-4988

Cartwright, J.E.; Holden, D.P.& Whitley, G.S. (1999). Hepatocyte growth factor regulates human trophoblast motility and invasion: a role for nitric oxide, *Br J Pharmacol*, Vol.128, No.1, pp. 181-189

Carty, D.M.; Delles, C.& Dominiczak, A.F. (2010) Preeclampsia and future maternal health, *J Hypertens*, Vol.28, No.7, pp. 1349-1355

Catalano, R.D.; Lannagan, T.R.; Gorowiec, M. et al. (2010) Prokineticins: novel mediators of inflammatory and contractile pathways at parturition?, *Mol Hum Reprod*, Vol.16, No.5, pp. 311-319

Charnock-Jones, D.S.; Kaufmann, P.& Mayhew, T.M. (2004). Aspects of human fetoplacental vasculogenesis and angiogenesis. I. Molecular regulation, *Placenta*, Vol.25, No.2-3, pp. 103-113

Cook, I.H.; Evans, J.; Maldonado-Perez, D. et al. Prokineticin-1 (PROK1) modulates interleukin (IL)-11 expression via prokineticin receptor 1 (PROKR1) and the calcineurin/NFAT signalling pathway, *Mol Hum Reprod*, Vol.16, No.3, pp. 158-169

Cross, J.C.; Werb, Z.& Fisher, S.J. (1994). Implantation and the placenta: key pieces of the development puzzle, *Science*, Vol.266, No.5190, pp. 1508-1518

Dekker, G.A. (1999). Risk factors for preeclampsia, *Clin Obstet Gynecol*, Vol.42, No.3, pp. 422-435

Dellian, M.; Witwer, B.P.; Salehi, H.A. et al. (1996). Quantitation and physiological characterization of angiogenic vessels in mice: effect of basic fibroblast growth factor, vascular endothelial growth factor/vascular permeability factor, and host microenvironment, *Am J Pathol*, Vol.149, No.1, pp. 59-71

Denison, F.C.; Battersby, S.; King, A.E. et al. (2008). Prokineticin-1: a novel mediator of the inflammatory response in third-trimester human placenta, *Endocrinology*, Vol.149, No.7, pp. 3470-3477

Dode, C.; Teixeira, L.; Levilliers, J. et al. (2006). Kallmann syndrome: mutations in the genes encoding prokineticin-2 and prokineticin receptor-2, *PLoS Genet*, Vol.2, No.10, pp. e175

Dorsch, M.; Qiu, Y.; Soler, D. et al. (2005). PK1/EG-VEGF induces monocyte differentiation and activation, *J Leukoc Biol*, Vol.78, No.2, pp. 426-434

Evans, J.; Catalano, R.D.; Brown, P. et al. (2009). Prokineticin 1 mediates fetal-maternal dialogue regulating endometrial leukemia inhibitory factor, *FASEB J*, Vol.23, No.7, pp. 2165-2175

Evans, J.; Catalano, R.D.; Morgan, K. et al. (2008). Prokineticin 1 signaling and gene regulation in early human pregnancy, *Endocrinology*, Vol.149, No.6, pp. 2877-2887

Fisher, S.J. (2004). The placental problem: linking abnormal cytotrophoblast differentiation to the maternal symptoms of preeclampsia, *Reprod Biol Endocrinol*, Vol.2, pp. 53

Fraser, H.M.; Bell, J.; Wilson, H. et al. (2005). Localization and quantification of cyclic changes in the expression of endocrine gland vascular endothelial growth factor in the human corpus luteum, *J Clin Endocrinol Metab*, Vol.90, No.1, pp. 427-434

Genbacev, O.; Jensen, K.D.; Powlin, S.S. et al. (1993). In vitro differentiation and ultrastructure of human extravillous trophoblast (EVT) cells, *Placenta*, Vol.14, No.4, pp. 463-475

Graham, C.H.; Hawley, T.S.; Hawley, R.G. et al. (1993). Establishment and characterization of first trimester human trophoblast cells with extended lifespan, *Exp Cell Res,* Vol.206, No.2, pp. 204-211

Graham, C.H.& Lala, P.K. (1991). Mechanism of control of trophoblast invasion in situ, *J Cell Physiol,* Vol.148, No.2, pp. 228-234

Grill, S.; Rusterholz, C.; Zanetti-Dallenbach, R. et al. (2009). Potential markers of preeclampsia--a review, *Reprod Biol Endocrinol,* Vol.7, pp. 70

Hoffmann, P.; Feige, J.J.& Alfaidy, N. (2007). Placental expression of EG-VEGF and its receptors PKR1 (prokineticin receptor-1) and PKR2 throughout mouse gestation, *Placenta,* Vol.28, No.10, pp. 1049-1058

Hoffmann, P.; Feige, J.J.& Alfaidy, N. (2006). Expression and oxygen regulation of endocrine gland-derived vascular endothelial growth factor/prokineticin-1 and its receptors in human placenta during early pregnancy, *Endocrinology,* Vol.147, No.4, pp. 1675-1684

Hoffmann, P.; Saoudi, Y.; Benharouga, M. et al. (2009). Role of EG-VEGF in human placentation: Physiological and pathological implications, *J Cell Mol Med,* Vol.13, No.8B, pp. 2224-2235

Hoogerwerf, W.A. (2006). Prokineticin 1 inhibits spontaneous giant contractions in the murine proximal colon through nitric oxide release, *Neurogastroenterol Motil,* Vol.18, No.6, pp. 455-463

Huppertz, B.& Peeters, L.L. (2005). Vascular biology in implantation and placentation, *Angiogenesis,* Vol.8, No.2, pp. 157-167

Ilekis, J.V.; Reddy, U.M.& Roberts, J.M. (2007). Preeclampsia--a pressing problem: an executive summary of a National Institute of Child Health and Human Development workshop, *Reprod Sci,* Vol.14, No.6, pp. 508-523

Irgens, L.M. (2007). Commentary: on the clinical prediction of pre-eclampsia and its enigmatic aetiology, *Int J Epidemiol,* Vol.36, No.2, pp. 420-421

Irving, J.A.& Lala, P.K. (1995). Functional role of cell surface integrins on human trophoblast cell migration: regulation by TGF-beta, IGF-II, and IGFBP-1, *Exp Cell Res,* Vol.217, No.2, pp. 419-427

Jauniaux, E.; Watson, A.L.; Hempstock, J. et al. (2000). Onset of maternal arterial blood flow and placental oxidative stress. A possible factor in human early pregnancy failure, *Am J Pathol,* Vol.157, No.6, pp. 2111-2122

King, A.; Burrows, T.& Loke, Y.W. (1996a). Human uterine natural killer cells, *Nat Immun,* Vol.15, No.1, pp. 41-52

King, A.; Jokhi, P.P.; Burrows, T.D. et al. (1996b). Functions of human decidual NK cells, *Am J Reprod Immunol,* Vol.35, No.3, pp. 258-260

Kingdom, J.; Huppertz, B.; Seaward, G. et al. (2000). Development of the placental villous tree and its consequences for fetal growth, *Eur J Obstet Gynecol Reprod Biol,* Vol.92, No.1, pp. 35-43

Kirkegaard, I.; Henriksen, T.B.& Uldbjerg, N. (2011). Early fetal growth, PAPP-A and free beta-hCG in relation to risk of delivering a small-for-gestational age infant, *Ultrasound Obstet Gynecol,* Vol.37, No.3, pp. 341-347

Kisliouk, T.; Levy, N.; Hurwitz, A. et al. (2003). Presence and regulation of endocrine gland vascular endothelial growth factor/prokineticin-1 and its receptors in ovarian cells, *J Clin Endocrinol Metab,* Vol.88, No.8, pp. 3700-3707

Krantz, D.; Goetzl, L.; Simpson, J.L. et al. (2004). Association of extreme first-trimester free human chorionic gonadotropin-beta, pregnancy-associated plasma protein A, and nuchal translucency with intrauterine growth restriction and other adverse pregnancy outcomes, *Am J Obstet Gynecol*, Vol.191, No.4, pp. 1452-1458

LeCouter, J.; Kowalski, J.; Foster, J. et al. (2001). Identification of an angiogenic mitogen selective for endocrine gland endothelium, *Nature*, Vol.412, No.6850, pp. 877-884

LeCouter, J.; Lin, R.; Tejada, M. et al. (2003). The endocrine-gland-derived VEGF homologue Bv8 promotes angiogenesis in the testis: Localization of Bv8 receptors to endothelial cells, *Proc Natl Acad Sci U S A*, Vol.100, No.5, pp. 2685-2690

Levine, R.J.; Maynard, S.E.; Qian, C. et al. (2004). Circulating angiogenic factors and the risk of preeclampsia, *N Engl J Med*, Vol.350, No.7, pp. 672-683

Li, H.; Gu, B.; Zhang, Y. et al. (2005). Hypoxia-induced increase in soluble Flt-1 production correlates with enhanced oxidative stress in trophoblast cells from the human placenta, *Placenta*, Vol.26, No.2-3, pp. 210-217

Li, M.; Bullock, C.M.; Knauer, D.J. et al. (2001). Identification of two prokineticin cDNAs: recombinant proteins potently contract gastrointestinal smooth muscle, *Mol Pharmacol*, Vol.59, No.4, pp. 692-698

Licht, P.; Fluhr, H.; Neuwinger, J. et al. (2007). Is human chorionic gonadotropin directly involved in the regulation of human implantation?, *Mol Cell Endocrinol*, Vol.269, No.1-2, pp. 85-92

Licht, P.; Russu, V.& Wildt, L. (2001). On the role of human chorionic gonadotropin (hCG) in the embryo-endometrial microenvironment: implications for differentiation and implantation, *Semin Reprod Med*, Vol.19, No.1, pp. 37-47

Lin, D.C.; Bullock, C.M.; Ehlert, F.J. et al. (2002). Identification and molecular characterization of two closely related G protein-coupled receptors activated by prokineticins/endocrine gland vascular endothelial growth factor, *J Biol Chem*, Vol.277, No.22, pp. 19276-19280

Lin, R.; LeCouter, J.; Kowalski, J. et al. (2002). Characterization of endocrine gland-derived vascular endothelial growth factor signaling in adrenal cortex capillary endothelial cells, *J Biol Chem*, Vol.277, No.10, pp. 8724-8729

Lysiak, J.J.; Han, V.K.& Lala, P.K. (1993). Localization of transforming growth factor alpha in the human placenta and decidua: role in trophoblast growth, *Biol Reprod*, Vol.49, No.5, pp. 885-894

Malassine, A.& Cronier, L. (2002). Hormones and human trophoblast differentiation: a review, *Endocrine*, Vol.19, No.1, pp. 3-11

Maldonado-Perez, D.; Evans, J.; Denison, F. et al. (2007). Potential roles of the prokineticins in reproduction, *Trends Endocrinol Metab*, Vol.18, No.2, pp. 66-72

Martin, C.; Balasubramanian, R.; Dwyer, A.A. et al. The role of the prokineticin 2 pathway in human reproduction: evidence from the study of human and murine gene mutations, *Endocr Rev*, Vol.32, No.2, pp. 225-246

Masuda, Y.; Takatsu, Y.; Terao, Y. et al. (2002). Isolation and identification of EG-VEGF/prokineticins as cognate ligands for two orphan G-protein-coupled receptors, *Biochem Biophys Res Commun*, Vol.293, No.1, pp. 396-402

McMaster, M.T.; Zhou, Y.& Fisher, S.J. (2004). Abnormal placentation and the syndrome of preeclampsia, *Semin Nephrol*, Vol.24, No.6, pp. 540-547

Murray, J.D. (2003). On the mechanochemical theory of biological pattern formation with application to vasculogenesis, *C R Biol*, Vol.326, No.2, pp. 239-252

Myatt, L.& Miodovnik, M. (1999). Prediction of preeclampsia, *Semin Perinatol*, Vol.23, No.1, pp. 45-57

Nagamatsu, T.; Fujii, T.; Kusumi, M. et al. (2004). Cytotrophoblasts up-regulate soluble fms-like tyrosine kinase-1 expression under reduced oxygen: an implication for the placental vascular development and the pathophysiology of preeclampsia, *Endocrinology,* Vol.145, No.11, pp. 4838-4845

Negri, L.; Lattanzi, R.; Giannini, E. et al. (2005). Biological activities of Bv8 analogues, *Br J Pharmacol,* Vol.146, No.5, pp. 625-632

Ngan, E.S.; Lee, K.Y.; Yeung, W.S. et al. (2006). Endocrine gland-derived vascular endothelial growth factor is expressed in human peri-implantation endometrium, but not in endometrial carcinoma, *Endocrinology,* Vol.147, No.1, pp. 88-95

Pasquali, D.; Rossi, V.; Staibano, S. et al. (2006). The endocrine-gland-derived vascular endothelial growth factor (EG-VEGF)/prokineticin 1 and 2 and receptor expression in human prostate: Up-regulation of EG-VEGF/prokineticin 1 with malignancy, *Endocrinology,* Vol.147, No.9, pp. 4245-4251

Rao, C.V.& Lei, Z.M. (2007). The past, present and future of nongonadal LH/hCG actions in reproductive biology and medicine, *Mol Cell Endocrinol,* Vol.269, No.1-2, pp. 2-8

Redman, C.W.& Sargent, I.L. (2005). Latest advances in understanding preeclampsia, *Science,* Vol.308, No.5728, pp. 1592-1594

Rodgers, G.M. (1988). Hemostatic properties of normal and perturbed vascular cells, *FASEB J,* Vol.2, No.2, pp. 116-123

Salker, M.; Teklenburg, G.; Molokhia, M. et al. Natural selection of human embryos: impaired decidualization of endometrium disables embryo-maternal interactions and causes recurrent pregnancy loss, *PLoS One,* Vol.5, No.4, pp. e10287

Schaffer, L.; Scheid, A.; Spielmann, P. et al. (2003). Oxygen-regulated expression of TGF-beta 3, a growth factor involved in trophoblast differentiation, *Placenta,* Vol.24, No.10, pp. 941-950

Shaw, J.L.; Denison, F.C.; Evans, J. et al. (2010) Evidence of prokineticin dysregulation in Fallopian tube from women with ectopic pregnancy, *Fertil Steril,*

Shi, Q.J.; Lei, Z.M.; Rao, C.V. et al. (1993). Novel role of human chorionic gonadotropin in differentiation of human cytotrophoblasts, *Endocrinology,* Vol.132, No.3, pp. 1387-1395

Sibai, B.; Dekker, G.& Kupferminc, M. (2005). Pre-eclampsia, *Lancet,* Vol.365, No.9461, pp. 785-799

Soga, T.; Matsumoto, S.; Oda, T. et al. (2002). Molecular cloning and characterization of prokineticin receptors, *Biochim Biophys Acta,* Vol.1579, No.2-3, pp. 173-179

Stewart, P.A.& Wiley, M.J. (1981). Developing nervous tissue induces formation of blood-brain barrier characteristics in invading endothelial cells: a study using quail--chick transplantation chimeras, *Dev Biol,* Vol.84, No.1, pp. 183-192

Strickland, S.& Richards, W.G. (1992). Invasion of the trophoblasts, *Cell,* Vol.71, No.3, pp. 355-357

Tiberi, F.; Tropea, A.; Apa, R. et al. (2010) Prokineticin 1 mRNA expression in the endometrium of healthy women and in the eutopic endometrium of women with endometriosis, *Fertil Steril,* Vol.93, No.7, pp. 2145-2149

Wells, M. (2007). The pathology of gestational trophoblastic disease: recent advances, *Pathology,* Vol.39, No.1, pp. 88-96

Winkler, M. (2003). Role of cytokines and other inflammatory mediators, *BJOG,* Vol.110 Suppl 20, pp. 118-123

Zygmunt, M.; Herr, F.; Keller-Schoenwetter, S. et al. (2002). Characterization of human chorionic gonadotropin as a novel angiogenic factor, *J Clin Endocrinol Metab,* Vol.87, No.11, pp. 5290-5296

14

The Morphology of Villous Capillary Bed in Normal and Diabetic Placenta

Marie Jirkovská
Charles University in Prague, First Faculty of Medicine, Czech Republic

1. Introduction

The functional competence of each organ depends markedly on characteristics of its capillary bed, i.e. volume, structure of the capillary wall, rate of the blood flow, spatial arrangement and relationship to the neighboring structural components of the organ (e.g. epithelium, muscle tissue). The knowledge of the structure, quantity, arrangement and features of microvascular bed of the organ is necessary for the complete understanding of its functions. It is obvious that those characteristics are markedly different among organs (e.g. kidney, liver, endocrine glands, brain, etc.).

In adult organism, the capillary bed of the majority of organs is stable. Active physiological angiogenesis is rare, nevertheless it takes place in some organs of fertile women, and manifests itself either by repeated formation of capillaries in corpus luteum and endometrium or by enlargement of placental capillary bed during pregnancy.

Optimal function of capillaries depends on the appropriate structure of the capillary wall. The microvascular bed, on the other hand, is involved in systemic diseases like hypertension and diabetes mellitus, and its disturbances and damages caused by pathological processes manifest themselves by clinical symptoms.

Maternal diabetes mellitus represents a serious illness threatening both the mother and fetus by serious complications. Metabolic disorders associated with maternal diabetes, however, influence not only the growth and development of fetus, but may have also long-term effects. Its incidence grows with the age of pregnant women. In developed countries, the age of parity of the women shifted to or rather behind their thirtieth year, and therefore the research of maternal diabetes is nowadays particularly topical.

Placenta, which is interposed between mother and fetus, mediates and modifies the influence of maternal diabetes on fetus. It is obvious that placental structure reflects the changed maternal milieu. Placental capillaries play a key role in the transfer of oxygen, nutrients and metabolites between mother and fetus, and any change of their function may have negative effect on fetal well-being. This chapter summarizes the knowledge regarding structural aspects of placental capillary bed in normal human placentas and in placentas from pregnancies complicated by maternal diabetes.

2. Placental capillary bed

Placenta is an organ ensuring and regulating the development of individual *in utero*. Unlike other organs it exists during a short time, holds, either transitorily or continually, the function of developing fetal organs, and is quite unique because of the continual growth and development of its morphology and functional capacity during the whole time of its existence. It fulfils numerous functions, e.g. the bidirectional transport between mother and fetus, secretion of many hormones and other regulating molecules, and so forth. In all those functions its circulatory system, and in particular its capillaries, play very important role.

2.1 Development of the placental vascular bed

In human hemochorial placenta, the fetal blood running through umbilical arteries enters the arteries of the chorionic plate and continues through the vessels of ramified tree-like villi outgrowing from the chorionic plate and (except anchoring villi) floating in maternal blood in the intervillous space. With advanced branching, the villous diameter as well as the diameter of villous vessels gradually decreases, and the thickness and structure of the vascular wall change as well.

Placental villi originate from trophoblast (consisting of external syncytiotrophoblast and internal cytotrophoblast) and extra-embryonic mesenchyme. In connection with the formation of embryonic circulatory system, the vessels start to differentiate within the villous mesenchyma in the 3rd week. Those villi called tertiary or mesenchymal villi repeatedly branch out, and are forerunners of other villous types. From the 6th week to the end of 2nd trimester, a part of mesenchymal villi differentiates into immature intermediate villi. During the first and second trimester, further growth and branching of those villi give rise to the furcated stem villi. Numerous mesenchymal villi appear at the tips of stem villi at the beginning of the third trimester. They are precursor villi of mature intermediate villi, which branch subsequently into terminal villi. At the end of pregnancy, terminal villi represent more than one half (55%) of the total number of villi (Castellucci et al. 1990; Benirschke & Kaufmann, 1995; Kingdom et al., 2000; Challier et al., 2001).

The development of placental villous vessels takes place during the whole pregnancy and comprises two periods, vasculogenesis and angiogenesis. Vasculogenesis takes place in the first and second trimester. During this period, the cords of vascular cells differentiate from mesenchymal cells of the villous core and form vascular lumina by dehiscence. Mesenchymal cells are the source of cells for elongation and widening of vessels and give rise also to perivascular cells - pericytes. In stem villi, the vessels become arteries and veins, and smooth muscle cells, myofibroblasts and fibroblasts of their wall are recruited from the villous stroma as well. Angiogenesis, on the other hand, prevails during the third trimester. In this process, new capillaries form by sprouting of already existing villous vessels, and emerging mature intermediate and terminal villi are vascularized this way (Demir et al., 1989). In the normal term placenta, the estimated total length and surface area of villous capillaries are 550 km and 15 m^2 respectively (Burton & Jauniaux, 1995). They contain approximately 25% of fetoplacental blood volume (Luckhardt et al. 1996).

2.2 Structure of the capillary wall in normal and diabetic placentas

The placenta is interposed between mother and fetus. As described above, both the chorionic plate and chorionic villi are derivatives of embryonic structures, and fetal blood circulates in their vessels. Therefore the placenta and through it the fetus are in contact with all changes, anomalies and irregularities of maternal organism, and the reaction of the fetus on changed conditions of its environment demonstrates itself in placental structure.

Diabetes mellitus represents a serious complication of pregnancy. Maternal diabetes mellitus threatens the pregnant mothers by development of serious complications based on diabetic microangiopathy, e.g. retinopathy, nephropathy, neuropathy, and enhances the risk of congenital defects, macrosomia and perinatal morbidity and mortality of infants. Various forms of diabetes complicate 3-5% of pregnancies. Type 1 diabetes (pregestational onset, insulin-dependent) represents about 10% of the total, the remainder is in the main gestational diabetes, for other forms, e.g. type 2, are rare (Hájek et al., 2004).

2.2.1 Light microscopy

Maternal diabetes mellitus changes structural features of the placenta. As shown using quantitative method, the consistent organization of villi inside the cotyledon, i.e. occurrence of shorter villi in the centre and longer villi in periphery, is disrupted, and villi (and villous vessels, as deduced by authors) are more branched in diabetic placentas (Bjork & Persson, 1984). The analysis performed by scanning electron microscopy revealed hypo- and hyper-ramified villi in diabetic placentas as compared with normal ones (Honda et al., 1992).

The placental capillary bed is located predominantly in terminal villi, which diameter is 30 - 80 μm in the normal placenta. They are covered by trophoblast consisting of a continual layer of syncytiotrophoblast and sparse cytotrophoblastic cells underneath. Trophoblast is separated by trophoblastic basal lamina from the villous core. It consists of the small amount of loose connective tissue and villous capillaries. Capillaries, lying mostly under trophoblast, display very variable diameter, the majority of them is sinusoidally dilated. Trophoblast covering capillaries is often reduced to a thin nuclei-free cytoplasmic layer of syncytiotrophoblast, which form with the capillary wall a vasculosyncytial membrane. The mean thickness of the barrier between maternal and fetal blood is about 4 μm in normal term placenta, (Mayhew et al, 1984; Burton et al, 1987), nevertheless markedly thinner vasculosyncytial membranes are considered as the sites of preferential transport (fig. 1).

Conventional light microscopic examination does not show striking and typical morphological differences between normal and diabetic placentas, nevertheless certain pathological changes are observable especially in terminal villi. Although a little amount of pathological forms of terminal villi may be found also in placentas from uncomplicated pregnancies, a variable proportion of pathologicaly changed villi appears in each diabetic placenta despite the type of diabetes (Fox & Sebire, 2008). One of structural changes concerns the villous size. It looks more variable at first glance, and as shown by measurement, the mean diameter of villi is greater in diabetic placenta (Emmrich & Müller, 1974). Based on the appearance of villi looking similar to villi from earlier stages of gestation, and on decreased formation of terminal villi, a delayed villous maturation is commonly diagnosed in diabetic placenta. A lot of signs, i.e. more frequent syncytial knots, more prominent cytotrophoblastic cells, more numerous mesenchymal cells in the stroma of some villi, villi displaying stromal oedema or stromal fibrosis, and changed amount, diameter and distribution of villous capillaries may occur and are reported as (of course nonspecific) attributes of placental structure in maternal diabetes (Semmler et al., 1982; Semmler &

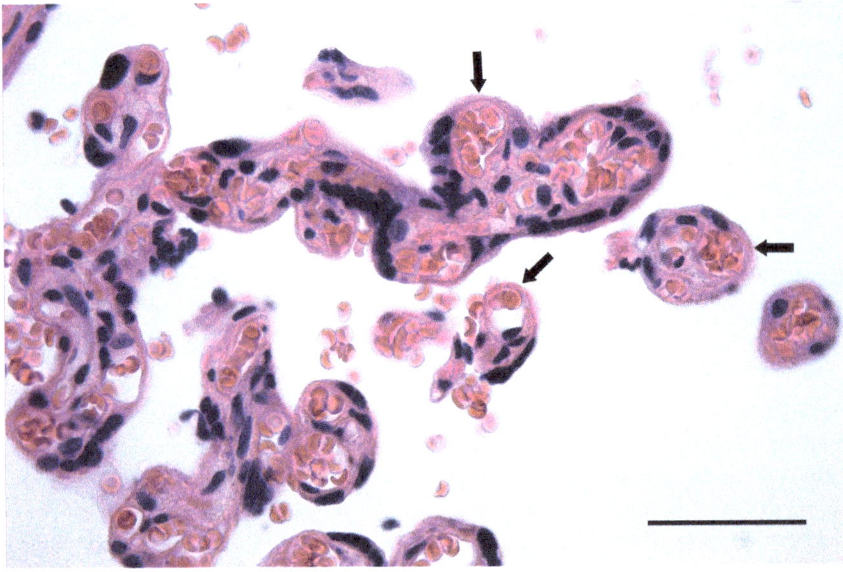

Fig. 1. The picture shows terminal villi of normal human term placenta. Sinusoidally dilated capillaries are in a very tight relationship with trophoblast, arrows indicate vasculosyncytial membranes. Bar = 100 μm.

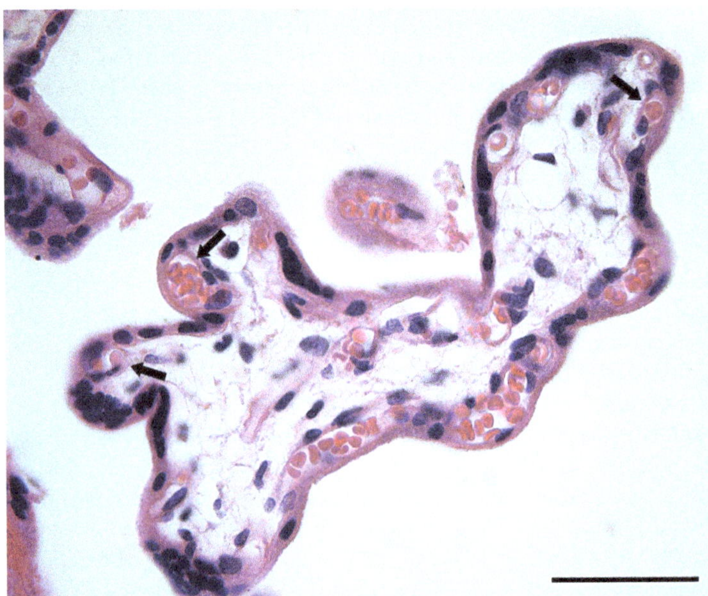

Fig. 2. Hypovascular terminal villi of diabetic term placenta. In the villi of greater diameter and more voluminous stroma (compare with fig. 1), thin capillaries run closely to the trophoblast, in several places as if embedded into it (arrows). Bar = 100 μm.

Emmrich, 1989; Madazli et al., 2008; Higgins et al., 2011). As demonstrated on the production of some placental proteins (e.g. placental alkaline phosphatase, placental lactogen), structural immaturity is associated with concomitant functional immaturity (Greco et al. 1989).

There are two forms of pathological villi differing from normal placental villi in the amount, diameter and distribution of villous capillaries. One form is characterized by sparse capillaries of small diameter located preferentially in a very tight relation to trophoblast, so that large proportion of capillary wall is surrounded by thin nuclei-free layer of syncytiotrophoblast. Voluminous stroma consists of markedly loose meshwork of connective tissue (fig. 2).

In the other type, the capillary profiles are conspicuously numerous, their lumina look often extremely wide, and only small amount of loose stroma is discernible (fig. 3). The thickness of villous trophoblast is markedly reduced, and a thin nuclei-free layer of syncytiotrophoblast covers the majority of capillaries. These hypervascularized villi occur focally in the placenta, and if their frequency meets the Altshuler´s rule (the presence of more than 10 vascular profiles in more than 10 villi in more than 10 areas of 3 non-infarcted placental areas), this finding is called placental chorangiosis. It is associated with increased risk of adverse perinatal outcomes (Altshuler, 1984).

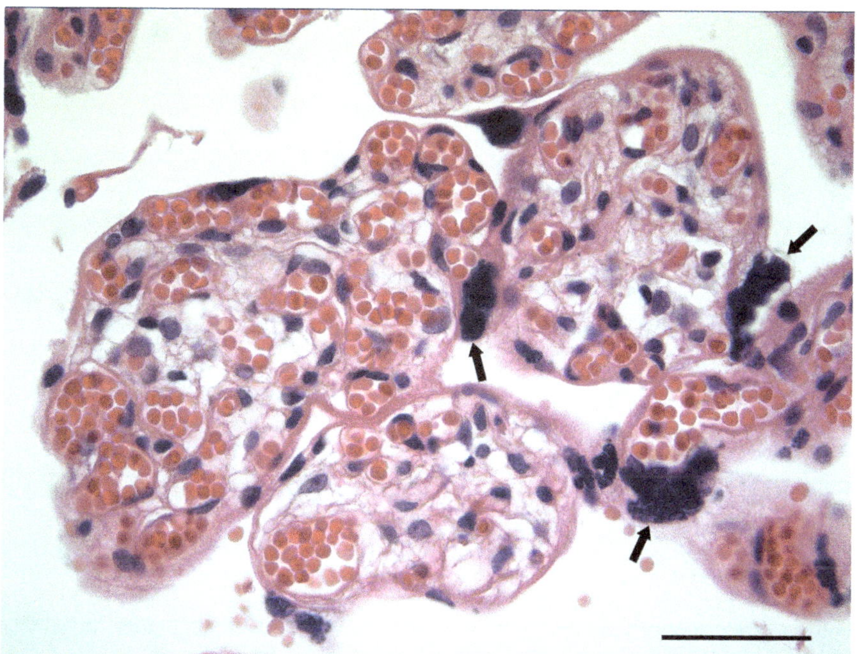

Fig. 3. Hypervascular terminal villi of diabetic term placenta. In the villi of large diameter (compare with fig. 1), very numerous capillary profiles of variable diameter occur in a small amount of stromal connective tissue. Thin trophoblastic layer is nearly completely free of nuclei, which are concentrated in prominent groups (arrows). Bar = 100 μm.

2.2.2 Utrastructure of the placental capillary wall

The structure of the wall of placental capillaries is consistent with its function, i.e. regulator of the bidirectional transport between mother and fetus and component of placental barrier. The capillary wall consists of endothelial cells and pericytes. The endothelium is of the continuous type. Individual endothelial cells are connected each to other with tight and adherent junctions ensuring cell-to-cell adhesion and regulating capillary permeability (Leach & Firth, 1992; Eaton et al., 1993). The abluminal surface is covered by basal lamina, which is divided into two layers where the cell bodies and projections of pericytes are interposed. In that part of capillary wall adjacent to the trophoblast, the pericyte projections are usually missing, and basal laminas of trophoblast and endothelium may fuse. In many instances only thin nuclei-free layer of syncytiotrophoblast covers the capillary, and those segments correspond to vasculosyncytial membranes (fig. 4).

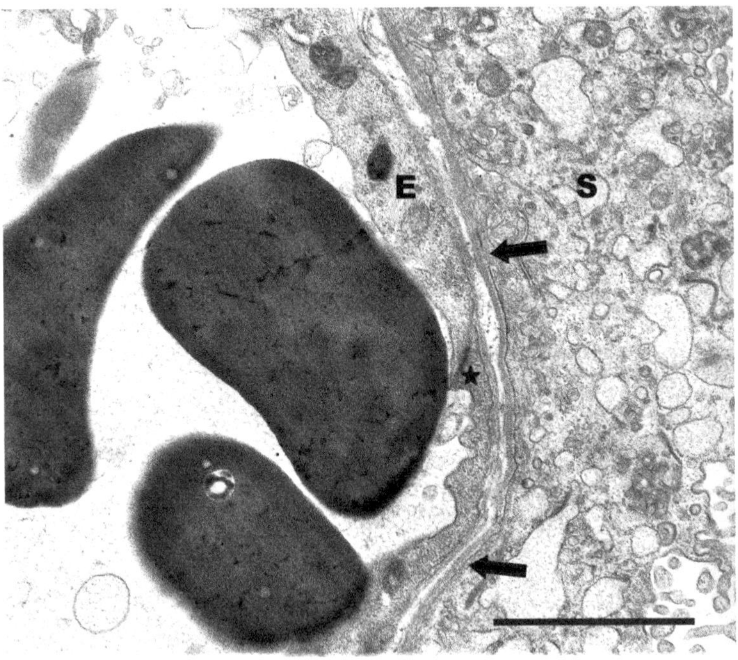

Fig. 4. A part of the capillary wall lying in a tight relationship to the syncytiotrophoblast at the site of vasculosyncytial membrane. No projections of pericytes are interposed between endothelium (E) and syncytiotrophoblast (S), which basal laminas tend here and there to fuse (arrows). Asterisk = adherent junction between endothelial cells. Bar = 2 μm.

Pinocytotic and other vesicles and large amount of fine filaments dominate the submicroscopic picture of typical thin endothelium. In some instances, the endothelial cells are prominent or bulging into the lumen, so that some capillaries may have a slit-like lumen only. The peripherally arranged heterochromatin and nucleoli in nuclei together with organelles (granular endoplasmic reticulum, Golgi aparatus) occurring in cytoplasma indicate an active cellular stage probably associated with current angiogenesis (fig. 5).

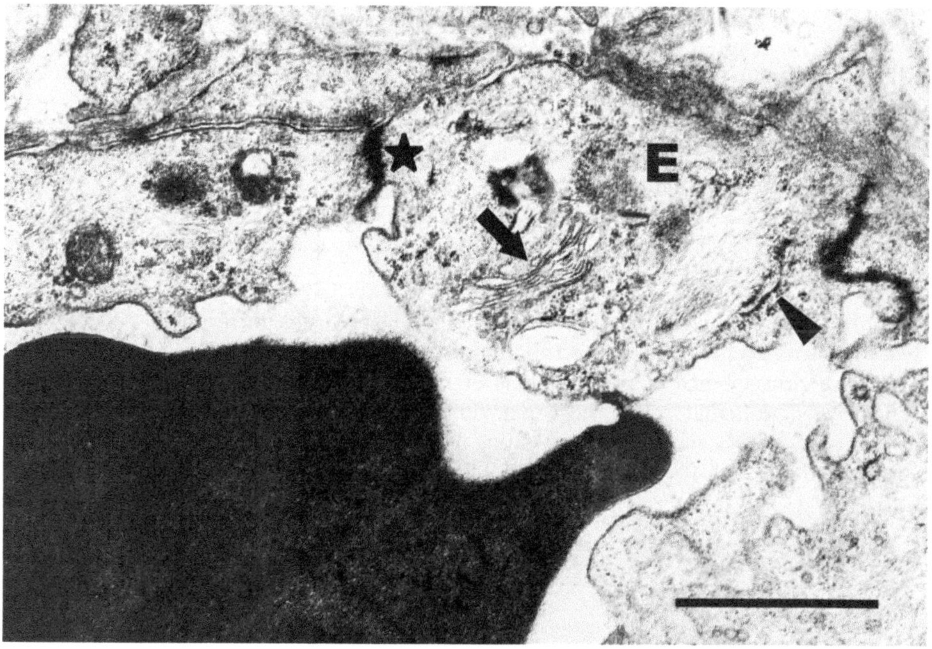

Fig. 5. Golgi apparatus (arrow) and granular endoplasmic reticulum (arrowhead) appearing in capillary endothelium (E) of term placenta. Asterisk = adherent junction between endothelial cells. Bar = 1 μm.

The phenotype of placental microvascular endothelium is characterized by expression of numerous molecules, e.g. von Willebrand factor, endothelial and inducible nitric oxide synthases, caveolin 1, CD 31, CD 34, ICAM 1, PECAM 1 (Dye et al., 2001), and differs from the endothelium of placental macrovessels (Lang et al., 2003). As reported in a current paper, the expression of some of them, in particular the nitric oxide synthase, is modified by maternal diabetes (Sobrevia et al., 2011).

Only little attention was paid to placental capillary pericytes up to the present, even in otherwise exhaustive papers dealing with the villous ultrastructure (e.g. Haust, 1981). According to some authors, pericytes do not display different structure in normal and diabetic placentas (Kacemi et al., 1999), although certain differences of the shape of their cytoplasmic projections were described in pathological placentas including those from pregnancies complicated by maternal diabetes (Jones & Desoye, 2010). Vimentin and smooth muscle actin, but no desmin were demonstrated in the cytoplasm of pericytes in normal as well as diabetic placentas (Kučera et al., 2010).

Being a component of placental capillaries, pericytes have a potential to react on changes of placental environment in maternal organism, e.g. hypoxia. To date, this topic was studied in two papers comparing the pericyte coverage between placentas from lowland and high altitudes, and between normal and diabetic placentas. Placental capillaries from high altitudes were found less covered by pericytes than those from lowland (Zhang et al. 2002). It is evident, that such decrease of thickness of the barrier separating maternal and fetal blood is an appropriate adaptation on low oxygen pressure. On the other hand, no difference was found in perivascular cell coverage between normal placentas and placentas in type 1 diabetes as well as between placentas of diabetic mother with normal and pathological levels of glycated hemoglobin (Kučera et al., 2010).

Although the basic structure of villous capillaries is similar, the comparison of capillaries of normal and diabetic placentas has shown further certain differences. For instance, glycogen granules are commonly found in capillary endothelium of normal placentas. In the villi of diabetic placentas, a higher content of glycogen deposits was described in endothelial cells and pericytes (and also stromal cells) of diabetic villi (Haust, 1981; Asmussen, 1982; Jones & Desoye, 1993).

A more frequent incidence of extravascular red blood cells in terminal villi of diabetic placentas was documented by electron microscopy (Okudaira et al., 1966; see also fig. 6). It may be a consequence of perturbations of molecules forming adherent junctions at the contact of endothelial cells. Those junctions were found less stable in placentas from pregnancies complicated by both gestational and type 1 diabetes mellitus (Babawale et al. 2000; Leach et al., 2004).

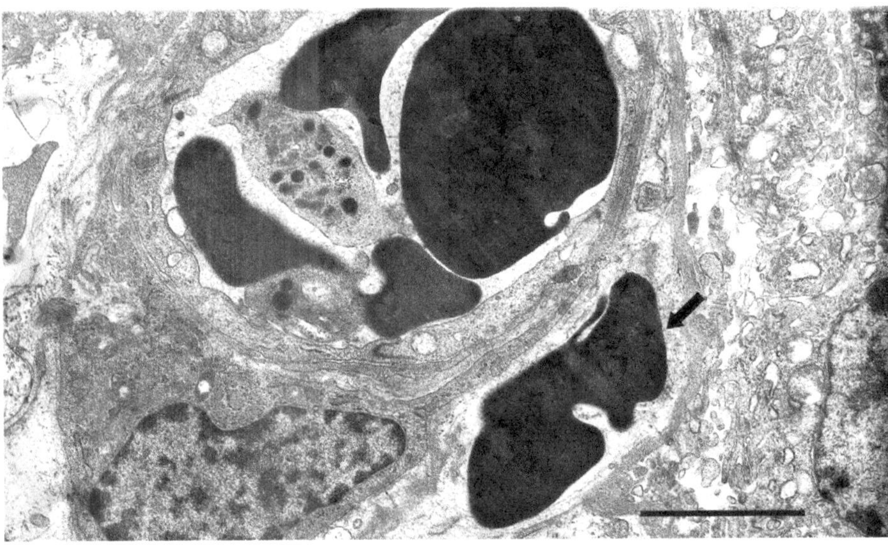

Fig. 6. Extravascular erythrocytes (arrow) are regularly found in diabetic term placenta. Bar = 2 μm.

2.2.3 Capillary basal lamina

The capillary basal lamina may be a compact layer surrounding the capillary (fig. 4), or appears in several loosely arranged stripes of basal lamina material in the neighborhood of capillaries. The latter may be found in normal placentas too, but is described as more frequent in diabetic villi (Okudaira et al., 1966; Jones & Fox, 1976; Asmussen, 1982; see also fig. 7). It is not quite easy to explain the origin of such arrangement, but taking into account that placental capillaries are dynamic structures, we assume that angiogenesis and apoptosis regulate their amount and volume.

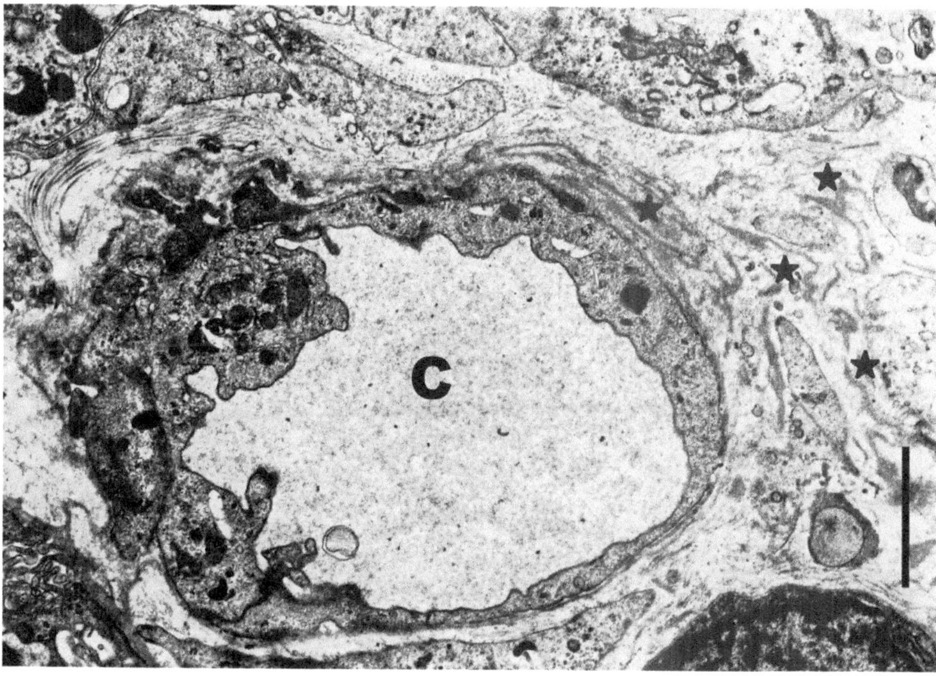

Fig. 7. Loosely arranged strips of the material of basal lamina (asterisks) occur in the neighborhood of diabetic placental capillary (C). Bar = 2 μm.

As documents the occurrence of apoptotic marker caspase 3, apoptosis takes place in placental capillary bed and manifests itself either in individual endothelial cells and pericytes or in larger patches of capillary wall (fig. 8). Stripes of basal lamina material may be probably the only residuals of previous segments of capillary wall. The only quantitative study comparing apoptosis in villous capillaries has shown that the apoptotic activity in the capillary bed of diabetic placentas seems to be higher, but the difference between normal and diabetic placentas as well as between placentas of diabetic mothers with normal and increased levels of glycated hemoglobin was not found statistically significant (Kučera et al., 2011).

Diabetes mellitus has been linked to accelerated microangiopathy, and thickenning of the capillary basal lamina has been considered as its manifestation. In descriptive studies based on qualitative electron microscopic analysis, discrepant opinions were reported regarding the thickness of the capillary basal lamina in diabetic placenta. However, only the measurements have shown that the mean thickness of capillary basal lamina is significantly lower in placentas of mothers suffering from type 1 diabetes mellitus (Emmrich et al., 1976; Jirkovská, 1991). In order to explain this phenomenon we have to take into account that placental capillaries belong to the fetoplacental circulation. Fetal pancreas produces sufficient amount of insulin, and thus fetus is not a diabetic. Therefore, no reason exists for development of diabetic microangiopathy in fetoplacental microvessels. The lower mean thickness of capillary basal lamina, on the other hand, may be a consequence of higher proportion of newly formed capillaries. Enhanced angiogenesis has been repeatedly documented in the villi of diabetic placentas in studies applying quantitative morphological methods (see further).

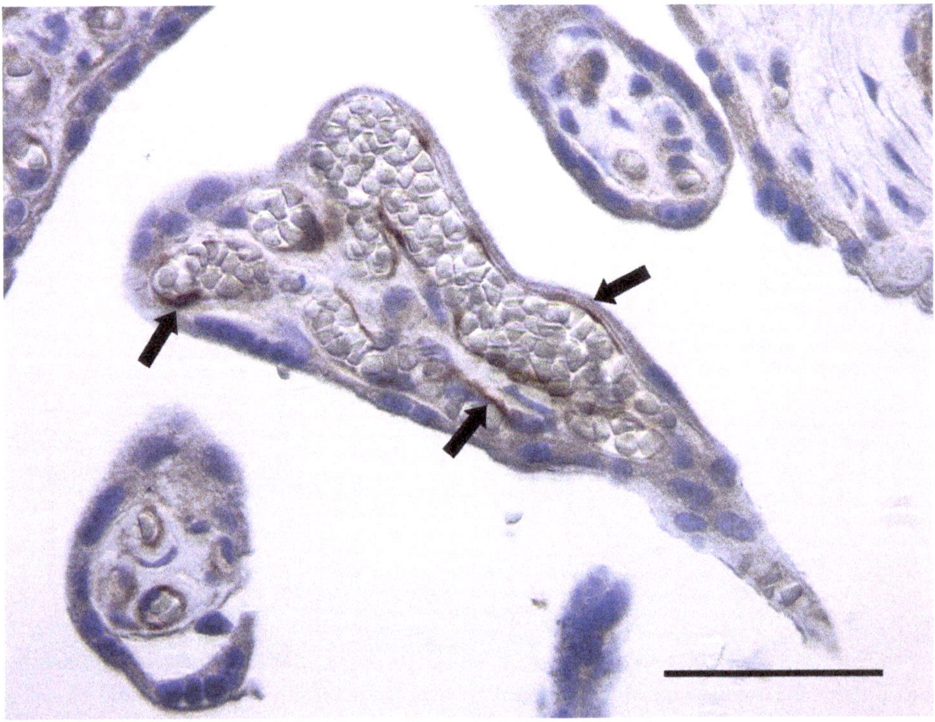

Fig. 8. Apoptosis in the villous capillary wall in diabetic placenta demonstrated by the occurrence of caspase 3 (arrows indicate brown reaction product). Bar = 100 μm.

2.3 Quantitative comparison of structural differences between normal and diabetic placentas

The quantitative approach to the explanation of the connections of placental morphology and function surely deserves our attention too. The effort to quantify histological structure of placenta and to compare normal organs and organs associated with pathologies of pregnancy brought a lot of useful information and enhanced our understanding of placental function. On the other hand, due to the progress in the treatment of maternal diabetes and the evolution of methodology used for such studies in the past four decades, results of those studies are often hardly comparable because of heterogeneous severity of diabetes, different standards of treatment of pregnant diabetic women, metabolic control achieved during pregnancy in examined diabetic mothers, different strategies of tissue sampling and processing, and different designs and methods of evaluation.

A simple microscopic evaluation performed mostly by a pathologist blinded to clinical data belongs to the traditional approaches. Two studies applying this method considered the decreased proportion of the vascular component in diabetic placental villi as indicative for more severe placental maturation disorders, and the occurrence of signs of placental maturation disorders as dependent on the quality of metabolic control (Semmler et al., 1982; Semmler & Emmrich, 1989). Results of the study, published in a more recent paper, were obtained using similar method. The authors concluded that villous immaturity and chorangiosis are increased in placentas in type 1 diabetes associated with both the large-for-gestational- age and appropriate-for-gestational-age infants (Evers et al. 2003).

Another approach, how to quantify the structure, is morphometry and stereology. Here are applied objective methods of measurement in order to either assess different parameters, e.g. villous calibre, trophoblast thickness, number and size of fetal vessels, or to estimate total numbers, volumes, surface areas, etc. A lot of articles dealing with quantification of placental structure are available in the literature, and many of them pay the attention to the comparison of parameters between normal and various types of diabetic placenta.

In addition to the already mentioned papers, further results of quantitative studies of diabetic placenta are presented as follows.

The total placental surface area, a key parameter of placental transport capacity, was estimated as greater in diabetic placentas (17.3 m^2) then in controls (11.4 m^2) as well as the proportion of parenchymal components (including capillaries) was found higher in diabetic placentas (Boyd et al. 1986).

In their studies, Geppert et al. (1982) and Jirkovská et al. (1994) have found significantly lower vascularization of the placental villi (defined as the area of capillary cross-sections within the villus divided by the area of the villous cross-section) in examined diabetic placentas. On the contrary, Teasdale found greater total capillary surface areas and more numerous capillary profiles per unit area in placentas of pregnant mothers suffering from both the gestational and type 1 diabetes (Teasdale, 1981; Teasdale, 1983; Teasdale, 1985).

Various placental parameters were compared, and quantitative structural changes of diabetic placentas were reported in other studies. The attention was paid of course to placental vascular bed, especially to villous capillaries. The greater total volume, length, surface area and mean diameter of capillaries have been reported in placentas in type 1 diabetes as well as in gestational diabetes, and those parameters were found also dependent on the sex of newborn, i.e. greater in placentas of male fetuses (Mayhew et al., 1993; Mayhew et al., 1994). Those findings were corroborated in later study (Mayhew, 2002). On the contrary, some authors (Jauniaux & Burton, 2006; Nelson et al., 2009) have found no differences of total capillary volumes and capillary surface areas between control and diabetic placentas. To date newest article reports greater placental capillary volumes, lengths and surface areas in type 1 and type 2 of maternal diabetes (Higgins et al. 2011).

Based on these, although rather ambiguous data, we may conclude after all that the angiogenesis is more active in diabetic placenta.

2.4 The spatial organization of villous capilary bed

2.4.1 The three-dimensional arrangement

In the placenta, the capillary bed play a key role in maternofetal transport, and thus acts as a decisive factor in the appropriate intrauterine development of fetus. Fetal blood runs in fetoplacental capillaries, but unlike other organs, the oxygen is not extracted there from erythrocytes. To the contrary, it diffuses through trophoblast and capillary wall, and binds fetal hemoglobin. It is obvious that the amount of oxygen available for oxygenation of fetal hemoglobin depends on many factors, the oxygen concentration in maternal blood, the total surface areas of trophoblast and capillary wall, and the thickness of placental barrier being the main. The proper blood flow in placental microvessels and macrovessels then ensures that the fetus obtains adequate amount of oxygen and nutrients. As the blood flow follows other physical principles in macrovessels than in microvessels, the correct understanding of features and function of placental microvascular bed, in particular capillaries, requires knowledge on its dimensions and spatial arrangement.

Some papers dealing with spatial organization of placental villous microvessels have been published in last five decades, but their paucity gives evidence that such study is quite a task. Moreover, their results are hardly comparable because of placental material of different stages of gravidity taken into study and various technical tools used.

Two of authors dealing with this subject applied injections of dye solutions into placental vessels and documented their distribution by photomicrographs (Crawford, 1956; Boe, 1969). Based on their findings, they created quite different schemes of villous capillary bed. According to Crawford´s conclusion, the long non-branched capillary runs garland-like through series of terminal villi and forms hairpin-like loops inside them (fig.9). The author does not describe sinusoidal dilations of capillaries.

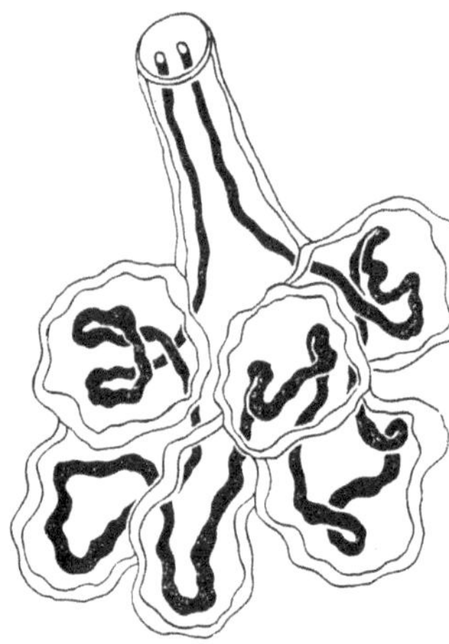

Fig. 9. The arrangement of villous capillaries according to Crawford (from Crawford, J.M. (1956). The foetal placental circulation. IV. The anatomy of the villus and its capillary structure. *J Obstet Gynaecol Br Emp, Vol.* 63, No. 4, pp. 548-552, John Wiley and Sons Ltd., with permission).

To the contrary, Boe demonstrated capillaries in densely arranged terminal branches of chorionic villi in the placenta at the end of first trimester. Their dense webby villous capillary networks connect dense, richly branched paravascular capillaries of so called immature intermediate villus. Segments of paravascular capillaries running at the base of terminal branches act as arterial-venous shunts. In accordance with other authors (Crawford, 1956; Arts, 1961), Boe considered the terminal villus as independent circulatory unit (fig. 10).

Unlike Boe´s scheme, the Arts´s (Arts, 1961) model of vessels in mature intermediate and terminal villi, based on the analysis of corrosive casts, is poor in paravascular capillary

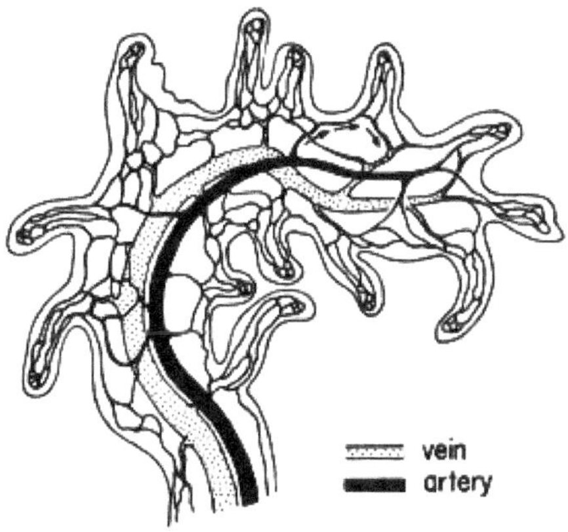

Fig. 10. The Boe´s model of the arrangement of placental microvascular bed (from Boe, F. (1969) Studies on the human placenta. III. Vascularization of the young foetal placenta. A. Vascularization of the chorionic villus. *Acta Obstet Gynecol Scand,* Vol. 48, No. 2, pp. 159-166, John Wiley and Sons Ltd., with permission).

network. Capillaries of terminal villi arise directly from arteries. Their segments are arranged parallel to the axis of villus and interconnected with short connections. The blood leaving terminal villi runs directly into veins. The sinusoidally dilated capillary segments are interpreted as sections of lower blood pressure and slow blood flow, which are favourable for materno-fetal transport (fig. 11).

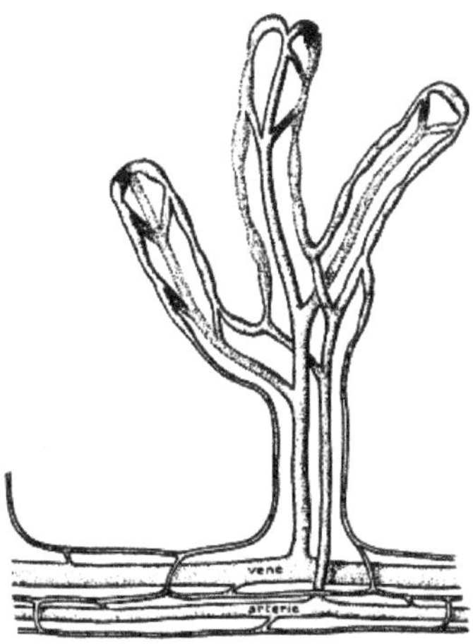

Fig. 11. A schematic representation of the vascular bed of mature intermediate and terminal villi according to Arts (from Arts, N.F.T. (1961) Investigations on the vascular system of the placenta. I. General introduction and the fetal vascular system. *Am J Obst Gynec,* Vol. 82, No. 1, pp. 147-158, Elsevier, with permission).

The analysis of corrosive preparations by scanning electron microscope showed the arrangement of villous capillaries more precisely, however due to the method, the relationships of capillaries and other tissues forming the villus were not preserved (Leiser et al., 1985; Kaufmann et al., 1985; Akiba et al., 1987; Burton, 1987).

Another model of placental microvascular bed was based on scanning electron microscopy of corrosive casts combined with physical 3D reconstruction from photomicrographs of serially cut histological sections of placental villi (Leiser et al., 1985; Kaufmann et al., 1985). This model represents a mature intermediate villus and its branches - terminal villi, and their vessels. The capillaries of terminal villi are predominantly represented by sinusoidally dilated U-like capillary loops, which branches are only seldom interconnected with a short capillary segment. No arterial-venous shunts were shown, but signs of current angiogenesis in human term placenta, i.e. blind capillary sprouts, were described in this study for the first time. The wavy course of long and rarely branched capillaries running through serially arranged terminal villi suggests to a certain degree the Crawford´s scheme.

As documented above, the successful representation of three-dimensional structure depends on the methods available. Nevertheless, regardless the technical progress, the making of 3D reconstruction of any biological object is very laborious and time consuming in any case. Usually it consists of serial sectioning of the object, appropriate staining of sections, acquisition of images by a microscope, alignment of images, generation and conversions of initial data, and application of relevant 3D rendering software. Many of those steps may create artifacts. The application of confocal microscopy eliminates problems with the alignment of serial physical sections, as it enables to acquire series of perfectly aligned optical sections inside thick physical section (fig. 12). Due to its advantages, the confocal laser scanning microscope has been used repeatedly for acquisition of initial data for 3D reconstruction of organ microvessels, e.g. for analysis of microvascular bed of human liver (Oikawa et al., 1999), for developmental study of vascular bed during the morphogenesis of intestinal villi (Hashimoto et al. 1999) or for studies on spatial organization of chick mesonephros (Jirkovská et al., 2001; Jirkovská et al., 2005).

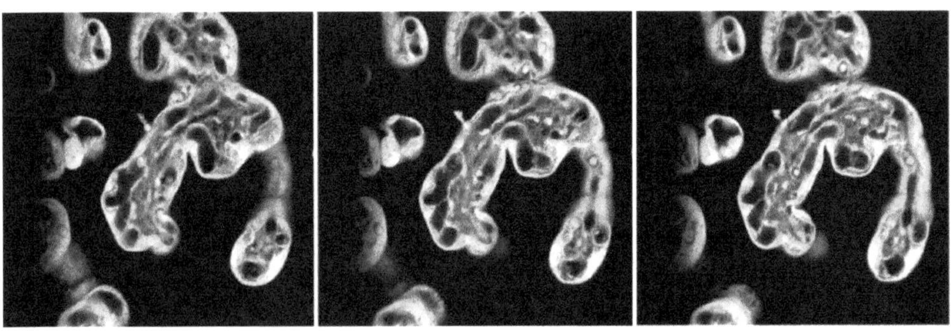

Fig. 12. Three perfectly aligned serial confocal optical sections of placental villi were taken 2 μm apart. Note very well discernible villous structure after fixation in a fixative with added eosin.

Confocal microscopy was also a key method used in our studies of villous capillary bed in normal and diabetic placenta. Its application together with the appropriate software enabled to create 3D reconstructions of sufficient amount of villi, and thus to visualize various arrangements of villous capillaries.

As shown in pictures of three-dimensionally reconstructed villous capillaries, their size, shape and arrangement displays great variability. Two simplest types represent a U-like loop and a Y-like bifurcation. Capillary segments of those beds are usually slightly wavy, and their course is more or less parallel with the axis of villus. In more complicated beds, the longitudinally oriented segments are interconnected with short connections. For the purpose of topological description, they are called "redundant", as they can be removed without disconnecting the villous capillary bed. It is evident that they are by no means redundant from the functional point of view (fig. 13).

Individual terminal villi, arising from the mature intermediate villi, are usually of cylindrical shape, and their capillaries arise from the vascular bed of mature intermediate villi. Terminal villi may also form cluster-like structures, and their capillaries are interconnected so that they form complicated capillary networks (fig. 14).

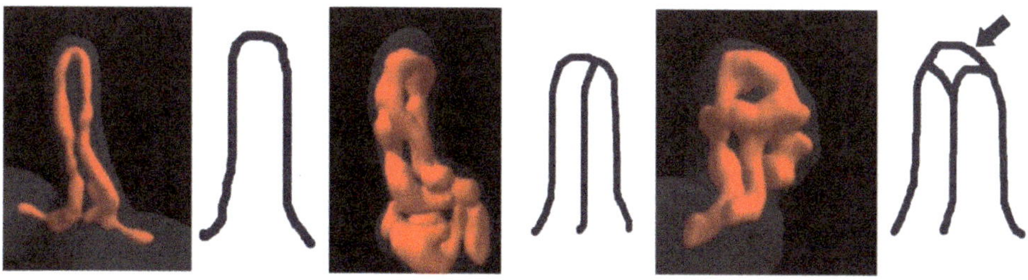

Fig. 13. Three-dimensional reconstructions and topological schemes of the U-like and Y-like villous capillaries, and of a capillary bed containing one redundant connection (arrow).

Terminal villi of more complicated shape originate from the pre-existing villus by a trophoblast protrusion driven by angiogenesis Their capillary bed originates from the capillary bed of pre-existing villus and is complex (fig. 15).

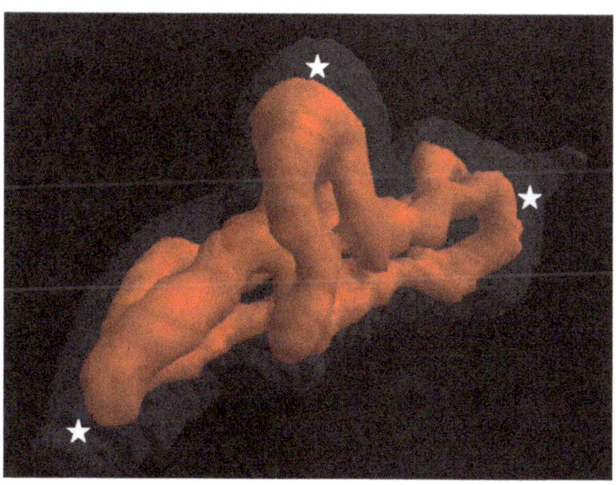

Fig. 14. An example of three villi (asterisks) in a cluster, and their interconnected capillaries.

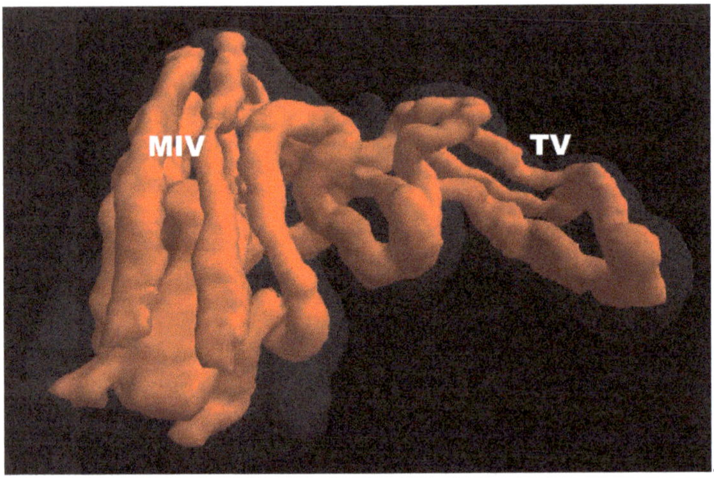

Fig. 15. A branched terminal villus (TV), which complex capillary bed is supplied from vessels of the mature intermediate villus (MIV).

The used methods of confocal microscopy and 3D reconstruction enabled us also to demonstrate that placental villous capillaries grow by elongation as well as by sprouting of pre-existing capillaries until term (Jirkovská et al, 1998; Jirkovská et al., 2002, Karen et al, 2003; Jirkovská et al., 2008). This finding challenged the hypothesis, expressed by some authors, that placental angiogenesis shifts from the sprouting to the elongating angiogenesis after the 25th week of gestation (Kaufmann et al., 1985; Mayhew, 2002 a; Mayhew, 2002 b).

In diabetic placentas, the spatial organization of villous capillaries was found mostly similar to the normal placenta, but there were some differences concerning shapes of villi. As shows the example in fig. 16, the mature terminal villi of normal placentas are long and slender. Their capillaries have straight or slightly waved course and are usually branched. They are arranged tightly and parallel to the villous axis.

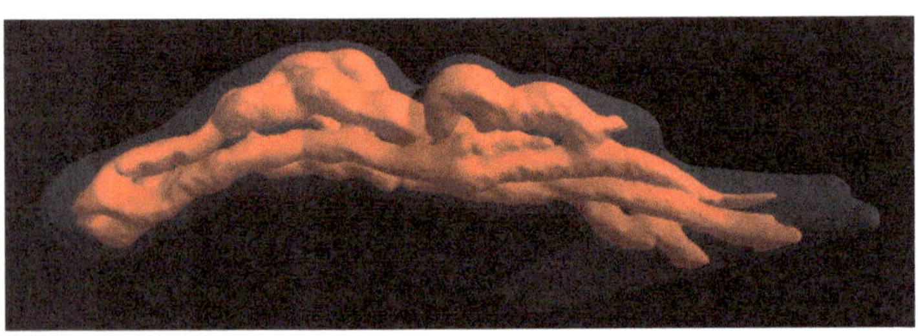

Fig. 16. Three-dimensional reconstruction of a normal placental terminal villus shows tightly arranged parallelly oriented villous capillaries.

Pathological forms of villi in diabetic placenta are rather of round shape. In hypovascularized villi, the 3D reconstruction revealed a conspicuously wavy course of thin capillaries (fig. 17), whereas hypervascularized villi displayed markedly wavy course of extremely distended capillary segments (fig. 18).

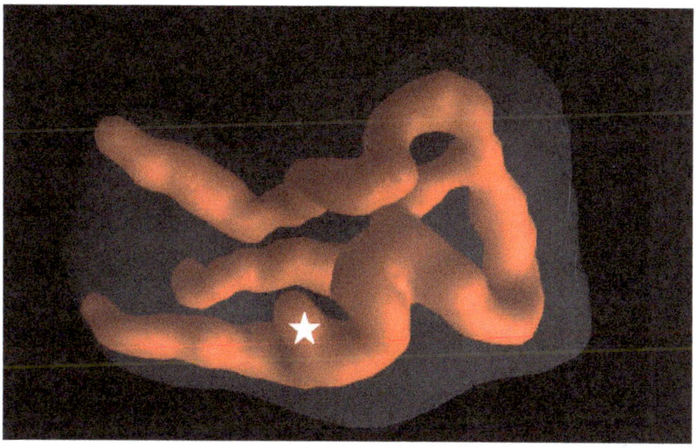

Fig. 17. Three-dimensional reconstruction of a hypovascularized villus of diabetic placenta. The capillaries are conspicuously wavy, asterisk indicates a capillary sprout.

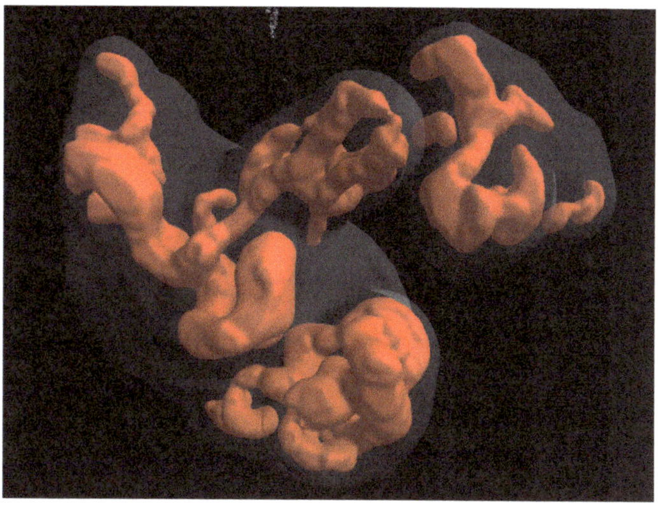

Fig. 18. Three-dimensional reconstruction of a hypervascularized villus of diabetic placenta shows capillaries of wavy course and often very large diameter.

2.4.2 The branching of villous capillaries in normal and diabetic placentas

As mentioned above, the majority of papers regarding quantitative comparison of capillary bed in normal and diabetic term placenta documented that maternal diabetes enhances placental angiogenesis. However, they gave no information on its consequences for spatial arrangement of capillaries.

The use of confocal microscope made possible not only to demonstrate spatial arrangement of villous capillaries, but also to perform quantitative analysis of the capillary branching in ample numbers of villi from normal and diabetic placentas using methods of topological schemes (fig. 13). These schemes of various forms of villous capillary beds were statistically analyzed, and mean numbers of redundant connections per villus and ratios of villous capillary beds without and with redundant connections were finally summarized in table 1. The results achieved in control placentas were significantly different from results achieved in placentas from pregnancies complicated by both gestational diabetes (Jirkovská et al., 2002) or type 1 diabetes (unpublished data). On the other hand, the results obtained in diabetic groups showed no significant differences.

These data indicate that enhanced capillary branching is a common manifestation of maternal diabetes in placental structure. This way, by means of placenta, the fetus probably reacts on adverse intrauterine environment caused by maternal metabolic disorder. It threatens the fetus above all by hypoxia (Mayhew et al., 2004), and the formation of new capillary segments represents undoubtedly a compensatory mechanism. Those new segments not only enlarge the capillary surface area, but their growth is also a driving force of the formation of new villi, and thus enlargement of the area of syncytiotrophoblast. The fact that the quantitative data concerning capillary branching are similar in both diabetic groups suggests that both types of maternal diabetes are equally serious from the fetal point of view, although the gestational diabetes represents only a transitory metabolic disorder for the mother.

Group (number of placentas)	Control (9)	GDM (11)	DM 1 (7)
Mean number of connections per villus	0,229 ± 0,092	0,449 ± 0,114 *	0,505 ± 0,278 *
Ratio of villi without connections	0,817 ± 0,087	0,632 ± 0,044*	0,596 ± 0,167 *
Ratio of villi with one connection	0,184 ± 0,083	0,308 ± 0,074	0,284 ± 0,144
Ratio of villi with two connections	0,002 ± 0,004	0,062 ± 0,043*	0,063 ± 0,058 *
Ratio of villi with three or more connections	0,00	0,017 ± 0,023	0,021 ± 0,044

Table 1. Summarized results of the analysis of villous capillary branching in control placentas and placentas from pregnancies complicated by gestational (GDM) or type 1 diabetes mellitus (DM 1). * = the value is significantly different from the control group.

3. Conclusion

The aim of this chapter was to summarize the knowledge regarding structural differences of the capillary bed of normal and diabetic term placenta. This overview comprises data obtained by conventional light microscopy and electron microscopy, by methods of quantitative morphology with emphasis on morphometry and stereology, and by methods based on confocal microscopy. It has been shown that structural differences between normal and diabetic placenta demonstrate themselves in higher degree of immaturity of diabetic villi, in different degree of villous capillarization, in different diameter of capillaries, and in the occurrence of basal lamina material and extravascular erythrocytes in the villous stroma. Three-dimensional reconstruction of villous capillaries revealed markedly waved thin capillaries in hypovascularized diabetic villi and markedly waved capillaries with conspicuously dilated segments in hypervascularized diabetic villi, as compared with villous capillaries of normal placenta. The majority of structural differences are of quantitative nature. It demonstrates itself in larger diameter of villi, in thinner capillary basal lamina, and in more branched capillaries of terminal villi. All this knowledge might and should be a challenge for further research, e.g. of functional consequences and molecular mechanisms leading to those structural changes.

4. Acknowledgments

This work was supported by the Grant Agency of the Czech Republic, project number 304/09/0733.

5. References

Akiba, K., Kuwabara, Y., Mizuno, M. & Fukuda, S. (1987). Semiquantitative study of the vascularisation of human term placenta using scanning electron microscopy. *J Clin Electron Microsc*, Vol. 20, pp. 5-6

Altshuler, G. (1984). Chorangiosis: an important placental sign of neonatal morbidity and mortality. *Arch Pathol Lab Med*, Vol. 108, No. 1, pp.71-74, ISSN 0003-9985

Arts, N.F.T. (1961) Investigations on the vascular system of the placenta. I. General introduction and the fetal vascular system. *Am J Obst Gynec*, Vol. 82, No. 1, pp. 147-158, ISSN 0002-9378

Asmussen, I. (1982). Ultrastructure of the villi and fetal capillaries of the placentas delivered by non-smoking diabetic women (White group D). *Acta Path Microbiol Immunol Scand Sect A*, Vol. 90, No. 2, pp. 95-101, ISSN 0365-4184

Babawale, M.O., Lovat, S., Mayhew, T.M., Lammiman, M.J., James, D.K. & Leach, L. (2000). Effects of gestational diabetes on junctional adhesion molecules in human term placental vasculature. *Diabetologia*, Vol. 43, No. 9, pp. 1185-1196, ISSN 0012-186X

Benirschke, K. & Kaufmann, P. (1995). *The Pathology of the Human Placenta* (3rd edition), Springer Verl., ISBN 0-387-94335-8, New York

Björk, O. & Persson, B. (1984). Villous structure in different parts of the cotyledon in placentas of insulin-dependent diabetic women. *Acta Obstet Gynecol Scand*, Vol. 63, No. 1, pp. 37-43, ISSN 0001-6349

Boe, F. (1969). Studies on the human placenta. III. Vascularization of the young foetal placenta. A. Vascularization of the chorionic villus. *Acta Obstet Gynecol Scand*, Vol. 48, No. 2, pp. 159-166, ISSN 0001-6349

Boyd, P.A., Scott, A. & Keeling, J.W. (1986). Quantitative structural studies on placentas from pregnancies complicated by diabetes mellitus. *Br J Obstet Gynaecol*, 93, pp. 31-35, ISSN 0306-5456

Burton, G.J. (1987). The fine structure of the human placenta villus as revealed by scanning electron microscopy. *Scanning Microsc*, Vol. 1, No. 4, pp. 1811-1828

Burton, G.J., Ingram, S.C. & Palmer, M.E. (1987). The influence of mode of fixation on morphometrical data derived from terminal villi in the human placenta at term: a comparison of immersion and perfusion fixation. *Placenta*, Vol. 8, No. 1, pp. 37-51, ISSN 0143-4004

Burton, G.J. & Jauniaux, E. (1995). Sonographic, stereological and Doppler flow velocimetric assessments of placental maturity. *Br J Obstet Gynaecol*, Vol. 102, No. 10, pp. 818 - 825, ISSN 0306-5456

Castellucci, M., Scheper, M., Scheffen, I., Celona, A. & Kaufmann, P. (1990). The development of the human placental villous tree. *Anat Embryol,* Vol. 181, No. 2, pp. 117-128, ISSN 0340-2061

Challier, J.C., Vervelle, C. & Uzan, S. (2001). Ontogenesis of villi and fetal vessels in the human placenta. *Fet Diagn Ther,* Vol. 16, No. 4, pp. 218-226, ISSN 1015-3837

Crawford, J.M. (1956). The foetal placenta circulation. IV. The anatomy of the villus and its capillary structure. *J Obstet Gynaecol Br Emp, Vol.* 63, No. 4, pp. 548-552, ISSN 0144-3615

Demir, R., Kaufmann, P., Castellucci, M., Erbengi, T. & Kotowski, A. (1989). Fetal vasculogenesis and angiogenesis in human placental villi. *Acta Anat,* Vol. 136, No. 3, pp. 190-203, ISSN 0001-5180

Dye, J.F., Jablenska, R., Donnelly, J.L., Lawrence, L., Leach, L., Clark, P. & Firth, J.A. (2001). Phenotype of the endothelium in the human term placenta. *Placenta,* Vol. 22, No. 1, pp. 32-43, ISSN 0143-4004

Eaton, B.M., Leach, L. & Firth, J.A. (1993). Permeability of fetal villous microvasculature in the isolated perfused term human placenta. *J Physiol (Lond),* 463, pp. 141-155, ISSN 0022-3751

Emmrich, P. & Müller, G. (1974) The size of chorionic villi in the placenta of diabetics. *Zentralbl Allg Pathol,* Vol. 118, No. 6, pp. 504-509, ISSN 0044-4030

Emmrich, P., Fuchs, U., Heinke, P., Jutzi, E. & Gődel, E. (1976). Epithelial and capillary basal laminae of the placenta in maternal diabetes mellitus. *Lab Invest,* Vol. 35, No. 1, pp. 87-92, ISSN 0023-6837

Evers, I.M., Nikkels, P.G.J., Sikkema, J.M. & Visser, G.H.A. (2003). Placental pathology in women with type 1 diabetes and in a control group with normal and large-for-gestational-age infants. *Placenta,* Vol. 24, No. 8-9, pp. 819-825, ISSN 0143-4004

Fox, H. & Sebire, N.J. (2008). *Pathology of the Placenta* (3rd edition), Saunders-Elsevier, ISBN 978-1-4160-2592-4

Geppert, M., Peters, F.D. & Geppert, J. (1982). Zur Histomorphometrie der Zottenvaskularisation von Plazenten diabetischer Mütter. *Geburtsh Frauenheilk,* Vol. 42, No. 8, pp. 628-632, ISSN 0016-5751

Greco, M.A., Kamat, B.R. & Demopoulos, R.I. (1989). Placental protein distribution in maternal diabetes mellitus: an immunocytochemical study. *Pediatr Pathol,* Vol. 9, No. 6, pp. 679-690

Hájek, Z., (Ed.) (2004). *Rizikové a patologické těhotenství (High-risk and Pathological Pregnancy, in Czech),* Grada Publishing a.s., ISBN 80-247-0418-8, Prague, Czech Republic

Hashimoto, H., Ishikawa, H. & Kusakabe, M. (1999). Development of vascular networks during the morphogenesis of intestinal villi in the fetal mouse. *Acta Anat Nippon,* Vol. 74, No. 5, pp. 567-576

Haust, M.D. (1981). Maternal diabetes mellitus - effects on the fetus and placenta, In: *Perinatal Diseases,* Naeye, R.L. & Kissane, J. (Eds.), pp. 201-285, Williams and Wilkins, Baltimore, U.S.A.

Higgins, M., Felle, P., Mooney, E.E., Bannigan, J. & McAuliffe, F.M. (2011). Stereology of the placenta in type 1 and 2 diabetes. *Placenta,* Vol. 32, No. 8, pp. 564-569, ISSN 0143-4004

Higgins, M.F., McAuliffe, F.M. & Mooney, E. (2011). Clinical associations with a placental diagnosis of delayed villous maturation: A retrospective study. *Pediatr Dev* Pathol, Feb 17 [Epub ahead of print], ISSN 1093-5266

Honda, M., Toyoda, C., Nakabayashi, M. & Omori, Y. (1992). Quantitative investigations of placental terminal villi in maternal diabetes mellitus by scanning and transmission electron microscopy. *Tohoku J Exp Med,* Vol. 167, No. 4, pp. 247-257, ISSN 0040-8727

Jauniaux, E. & Burton, G.J. (2006). Villous histomorphometry and placental bed biopsy in diabetic pregnancies. *Placenta,* Vol. 27, No. 4-5, pp. 468-474, ISSN 0143-4004

Jirkovská, M. (1991). Comparison of the thickness of the capillary basement membrane of the human placenta under normal conditions and in type I diabetes. *Funct Dev Morphol,* Vol. 1, No. 3, pp. 9-16

Jirkovská, M., Šmídová, J. & Frýda, T. (1994). Morphometric analysis of the vascularization of the terminal villi in normal and diabetic placenta. *Acta Stereol,* Vol. 13, No. 1, pp. 43-47, ISSN 0351-580X

Jirkovská, M., Kubínová, L., Krekule, I. & Hach, P. (1998). Spatial arrangement of fetal placental capillaries in terminal villi: a study using confocal microscopy. *Anat Embryol,* Vol. 197, No. 4, pp. 63-272, ISSN 0340-2061

Jirkovská, M,. Janáček, J., Jirsová, Z., Kubínová, L. & Zemanová, Z. (2001). Spatial arrangement of peritubular vascular bed in chick mesonephros. *Image Anal Stereol,* 20 (Suppl 1), pp. 338-341, ISSN 1580-3139

Jirkovská, M., Náprstková, I., Janáček, J., Kučera, T., Macášek, J., Karen, P. & Kubínová, L. (2005). Three-dimensional reconstructin from non-deparaffinized tissue sections. *Anat Embryol,* Vol. 210, No. 3, pp. 163-173, ISSN 0340-2061

Jirkovská, M., Kubínová, L., Janáček, J., Moravcová, M., Krejčí, V., Karen, P. (2002). Topological properties and spatial organization of villous capillariers in normal and diabetic placentas. *J Vasc Res,* Vol. 39, No. 3, pp. 268-278, ISSN 1018-1172

Jirkovská, M., Janáček, J., Kaláb, J. & Kubínová, L. (2008). Three-dimensional arrangement of the capillary bed and its relationship to microrheology in the terminal villi of normal term placenta. *Placenta,* Vol. 29, No. 10, pp. 892-897, ISSN 0143-4004

Jones, C.J. & Fox, H. (1976). Placental changes in gestational diabetes. An ultrastructural study. *Obstet Gynecol,* Vol. 48, No. 3, pp. 274-280, ISSN 0029-7844

Jones, C.J.P. & Desoye, G. (1993). Glycogen distribution in the capillaries of the placental villus in normal, overt and gestational diabetic pregnancy. *Placenta,* Vol. 14, No. 5, pp. 505-517,

Jones, C.J.P. & Desoye, G. (2010). A new possible function for placental pericytes. *Placenta,* Vol. 31, No. 9, Abstracts for the forthcoming International Federation of Placenta Associations Meeting 2010, p.A.18, ISSN 0143-4004

Kacemi, A., Vervelle, C., Uzan, S. & Challier, J.C. (1999). Immunostaining of vascular, perivascular cells and stromal components in human placental villi. *Cell Mol Biol (Noisy-le-grand),* Vol. 45, No. 1, pp. 101-113, ISSN 0145-5680

Karen, P., Jirkovská, M., Tomori, Z., Demjénová, E., Janáček, J. & Kubínová, L. (2003). Three-dimensional computer reconstruction of large tissue volumes based on composing series of high- resolution confocal images by GlueMRC and LinkMRC software. *Microsc Res Tech*, Vol. 62, No. 5, pp. 415-422, 1 ISSN 059-910X

Kaufmann, P., Bruns, U., Leiser, R., Luckhardt, M. & Winterhager, E. (1985). The fetal vascularisation of term human placental villi. II. Intermediate and terminal villi. *Anat Embryol*, Vol. 173, No. 2, pp. 203-214, ISSN 0340-2061

Kingdom, J., Huppertz, B., Seaward, G. & Kaufmann, P. (2000). Development of the placental villous tree and its consequence for fetal growth. *Eur J Obstet Gynecol Reprod Biol*, Vol. 92, No. 1, pp. 35-43, ISSN 0301-2115

Kučera, T., Vyletěl, I., Moravcová, M., Krejčí, V., Žižka, Z. & Jirkovská, M. (2010). Pericyte coverage of fetoplacental vessels in pregnancies complicated by type 1 diabetes mellitus. *Placenta*, Vol. 31, No. 12, pp. 1120-1122, ISSN 0143-4004

Kučera,T., Jadrníček, M., Niedobová, V., Žižka, Z., Krejčí, V., Moravcová, M. & Jirkovská, M. (2011). Apoptosis in placental vasculature in pregnancies complicated by diabetes mellitus type I. *Placenta*, Vol. 32, No. 9, Abstracts of the IFPA Meeting 2011, p. A16, ISSN 0143-4004

Lang, I., Pabst, M.A., Hiden, U., Blaschitz, A., Dohr, G., Hahn, T., & Desoye, G. (2003). Heterogeneity of microvascular endothelial cells isolated from human term placenta and macrovascular umbilical vein endothelial cells. *Eur J Cell Biol*, Vol. 82, No. 4, pp. 163-173, ISSN 0171-9335

Leach, L. & Firth, J.A. (1992). Fine structure of the paracellular junctions of terminal villous capillaries in the perfused human placenta. *Cell Tiss Res*, Vol. 268, No. 3, pp. 447-452, ISSN 0302-766X

Leach, L., Gray, C., Staton, S., Babawale, M.O., Gruchy, A., Foster, C., Mayhew, T.M., & James, D.K. (2004). Vascular endothelial cadherin and β-catenin in human fetoplacental vessels of pregnancies complicated by Type 1 diabetes: associations with angiogenesis and perturbed barrier function. *Diabetologia*, Vol. 47, No. 4, pp. 695-709, ISSN 0012-186X

Leiser, R., Luckhardt, M., Kaufmann, P., Winterhager, E. & Bruns, U. (1985). The fetal vascularisation of term human placental villi. I. Peripheral stem villi. *Anat Embryol*, Vol. 173, No. 1, pp. 71-80, ISSN 0340-2061

Luckhardt, M., Leiser, R., Kingdom, J., Malek, A., Sager, R., Kaisig, C. & Schneider, H. (1996). Effect of physiologic perfusion-fixation on the morphometrically evaluated dimensions of the term placental cotyledon. *J Soc Gynecol Invest*, Vol. 3, No. 4, pp. 166-171, ISSN 1071-5576

Madazli, R., Tuten, A., Calay, Z., Uzun, H., Uludag, S., & Ocak, V. (2008). The incidence of placental abnormalities, maternal and cord plasma malondialdehyde and vascular endothelial growth factor levels in women with gestational diabetes mellitus and nondiabetic controls. *Gynecol Obstet Invest*, Vol. 65, No. 4, pp. 227-232, ISSN 0378-7346

Mayhew, T.M., Joy, C.F, Haas, J.D. (1984). Structure-function correlation in the human placenta: the morphometric diffusing capacity for oxygen at full term. *J Anat*, Vol. 139, No. 4, pp. 691-708, ISSN 0021-8782

Mayhew, T.M., Sørensen, F.B., Klebe, J.G. & Jackson, M.R. (1993). The effects of mode of delivery and sex of newborn on placental morphology in control and diabetic pregnancies. *J Anat*, Vol. 183, No. 3, pp. 545-552, ISSN 0021-8782

Mayhew, T.M., Sørensen, F.B., Klebe, J.G., Jackson, M.R. (1994). Growth and maturation of villi in placentae from well-controlled diabetic women. *Placenta*, Vol. 15, No. 1, pp. 57-65, ISSN 0143-4004

Mayhew, T.M. (2002 a). Enhanced fetoplacental angiogenesis in pre-gestational diabetes mellitus: the extra growth is exclusively longitudinal and not accompanied by microvascular remodelling. *Diabetologia*, Vol. 45, No. 10, pp. 1434-1439, ISSN 0012-186X

Mayhew, T. M. (2002 b). Fetoplacental angiogenesis during gestation is biphasic, longitudinal and occurs by proliferation and remodelling of vascular endothelial cells. *Placenta*, Vol. 23, No. 10, pp. 742-750, ISSN 0143-4004

Mayhew, T.M., Charnock-Jones, D.S. & Kaufmann, P. (2004). Aspects of human fetoplacental vasculogenesis and angiogenesis. III. Changes in complicated pregnancies. *Placenta*, Vol. 25, No. 2-3, pp. 127-139, ISSN 0143-4004

Nelson, S.M., Coan, P.M., Burton, G.J. & Lindsay, R.S. (2009). Placental structure in type 1 diabetes: relation to fetal insulin, leptin and IGF-I. *Diabetes*, Vol. 58, No. 11, pp. 2634-2641, ISSN 0012-1797

Oikawa, H., Masuda, T., Yashima, A. & Satodate, R. (1999). Blood-flow route from the hepatic artery and portal vein to the sinusoid in normal human liver observed by confocal laser scanning microscopy. *Analytical and Quantitative Cytology and Histology*, Vol. 21, No. 3, pp. 255-261

Okudaira, Y., Hirota, K., Cohen, S. & Strauss, L. (1966). Ultrastructure of the human placenta in maternal diabetes mellitus. *Lab Invest*, Vol. 15, No. 5, pp. 910-926, ISSN 0023-6837

Semmler, K., Emmrich, P., Fuhrmann, K., & Gödel, E. (1982). Reifungsstörungen der Plazenta in Relation zur Qualiät der metabolischen Kontrolle während der Schwangerschaft beim insulinpflichtigen und Gestationsdiabetes. Zbl Gynäkol, Vol. 104, No. 23, pp. 1494-1502, ISSN 0044-4197

Semmler, K. & Emmrich, P. (1989). Morphologie der Plazenta in Relation zur Glykämielage in der Schwangerschaft beim Diabetes mellitus. *Z Geburtsh Perinat*, Vol. 193, No. 3, pp. 124-128, ISSN 0300-5577

Sobrevia, L., Abarzúa, F., Nien, J.K., Salomón, C., Westermeier, F., Puebla, C., Cifuentes, F., Guzmán-Gutiérrez, E., Leiva, A. & Casanello, P. (2011). Review: Differential placental macrovascular and microvascular endothelial dysfunction in gestational diabetes. *Placenta*, 32, Supplement B, Trophoblast Research, 25, S159-S164, ISSN 0143-4004

Teasdale, F. (1981). Histomorphometry of the placenta of the diabetic women: class A diabetes mellitus. *Placenta*, Vol. 2, No. 3, pp. 241-252, ISSN 0143-4004

Teasdale, F. (1983). Histomorphometry of the human placenta in class B diabetes mellitus. *Placenta*, Vol. 4, No. 1, pp. 1-12, ISSN 0143-4004

Teasdale, F. (1985). Histomorphometry of the human placenta in class C diabetes mellitus. *Placenta*, Vol. 6, No. 1, pp. 69-82, ISSN 0143-4004

Zhang, E.G., Burton G.J., Smith S.K. & Charnock-Jones, D.S. (2002). Placental vessel adaptation during gestation and to high altitude: changes in diameter and perivascular cell coverage. *Placenta*, Vol. 23, No. 10, pp. 751-762, ISSN 0143-4004

Part 5

Transport Across the Placental Barrier

15

Placental Transport of Thyroid Hormone and Iodide

Kerry Richard, Huika Li, Kelly A. Landers,
Jatin Patel and Robin H. Mortimer
Royal Brisbane and Women's Hospital and The University of Queensland, Australia

1. Introduction

1.1 The thyroid gland

The major role of the thyroid is to synthesise and secrete thyroid hormones (TH). It does this by a complex process that begins with extraction of iodide from circulating blood via the sodium iodide symporter (NIS) (Dai, et al. 1996). Intracellular iodide is oxidised, under the influence of a thyroperoxidase leading to iodination of the amino acid tyrosine on the abundant thyroglobulin that occupies thyroid follicles. Iodinated tyrosines are combined to form thyroxine (4 iodine atoms, T_4) and triiodothyronine (3 iodine atoms, T_3). Both T_4 and T_3 are secreted from the thyroid gland and circulate bound to a family of thyroid binding proteins so that only a tiny fraction of T_4 and T_3 remain unbound (Benvenga 2005). T_4 is avidly taken up by liver and deiodinated by a type 1 deiodinase (D1) (Bianco, et al. 2002) to the biologically more active T_3 and the biologically inactive reverse T_3 (rT_3). Most circulating T_3 is of hepatic origin. T_4, and to a lesser extent T_3 feed back at the pituitary level. Intrapituitary T_4 is deiodinated to T_3 by a Type 2 deiodinase (D2) and this together with T_3 from the circulation inhibits synthesis and secretion of thyroid stimulating hormone (TSH), also known as thyrotropin (Shupnik, et al. 1985). TSH is a highly glycosylated protein with alpha and beta chains and is under the tonic control of the inhibitory hypothalamic hormone somatostatin (Weeke, et al. 1975) and the stimulatory thyrotropin releasing hormone (TRH) (Shupnik, et al. 1986). TSH via thyroid cell membrane TSH receptors stimulates iodide uptake (Levy, et al. 1997) and TH synthesis and secretion. Serum TH levels are controlled by the pituitary feedback mechanism.

1.2 Thyroxine (T_4)

The thyroid gland is the only known source of T_4 in the body (Chopra 1996). T_4 is the most abundant iodothyronine in the circulation, present at around twenty times the concentration of T_3, up to one hundred times more than rT_3 and more than one thousand times the concentration of any other iodothyronine derivative. Iodine constitutes about 65% (by weight) of the T_4 molecule and T_4 accounts for up to 90% of protein bound iodine in serum. The extent of overall protein binding is great, such that the serum free T_4 concentration is usually less than 0.1% of total T_4 concentration. The major TH binding proteins are; thyroxine binding globulin (TBG), transthyretin (TTR) and albumin as well as several minor carriers. The less biologically active T_4 is largely deiodinated in peripheral tissues to the bioactive form of TH, T_3 (Figure 1). Alternatively, T_4 may be converted to the inactive metabolite, rT_3. Both T_3 and rT_3 can be further metabolised in peripheral tissues to 3,3'-diiodothyronine (T_2).

1.3 3,5,3'-triiodothyronine (T_3)

T_3 was first discovered in human serum in 1951 (Gross and Leblond 1951) and was found to be several times more biologically potent than T_4 in producing the classic effects of THs (Gershengorn, et al. 1979). T_3 is formed by the removal of an iodine atom, by deiodinase enzymes, from the phenolic ring of T_4 (Figure 1). Like T_4, T_3 in serum is bound to TBG, TTR and albumin. As indicated above the main source of T_3 is peripheral conversion from T_4 in addition to some limited direct thyroid gland secretion.

1.4 3,3',5'-triiodothyronine (rT_3)

Reverse T_3 (rT_3) differs from T_3 in that iodine is removed from the inner or tyrosyl ring of T_4 rather than the outer or phenolic ring (Chopra 1996) (Figure 1). rT_3 was first found in the blood of rats in 1956, it has little or no activity when administered to animals and its metabolism is extremely rapid. The main source of rT_3 is inner-ring deiodination of T_4 in peripheral tissue, predominantly liver (Chopra, et al. 1975).

1.5 other thyronine derivatives

Besides T_4, T_3 and rT_3 several other thyronine derivatives are found in serum. These include three diiodothyronines (3,3'-T_2, 3',5-T_2 and 3',5'-T_2), two monoiodothyronines (3'-T_1 and 3-T_1) and two acetic acid analogues of T_4 (tetrac) and T_3 (triac) as well as the sulfate and glucuronide conjugates of T_4, T_3 and rT_3. Sulfate conjugates of iodothyronines are more actively deiodinated than the parent iodothyronine and sulfated T_3 loses its affinity for the thyroid receptor (Visser 1994).

1.6 Thyroid hormone receptors

Thyroid hormones act by binding to specific nuclear receptors that interact with DNA causing activation or repression of transcription (Tata and Widnell 1966). In the 1960s it was noted that nuclear RNA transcription preceded many of the physiological effects of T_3 and this led to the discovery of high affinity nuclear receptors for T_3 (Oppenheimer, et al. 1972; Samuels and Tsai 1973). The cloning from many species of multiple cDNAs encoding proteins with the characteristics of TH receptors (TR) brought about the realisation that there is a family of TRs (Evans 1988). These have molecular weights of 50 to 55kDa and bind T_3 with high affinities (Sap, et al. 1986; Weinberger, et al. 1986). The TR isoforms have substantial amino acid sequence homology with the steroid hormone receptors (Evans 1988). Levels of nuclear TRs correlate well with the developmental and tissue specific effects of T_3 (Chan, et al. 2002).

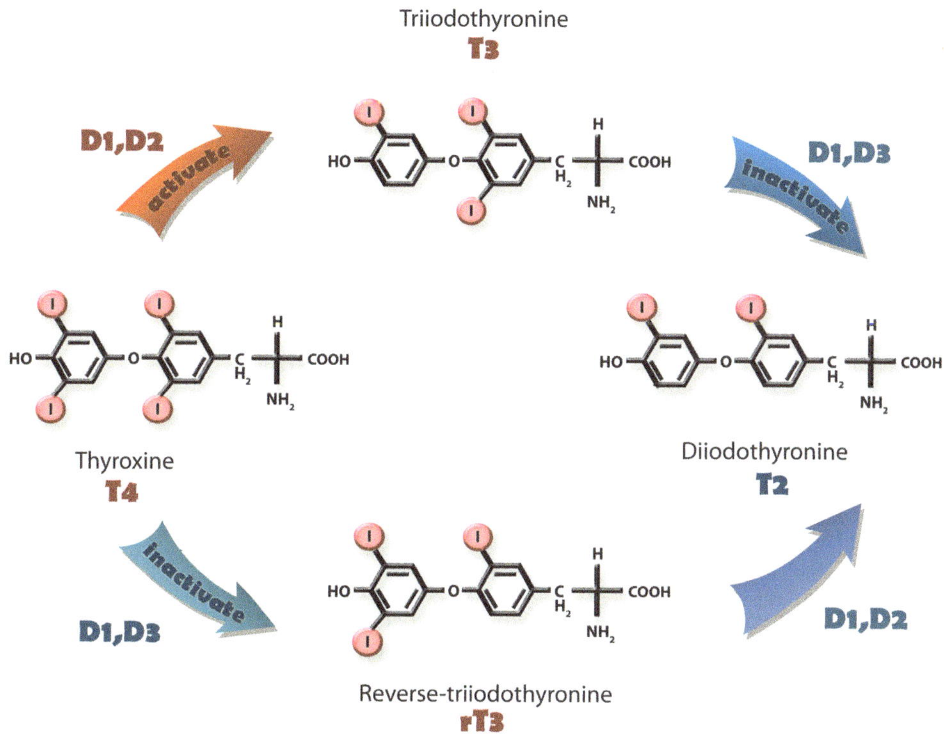

Fig. 1. Deiodination pathways of the thyroid hormones. D1, Deiodinase Type 1; D2, Deiodinase Type 2; D3, Deiodinase Type 3

2. Thyroid hormone and iodide are required for normal fetal development

2.1 Mild maternal thyroid dysfunction and impaired neuro-cognitive function in the offspring

There is now ample evidence that even mild maternal hypothyroidism is associated with impaired fetal neuro-cognitive outcome. World wide, the most common cause of maternal hypothyroidism is iodine deficiency (Andersson, et al. 2010; Pharoah and Connolly 1991). Severe iodine deficiency is well known to cause severe mental retardation, neuro-muscular impairment and short stature, a syndrome known as cretinism. While cretinism was described hundreds of years ago, the link between milder degrees of iodine deficiency and reduced intelligence of the offspring was first described described in the Himalayas in the early 20th century. Subsequent work in the highlands of Papua New Guinea by Pharoah confirmed the link between milder degrees of iodine deficiency and reduced neuro-cognitive function and provided evidence of correlations between reduced maternal T_4 (but not T_3) levels and reduced intelligence and coordination (Pharoah and Connolly 1991). A small, more recent Italian study (Vermiglio, et al. 2004) confirmed reduced IQ levels and a high incidence of attention deficit disorder in offspring of women from an area of moderate iodine deficiency. There was a strong inverse correlation between maternal mid gestation free T_4 (FT_4) and offspring IQ. A Spanish study emphasised the importance of early iodine supplementation in preventing neurological damage (Berbel, et al. 2009).

A link between mild maternal hypothyroidism and impaired intellectual development of offspring was suggested in the 1960s. Over several years, from the late 1960s to the 1970s Man and co-workers published data from 1349 women whose serum T_4 was estimated by measuring butanol-extractable iodine during early and late pregnancy (Man, et al. 1991); three percent were hypothyroxinemic. Developmental and intellectual outcomes of progeny of 210 euthyroxinemic women, 15 hypothyroxinemic women adequately treated with thyroxine and 21 women inadequately treated with T_4 were compared at eight months, four and seven years of age. Mothers were well matched for intelligence, years of education and chronological age. At each age children of mothers with inadequately treated hypothyroidism had lower mean developmental and intellectual scores.

Subsequent studies using more precise measurements of TH status have yielded similar results. Haddow and co-workers (Haddow 1999) measured TSH levels in stored blood taken from over 25,000 pregnant women. Seventy-five women (0.3%) had levels at or above the 99.7th percentile; 47 were contacted and agreed to allow neuropsychological testing of their children at seven to nine years of age. Children of an additional 15 women with serum TSH levels between the 98th and 99.6th percentiles were also tested; 77 % of these 62 women had positive thyroid antibodies (markers of potential autoimmune thyroid disease). Results were compared with those of 124 women with normal thyroid function (14% of whom had positive antithyroid antibodies) and demonstrated significantly ($p=0.06$) reduced full-scale IQ scores, reduced verbal IQ scores ($p=0.06$) and word discrimination ($p=0.01$).

Children of women with normal thyroid stimulating hormone (TSH) levels but FT_4 levels less than the 10th percentile during early pregnancy (i.e. technically normal thyroid function) had significantly lower Bayley Psychomotor Development Index scores at ten months of age than children of women with higher FT_4 levels. Mothers with FT_4 levels below the 10th percentile had a significantly higher incidence of positive antithyroid antibodies (Pop, et al. 1999).

These, and other (Ghassabian, et al. 2011; Klein, et al. 2001; Kooistra, et al. 2006; Li, et al. 2010), clinical studies provide strong evidence of a relationship between reduced or low normal early pregnancy FT_4 levels and neuro-cognitive functioning of offspring. This relationship holds whether maternal thyroid dysfunction results from iodine deficiency or autoimmune thyroid disease. These findings suggest that maternal thyroxine is required for early fetal brain development and that maternal TH crosses the placental barrier.

2.2 Maternal hypothyroxinemia

Under normal circumstances maternal FT_4 levels rise in the mid first trimester in response to a surge in maternal human chorionic gonadotropin (hCG) levels (Fisher 1983) (Figure 2). HCG is a double chain glycosylated protein secreted by placenta from early pregnancy that shares a common alpha subunit with TSH. The beta subunits of each hormone and their cell membrane receptors are also significantly homologous. HCG stimulates the normal maternal thyroid via the TSH receptor to synthesise and secrete TH. Very high hCG levels as are seen in women with excessive pregnancy induced vomiting (hyperemesis) and women with placental malignancy (choriocarcinoma) can cause maternal hyperthyroidism. As normal pregnancy progresses hCG levels fall and this is reflected in falling FT_4 levels (Figure 2). Impairment of maternal TH secreting capacity from iodine deficiency or autoimmune thyroid disease can blunt the physiological first trimester surge in maternal TH secretion, or if more severe can result in maternal hypothyroidism.

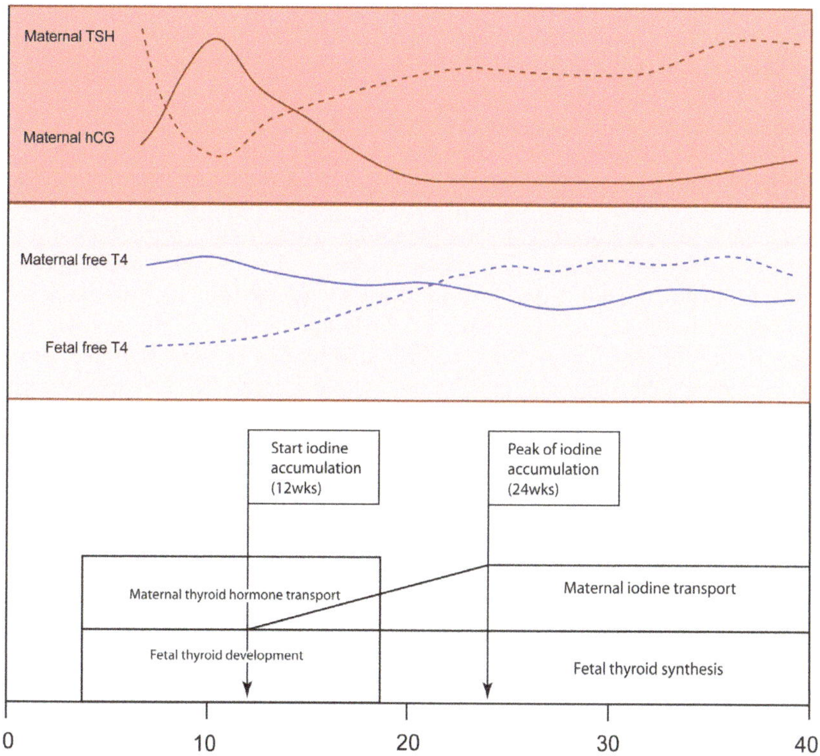

Fig. 2. Ontogenic changes in maternal and fetal thyroid gland and hormone function (compiled with data from (Fisher 1983; Fuse 1996)). hCG, human chorionic gonadotropin; TSH, thyroid stimulating hormone/thyrotropin; T_4, thyroxine.

Mild iodine deficiency is prevalent in many parts of the world, including some European countries, the USA and Australia and as discussed above is a common cause of maternal hypothyroxinemia. Iodine deficiency can be exacerbated by maternal smoking, which increases blood thiocyanate levels. Thiocyanate competitively blocks the sodium iodide cell membrane symporter (NIS) responsible for transfer of iodide into maternal and fetal thyroid and for materno-fetal transfer of iodide by the placenta (Manley, et al. 2005) . Thyroid autoimmunity is common in pregnant women. Autoimmune thyroid disease (AITD) is associated with autoantibodies to thyroperoxidase (TPO). This enzyme oxidises iodine in the presence of hydrogen peroxide, facilitating iodination of tyrosine and synthesis of TH. Enzyme activity is blocked by anti-TPO autoantibodies. About 10% of pregnant women have positive anti-thyroperoxidase antibodies at 14 weeks gestation and about 2.5% have asymptomatic hypothyroidism (Lazarus 2005).

2.3 Ontogeny of the human fetal hypothalamic-pituitary-thyroid axis

The thyroid gland is the first endocrine organ to develop in man where it originates as a thickening in tissue destined to become the tongue (Fuse 1996). This bud descends to the level of the larynx, forming two lobes connected by an isthmus. Recognisable thyrocytes are present by the end of 7 weeks gestation but mature thyroid follicles containing colloid do not appear until after 13.5 weeks gestation. The fetal thyroid appears to be able to accumulate iodine by about 12 weeks gestation (Figure 2). Iodine concentrating capacity increases from about 12 weeks, reaching a peak at about 24 weeks gestation. T_4 is synthesised by about 19 weeks gestation (Fuse 1996) (Figure 2).

The pituitary gland has two separate origins, the glandular component (appearing in the developing mouth at about 3 weeks gestation) and the neural primordium (extending from the hypothalamus about 5.5 weeks). The glandular primordium forms Rathke's Pouch, which loses its connection with the oral cavity by about 8.5 weeks. This adenohypophyseal primordium forms the anterior pituitary and forms a close association with the developing neural structure forming the neurohypophysis. Cells staining for the alpha subunit of TSH can be seen from 8-12 weeks gestation. The beta subunit can be identified by 13-15 weeks gestation. Immunoreactive TSH can be identified in fetal serum by 12 weeks gestation but levels are low until a rapid increase at 18-22 weeks.

These data suggest that while the fetal thyroid can concentrate iodine and synthesise TH in the late first trimester. TSH regulated TH secretion may not occur until as late as 18-20 weeks gestation (Figure 2).

2.4 Feto-maternal transfer of iodide and thyroid hormones

2.4.1 Iodide

Detectable iodine in the amniotic fluid of pregnant rabbits fed potassium iodide was reported in 1859 and in 1872 similar results were reported in man (quoted by (Gersten 1954). Transfer of radioiodine from the maternal to fetal circulations of the guinea pig was reported in 1955 (Logothetopoulos and Scott 1955) who noted that transport was blocked by sodium thiocyanate, suggesting an active transport process. In thyroid iodide is transferred from blood to the thyroid cell by the sodium iodide symporter (NIS) and iodide efflux from the thyrocyte is mediated by another transporter called Pendrin. NIS (Bidart, et al. 2000; Mitchell, et al. 2001) and Pendrin (Bidart et al. 2000) have been reported in trophoblasts and functional studies in a trophoblast cell line suggest that these are responsible for iodide influx and efflux in placenta (Manley et al. 2005). Sodium thiocyanate is a powerful inhibitor of NIS. Recently SLC5A6, a placental sodium/multivitamin transporter has been identified as an iodide transporter (de Carvalho and Quick 2011) but its role in placental iodide transfer is as yet unclear.

2.4.2 Thyroid hormone

Early human studies suggested that there was significant materno-fetal transfer of TH (Raiti, et al. 1967) and this was supported by detection of significant amounts of TH in cord blood of infants unable to synthesise TH (Vulsma, et al. 1989). Investigation of transfer of T_4 in the isolated perfused human placenta demonstrated that the abundant type 3 deiodinase (D3) significantly limited transfer so that the fetal circuit T_4 reached only 0.008% of maternal levels. Inhibition of D3 by iopanoic acid increased fetal T_4 levels to 30% of those in the maternal circuit (Mortimer, et al. 1996). Membrane TH transporters were demonstrated in human trophoblasts and choriocarcinoma cell lines (Mitchell, et al. 1992) mediating uptake and efflux of TH. The identities of these transporters were subsequently ascertained.

There is now clear evidence of THs in fetal serum, coelomic and amniotic fluid and brain in early pregnancy, a time when the fetal thyroid gland has not yet developed the capacity to secrete TH (Calvo, et al. 2002). These studies were done in human tissues obtained from fetuses as early as 5-6 weeks gestation. The early feto-placental unit (up to 12-13 weeks gestation) consists of the fetus floating in amniotic fluid (AF) within an amniotic sac. This in turn is contained within an exocoelomic cavity containing coelomic fluid (CF) in which floats a prominent secondary yolk sac. The yolk sac, an extension of the fetal gastrointestinal tract and circulation, secretes and resorbs a variety of proteins. The CF is contained within a uterus lined by the early placenta. The early placenta is poorly vascularised, relatively hypoxic and covers the surface of the chorionic sac. The CF is protein rich, containing albumin and TTR whereas AF is essentially a low protein ultrafiltrate of maternal serum containing placental and yolk sac secretory products. Its volume is increased by urine secreted by the developing fetal kidneys.

With increasing gestational age, the yolk sac and the majority of the placenta regress and the exocoelomic cavity is largely obliterated by an expanding amniotic sac. The placenta forms a circumscribed disc-like structure and trophoblasts, the epithelial cells that mediate materno-fetal exchange, invade the uterine vasculature. This allows development of a mature maternal and fetal circulation within the placenta and a rise in placental oxygen levels. There is increasing evidence that the changing oxygen levels within the developing placenta have major effects on trophoblast function (Patel, et al. 2010b).

Human studies have provided considerable insight into TH levels in fetal serum (FS), CF and AF. It is clear that maternal TH crosses the placenta, entering the human embryonic cavities and fetal blood well before the fetal thyroid is secreting its own TH (Calvo et al. 2002; Contempre B 1993) (Figure 3). Total T_4 was detectable in several sets of CF fluid obtained between 5.8 and 11 weeks gestation, with set means ranging from 950 to 1280 pmol/litre. Total T_3 levels were very much lower (2.50 to 2.82 pmol/litre). rT_3 levels were high, ranging from 2.1 to 5.48 nmol/liter. T_4, T_3 and rT_3 were also found in AF sampled from 8 weeks on. Total T_4 ranged from 63 to 2041 pmol/litre, whereas total T_3 was 6 to 12 pmol/litre. rT_3 levels were again relatively high at 210 to 3430 pmol/litre. The high ratios of rT_3 to T_4 suggest active Type 3 deiodination (see below). The yolk sac synthesises and secretes the T_4 binding protein TTR and low levels of TTR were detected in CF from 7 weeks gestation, increasing with increasing gestational age. Mean free T_4 levels of 2.5 to 2.82 pmol/litre could be estimated in CF. Mean FT_4 in AF ranged from 6.45 to 20.43 pmol/litre.

These TH levels, expressed as a percentage of corresponding maternal levels in early pregnancy, are shown in Figure 3. Although fetal total T_4 is only about 5% of maternal levels and CF and AF levels are less than 1% of maternal values, free T_4 levels are much higher (approaching maternal levels) in these compartments due to very low TBG levels (Calvo et al. 2002).

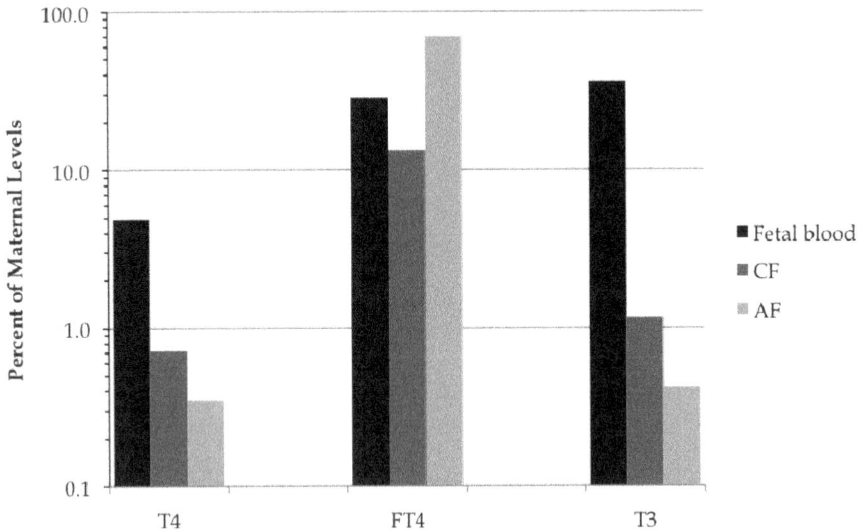

Fig. 3. Levels of total and free T_4 and total T_3 in first trimester fetal blood, coelomic (CF) and amniotic (AF) fluids as a percentage of maternal levels in the first trimester. (Data from (Calvo et al. 2002)).

Maternal T_4 and FT_4 levels increase during the first and second trimester. T_4 levels in CF correlate with those in maternal serum and in the second trimester fetal blood levels also correlate with maternal values. Interestingly T_3 and free T_3 levels in CF do not correlate with maternal levels (Calvo et al. 2002). These data strongly argue for significant transfer of maternal THs to the coelomic and amniotic fluids and into the fetal circulation. The significant gradient of total T_4 from maternal to fetal circulations and high levels of rT_3 in CF and AH suggest that active conversion of T_4 to rT_3 by D3 in placenta, placental membranes and the fetus strongly modulates fetal T_4 supply. Despite this fetal T_4 levels are strongly determined by maternal levels.

There is also strong clinical evidence that, at least in the presence of a hypothyroid fetus, transfer of maternal T_4 to the fetus continues throughout pregnancy. In 1989 Vulsma and colleagues reported that cord blood T_4 levels from infants with complete thyroid agenesis or a complete defect in organification of iodine and capacity to synthesise TH had T_4 levels of 30 - 75 nmol/liter, which must have been of maternal origin (Vulsma et al. 1989). Placental D3 levels appear normal in these infants (Koopdonk-Kool, et al. 1996).

2.5 Thyroid hormone and development of the fetal brain

Although fetal serum T_3 levels are very low at that time, T_3 and TH receptors have been identified in human fetal brain as early as 9 weeks gestation (Bernal and Pekonen 1984; Chan et al. 2002). Brain T_3 is locally produced by Type 2 deiodination of T_4 and rat studies indicate that brain T_3 in the hypothyroid rat fetus cannot be replenished by maternal T_3 administration but requires maternal T_4. T_4 enters brain via the cerebral circulation but a significant proportion also appears to be transferred through the choroid plexus, a potent source of cerebro-spinal fluid (CSF) transthyretin (TTR). TTR represents about 20% of CSF protein and is the major TH transporter in CSF. Membrane TH transporters, notably monocarboxylate transporter (MCT) 8, are important mediators of neuronal T_3 uptake. Intracellular T_3 is translocated to the cell nucleus where it binds to TRs and, following homodimerisation or heterodimerisation with retinoic acid receptors, it binds to TH response elements present in many genes, positively or negatively regulating them. T_3 has major effects on neurogenesis, cell migration and myelination in the developing brain (Patel, et al. 2011).

3. Placental regulation of thyroid hormone transfer

3.1 Iodothyronine deiodinases

The deiodinases play an important role in coordinating TH action during vertebrate development and they regulate TH action within selected tissues during development and adulthood. Three deiodinases have been identified, deiodinase type 1 (D1), deiodinase type 2 (D2) and deiodinase type 3 (D3), and all are integral membrane proteins and are selenoenzymes that have regions of high homology surrounding the selenocysteine residue at the active site (Bianco and Larsen 2005). Interestingly, the deiodinases differ in tissue distribution, substrate specificities, catalytic profile, physiological functions and regulation. Of the three deiodinating enzymes, only D2 and D3 have been identified in the placenta (Koopdonk-Kool et al. 1996). Placental D3 activity is much greater (~200 times in first trimester and ~400 times at term) than D2 activity, however the activity and expression of both D2 and D3 falls as gestation progresses (Chan, et al. 2003; Koopdonk-Kool et al. 1996; Stulp, et al. 1998). D2 is an outer ring deiodinase (Nelson, et al.) found primarily in brain, pituitary, brown adipose tissue, thyroid and placenta with a preference for $T_4 > rT_3$ as a substrate (Figure 1). D2 converts the biologically inactive T_4 to the active T_3. Conversely, D3 catalyses inner ring deiodination (IRD) of T_4 and T_3 and is mainly present in placenta, brain and skin with T_3 being the preferred substrate over T_4 (Figure 1) (Gereben, et al. 2008). D3 inactivates T_3 to T_2 or T_4 to rT_3. T_2 and rT_3 were previously considered inactive metabolites because they do not bind TH receptors, however more recently rT_3 has been implicated in actin polymerisation (Farwell, et al. 2005) and T_2 in stimulation of mitochondrial respiration (O'Reilly and Murphy 1992).

D2 and D3 have been found to be present in the placenta throughout gestation (Chan et al. 2003). D2 has been localised to the villous cytotrophoblasts cells in the first trimester with expression in villous syncytiotrophoblasts (ST) variable and weak. In contrast, D3 has been localised to the villous ST cells and syncytial sprouts with expression in villous CTs focal and weak. In the third trimester villous ST expressed D2 and D3, whilst villous CTs were stronger for D2 than D3 (Chan et al. 2003). The localisation of the deiodinases suggests that they may regulate the amount of maternal TH reaching fetal circulation. D3 localised to the villous ST layer, which is in direct contact with the maternal circulation can protect the fetus from excessive maternal TH.

3.2 Placental TH membrane transporters

TH membrane transporters mediate cellular uptake and efflux of TH (Hennemann, et al. 2001; Visser, et al. 2008). Trophoblast membrane transport of TH was first reported in 1992 by Mitchell et al, using the human placenta choriocarcinoma cell line, JAR (Mitchell et al.

1992). Since this time significant findings in placental TH transporters have been made. TH transporters identified in the human placenta to date include the monocarboxylate transporters MCT8 (Chan, et al. 2006) & MCT10 (Friesema, et al. 2008), L-type amino acid transporters LAT1 (Okamoto, et al. 2002) and LAT2 (Park, et al. 2005) and organic anion transporting polypeptides OATP1A2 (Patel, et al. 2003) and OATP4A1 (Patel et al. 2003) (Sato, et al. 2003). However, their individual contribution to placental TH transport has yet to be elucidated.

3.2.1 MCT8 & MCT10

Freisema et al identified MCT8 as a TH transporter with a preference for T_3 over T_4 (Friesema, et al. 2003). Both MCT8 and MCT10 mRNAs have been identified in placenta however it is only recently that both mRNAs were identified in early human placenta (from 6 weeks gestation) and both increased in expression throughout pregnancy (Loubiere, et al. 2010). Immunohistochemical studies have localised MCT8 and MCT10 proteins to villous ST, CT and extra villous trophoblasts (EVTs) in first trimester placental tissue, with marked immunostaining of MCT10 in the CT layer (Chan et al. 2006; Loubiere et al. 2010). Both proteins localised to villous STs in term placental tissue.

3.2.2 OATP1A2 & OATP4A1

The expression of OATP1A2 and OATP4A1 in placenta and their ability to mediate transport of T_4, T_3 and rT_3 have implicated both proteins as TH transport mechanisms in the placenta (Patel et al. 2003; Sato et al. 2003). RT-PCR analysis revealed OATP1A2 mRNA increases in human placental tissue throughout gestation, whilst OATP4A1 decreases to mid-gestation followed by an increase towards term. Western blotting results suggest no significant change in both proteins throughout gestation.

OATP1A2 and OATP4A1 proteins have been localised to villous STs in the first trimester with OATP1A2 also found moderately strong in villous CT and extra villous trophoblasts (EVTs). In term tissue both proteins revealed diffuse, weak expression, with OATP4A1 preferentially localised to the apical surface in STs (Loubiere et al. 2010; Sato et al. 2003).

3.2.3 LAT1 & LAT2

LAT1 protein has been localised to the ST layer in placenta and LAT2 to the apical and basal membranes of ST at term (Hoeltzli and Smith 1989; Lewis, et al. 2007; Okamoto et al. 2002; Ritchie and Taylor 2001). Localisation of the proteins throughout gestation has yet to be elucidated. A more recent study of LAT1 mRNA expression in human placenta revealed that it increases with gestation, whilst LAT2 did not alter.

Considering in the first trimester STs are in direct contact with maternal blood, MCT8, OATP4A1 and LAT1 may be the key transporters for TH uptake from the maternal circulation as they are preferentially localised to the apical membrane of STs (Chan et al. 2006; Ritchie and Taylor 2001; Sato et al. 2003), whilst OATP4A1 and LAT2 may play more prominent roles later in gestation. TH membrane transporters in the placenta most likely act in concert to regulate the passage of TH transported from the maternal to the fetal circulation throughout gestation.

3.3 Placental TH binding proteins

Thyroid hormone is extremely hydrophobic and carried in serum bound to three hepatically secreted binding proteins, thyroxine binding globulin (TBG), transthyretin (TTR) and albumin (Schussler 2000). Previously our group has described the synthesis of the TH binding proteins TTR and albumin by human placenta (McKinnon, et al. 2005).

3.3.1 Transthyretin (TTR)

Studies have reported high levels of TTR in fetal serum as early as 13 wks gestation (Fryer, et al. 1993) and considering little TTR mRNA is detectable in fetal liver at this time (Jacobsson 1989) we propose that the fetal TTR present may be of placental origin. Using placental explants and the choriocarcinoma cell line JEG3, we demonstrated that TTR was not only synthesised (McKinnon et al. 2005) but also secreted mainly through the apical cell membrane of these cells (Landers, et al. 2009).

We have also shown internalisation of TTR by placental explants and JEG3 cells which increased in the presence of T_4 (Landers et al. 2009). This increased internalization occurred under TTR: T4 ratios that favoured TTR tetramer formation (Landers et al. 2009) Similar increases have been described in astrocytoma cells (Divino and Schussler 1990b). Cross-linking studies of TTR bound to ^{125}I-T_4 suggest that TTR-T_4 is internalised by JEG3 cells as a TTR-T_4 complex. However, further research is required to confirm this finding and elucidate the mechanisms by which TTR or TTR-T_4 is internalised by the placenta. The protective role of TTR was postulated when binding of TTR to T_4 in placental cytosol was inhibited by addition of mefanamic acid, resulting in an increase in T_4 deiodination as determined by HPLC (McKinnon et al. 2005). The exact mechanisms of this are yet to be confirmed. TTR internalisation has previously been observed in ependymoma cells (Kuchler-Bopp, et al. 2000), chicken oocytes (Vieira, et al. 1995) and kidney proximal tubules (Sousa, et al. 2000) via megalin-mediated endocytosis. Receptor-mediated uptake of TTR was first described in HepG2 cells, primary rat hepatocytes, renal adenocarcinoma cells, neuroblastoma and transformed lung cells (Divino and Schussler 1990a). Similarly apical secretion of TTR has been described in the choroid plexus (Dickson 1986) and retinal pigment epithelium (Jaworowski, et al. 1995). Apical secretion of TTR by trophoblast cells into what would be the maternal circulation would increase local serum TTR concentrations at the surface of trophoblast cells. We propose that this would result in increased binding of maternal T_4 to placental TTR where TTR may serve to protect T_4 from deiodination and deliver T_4 or the TTR-T_4 complex to trophoblast cells of the placenta for eventual delivery to fetal circulation.

Many chemicals, including a variety of environmental pollutants, bind to TTR and displace T_4. These agents can cross the placenta and interfere with fetal thyroid function (Koopman-Esseboom, et al. 1994). Their role in interfering with TTR TH transfer is however yet to be investigated.

3.3.2 Albumin

There is an abundance of albumin during human pregnancy that comes into direct contact with the trophoblast cell layer. Early studies have demonstrated that maternal albumin is internalised by placental explants and in the syncytiotrophoblast layer the protein is either apically recycled into the maternal circulation or degraded (Lambot, et al. 2006). The exact role albumin plays at the trophoblast surface remains unclear and requires further investigation particularly in first trimester tissue and in the presence of TH. Furthermore, the fate of albumin synthesized by placenta (McKinnon et al. 2005) is also of interest as, like TTR, it may also play a protective role for TH and aid in the transport of TH to fetal circulation.

4. Placental regulation of Iodide transport

4.1 Iodide transporters

It has been long recognised that maternal iodide crosses the placenta to the fetal circulation (Logothetopoulos and Scott 1956). Two transporters carry out placental iodide transport from the maternal to the fetal circulation: the sodium-iodide symporter (NIS) and Pendrin. Both transporters were first described in thyroid (Dai et al. 1996) followed by placenta (Mitchell et al. 2001) and kidney (Spitzweg, et al. 2001). NIS is a membrane-bound glycoprotein and the fifth member of the solute carrier family (SLC5A5)(Dohan, et al. 2003). As its name suggests, NIS simultaneously takes up two Na+ and one I- ion from extracellular fluid (i.e. blood) into cells (Figure 4). This process is an active transport powered by the sodium gradient across the cell membrane generated by sodium potassium pumps, (Na+/K+ ATPase). Pendrin is an anion exchanger, encoded by the Pendred syndrome gene (PDS) (Manley et al. 2005; Royaux, et al. 2001; Scott and Karniski 2000) activated by high concentration of intracellular iodide (Yoshida, et al. 2004). Pendrin activity is dependent on NIS transporting iodide into the cells (Figure 4).

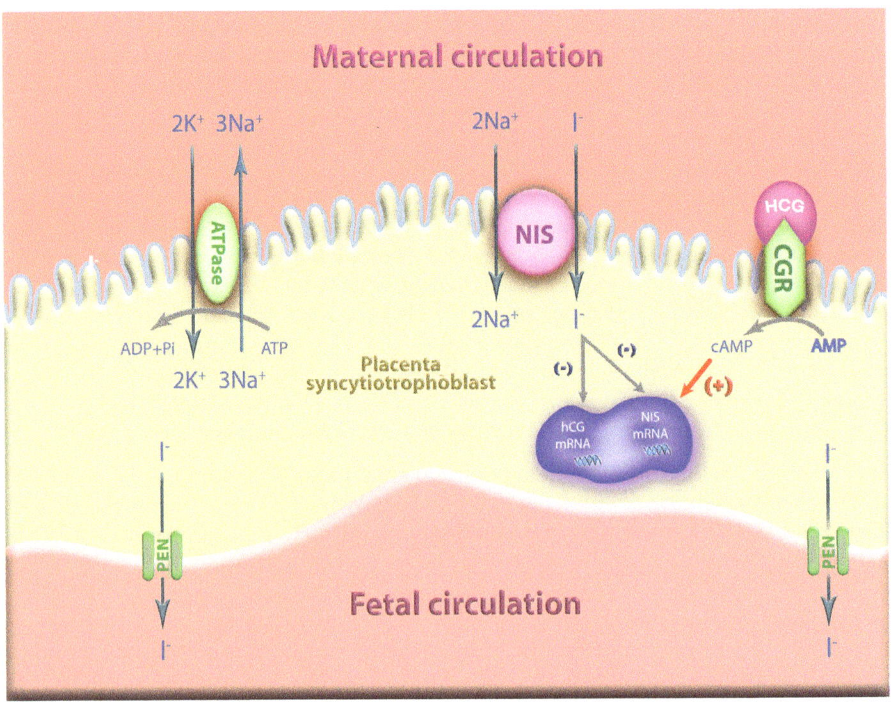

Fig. 4. Regulation of iodide transport across placental syncytiotrophoblast. NIS, sodium iodide symporter; PEN, Pendrin; hCG, human chorionic gonadotropin; CGR, chorionic gonadotropin receptor.

The physiological functions of these two transporters are similar in placenta and thyroid. In thyroid gland, NIS is localised at the basal membrane of thyrocytes and takes up iodide from the blood stream into the cells (Caillou, et al. 1998; Castro, et al. 1999; Dai et al. 1996; Royaux, et al. 2000; Yoshida, et al. 2002). Pendrin is expressed on the apical membrane of thyrocytes and releases iodide into thyroid follicles for TH synthesis (Dohan and Carrasco 2003; Mian, et al. 2001; Spitzweg, et al. 2000). In placenta, NIS is localised to the apical membrane (maternal side) of syncytiotrophoblasts, which directly contacts with maternal blood and influxes iodide into the cells (Figure 4). Conversely, Pendrin is located in the basal membrane (fetal side) of syncytiotrophoblasts and effluxes iodide into the extracellular space (Bidart et al. 2000; Manley et al. 2005; Mitchell et al. 2001). Mutations of NIS have been found in patients previously found to have congenital hypothyroidism due to an iodide transport defect. Some of these NIS mutations have been confirmed to cause failure of membrane targeting (Kosugi, et al. 1999; Kosugi, et al. 1998; Matsuda and Kosugi 1997; Pohlenz, et al. 2000). Pendred syndrome, a recessively inherited disorder causing congenital deafness and thyroid goitre is caused by a genetic defect in the PDS gene (Everett, et al. 1997; Kopp, et al. 1999; Royaux et al. 2000; Taylor, et al. 2002).

4.2 Cell model for study of placental iodide transport

During development of the human placenta, cytotrophoblasts fuse to form multinucleated syncytiotrophoblasts that form the surface of the placental villi and are directly bathed in maternal blood. Syncytiotrophoblast cells conduct maternal-fetal nutrient and gas exchange and have a distinct endocrine function to produce and secrete pregnancy hormones such as hCG and placental lactogen. BeWo cells are a human trophoblast-derived choriocarcinoma cell line that shares many features with primary trophoblasts in culture. They form a well-differentiated monolayer, undergo syncytialization and, secrete hCG (Bode, et al. 2006; Liu, et al. 1997; Sullivan 2004). They have been used widely in placental transport studies, e.g. glucose (Antony, et al. 2007; Araujo, et al. 2008; Baumann, et al. 2007; Di Simone, et al. 2009; Mark and Waddell 2006), amino acid (Jones, et al. 2006a, b; Novak, et al. 2006), iron (Danzeisen and McArdle 1998; Gambling, et al. 2001), fatty acid (Johnsen, et al. 2009; Tobin, et al. 2009), and drug and toxicity studies (Araujo, et al. 2009; Hirano, et al. 2008; Magnarin, et al. 2008; Prouillac, et al. 2009). BeWo cells express both of the iodide transporters, NIS and Pendrin (Manley et al. 2005). NIS proteins are located in the apical membrane of polarized BeWo cells while Pendrin is located to the basolateral membrane. BeWo cells demonstrate significant uptake and efflux of iodide, with kinetic and inhibitory characteristics consistent with these transporters (Li, et al. 2007; Manley et al. 2005). The human JAr placental choriocarcinoma cell line has also been used in iodide transport studies but radio-labelled iodide (I^{125}) uptake was dependent on the presence of exogenous hCG in the culture medium (Arturi, et al. 2002a) limiting their use in many studies. The JEG-3 cell line also expresses both NIS and Pendrin, however JEG-3 cells do not take up measureable amounts of I^{125}, even after hCG treatment, since the NIS protein is not localized to the apical membrane (unpublished observation). Primary trophoblasts and placental explant cultures might appear to be the ideal model for iodide transport studies, but due to variations in sample quality and low NIS expression their use is limited. Clearly, BeWo cells possess the physiological properties required and are the best cell model for studies of iodide transport.

4.3 Regulation of placental iodide transport

In thyroid follicular cells, NIS is regulated by serum levels of the pituitary derived TSH (Ajjan, et al. 1998; Kogai, et al. 1997; Saito, et al. 1997). However, unlike thyroid, placental syncytiotrophoblasts not only express NIS but also produce hCG. NIS expression and iodide uptake is increased in Jar cells exposed to hCG, and withdrawing hCG from the culture medium, leads to decreased NIS expression and iodide uptake (Arturi et al. 2002a). In BeWo cells NIS mRNA and membrane protein is up-regulated by hCG, and is accompanied by increased levels of iodide uptake (Li et al. 2007). Clearly hCG is an important regulator of placental iodide transport. In thyroid, hCG can stimulate NIS expression, subsequently increasing iodide uptake and TH synthesis and secretion (Arturi, et al. 2002b; Kraiem, et al. 1994).

An inhibitory effect of excess iodide on iodide organification in the normal thyroid (Wolff-Chaikoff effect) was reported by Wolff and Chaikoff in 1949 (Wolff, et al. 1949). Following the discovery of NIS, persuasive evidence suggested that the inhibitory effect of iodide is associated with a decrease in NIS mRNA and protein levels, subsequently reducing iodide transport to the thyroid (Eng, et al. 1999; Eng PH 2001; Glatt, et al. 2005). In iodine deficient rats, NIS mRNA is up regulated in fetal thyroid, as well as in the placenta (Schroder-van der Elst, et al. 2001). In BeWo cells iodide also caused a significant decrease in NIS mRNA and apical membrane protein, followed by a decrease in levels of iodide uptake (Li et al. 2007). These studies suggest that self-regulation of iodide uptake by intracellular iodide occurs in thyroid and placenta. In BeWo cells, iodide decreases hCG mRNA expression and protein secretion. Interestingly cord blood TH levels in neonates of mothers with moderate iodine deficiency and hypothyroxinemia are significantly higher than maternal levels (Glinoer 1997; Glinoer, et al. 1992). Although no measurements of serum inorganic iodine concentrations were made in these cases it is tempting to hypothesise that in the face of moderate maternal iodide deficiency up-regulated placental NIS expression and increased materno-fetal placental iodide transport may allow the fetus to maintain normal TH levels. Excessive maternal iodide intake may, on the other hand, down-regulate NIS expression in placenta and reduce iodide transport to the fetus.

5. Importance of oxygen in placental thyroid hormone and iodide transport

5.1 Changes in placental oxygen concentration through gestation

The adaptive processes of the developing placenta have long been studied demonstrating that under rapid physiological changes specific genes and associated proteins are affected, leading to altered nutrient, hormone and waste exchange between the mother and fetus. Many of these physiological changes relate to changing oxygen concentrations in the placenta that relate to placental vascularisation by the end of the first trimester of pregnancy. In the first trimester, EVT cells invade into the decidua, occluding uterine spiral arteries (Jauniaux, et al. 2003). This restricts blood flow into the intervillous space (IVS) resulting in a low oxygen environment that is essential for placental and embryonic development (Burton, et al. 1999; Genbacev, et al. 1997; Huppertz and Peeters 2005; Osol and Mandala 2009). Measurements with oxygen sensitive probes during ultrasonography at 8 weeks gestation have established that the oxygen concentration within the IVS is <20 mmHg or 3-5% O_2 (Rodesch, et al. 1992). Oxygen concentrations within the underlying maternal decidua are approximately 60 mmHg or 8-10% O_2. Between weeks 11-12 of gestation, uterine spiral arterioles become patent, allowing significant maternal blood flow and increasing oxygen levels (Carter 2009; Jauniaux, et al. 2000; Rodesch et al. 1992). Recent in vitro studies have demonstrated the capacity of EVTs to initiate apoptosis of vascular smooth muscle cells (VSMC) and endothelial cells. This may represent the mechanism of the physiological modification of the uterine spiral arterioles that leads to the increased vascular compliance and circumference of early pregnancy (Ashton, et al. 2005; Harris, et al. 2006; Moffett-King 2002; Zygmunt, et al. 2003). The resulting increased blood flow and growth of the vascular and capillary network meets the demands of the growing fetus (Burton 2009).

Many placental transport processes are regulated by low oxygen levels, including hormonal, glucose, amino acid (system A - a sodium dependant transport process of amino acids) and iodide transporters. Here we describe potential placental adaptations to T_4 uptake through regulation of TTR expression and iodide uptake through regulation of the NIS cell membrane transporter.

5.2 Low oxygen in the placenta and NIS expression and function

As described earlier, placental iodide transport to the developing fetus is essential to allow the fetal thyroid to produce TH from about week 12 of gestation. We have demonstrated down regulation of mRNA and protein expression of the NIS transporter in human BeWo placental cells cultured at 1% oxygen in comparison to controls cultured at 8% oxygen (Li, et al. 2011). A significant reduction in iodide uptake in cells cultured at low oxygen was also observed (Li et al. 2011). This suggests that the increasing oxygenation of the placenta at about 12 weeks gestation may up regulate NIS expression leading to increased iodide transport at a time when the developing fetal thyroid requires maternal iodide. hCG expression measured in the same study mirrored the expression of NIS. hCG regulates Pax8, an essential protein that must bind to the NIS promoter and enhancer region to up regulate NIS transcription (Schmitt, et al. 2001). This highlights the complexity of placental NIS expression, with oxygen concentrations and hormonal expression both playing a role in NIS regulation.

5.3 Low oxygen, the placenta and transthyretin (TTR) expression and function

As described above, the low oxygen environment within the placenta clearly regulates a number of important genes including those related to specific transport processes. Recently, our group demonstrated that low oxygen levels up-regulate expression, secretion and re-uptake of TTR (Patel, et al. 2010a). Human placental JEG-3 and primary trophoblast cells cultured under low oxygen conditions (1-3% O_2), showed an increase in TTR mRNA and protein expression. Using fluorescent and ^{125}I labelled TTR, increased up-take into trophoblast cells was observed using the same low oxygen culture conditions. The uptake studies were conducted in the presence of excess T_4 which causes TTR tetramerisation, a process that appears critical for significant TTR uptake by cells (Landers et al. 2009). This study was the first to demonstrate physiological regulation of trophoblast TTR uptake. Although speculative at this stage, this could suggest increased transplacental delivery of thyroxine (T_4) during the first trimester of pregnancy, when fetal requirement for maternal T_4 is higher (as detailed earlier in this chapter) and when a physiological low oxygen environment is present.

Increased concentrations of placental TTR protein have been demonstrated in patients with preeclampsia (Gharesi-Fard, et al. 2010). This increased TTR expression probably relates to placental hypoxia, which is common in pre-eclampsia, but further investigation of TTR in the cause and/or diagnosis of pre-eclampsia is warranted.

6. Conclusion

Adequate supplies of maternal TH and iodide are essential for normal fetal brain development, with TH critical in the first trimester and iodide from the second trimester on. It is increasingly apparent that even very mildly reduced maternal T_4 levels may impair the offspring's neuro-cognitive function. Impaired maternal thyroid function from iodine deficiency or autoimmune thyroid disease is common and may represent a major public health issue. The mechanisms underlying materno-fetal transport of iodide and TH are slowly being unravelled. NIS and Pendrin mediate iodide transfer in placenta, as they do in the thyroid gland. HCG, iodide and placental oxygen levels regulate placental NIS. NIS transport is blocked by thiocyanate, a component of tobacco smoke, which may exacerbate marginal iodide deficiency in smoking mothers.

TH transfer appears to involve trophoblast membrane TH transporters but the important role of placental TTR requires further evaluation. There is increasing evidence that placental TTR participates in a shuttle in which TTR secreted by the apical trophoblast membrane is taken up by the trophoblast. This shuttle appears to be involved in TH transfer but whether this is by carriage of TH across the placenta, delivery of TH to the membrane transporters or both is as yet unclear. The low placental oxygen level of early pregnancy up regulates both TTR expression and reuptake. Many agents interfere with T_4 binding to TTR and impair fetal thyroid function but a role in interfering with placental transfer of TH is yet to be studied. Placental D3, which converts T_4 to the biologically inactive rT_3, is an important modulator of TH transfer. The interaction of TTR, if any, with the deiodinase requires investigation.

Lastly, TTR is up regulated in placentas of women with pre-eclampsia. While this may be the effect of placental hypoxia, which is prevalent in this condition, its role as a marker of pre-eclampsia deserves further attention.

7. Acknowledgements

We would like to thank Mimi Kersting for help with preparing figures.

8. References

Ajjan RA, Kamaruddin NA, Crisp M, Watson PF, Ludgate M & Weetman AP 1998 Regulation and tissue distribution of the human sodium iodide symporter gene. *Clin Endocrinol (Oxf)* 49 517-523.

Andersson M, de Benoist B & Rogers L 2010 Epidemiology of iodine deficiency: Salt iodisation and iodine status. *Best Pract Res Clin Endocrinol Metab* 24 1-11.

Antony N, Bass JJ, McMahon CD & Mitchell MD 2007 Myostatin regulates glucose uptake in BeWo cells. *Am J Physiol Endocrinol Metab* 293 E1296-1302.

Araujo JR, Goncalves P & Martel F 2008 Modulation of glucose uptake in a human choriocarcinoma cell line (BeWo) by dietary bioactive compounds and drugs of abuse. *J Biochem* 144 177-186.

Araujo JR, Goncalves P & Martel F 2009 Effect of cannabinoids upon the uptake of folic acid by BeWo cells. *Pharmacology* 83 170-176.

Arturi F, Lacroix L, Presta I, Scarpelli D, Caillou B, Schlumberger M, Russo D, Bidart JM & Filetti S 2002a Regulation by human chorionic gonadotropin of sodium/iodide symporter gene expression in the JAr human choriocarcinoma cell line. *Endocrinology* 143 2216-2220.

Arturi F, Presta I, Scarpelli D, Bidart JM, Schlumberger M, Filetti S & Russo D 2002b Stimulation of iodide uptake by human chorionic gonadotropin in FRTL-5 cells: effects on sodium/iodide symporter gene and protein expression. *Eur J Endocrinol* 147 655-661.

Ashton SV, Whitley GS, Dash PR, Wareing M, Crocker IP, Baker PN & Cartwright JE 2005 Uterine spiral artery remodeling involves endothelial apoptosis induced by extravillous trophoblasts through Fas/FasL interactions. *Arterioscler Thromb Vasc Biol* 25 102-108.

Baumann MU, Zamudio S & Illsley NP 2007 Hypoxic upregulation of glucose transporters in BeWo choriocarcinoma cells is mediated by hypoxia-inducible factor-1. *Am J Physiol Cell Physiol* 293 C477-485.

Benvenga S 2005 Thyroid hormone transport proteins and the physiology of hormone binding. In *The Thyroid; A Fundamental and Clinical Text,* pp 97 - 108. Ed U Braverman L.E., R.D. Philadelphia: Lippincott Williams and Wilkins.

Berbel P, Mestre JL, Santamaria A, Palazon I, Franco A, Graells M, Gonzalez-Torga A & de Escobar GM 2009 Delayed neurobehavioral development in children born to pregnant women with mild hypothyroxinemia during the first month of gestation: the importance of early iodine supplementation. *Thyroid* 19 511-519.

Bernal J & Pekonen F 1984 Ontogenesis of the nuclear 3,5,3'-triiodothyronine receptor in the human fetal brain. *Endocrinology* 114 677-679.

Bianco AC & Larsen PR 2005 Cellular and structural biology of the deiodinases. *Thyroid* 15 777-786.

Bianco AC, Salvatore D, Gereben B, Berry MJ & Larsen PR 2002 Biochemistry, cellular and molecular biology, and physiological roles of the iodothyronine selenodeiodinases. *Endocr Rev* 23 38-89.

Bidart JM, Lacroix L, Evain-Brion D, Caillou B, Lazar V, Frydman R, Bellet D, Filetti S & Schlumberger M 2000 Expression of Na+/I- symporter and Pendred syndrome genes in trophoblast cells. *J Clin Endocrinol Metab* 85 4367-4372.

Bode CJ, Jin H, Rytting E, Silverstein PS, Young AM & Audus KL 2006 In vitro models for studying trophoblast transcellular transport. *Methods Mol Med* 122 225-239.

Burton GJ 2009 Oxygen, the Janus gas; its effects on human placental development and function. *J Anat* 215 27-35.

Burton GJ, Jauniaux E & Watson AL 1999 Maternal arterial connections to the placental intervillous space during the first trimester of human pregnancy: the Boyd collection revisited. *Am J Obstet Gynecol* 181 718-724.

Caillou B, Troalen F, Baudin E, Talbot M, Filetti S, Schlumberger M & Bidart JM 1998 Na+/I- symporter distribution in human thyroid tissues: an immunohistochemical study. *J Clin Endocrinol Metab* 83 4102-4106.

Calvo RM, Jauniaux E, Gulbis B, Asuncion M, Gervy C, Contempre B & Morreale de Escobar G 2002 Fetal tissues are exposed to biologically relevant free thyroxine concentrations during early phases of development. *J Clin Endocrinol Metab* 87 1768-1777.

Carter AM 2009 Evolution of factors affecting placental oxygen transfer. *Placenta* 30 Suppl A S19-25.

Castro MR, Bergert ER, Beito TG, McIver B, Goellner JR & Morris JC 1999 Development of monoclonal antibodies against the human sodium iodide symporter: immunohistochemical characterization of this protein in thyroid cells. *J Clin Endocrinol Metab* 84 2957-2962.

Chan S, Kachilele S, Hobbs E, Bulmer JN, Boelaert K, McCabe CJ, Driver PM, Bradwell AR, Kester M, Visser TJ, et al. 2003 Placental iodothyronine deiodinase expression in normal and growth-restricted human pregnancies. *J Clin Endocrinol Metab* 88 4488-4495.

Chan S, Kachilele S, McCabe CJ, Tannahill LA, Boelaert K, Gittoes NJ, Visser TJ, Franklyn JA & Kilby MD 2002 Early expression of thyroid hormone deiodinases and receptors in human fetal cerebral cortex. *Brain Res Dev Brain Res* 138 109-116.

Chan SY, Franklyn JA, Pemberton HN, Bulmer JN, Visser TJ, McCabe CJ & Kilby MD 2006 Monocarboxylate transporter 8 expression in the human placenta: the effects of severe intrauterine growth restriction. *J Endocrinol* 189 465-471.

Chopra IJ 1996 Nature, Source and Relative Significance of Circulating Thyroid Hormones. In *Werner and Ingbar's The Thyroid*, pp 111-124. Ed U Braverman L.E., R.D. Philadelphia: Lippincott Williams.

Chopra IJ, Sack J & Fisher DA 1975 3,3',5'-Triiodothyronine (reverse T3) and 3,3',5-triiodothyronine (T3) in fetal and adult sheep: studies of metabolic clearance rates, production rates, serum binding, and thyroidal content relative to thyroxine. *Endocrinology* 97 1080-1088.

Contempre B JE, Calvo R, Jurkovic D, Campbell S, de Escobar GM 1993. *Journal of Clinical Endocrinology and Metabolism* 77 1719-1722.

Dai G, Levy O & Carrasco N 1996 Cloning and characterization of the thyroid iodide transporter. *Nature* 379 458-460.

Danzeisen R & McArdle HJ 1998 Copper and iron interactions in a placental cell line (BeWo). *Biochem Soc Trans* 26 S99.

de Carvalho FD & Quick M 2011 Surprising substrate versatility in SLC5A6: Na+-coupled I- transport by the human Na+/multivitamin transporter (hSMVT). *J Biol Chem* 286 131-137.

Di Simone N, Di Nicuolo F, Marzioni D, Castellucci M, Sanguinetti M, D'Lppolito S & Caruso A 2009 Resistin modulates glucose uptake and glucose transporter-1 (GLUT-1) expression in trophoblast cells. *J Cell Mol Med* 13 388-397.

Dickson PW AA, Marley PD, Bannister D, Schreiber G 1986 Rat choroid plexus specializes in the synthesis and the secretion of transthyretin (prealbumin). Regulation of transthyretin synthesis in choroid plexus is independent from that in liver. *The Journal of Biological Chemistry* 261 3475-3478.

Divino CM & Schussler GC 1990a Receptor-mediated uptake and internalization of transthyretin. *J Biol Chem* 265 1425-1429.

Divino CM & Schussler GC 1990b Transthyretin receptors on human astrocytoma cells. *J Clin Endocrinol Metab* 71 1265-1268.

Dohan O & Carrasco N 2003 Advances in Na(+)/I(-) symporter (NIS) research in the thyroid and beyond. *Mol Cell Endocrinol* 213 59-70.

Dohan O, De la Vieja A, Paroder V, Riedel C, Artani M, Reed M, Ginter CS & Carrasco N 2003 The sodium/iodide Symporter (NIS): characterization, regulation, and medical significance. *Endocr Rev* 24 48-77.

Eng PH, Cardona GR, Fang SL, Previti M, Alex S, Carrasco N, Chin WW & Braverman LE 1999 Escape from the acute Wolff-Chaikoff effect is associated with a decrease in thyroid sodium/iodide symporter messenger ribonucleic acid and protein. *Endocrinology* 140 3404-3410.

Eng PH CG, Previti MC, Chin WW, Braverman LE 2001. *European Journal of Endocrinology* 144 139-144.

Evans RM 1988 The steroid and thyroid hormone receptor superfamily. *Science* 240 889-895.

Everett LA, Glaser B, Beck JC, Idol JR, Buchs A, Heyman M, Adawi F, Hazani E, Nassir E, Baxevanis AD, et al. 1997 Pendred syndrome is caused by mutations in a putative sulphate transporter gene (PDS). *Nat Genet* 17 411-422.

Farwell AP, Dubord-Tomasetti SA, Pietrzykowski AZ, Stachelek SJ & Leonard JL 2005 Regulation of cerebellar neuronal migration and neurite outgrowth by thyroxine and 3,3',5'-triiodothyronine. *Brain Res Dev Brain Res* 154 121-135.

Fisher DA 1983 Maternal-fetal thyroid function in pregnancy. *Clin Perinatol* 10 615-626.

Friesema EC, Ganguly S, Abdalla A, Manning Fox JE, Halestrap AP & Visser TJ 2003 Identification of monocarboxylate transporter 8 as a specific thyroid hormone transporter. *J Biol Chem* 278 40128-40135.

Friesema EC, Jansen J, Jachtenberg JW, Visser WE, Kester MH & Visser TJ 2008 Effective cellular uptake and efflux of thyroid hormone by human monocarboxylate transporter 10. *Mol Endocrinol* 22 1357-1369.

Fryer AA, Jones P, Strange R, Hume R & Bell JE 1993 Plasma protein levels in normal human fetuses: 13 to 41 weeks' gestation. *Br J Obstet Gynaecol* 100 850-855.

Fuse Y 1996 Development of the hypothalamic-pituitary-thyroid axis in humans. *Reprod Fertil Dev* 8 1-21.

Gambling L, Danzeisen R, Gair S, Lea RG, Charania Z, Solanky N, Joory KD, Srai SK & McArdle HJ 2001 Effect of iron deficiency on placental transfer of iron and expression of iron transport proteins in vivo and in vitro. *Biochem J* 356 883-889.

Genbacev O, Zhou Y, Ludlow JW & Fisher SJ 1997 Regulation of human placental development by oxygen tension. *Science* 277 1669-1672.

Gereben B, Zavacki AM, Ribich S, Kim BW, Huang SA, Simonides WS, Zeold A & Bianco AC 2008 Cellular and molecular basis of deiodinase-regulated thyroid hormone signaling. *Endocr Rev* 29 898-938.

Gershengorn MC, Geras E, Marcus-Samuels BE & Rebecchi MJ 1979 Receptor affinity and biological potency of thyroid hormones in thyrotropic cells. *Am J Physiol* 237 E142-146.

Gersten J 1954 The transfer of radioiodine across placenta and breast. *The Ohio Journal of Science* 54 161.

Gharesi-Fard B, Zolghadri J & Kamali-Sarvestani E 2010 Proteome differences of placenta between pre-eclampsia and normal pregnancy. *Placenta* 31 121-125.

Ghassabian A, Bongers-Schokking JJ, Henrichs J, Jaddoe VW, Visser TJ, Visser W, SM DEMK-S, Hooijkaas H, Steegers EA, Hofman A, et al. 2011 Maternal thyroid function during pregnancy and behavioral problems in the offspring: the generation R study. *Pediatr Res* 69 454-459.

Glatt CM, Ouyang M, Welsh W, Green JW, Connor JO, Frame SR, Everds NE, Poindexter G, Snajdr S & Delker DA 2005 Molecular characterization of thyroid toxicity: anchoring gene expression profiles to biochemical and pathologic end points. *Environ Health Perspect* 113 1354-1361.

Glinoer D 1997 The regulation of thyroid function in pregnancy: pathways of endocrine adaptation from physiology to pathology. *Endocr Rev* 18 404-433.

Glinoer D, Delange F, Laboureur I, de Nayer P, Lejeune B, Kinthaert J & Bourdoux P 1992 Maternal and neonatal thyroid function at birth in an area of marginally low iodine intake. *J Clin Endocrinol Metab* 75 800-805.

Gross J & Leblond CP 1951 The presence of free iodinated compounds in the thyroid and their passage into the circulation. *Endocrinology* 48 714-725.

Haddow JE PG, Allan WC, Williams JR, Knight GJ, Gagnon J, O'Heir CE, Mitchell ML, Hermos RJ, Waisbren SE, Faix JD, Klein RZ 1999. *New England Journal of Medicine* 341 549-555.

Harris LK, Keogh RJ, Wareing M, Baker PN, Cartwright JE, Aplin JD & Whitley GS 2006 Invasive trophoblasts stimulate vascular smooth muscle cell apoptosis by a fas ligand-dependent mechanism. *Am J Pathol* 169 1863-1874.

Hennemann G, Docter R, Friesema EC, de Jong M, Krenning EP & Visser TJ 2001 Plasma membrane transport of thyroid hormones and its role in thyroid hormone metabolism and bioavailability. *Endocr Rev* 22 451-476.

Hirano T, Yasuda S, Osaka Y, Asari M, Kobayashi M, Itagaki S & Iseki K 2008 The inhibitory effects of fluoroquinolones on L-carnitine transport in placental cell line BeWo. *Int J Pharm* 351 113-118.

Hoeltzli SD & Smith CH 1989 Alanine transport systems in isolated basal plasma membrane of human placenta. *Am J Physiol* 256 C630-637.

Huppertz B & Peeters LL 2005 Vascular biology in implantation and placentation. *Angiogenesis* 8 157-167.

Jacobsson B 1989 Localization of transthyretin-mRNA and of immunoreactive transthyretin in the human fetus. *Virchows Arch A Pathol Anat Histopathol* 415 259-263.

Jauniaux E, Gulbis B & Burton GJ 2003 The human first trimester gestational sac limits rather than facilitates oxygen transfer to the foetus--a review. *Placenta* 24 Suppl A S86-93.

Jauniaux E, Watson AL, Hempstock J, Bao YP, Skepper JN & Burton GJ 2000 Onset of maternal arterial blood flow and placental oxidative stress. A possible factor in human early pregnancy failure. *Am J Pathol* 157 2111-2122.

Jaworowski A, Fang Z, Khong TF & Augusteyn RC 1995 Protein synthesis and secretion by cultured retinal pigment epithelia. *Biochim Biophys Acta* 1245 121-129.

Johnsen GM, Weedon-Fekjaer MS, Tobin KA, Staff AC & Duttaroy AK 2009 Long-chain polyunsaturated fatty acids stimulate cellular fatty acid uptake in human placental choriocarcinoma (BeWo) cells. *Placenta* 30 1037-1044.

Jones HN, Ashworth CJ, Page KR & McArdle HJ 2006a Cortisol stimulates system A amino acid transport and SNAT2 expression in a human placental cell line (BeWo). *Am J Physiol Endocrinol Metab* 291 E596-603.

Jones HN, Ashworth CJ, Page KR & McArdle HJ 2006b Expression and adaptive regulation of amino acid transport system A in a placental cell line under amino acid restriction. *Reproduction* 131 951-960.

Klein RZ, Sargent JD, Larsen PR, Waisbren SE, Haddow JE & Mitchell ML 2001 Relation of severity of maternal hypothyroidism to cognitive development of offspring. *J Med Screen* 8 18-20.

Kogai T, Endo T, Saito T, Miyazaki A, Kawaguchi A & Onaya T 1997 Regulation by thyroid-stimulating hormone of sodium/iodide symporter gene expression and protein levels in FRTL-5 cells. *Endocrinology* 138 2227-2232.

Kooistra L, Crawford S, van Baar AL, Brouwers EP & Pop VJ 2006 Neonatal effects of maternal hypothyroxinemia during early pregnancy. *Pediatrics* 117 161-167.

Koopdonk-Kool JM, de Vijlder JJ, Veenboer GJ, Ris-Stalpers C, Kok JH, Vulsma T, Boer K & Visser TJ 1996 Type II and type III deiodinase activity in human placenta as a function of gestational age. *J Clin Endocrinol Metab* 81 2154-2158.

Koopman-Esseboom C, Morse DC, Weisglas-Kuperus N, Lutkeschipholt IJ, Van der Paauw CG, Tuinstra LG, Brouwer A & Sauer PJ 1994 Effects of dioxins and polychlorinated biphenyls on thyroid hormone status of pregnant women and their infants. *Pediatr Res* 36 468-473.

Kopp P, Arseven OK, Sabacan L, Kotlar T, Dupuis J, Cavaliere H, Santos CL, Jameson JL & Medeiros-Neto G 1999 Phenocopies for deafness and goiter development in a large inbred Brazilian kindred with Pendred's syndrome associated with a novel mutation in the PDS gene. *J Clin Endocrinol Metab* 84 336-341.

Kosugi S, Bhayana S & Dean HJ 1999 A novel mutation in the sodium/iodide symporter gene in the largest family with iodide transport defect. *J Clin Endocrinol Metab* 84 3248-3253.

Kosugi S, Sato Y, Matsuda A, Ohyama Y, Fujieda K, Inomata H, Kameya T, Isozaki O & Jhiang SM 1998 High prevalence of T354P sodium/iodide symporter gene mutation in Japanese patients with iodide transport defect who have heterogeneous clinical pictures. *J Clin Endocrinol Metab* 83 4123-4129.

Kraiem Z, Sadeh O, Blithe DL & Nisula BC 1994 Human chorionic gonadotropin stimulates thyroid hormone secretion, iodide uptake, organification, and adenosine 3',5'-monophosphate formation in cultured human thyrocytes. *J Clin Endocrinol Metab* 79 595-599.

Kuchler-Bopp S, Dietrich JB, Zaepfel M & Delaunoy JP 2000 Receptor-mediated endocytosis of transthyretin by ependymoma cells. *Brain Res* 870 185-194.

Lambot N, Lybaert P, Boom A, Delogne-Desnoeck J, Vanbellinghen AM, Graff G, Lebrun P & Meuris S 2006 Evidence for a clathrin-mediated recycling of albumin in human term placenta. *Biol Reprod* 75 90-97.

Landers KA, McKinnon BD, Li H, Subramaniam VN, Mortimer RH & Richard K 2009 Carrier-mediated thyroid hormone transport into placenta by placental transthyretin. *J Clin Endocrinol Metab* 94 2610-2616.

Lazarus JH 2005 Thyroid disorders associated with pregnancy: etiology, diagnosis, and management. *Treat Endocrinol* 4 31-41.

Levy O, Dai G, Riedel C, Ginter CS, Paul EM, Lebowitz AN & Carrasco N 1997 Characterization of the thyroid Na+/I- symporter with an anti-COOH terminus antibody. *Proc Natl Acad Sci U S A* 94 5568-5573.

Lewis RM, Glazier J, Greenwood SL, Bennett EJ, Godfrey KM, Jackson AA, Sibley CP, Cameron IT & Hanson MA 2007 L-serine uptake by human placental microvillous membrane vesicles. *Placenta* 28 445-452.

Li H, Landers K, Patel J, Richard K & Mortimer RH 2011 Effect of oxygen concentrations on sodium iodide symporter expression and iodide uptake and hCG expression in human choriocarcinoma BeWo cells. *Am J Physiol Endocrinol Metab* 300 E1085-1091.

Li H, Richard K, McKinnon B & Mortimer RH 2007 Effect of Iodide on Human Choriogonadotropin, Sodium-Iodide Symporter Expression, and Iodide Uptake in BeWo Choriocarcinoma Cells. *J Clin Endocrinol Metab* 92 4046-4051.

Li Y, Shan Z, Teng W, Yu X, Fan C, Teng X, Guo R, Wang H, Li J, Chen Y, et al. 2010 Abnormalities of maternal thyroid function during pregnancy affect neuropsychological development of their children at 25-30 months. *Clin Endocrinol (Oxf)* 72 825-829.

Liu F, Soares MJ & Audus KL 1997 Permeability properties of monolayers of the human trophoblast cell line BeWo. *Am J Physiol* 273 C1596-1604.

Logothetopoulos J & Scott RF 1955 Concentration of iodine-131 across the placenta of the guinea pig and the rabbit. *Nature* 175 775-776.

Logothetopoulos J & Scott RF 1956 Active iodide transport across the placenta of the guinea-pig, rabbit and rat. *J Physiol* 132 365-371.

Loubiere LS, Vasilopoulou E, Bulmer JN, Taylor PM, Stieger B, Verrey F, McCabe CJ, Franklyn JA, Kilby MD & Chan SY 2010 Expression of thyroid hormone transporters in the human placenta and changes associated with intrauterine growth restriction. *Placenta* 31 295-304.

Magnarin M, Rosati A, De Iudicibus S, Bartoli F & Decorti G 2008 Role of ABC Transporters in the BeWo Trophoblast Cell Line. *Toxicol Mech Methods* 18 763-769.

Man EB, Brown JF & Serunian SA 1991 Maternal hypothyroxinemia: psychoneurological deficits of progeny. *Ann Clin Lab Sci* 21 227-239.

Manley SW, Li H & Mortimer RH 2005 The BeWo choriocarcinoma cell line as a model of iodide transport by placenta. *Placenta* 26 380-386.

Mark PJ & Waddell BJ 2006 P-glycoprotein restricts access of cortisol and dexamethasone to the glucocorticoid receptor in placental BeWo cells. *Endocrinology* 147 5147-5152.

Matsuda A & Kosugi S 1997 A homozygous missense mutation of the sodium/iodide symporter gene causing iodide transport defect. *J Clin Endocrinol Metab* 82 3966-3971.

McKinnon B, Li H, Richard K & Mortimer R 2005 Synthesis of thyroid hormone binding proteins transthyretin and albumin by human trophoblast. *J Clin Endocrinol Metab* 90 6714-6720.

Mian C, Lacroix L, Alzieu L, Nocera M, Talbot M, Bidart JM, Schlumberger M & Caillou B 2001 Sodium iodide symporter and pendrin expression in human thyroid tissues. *Thyroid* 11 825-830.

Mitchell AM, Manley SW, Morris JC, Powell KA, Bergert ER & Mortimer RH 2001 Sodium iodide symporter (NIS) gene expression in human placenta. *Placenta* 22 256-258.

Mitchell AM, Manley SW & Mortimer RH 1992 Membrane transport of thyroid hormone in the human choriocarcinoma cell line, JAR. *Mol Cell Endocrinol* 87 139-145.

Moffett-King A 2002 Natural killer cells and pregnancy. *Nat Rev Immunol* 2 656-663.

Mortimer RH, Galligan JP, Cannell GR, Addison RS & Roberts MS 1996 Maternal to fetal thyroxine transmission in the human term placenta is limited by inner ring deiodination. *J Clin Endocrinol Metab* 81 2247-2249.

Nelson HS, Oppenheimer J, Buchmeier A, Kordash TR & Freshwater LL 1996 An assessment of the role of intradermal skin testing in the diagnosis of clinically relevant allergy to timothy grass. *J Allergy Clin Immunol* 97 1193-1201.

Novak D, Quiggle F & Haafiz A 2006 Impact of forskolin and amino acid depletion upon System A activity and SNAT expression in BeWo cells. *Biochimie* 88 39-44.

O'Reilly I & Murphy MP 1992 Studies on the rapid stimulation of mitochondrial respiration by thyroid hormones. *Acta Endocrinol (Copenh)* 127 542-546.

Okamoto Y, Sakata M, Ogura K, Yamamoto T, Yamaguchi M, Tasaka K, Kurachi H, Tsurudome M & Murata Y 2002 Expression and regulation of 4F2hc and hLAT1 in human trophoblasts. *Am J Physiol Cell Physiol* 282 C196-204.

Oppenheimer JH, Koerner D, Schwartz HL & Surks MI 1972 Specific nuclear triiodothyronine binding sites in rat liver and kidney. *J Clin Endocrinol Metab* 35 330-333.

Osol G & Mandala M 2009 Maternal uterine vascular remodeling during pregnancy. *Physiology (Bethesda)* 24 58-71.

Park SY, Kim JK, Kim IJ, Choi BK, Jung KY, Lee S, Park KJ, Chairoungdua A, Kanai Y, Endou H, et al. 2005 Reabsorption of neutral amino acids mediated by amino acid transporter LAT2 and TAT1 in the basolateral membrane of proximal tubule. *Arch Pharm Res* 28 421-432.

Patel J, Landers K, Li H, Mortimer RH & Richard K 2010a Oxygen concentration regulates expression and uptake of transthyretin, a thyroxine binding protein, in JEG-3 choriocarcinoma cells. *Placenta* 32 128-133.

Patel J, Landers K, Li H, Mortimer RH & Richard K 2011 Thyroid hormones and fetal neurological development. *J Endocrinol* 209 1-8.

Patel J, Landers K, Mortimer RH & Richard K 2010b Regulation of hypoxia inducible factors (HIF) in hypoxia and normoxia during placental development. *Placenta* 31 951-957.

Patel P, Weerasekera N, Hitchins M, Boyd CA, Johnston DG & Williamson C 2003 Semi quantitative expression analysis of MDR3, FIC1, BSEP, OATP-A, OATP-C,OATP-D, OATP-E and NTCP gene transcripts in 1st and 3rd trimester human placenta. *Placenta* 24 39-44.

Pharoah PO & Connolly KJ 1991 Relationship between maternal thyroxine levels during pregnancy and memory function in childhood. *Early Hum Dev* 25 43-51.

Pohlenz J, Duprez L, Weiss RE, Vassart G, Refetoff S & Costagliola S 2000 Failure of membrane targeting causes the functional defect of two mutant sodium iodide symporters. *J Clin Endocrinol Metab* 85 2366-2369.

Pop VJ, Kuijpens JL, van Baar AL, Verkerk G, van Son MM, de Vijlder JJ, Vulsma T, Wiersinga WM, Drexhage HA & Vader HL 1999 Low maternal free thyroxine concentrations during early pregnancy are associated with impaired psychomotor development in infancy. *Clin Endocrinol (Oxf)* 50 149-155.

Prouillac C, Videmann B, Mazallon M & Lecoeur S 2009 Induction of cells differentiation and ABC transporters expression by a myco-estrogen, zearalenone, in human choriocarcinoma cell line (BeWo). *Toxicology* 263 100-107.

Raiti S, Holzman GB, Scott RL & Blizzard RM 1967 Evidence for the placental transfer of tri-iodothyronine in human beings. *N Engl J Med* 277 456-459.

Ritchie JW & Taylor PM 2001 Role of the System L permease LAT1 in amino acid and iodothyronine transport in placenta. *Biochem J* 356 719-725.

Rodesch F, Simon P, Donner C & Jauniaux E 1992 Oxygen measurements in endometrial and trophoblastic tissues during early pregnancy. *Obstet Gynecol* 80 283-285.

Royaux IE, Suzuki K, Mori A, Katoh R, Everett LA, Kohn LD & Green ED 2000 Pendrin, the protein encoded by the Pendred syndrome gene (PDS), is an apical porter of iodide in the thyroid and is regulated by thyroglobulin in FRTL-5 cells. *Endocrinology* 141 839-845.

Royaux IE, Wall SM, Karniski LP, Everett LA, Suzuki K, Knepper MA & Green ED 2001 Pendrin, encoded by the Pendred syndrome gene, resides in the apical region of renal intercalated cells and mediates bicarbonate secretion. *Proc Natl Acad Sci U S A* 98 4221-4226.

Saito T, Endo T, Kawaguchi A, Ikeda M, Nakazato M, Kogai T & Onaya T 1997 Increased expression of the Na+/I- symporter in cultured human thyroid cells exposed to thyrotropin and in Graves' thyroid tissue. *J Clin Endocrinol Metab* 82 3331-3336.

Samuels HH & Tsai JS 1973 Thyroid hormone action in cell culture: domonstration of nuclear receptors in intact cells and isolated nuclei. *Proc Natl Acad Sci U S A* 70 3488-3492.

Sap J, Munoz A, Damm K, Goldberg Y, Ghysdael J, Leutz A, Beug H & Vennstrom B 1986 The c-erb-A protein is a high-affinity receptor for thyroid hormone. *Nature* 324 635-640.

Sato K, Sugawara J, Sato T, Mizutamari H, Suzuki T, Ito A, Mikkaichi T, Onogawa T, Tanemoto M, Unno M, et al. 2003 Expression of organic anion transporting polypeptide E (OATP-E) in human placenta. *Placenta* 24 144-148.

Schmitt TL, Espinoza CR & Loos U 2001 Transcriptional regulation of the human sodium/iodide symporter gene by Pax8 and TTF-1. *Exp Clin Endocrinol Diabetes* 109 27-31.

Schroder-van der Elst JP, van der Heide D, Kastelijn J, Rousset B & Obregon MJ 2001 The expression of the sodium/iodide symporter is up-regulated in the thyroid of fetuses of iodine-deficient rats. *Endocrinology* 142 3736-3741.

Schussler GC 2000 The thyroxine-binding proteins. *Thyroid* 10 141-149.

Scott DA & Karniski LP 2000 Human pendrin expressed in Xenopus laevis oocytes mediates chloride/formate exchange. *Am J Physiol Cell Physiol* 278 C207-211.

Shupnik MA, Chin WW, Habener JF & Ridgway EC 1985 Transcriptional regulation of the thyrotropin subunit genes by thyroid hormone. *J Biol Chem* 260 2900-2903.
Shupnik MA, Greenspan SL & Ridgway EC 1986 Transcriptional regulation of thyrotropin subunit genes by thyrotropin-releasing hormone and dopamine in pituitary cell culture. *J Biol Chem* 261 12675-12679.
Sousa MM, Norden AG, Jacobsen C, Willnow TE, Christensen EI, Thakker RV, Verroust PJ, Moestrup SK & Saraiva MJ 2000 Evidence for the role of megalin in renal uptake of transthyretin. *J Biol Chem* 275 38176-38181.
Spitzweg C, Dutton CM, Castro MR, Bergert ER, Goellner JR, Heufelder AE & Morris JC 2001 Expression of the sodium iodide symporter in human kidney. *Kidney Int* 59 1013-1023.
Spitzweg C, Heufelder AE & Morris JC 2000 Thyroid iodine transport. *Thyroid* 10 321-330.
Stulp MR, de Vijlder JJ & Ris-Stalpers C 1998 Placental iodothyronine deiodinase III and II ratios, mRNA expression compared to enzyme activity. *Mol Cell Endocrinol* 142 67-73.
Sullivan MH 2004 Endocrine cell lines from the placenta. *Mol Cell Endocrinol* 228 103-119.
Tata JR & Widnell CC 1966 Ribonucleic acid synthesis during the early action of thyroid hormones. *Biochem J* 98 604-620.
Taylor JP, Metcalfe RA, Watson PF, Weetman AP & Trembath RC 2002 Mutations of the PDS gene, encoding pendrin, are associated with protein mislocalization and loss of iodide efflux: implications for thyroid dysfunction in Pendred syndrome. *J Clin Endocrinol Metab* 87 1778-1784.
Tobin KA, Johnsen GM, Staff AC & Duttaroy AK 2009 Long-chain polyunsaturated fatty acid transport across human placental choriocarcinoma (BeWo) cells. *Placenta* 30 41-47.
Vermiglio F, Lo Presti VP, Moleti M, Sidoti M, Tortorella G, Scaffidi G, Castagna MG, Mattina F, Violi MA, Crisa A, et al. 2004 Attention deficit and hyperactivity disorders in the offspring of mothers exposed to mild-moderate iodine deficiency: a possible novel iodine deficiency disorder in developed countries. *J Clin Endocrinol Metab* 89 6054-6060.
Vieira AV, Sanders EJ & Schneider WJ 1995 Transport of serum transthyretin into chicken oocytes. A receptor-mediated mechanism. *J Biol Chem* 270 2952-2956.
Visser TJ 1994 Role of sulfation in thyroid hormone metabolism. *Chem Biol Interact* 92 293-303.
Visser WE, Friesema EC, Jansen J & Visser TJ 2008 Thyroid hormone transport in and out of cells. *Trends Endocrinol Metab* 19 50-56.
Vulsma T, Gons MH & de Vijlder JJ 1989 Maternal-fetal transfer of thyroxine in congenital hypothyroidism due to a total organification defect or thyroid agenesis. *N Engl J Med* 321 13-16.
Weeke J, Hansen AP & Lundaek K 1975 Inhibition by somatostatin of basal levels of serum thyrotropin (TSH) in normal men. *J Clin Endocrinol Metab* 41 168-171.
Weinberger C, Thompson CC, Ong ES, Lebo R, Gruol DJ & Evans RM 1986 The c-erb-A gene encodes a thyroid hormone receptor. *Nature* 324 641-646.
Wolff J, Chaikoff IL & et al. 1949 The temporary nature of the inhibitory action of excess iodine on organic iodine synthesis in the normal thyroid. *Endocrinology* 45 504-513, illust.

Yoshida A, Hisatome I, Taniguchi S, Sasaki N, Yamamoto Y, Miake J, Fukui H, Shimizu H, Okamura T, Okura T, et al. 2004 Mechanism of iodide/chloride exchange by pendrin. *Endocrinology* 145 4301-4308.

Yoshida A, Taniguchi S, Hisatome I, Royaux IE, Green ED, Kohn LD & Suzuki K 2002 Pendrin is an iodide-specific apical porter responsible for iodide efflux from thyroid cells. *J Clin Endocrinol Metab* 87 3356-3361.

Zygmunt M, Herr F, Munstedt K, Lang U & Liang OD 2003 Angiogenesis and vasculogenesis in pregnancy. *Eur J Obstet Gynecol Reprod Biol* 110 Suppl 1 S10-18.

16

ABC Transporters in Human Placenta and Their Role in Maternal-Fetal Cholesterol Transfer: ABCA1 Candidate Target

Jayonta Bhattacharjee[1,2], Francesca Ietta[1], Roberta Romagnoli[1], Nicoletta Bechi[1], Isabella Caniggia[2] and Luana Paulesu[1]
[1]*Department of Physiology, University of Siena, Siena,*
[2]*Samuel Lunenfeld Research Institute, Mount Sinai Hospital, Toronto,*
[1]*Italy*
[2]*Canada*

1. Introduction

Placenta is the highly specialized organ of pregnancy, in association with the fetal membranes and amniotic fluids; placenta supports normal fetal growth and development. Primary function of the placenta in all species is to selective transfer of nutrients and waste products between mother and fetus. It participates in the transfer and metabolism of carbohydrates, amino acids, lipids, water, inorganic ions, minerals and vitamins. Respiratory gases also transfer between mother and fetus through placenta. Another important function of placenta is the endocrine function. Adequate nutrient transfer by placenta between mother and fetus during pregnancy is crucial for proper fetal growth and development. Among all nutrients, cholesterol is important as well for proper fetal growth. Embryo and fetal growth phase is the rapid cellular proliferative stage. In this phase, cells differentiate into various cell types. That's why; cells need all the substrates for their proper growth. As long as cells are proliferating, the important cellular structure such as membrane is also vital for the proliferative cells. One of the principal and key components of cell membrane is cholesterol. Cholesterol maintains membrane fluidity and lipid rich microdomain. Any alteration of cellular cholesterol content may lead to diverse complication in different metabolic processes. Cholesterol is the precursor of bile acids, steroid hormones and metabolic regulators such as oxysterols.

Cholesterol is also essential for both activation and propagation of Hedgehog signaling. Sonic Hedgehog (SHH) is responsible for patterning and development of the central nervous system (Porter et al., 1996; Martì & Bovolenta, 2002; Cooper et al., 2003). There are two routes by which cholesterol is available to the fetus, *de novo* synthesis and exogenous source. It has been believed that cholesterol required by the fetus is synthesized by *de novo* cholesterol synthesis by the fetus itself. The individual lacking *de novo* cholesterol synthesis may develop lethal congenital birth defects (Kelley, 2000; Herman, 2003). Convincing evidence shows that maternal cholesterol is a source of fetal cholesterol (Napoli et al., 1997; McConihay et al., 2001). *In vivo* studies in murine and *in vitro* assays using the choriocarcinoma cell line, BeWo have demonstrated that cholesterol is transported across the trophoblast cells (Schmid et al., 2003; Yoshida & Wada, 2005). ATP-Binding cassette transporter A1 (ABCA1) and ABCG1 are two important transporter involved in cellular cholesterol homeostasis. Recent studies have demonstrated the expression and localization of ABCA1 and ABCG1 in human placenta (Bhattacharjee et al., 2010; Stefulj et al., 2009). Functional involvement of these two transporters in maternal and fetal cholesterol transfer has not been elucidated till now. In this chapter, we will discuss the present knowledge of ABC transporters in human placenta and role of ATP binding cassette transporter A1 (ABCA1) and G1 (ABCG1) on maternal-fetal cholesterol transfer and metabolism through placenta.

2. Sources of fetal cholesterol

Cholesterol is obligatory for all tissues and cells to maintain normal structure and function. The rapidly growing tissues need a significant amount of cholesterol to maintain their cell membrane cholesterol unit, the structural unit of cell membrane. The embryo and fetus are continuously growing and increasing their mass more rapidly compared with adult tissues. In this growth phase, cholesterol, including all other nutrients are crucial for proper development. Cholesterol is available to the tissues by *de novo* synthesis and from exogenous source (i.e. from circulation/diet). It is available to the circulation mainly from diet. The fetal circulation receives maternal circulating cholesterol through placenta. Considering number of evidences show that fetus gets circulation from maternal cholesterol along with its own *de novo* synthesis (Napoli et al., 1997; McConihay et al., 2001). Fetal development includes two different period of growth one is from fertilization to eight week of gestation (embryo) and another is from ninth week of gestation to birth (fetus). At early development, blastocyst is formed by outer layer of trophoblast cells, which invade the endometrium and inner cell mass, and develops into embryo. During this period, maternal blood and remnants of cells digested from trophoblast invasion, immerse the conceptus is an important source of cholesterol (Woollett LA, 2008). Along with the progression of gestation, maternal blood flows into the lacunae of the uterus and forms uteroplacental circulation. The spiral arteries remain plugged in early gestation thus approximately between fourth and eight week of gestation, only small amount of maternal blood leak into the lacunae or intervillous space of the placenta (Burton et al., 1999; Hustin & Schaaps, 1987). At that period, intervillous space contains uterine gland secretion and tiny amount of maternal blood. The uterine glands secrete nutrients, including lipids, to the intervillous space as well (Burton et al., 2002; Hempstock et al., 2004). Thus intervillous space comprises maternal blood containing cholesterol-carrying lipoproteins, and uterine gland secretions, such as lipids and presumably cholesterol. The nutrients would be taken up by syncytiotrophoblasts, will exit through the basolateral side, and diffuse along the stromal channels to the extracoelomic cavity (Woollett, 2008). In an elegant review, Woollett (2008) has discussed the possible source of fetal cholesterol. The Secondary Yolk Sac (SYC) is floating in extracoelomic cavity, the transport of maternally derived nutrients, possibly from the uterine gland secretions and from the maternal circulation, to the embryo occurs through SYC (Enders & King, 1993; Hopkins et al., 1987; Lanford et al., 1991; Perda et al., 1994; Shi et al., 1985). The need for nutrition increases with the progression of gestation and necessitate a more efficient method of nutrient exchange. Thus, the mode of transport of maternally derived nutrition to the fetus becomes primarily hemotrophic as gestation progresses and the placenta becomes the primary route of transport (Woollett, 2008). The spiral arteries are present from the fourth week of gestation but become functional from eighth week of gestation. When the spiral arteries start functioning, the maternal blood enters into the intervillous space and bathes the syncytiotrophoblasts of the chorionic villi. Maternal nutrients are taken up by the syncytiotrophoblasts by receptor-mediated as well as receptor-independent processes. Once taken up, nutrients cross cells and pass through or between endothelial cells to enter into the fetal circulation (Woollett, 2008). The maternal blood within the intervillous space exchanges three to four times per minute, thus it is an excellent source of nutrients (including cholesterol) for the developing fetus.

3. Routes of maternal-fetal cholesterol transfer

We already know from different observations that maternal cholesterol is a source of fetal cholesterol (Napoli et al., 1997; McConihay et al., 2001). *In vivo* studies in murine and *in vitro* assays using the choriocarcinoma cell line, BeWo have demonstrated that cholesterol is transported across the trophoblast cells (Schmid et al., 2003; Yoshida Wada, 2005). The uptake and utilization of cholesterol by trophoblast through very low density lipoprotein (VLDL) receptor, low density lipoprotein receptor-related protein (LRP), LDL receptor, and Scavenger Receptor B 1 (SR-B1) have been reported (Wadsack et al., 2003; Wyne & Woollett, 1998). Placenta is composed of different cell types, including trophoblasts, endothelial cells, fibroblasts, as well as blood cells in the intervillous space and fetal vessels. But the actual barrier between maternal and fetal circulation is made up of trophoblast cells. In order to acquire maternal cholesterol by the fetus, cholesterol must be taken through the apical side of the placental trophoblast cells and exit through the basolateral side of the trophoblast layer to enter into the fetal circulation. Experimental evidence suggests that trophoblasts efflux cholesterol from cells like any other polarized cells (Woollett, 2005). So far three different mechanisms for cholesterol efflux have been proposed namely aqueous diffusion and protein independent pathway based on concentration gradient, SR-B1 mediated efflux and ABCA1 mediated efflux (Rothblat et al., 1999; Yancey et al., 2003). Apparently all the processes may occur in placenta through the basolateral membrane of trophoblast layer as placenta possesses SR-B1 (Wadsack et al., 2003) and ABCA1 (Langmann et al., 1999). ABCA1 is one of the efflux transporters highly expressed in human placenta (Langmann et al., 1999). It performs cholesterol and phospholipids efflux to lipid poor Apolipoprotein A-1 (ApoA-1), precursor of high density lipoprotein.

4. ABC transporters

The human genome consists of a total of 49 Adenosine-Triphosphate-Binding Cassette (ABC) genes belonging to seven subfamilies named ABCA, ABCB, ABCC, ABCD, ABCE, ABCF and ABCG. The placenta serves an important role as protective barrier as wells as in normal fetal development, where ABC transporter plays significant role. ATP-Binding cassette (ABC) transporters perform role in the distribution of nutrients and exchange of metabolites across the placenta. Until now, a number of ATP Binding cassette transporters have been found in human placenta. These include multidrug resistance gene product 1 (MDR1/ABCB1), also known as P-glycoprotein (P-gp), multidrug resistance associated protein (MRPs), Breast Cancer Resistance Protein (BCRP/ABCG2), the Multidrug Resistance-Associated Proteins (MRPs/ABCC1-6 and 7-11) and efflux transporter ABCA1 and ABCG1 (Bhattacharjee et al., 2010; Young et al., 2003). Recently, along with ABCA1, ABCG1 has also been detected in cholesterol efflux activities in human placenta (Stefulj et al., 2009; Aye et al., 2010).

4.1 ATP Binding cassette transporter G1 (ABCG1)

ABCG1 is the transporter responsible for cellular cholesterol efflux. Unlike ABCA1, ABCG1 promotes efflux of cholesterol and oxysterols to HDL whereas ABCA1 predominantly efflux to ApoA1. ABCG1 is expressed both in fetal capillaries and in the syncytiotrophoblast of the placenta (Stefulj et al., 2009; Aye et al., 2010).

4.2 Breast cancer-resistance protein (BCRP)/ABCG2

Breast cancer resistance protein (BCRP) is an ATP dependent transporter also known as mitoxantrone resistance-associated protein (Allikmets et al., 1998) is highly expressed in the placenta, as well as in the uterus (Langmann et al., 2003) and is localized on the apical surface of the chorionic villi syncytiotrophoblast (Litman et al., 2002). The substrate specificity of BCRP has not been elucidated completely. There is considerable overlap of substrates between BCRP and P-gp (Cooray et al., 2002). These include a variety of anti-cancer agents, organic cations and lipophilic conjugates (Sarkadi et al., 2004). The role of BCRP in placenta is not yet known precisely, but from its structure and localization in the placenta, it is assumed that BCRP functions as protective structure in removing cytotoxic drugs from the fetal tissues.

4.3 P-glycoprotein (P-gp/MDR1/ABCB1)

P-glycoprotein (P-gp) is the first and best characterized ABC transporter to be identified so far (Juliano & Ling, 1976). P-gp is expressed in human placenta from first trimester to term (Tanabe et al., 2001). It is localized on the apical membrane of placental syncytiotrophoblasts where it is involved in the extrusion of drug substances from placenta. P-gp is involved with protection of the fetus from entry of harmful substances to the fetus (Lankas et al., 1998; Smit et al., 1999; Ushigome et al., 2000; Samtani et al., 2004). P-gp has an extremely broad substrate specify. It transports lipophilic drugs that are neutral or cationic belongs to diverse therapeutic categories including antimicrobials (e.g. rifampin), antivirals (e.g. anti-HIV protease inhibitors), anti-arrhythmic (e.g. verapamil) and anti-neoplastics (e.g. vincristine).

4.4 Multidrug resistance gene products 1 and 3 (MDR1, 3) / (ABCB1, ABCB4)

Multidrug resistance gene products are expressed in placenta both in messenger RNA and protein levels (MacFarland et al., 1994). MDR1/ABCB1 is located at the apical surface of the placental syncytiotrophoblast membrane, where it is responsible for the efflux of substrates from trophoblast into the maternal plasma (Litman et al., 2001; Keppler et al., 1998; Bera et al., 2001). These transports actively extrude different substrates from the cytoplasm including different drugs. Typical substrates of this transporter include some hydrophobic or slightly charged compounds. The hydrophobic/cationic conjugates and drugs include estradiol glucuronide, glucocorticoids, dexamethasone, verapamil, nifedipine, digoxin, paclitaxel, etoposide, vinblastine, doxorubicin, protease inhibitors, fexofenadine, methadone, phenytoin, cyclosporine A, lovastatin etc.

4.5 Multi-drug-resistance associated proteins (MRPs)

Multidrug resistance associated proteins (MRPs) are another family of ATP dependent efflux transporter. There are eight known MRPs so far, six of which have been fully sequenced (Borst et al., 2000). Their size and function vary greatly among the transporters. It is primarily speculated that MRPs appear to efflux polar compounds and conjugated metabolites in particular unconjugated bilirubin and bile acids (Borst et al., 2000; Bodó et al., 2003). Although there are some controversies about the cellular localization of different MRPs in human placenta, most of the MRPs (MRP1-6, and MRP7) have been found in human placenta (Langmann et al., 2003; Litman et al., 2001; Keppler et al., 1998; Bera et al., 2001; Ozvegy et al., 2001; Sato et al., 2003; Pascolo et al., 2003). MRPs proteins are associated with the removal of glutathione (GSH), glucuronide or sulphate conjugated metabolites from cells (Mathias et al., 2005; St-Pierre et al., 2002). It has also been reported that some unmodified toxins and drugs are transported by the MRP family (Keppler et al., 1998; Nagashige et al., 2003). The specific roles of MRPs in placenta have not been defined, but they perform efflux of polar conjugates xenobiotics or metabolites of endogenous compounds (Pascolo et al., 2003; Leazer & Klaassen, 2003).

4.6 ABCA1

ABCA1 is a 2,261-amino-acid integral membrane protein that comprises two halves of similar structure (Fitzgerald et al., 2001). Each half has a transmembrane domain containing six helices and a nucleotide binding domain (NBD) with two conserved peptide motifs known as Walker A and Walker B, which are present in many proteins that utilize ATP, and a Walker C signature unique to ABC transporters (Dean et al., 2001). ABCA1 is predicted to have an NH2 terminus oriented into the cytosol and two large extracellular loops that are highly glycosylated and linked by one or more cysteine bonds (Dean et al., 2001; Bungert et al., 2001).

4.6.1 ABCA1 in cellular cholesterol efflux and reverse cholesterol transport

Cholesterol is the integral part of eukaryotic membranes and the precursor of bile acids and of all the steroid hormones. In humans, approximately two thirds of cholesterol is transported by low-density lipoproteins (LDLs) and ~20% by high-density lipoproteins (HDLs); the remaining cholesterol is carried by very low density lipoprotein (VLDL) particles (Attie, 2007). The risk of premature cardiovascular disease is positively correlated with LDL levels and negatively correlated with HDL levels (Attie, 2007). HDL functions as cholesterol acceptor and promotes cholesterol efflux from cells. The ability of HDL to deliver cholesterol to the liver, where it can be secreted into bile and then excreted in the feces, completes a pathway that has been termed 'reverse cholesterol transport' (Attie, 2007). Although ABCA1 was identified as having role in macrophage engulfment of apoptotic cells, the special role of ABCA1 in cholesterol efflux was evident in the year 1999. At 1999, several authors published articles that identified ABCA1 gene mutation in two HDL- deficiency syndromes: familial hypoalphalipoproteinemia and Tangier disease (Rust et al., 1999; Lawn et al., 1999). Since, ABCA1's cholesterol efflux is Apolipoprotein A1 (ApoA1) dependent, ABCA1/ApoA1 association is very important for proper cholesterol efflux. The association of ABCA1 and ApoA1 is not clear enough. Some studies suggest that apoA-1 binds to ABCA1 directly (Oram et al., 2000; Wang et al., 2000; Fitzgerald et al., 2002), whereas some suggest ApoA-1 binding to the cell surface results in a relatively static complex (Smith et al., 2002). An alternative mechanism recently proposed by Chambenoit et al. (2001) saying ApoA-1 initially binds to a lipid domain formed by ABCA1 activity, the "tethered" apoA-1 can then diffuse within the plane of the membrane until contacting ABCA1 (Chambenoit et al. 2001). Regardless of the nature of its interaction with the cell, apoA-1 has been shown to selectively remove cholesterol that would otherwise be used by Acyl-CoA:cholesterol acyltransferase (ACAT) for esterification/storage (Li et al., 1997). It would stand to reason that an important function of ABCA1 is to promote removal of excess cellular cholesterol which would otherwise be esterified and potentially lead to "foam cell" formation in macrophages. Therefore, two different models have been proposed for the process of apolipoprotein lipidation by ABCA1. The first model suggests that apolipoproteins interact with ABCA1 at the cell surface and excess cellular cholesterol is transported to the plasma membrane by a vesicular mechanism, possibly packaged in the Golgi (Oram, 2003). The second model is based on evidence suggesting that ApoA1 and ABCA1 interact at the cell surface and then internalized where lipidation actually takes place in the lumen of an endosome from which the cholesterol is taken (Takahashi and Smith, 1999; Santamarina-Fojo et al., 2001). ABCA1 has been shown to recycle between the plasma membrane and the endosomal/lysosomal compartments (Neufeld et al., 2001). However, this recycling may be involved in the regulation of ABCA1 degradation rather than its function (Oram, 2003). It should also be considered that both models are correct and contribute in some way to pre-β HDL particle formation. There is some evidence that ABCA1 is actually a phospholipid "pump" or "floppase" instead of moving cholesterol itself. One study was able to pharmacologically uncouple phospholipid from cholesterol removal (Fielding et al., 2000). This finding has led to a hypothesis that ABCA1 lipidates ApoA1 with phospholipid only and the newly formed pre-β HDL obtains cholesterol by diffusional means from cholesterol-rich lipid rafts or caveolae in a "two-step" mechanism (Fielding et al., 2000; Wang et al., 2001). Others have found that ABCA1 does not use caveolae or lipid raft cholesterol (Mendez et al., 2001). Interestingly, one group did report that ABCA1 promotes cholesterol removal from "lubrol rafts" (defined by the authors as lipid rafts soluble in Triton-X, but insoluble in the detergent lubrol) (Drobnik et al., 2002). ABCA1 activity has also been shown to increase outer plasma membrane leaflet phosphatidylserine(PS) exposure-leading to speculation that PS may play a role in ApoA1 binding and lipidation (Hamon et al., 2000; Chambenoit et al. 2001) . This result was more closely examined and PS was found not to mediate apoA1 binding or cholesterol removal (Smith, 2002). The increase in PS exposure is likely a side effect of prolonged, increased ABCA1 expression which can damage cell membranes (Oram, 2003). Although ABCA1 may function as a phospholipid translocase, it is feasible that cholesterol is still able to be moved with the phospholipid (Oram, 2002). ABCA1 mediated transport of other molecules have been discovered including α- tocophenol (Oram et al., 2001), ApoE (Von Eckardstein et al., 2001), and interleukin-1β (Zhou et al., 2002). P-glycoprotein, a close relative of ABCA1, is predicted to have a central pore or pocket of 3 nm in diameter (Higgins et al., 1997). An opening of this size would allow many molecules to be transported together. Therefore, considering the variety of molecules transported by ABCA1, it can be envisioned that ABCA1 functions by transporting lipophilic molecules complexes with phospholipid including cholesterol (Oram, 2002). Indeed, using a transfected cell line with an inducible ABCA1 promoter revealed that a "two-step" cholesterol removal mechanism is unlikely (Vaughan &Oram, 2003).

4.6.2 ABCA1 in cellular apoptosis and proliferation

Hamon et al (2000) provided evidence that several cellular functions are controlled by ABC1 (now said ABCA1). Optimal engulfment of cell corpses generated by apoptosis is hampered by lack of ABC1 function and enhanced by it's over expression. Very recently, Yvan-Charvet et al (2010) showed ABCA1, ABCG1, and HDL inhibit the proliferation of hematopoietic stem and multipotential progenitor cells (HSPCs). They suggested the proliferation of HSPCs is regulated by cholesterol efflux mechanisms involving LXRs, ABCA1, ABCG1, and HDL (Yvan-Charvet et al., 2010). In the same article, Yvan-Charvet et al (2010) speculated that increased membrane cholesterol content secondary to ABC transporter deficiency results in increased cell-surface expression of the common β subunit of the IL-3/GM-CSF receptor that, in turn leads to increased downstream Ras/Erk signaling and increased proliferative response to IL-3 and GM-CSF. In mammalian cells, cholesterol, glycolipids, and proteins are organized in lipid rafts in the plasma membrane. ABCA1 and ABCG1 transport excess cholesterol from plasma membrane to form HDL. In HPSCs, growth factor receptors are organized in lipid rafts to promote receptor signaling and consequently, cell proliferation and migration (Giebel et al., 2004). As cholesterol overload can cause havoc in cells, its concentration is regulated by several mechanisms. Excess cholesterol is removed by ATP binding cassette (ABC) transporters in the plasma membrane, which move cholesterol to extracellular HDL particles at the cell surface (Tall, 2008). Recently it was shown in HSPC cells that when cholesterol is removed from this type of cells, the membrane raft disassemble, receptor signaling (such as through the IL-3 receptor) is hampered, and receptor dependent outcomes such as cell proliferation are reduced (Yvan-Charvet et al., 2010; Hansson &Björkholm, 2010).

4.6.3 ABCA1 in inflammation

Until now, we have seen the function of ABCA1 in cellular cholesterol efflux, cellular apoptosis, proliferation and reverse cholesterol transport and as an important target for atherosclerosis treatment (Tall, 2008; Schmitz & Grandl, 2008). Several recent studies showed that ABCA1 is also involved in inflammation and/or immune response. Studies with ABCA1 knockout mice demonstrated the relationship between ABCA1 and inflammation (Yvan-Charvet et al., 2008; Koseki et al., 2007; Schmitz et al., 1999; Aiello et al., 2003; Zhu et al., 2008; Francone et al., 2005; McNeish et al., 2000; Christiansen-Weber et al., 2000). Although the precise mechanism that ABCA1 plays a key role in modulating inflammatory response remains to be elucidated, several studies shown that the cholesterol export activity of ABCA1 could account for its potent anti-inflammatory properties (Koseki et al., 2007; Zhu et al., 2008; Murphy et al., 2008; Tellier et al., 2008). ABCA1 has been also reported in the regulated secretion of macrophage migration inhibitor factor (MIF) (Flieger et al., 2003). MIF is the pleiotropic multifactorial cytokine with a mostly proinflammatory spectrum of action in the host immune response. MIF is a critical mediator of a number of immune and inflammatory conditions (Calandra & Bucala, 1996; Mitchell & Bucala, 2000; Lue et al., 2002).

4.6.4 ABCA1 in placenta

The existence of ABCA1 in human placenta was first identified by Langmann and his team in mRNA levels in the year of 1999. Thereafter, it received more attention when it is known that maternal cholesterol is an important source of fetal cholesterol and Christiansen-Weber et al (2000) showed ABCA1 malfunction resulted in sever placental malformation, structural abnormalities, intrauterine growth restriction and increased neonatal death. Until now there are few publications showing ABCA1 expression and localization in human placenta. We showed the expression and localization of ABCA1 at both first trimester and term human placenta (Bhattacharjee et al., 2010).

Western blotting and real time PCR analysis showed that ABCA1 is expressed both in first trimester and term placenta and its expression does not differ between first trimester and term placenta both in protein and mRNA levels (Figure 1). We also showed the localization of ABCA1 by immunohistochemistry and immunofluorescent staining both in first trimester and term placental tissues (Figure 2). We found that ABCA1 is more predominantly localized at the basolateral and infrequently at the apical part of the cytotrophoblast cell layer of first trimester human placenta (Bhattacharjee et al., 2010). It was also localized in some other cell types of the placenta including stromal and endothelial cells of chorionic villi. In term placenta, the localization was observed in few villous cytotrophoblast and endothelial cells of the placental vasculature. Although, we found a very punctuate staining in the syncytial layer of the placenta some other researchers showed the expression of ABCA1 in the syncytial layer of placental epithelial layer. Different sampling variation and different antibodies might be responsible for not being exact results. In a nut shell, from the

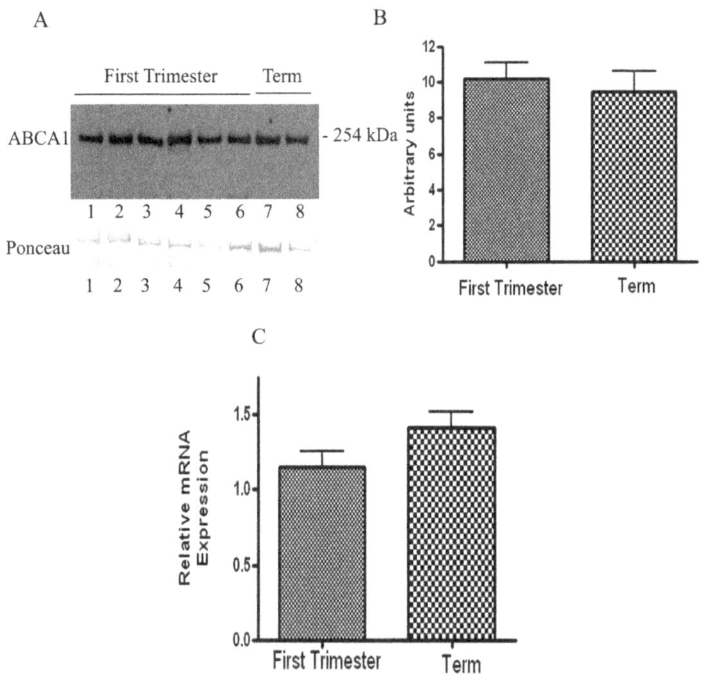

Fig. 1. Western blot and qRT-PCR analysis of ABCA1 in human placenta tissues. (A) Top, representative western blot analysis of ABCA1 protein at first trimester (lanes 1-6) and term human placenta (lanes 7-8) using mouse anti-human ABCA1 monoclonal antibody. Bottom, Membrane stained with ponceau S to assess total loaded protein in each lane. (B) The histogram represents densitometric measurement of western blot bands of first trimester and term placental tissues. (C) Quantification of ABCA1 mRNA in human placenta during the first trimester and term of gestation using qRT-PCR (Reproduced from Bhattacharjee et al., 2010 with the permission from Elsevier).

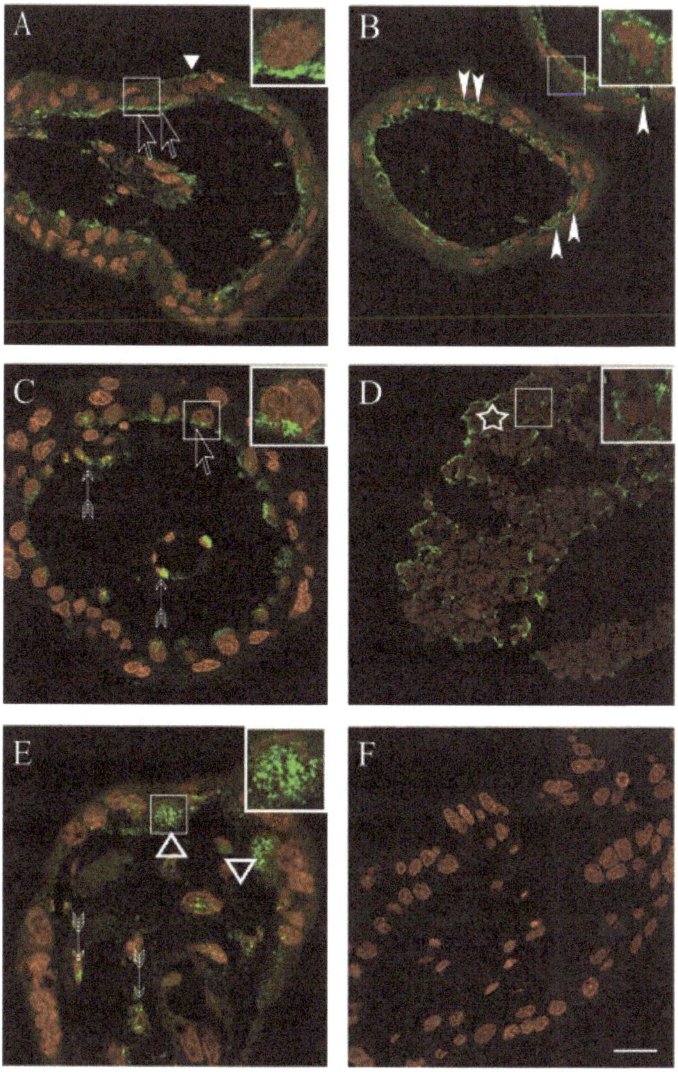

Fig. 2. Confocal laser scanning microscopic localization of ABCA1 using mouse anti-human ABCA1 monoclonal antibody in first trimester (A-D) and term (E) human placenta. Positive staining of ABCA1 is shown in green. Red staining represents nuclei (propidium iodide stained). In first trimester placenta, ABCA1 staining was found in the basolateral (windows pointers) and in the apical part (arrow heads) of villous cytotrophoblast cell membrane, rarely observed staining in syncytial brush border (triangle) and in endothelial cells (arrows) of the villous core (A-C). (D) ABCA1 positive staining in the cell membrane of most extravillous cytotrophoblast cells (star frame). In term placenta (E), diffuse ABCA1 positive staining in the cytotrophoblast cells (triangle frame). (F) Negative control in first trimester placenta. Inserts show the higher magnification of the selected part. Scale bar= 20 mm for all the images (Reproduced from Bhattacharjee et al., 2010 with the permission from Elsevier).

studies till now, it is evident that ABCA1 is expressed both in cytotrophoblast and syncytiotrophoblast layer of the placental along with hofbauer cells and endothetial cells of the placenta. These finding together support the role of ABCA 1 in feto-placental transport function. The different localization of ABCA1 in different cells types may have different functions, which remains to be elucidated.

In term placental tissues, ABCA1 is present in cytotrophoblast cells but diffuse in the whole cell without any specific localization. Some staining in the term placental cytotrophoblast cells suggests it to be in intracellular endocytic compartment. ABCA1 is actually a membrane transporter although its expression in the intracellular endocytic compartment has also been reported in different cell types (Hamon et al., 2000; Cooper et al., 2003)

4.6.5 Role of ABCA1 in Cholesterol transfer through human placenta

As placenta is the vital organ and a site for nutrient and waste exchange between mother and fetus, placental transport and metabolism of cholesterol and lipids are critical for the fetal development and its survival. Cholesterol is an integral part of cell membranes, precursor of steroid hormones such as progesterone and metabolic mediators such as oxysterol (Woollett, 2005). Cholesterol is essential for both activation and propagation of Hedgehog signaling (SHH), responsible for patterning and development of the central nervous system (Porter et al., 1996; Marti & Bovolenta, 2002; Cooper et al., 2003). There are two routes by which cholesterol is available to the fetus, the *de novo* synthesis and exogenous source. The individual lacking *de novo* cholesterol synthesis may develop lethal congenital birth defects (Kelley, 2000; Herman, 2003).

Dysfunction of ABCA1 in mice resulted in severe placental malformation with structural abnormalities, intrauterine growth retardation and increased neonatal death (Christiansen-Weber et al., 2000). Reduced expression of placental ABCA1 was observed in women with antiphospholipid syndrome (Albrecht et al., 2007) and ABCA1 was reported as a potential target for *in utero* therapy of Smith-Lemli-Opitz syndrome (Lindegaard et al., 2008). Recently, Stefulj et al. (2009) demonstrated the presence of ABCA1 in endothelial cells of term placenta and its involvement in cholesterol transfer towards fetal circulation. However, no information is available on the regulation of ABCA1 expression and its functions in human placenta.

By using florescent tagged cholesterol in first trimester placental explants as an *ex-vivo* model, we found that ABCA1 is significantly involved in cholesterol efflux in human placenta explants (Unpublished observation). Further functional studies are required to explore the role of ABCA1 in maternal fetal cholesterol transfer and metabolism. Recently, there are few studies showed that silencing of ABCA1 and pharmacological inhibition of ABCA1 by glyburide decreased cholesterol efflux to Apolipoprotein A-1 in cultured primary trophoblast cells (ApoA-1) (Aye et al., 2010). On the other hand they also showed that endogenous receptor induction by synthetic LXR α/β inducer have increased ABCA1 and enhanced cholesterol efflux to ApoA-1 (Aye et al., 2010).

Two mechanisms have been suggested to explain ABCA1-mediated cholesterol efflux to apoA-1 (Takahashi & Smith, 1999; Oram et al., 1991; Chen et al., 2001). The apoA-1 forms complexes with phospholipid and cholesterol at the cell surface in a process promoted by ABCA1 activity (Chen et al., 2001). Alternatively, apoA1 binds ABCA1 at the cell surface and the complex is subsequently internalized and targeted to late endosomes, where apoA1 picks up lipids. The apolipoprotein-ABCA1-lipid complexes are then resecreted from the cell by exocytosis (Chen et al., 2001). Azuma et al. (2009) have shown that apoA-1 internalizes inside the cell and colocalizes with the cell surface-derived ABCA1 on endosomal compartment contributing to HDL formation when excess lipoprotein-derived cholesterol has accumulated in cells.

Thus in light of our results we can speculate that at term of gestation, the pathway involving the internalization of apoA1/ABCA1 complex might prevail on the other one operating possibly at first trimester.

During the first trimester of pregnancy cholesterol is crucially important for both fetal and placenta development (Napoli et al., 1997). Along with *de novo* cholesterol synthesis, fetal plasma cholesterol concentration is significantly correlated with the maternal one and the significance is greatest in the fetuses that are less than 6 months old (Woollett, 2001) suggesting maternal cholesterol supply is crucially important during the earlier phases of development.

Although it is believed that maternal cholesterol level is correlated with fetal cholesterol , still now no direct evidence exists about the maternal cholesterol entrance through the placenta nor cholesterol trafficking and efflux by ABCA1 in human first trimester placenta. By using a chorioncarcinoma cell line Schmid et al (2003) have shown the ability of placental cells to transport maternal derived cholesterol. In the same study the ABCA1 mediated cholesterol efflux was not apparent, and despite multiple manipulations to up-regulate the expression of ABCA1, there was no increase of cholesterol efflux to exogenous apoA1.

Significant involvement of ABCA1 in cholesterol efflux at the maternal fetal interface has been recently demonstrated by several studies on endothelial and cytotrophoblast primary isolated cells from term placental tissues (Stefulj et al., 2009; Aye et al., 2010).

5. Other ABC transporters involved in cholesterol transfer

Many ABC transporters are involved in cholesterol homeostasis by participating transferring lipid molecules including cholesterol. Unlike ABCA1 and ABCG1, ABCG5 and ABCG8 expressed in liver, and function in the secretion of biliary cholesterol. ABCG5 and ABCG8 restrain cholesterol absorption in the lumen of the intestine by excreting absorbed cholesterol. These transporter help in the removal of excess cholesterol from the body and maintain cholesterol homeostasis. ABCG1 is also expressed in the brain along with placenta. ABCG1 and ABCG4 are expressed in the brain, function in cholesterol metabolism in the central nervous system (CNS) (Matsuo, 2010). ABCA2 has also been reported to be involved in cholesterol efflux. ABCA2 is also expressed in animal and human placenta but its role in placenta has not been studied precisely still now (Burke et al., 2009).

6. Conclusion and future explorations

Although cholesterol is the fundamental factor for normal fetal development, there is evidence suggesting that an excess of maternal cholesterol can have both acute and chronic detrimental effect to the fetus health. Maternal hypercholesterolemia is correlated with the fatty streaks aortas in the fetus that persist in childhood (Napoli et al., 1997). This fatty streak formation has been suggested as a programming mechanism target for the development of atherosclerosis later in life (Palinski et al., 2002). Considering the importance and detrimental efflux of cholesterol, cholesterol transferring pathway including ABC transporter can be a target for *in utero* therapy to control the anomalies derived from cholesterol deficiency or adequacy. In a recent study ABCA1 has been detected as a target for *in utero* therapy of Smith-Lemli-Opitz Syndrome (SLOS), a congenital anomaly due to error of cholesterol synthesis (Lindegaard et al., 2008).

In addition to its lipid export activity, it has been demonstrated that ABCA1 plays an important role in immune responses (Zhu et al., 2008; Tanc et al., 2009; Yvan-Charvet et al., 2010). Mice lacking ABCA1 have an enhanced inflammatory response to lipopolysaccharide (LPS) (McNeish et al., 2000). Incubating apoA-1 with activated ABCA1-expressing macrophages suppressed production of the inflammatory cytokines interleukin 1β (IL-1β), interleukin-6 (IL-6), and tumor necrosis factor-α (TNF-α) (Tanc et al., 2009). Thus the expression of ABCA1 in the villous and extravillous trophoblast may reflect additional functions other than those involved in cholesterol homeostasis. Our group has recently been demonstrated that 17 beta estradiol modulate placental MIF secretion by regulating the expression of ABCA1 transporter protein (Ietta et al., 2010).

Although ABCA1 and ABCG1 are involved in placental cholesterol efflux, this is more likely to occur by the involvement of other mechanisms along with simple diffusion such as via SR-B1, fatty acid-binding proteins (FABPs) and other transporters. Further studies on these transporters will clarify the complete placental cholesterol transfer mechanisms.

7. References

Aiello RJ, Brees D, Francone OL. 2003. ABCA1-deficient mice: insights into the role of monocyte lipid efflux in HDL formation and inflammation. *Arterioscler Thromb Vasc Biol*, 23(6):972-980.

Albrecht C, Soumian S, Tetlow N, Patel P, Sullivan MH, Lakasing L, Nicolaides K, Williamson C. 2007. Placental ABCA1 expression is reduced in primary antiphospholipid syndrome compared to pre-eclampsia and controls. *Placenta*, 28(7): 701-708.

Allikmets, Schriml LM, Hutchinson A, Romano-Spica V, Dean M. 1998. A human placenta-specific ATP-binding cassete gene (ABCP) on chromosome 4q22 that is involved in multidrug resistance. *Cancer Res*, 58(23): 5337-5339.

Attie AD. 2007. ABCA1: at the nexus of cholesterol, HDL and atherosclerosis. *Trends Biochem Sci*, 32(4):172-179.

Aye IL, Waddell BJ, Mark PJ, Keelan JA. 2010. Placental ABCA1 and ABCG1 transporters efflux cholesterol and protect trophoblasts from oxysterol induced toxicity. *Biochim Biophys Acta*, 1801(9):1013-1024.

Azuma Y, Takade M, Shin HW, Kioka N, Nakayama K, Ueda K. 2009. Retroendocytosis pathway of ABCA1/apoA-I contributes to HDL formation. *Genes Cells*, 14(2): 191-204.

Bera TK, Lee S, Salvatore G, Lee B, Pastan I. 2001. MRP8, a new member of ABC transporter superfamily, identified by EST database mining and gene prediction program, is highly expressed in breast cancer. *Mol Med*, 7(8): 509-516.

Bhattacharjee J, Ietta F, Giacomello E, Bechi N, Romagnoli R, Fava A, Paulesu L. 2010. Expression and localization of ATP binding cassette transporter A1 (ABCA1) in first trimester and term human placenta. *Placenta*, 31(5):423-430.

Bodó A, Bakos E, Szeri F, Váradi A, Sarkadi B. 2003 The role of multidrug transporters in drug availability, metabolism and toxicity. *Toxicol Lett*, 140-141: 133-143.

Borst P, Evers R, Kool M, Wijnholds J. 2000. A family of drug transporters: the multidrug resistance-associated proteins. *J Natl Cancer Inst*, 92: 1295-1302.

Bungert S, Molday LL, and Molday RS. 2001. Membrane topology of the ATP binding cassette transporter ABCR and its relationship to ABC1 and related ABCA transporters: identification of N-linked glycosylation sites. *J Biol Chem*, 276(26): 23539-23546.

Burton GJ, Jauniaux E, Watson AL. 1999. Maternal arterial connections to the placental intervillous space during the first trimester of human pregnancy: the Boyd Collection revisited. *Am J Obstet Gynecol*, 181(3):718–724

Burton GJ,Watson AL, Hempstock J, Skepper JN, Jauniaux E. 2002. Uterine glands provide histiotrophic nutrition for the human fetus during the first trimester of pregnancy. *J Clin Endocrinol Metab* 87(6):2954–2959.

Calandra T, Bucala R. 1996. Macrophage migration inhibitory factor: a counterregulator of glucocorticoid action and critical mediator of septic shock. *J Inflamm*, 47(1-2): 39-51.

Chambenoit O, Hamon Y, Marguet D, Rigneault H, Rosseneu M, Chimini G. 2001. Specific docking of apoliproprotein A-I at the cell surface requires a functional ABCA1 transporters. *J Biol Chem*, 276(13): 9955-9960.

Chen W, Sun Y, Welch C, Gorelik A, Leventhal AR, Tabas I, Tall AR. 2001. Preferential ATP-binding cassette transporter A1-mediated cholesterol efflux from late endosomes/lysosomes. *J Biol Chem*, 276(47): 43564-43569.

Christiansen-Weber TA, Voland JR, Wu Y, Ngo K, Roland BL, Nguyen S, Peterson PA, Fung-Leung WP. 2000. Functional loss of ABCA1 in mice causes severe placental malformation, aberrant lipid distribution, and kidney glomerulonephritis as well as high-density lipoprotein cholesterol deficiency. *Am J Pathol*, 157(3):1017-1029.

Cooper MK, Wassif CA, Krabowiak PA, Taipale J, Gong R, Kelley RI, Porter FD, Beachy PA. 2003 . A defective response to Hedgehog signaling in disorders of cholesterol biosynthesis. *Nat Genet*, 33(4):508-513.

Cooray HC, Blackmore CG, Maskell L and Barrand MA. 2002. Localisation of breast cancer resistance protein in microvessel endothelium of human brain. *Neuroreport*, 13 (16): 2059-2063.

Dean M, Hamon Y, Chimini G. 2001. The human ATP-binding cassette (ABC) transporter superfamily. *J Lipid Res*, 42(7): 1007-1017.

Drobnik W, Borsukova H, Böttcher A, Pfeiffer A, Liebisch G, Schütz GJ, Schindler H, Schmitz G. 2002. Apo AI/ABCA1-dependent and HDL3-mediated lipid efflux from compositionlly distinct cholesterol-based microdomains. *Traffic*, 3(4): 268-278.

Enders AC, King BF. 1993. Development of the human yolk sac. In *The Human Yolk Sac and Yolk Sac Tumors*, ed. FF Nogales, pp. 33–47. Springer-Verlag, ISBN 3540560319, 0387560319, Berlin, New York.

Fielding PE, Nagao K, Hakamata H, Chimini G, Fielding CJ. 2000. A two-step mechanism for free cholesterol and phospholipid efflux from human vascular cells to apolipoprotein A-1. *Biochemistry*, 39(46): 14113-14120.

Fitzgerald ML, Mendez AJ, Moore KJ, Andersson LP, Panjeton HA, Freeman MW. 2001. ATP-binding cassette transporter A1 contains an NH2-terminal signal anchor sequence that translocates the protein's first hydrophilic domain to the exoplasmic space. *J Biol Chem*, 276(18): 15137-15145.

Fitzgerald ML, Morris AL, Rhee JS, Andersson LP, Mendez AJ, Freeman MW. 2002. Naturally occurring mutations in the largest extracellular loops of ABCA1 can disrupt its direct interaction with apolipoprotein A-I. *J Biol Chem*, 277(36): 33178-33187.

Flieger O, Engling A, Bucala R, Lue H, Nickel W, Bernhagen J. 2003. Regulated secretion of macrophage migration inhibitory factor is mediated by a nonclassical pathway involving an ABC transporter. *FEBS Lett*, 551(1-3):78-86.

Francone OL, Royer L, Boucher G, Haghpassand M, Freeman A, Brees D, Aiello RJ. 2005. Increased cholesterol deposition, expression of scavenger receptors, and response to chemotactic factors in Abca1-deficient macrophages. *Arterioscler Thromb Vasc Biol*, 25(6):1198-1205.

Giebel B, Corbeil D, Beckmann J, Höhn J, Freund D, Giesen K, Fischer J, Kögler G, Wernet P. 2004. Segregation of lipid raft markers including CD133 in polarized human hematopoietic stem and progenitor cells. *Blood*, 104(8): 2332-2338.

Hamon Y, Broccardo C, Chambenoit O, Luciani MF, Toti F, Chaslin S, Freyssinet JM, Devaux PF, McNeish J, Marguet D, Chimini G. 2000. ABC1 promotes engulfment of apoptotic cells and transbilayer redistribution of phosphatidylserine. *Nat Cell Biol*, 2(7): 399-406.

Hansson GK, Björkholm M. Medicine. 2010. Tackling two diseases with HDL. *Science*, 328(5986):1641-1642.

Hempstock J, Cindrova-Davies T, Jauniaux E, Burton GJ. 2004. Endometrial glands as a source of nutrients, growth factors and cytokines during the first trimester of human pregnancy: a morphological and immunohistochemical study. *Reprod Biol Endocrinol* 2:58–72.

Herman GE. 2003. Disorders of cholesterol biosynthesis: prototypic metabolic malformation syndromes. *Hum Mol Genet*, 12 (Spec No 1):R75-88.

Higgins CF, Callaghan R, Linton KJ, Rosenberg MF, Ford RC. 1997. Structure of the multidrug resistance P-glycoprotein. *Semin Cancer Biol*, 8(3): 135-142.

Hopkins B, Brice AL, Schofield PN, Baralle FE, Graham CF. 1987. Identity of cells containing apolipoprotein B messenger RNA, in 6- to 12-week postfertilization human embryos. *Development* 100(1):83–93.

Hustin J, Schaaps JP. 1987. Echographic and anatomic studies of the maternotrophoblastic border during the first trimester of pregnancy. *Am J Obstet Gynecol*, 157(1):162–168.

Ietta F, Bechi N, Romagnoli R, Bhattacharjee J, Realacci M, Di Vito M, Ferretti C, Paulesu L. 2010. 17{beta}-Estradiol modulates the macrophage migration inhibitory factor secretory pathway by regulating ABCA1 expression in human first-trimester placenta. *Am J Physiol Endocrinol Metab*,298(3):E411-418.

Juliano RL, Ling V. 1976. A surface glycoprotein modulating drug permeability in Chinese hamster ovary cell mutants. *Biochem Biophys Acta* 455(1): 152-162.

Kelley RI. 2000. Inborn errors of cholesterol biosynthesis. *Adv Pediatr,* 47:1-53.

Keppler D, Leier I, Jedlitschky G, König J. 1998. ATP-dependent transport of glutathione S-conjugates by the multidrug resistance protein MRP1 and its apical isoform MRP2. *Chem Biol Interact,* 111-112: 153-161.

Koseki M, Hirano K, Masuda D, Ikegami C, Tanaka M, Ota A, Sandoval JC, Nakagawa-Toyama Y, Sato SB, Kobayashi T, Shimada Y, Ohno-Iwashita Y, Matsuura F, Shimomura I, Yamashita S. 2007. Increased lipid rafts and accelerated lipopolysaccharide-induced tumor necrosis factor-alpha secretion in Abca1-deficient macrophages. *J Lipid Res,* 48(2):299-306.

Lanford RE, Bronson DL, Estlack LE,Wians FH Jr. 1991. Plasma protein and apolipoprotein synthesis by human yolk sac carcinoma cells in vitro. *In Vivo Cell Dev Biol* 27A (3 Pt 1):205–210.

Langmann T, Klucken J, Reil M, Liebisch G, Luciani MF, Chimini G, Kaminski WE, Schmitz G. 1999. Molecular cloning of the human ATP-Binding cassette transporter 1 (hABC1): evidence for sterol-dependent regulation in macrophages. *Biochem Biophys Res Commun* 257(1):29-33.

Langmann, T, Mauerer R, Zahn A, Moehle C, Probst M, Stremmel W, Schmitz G. 2003. Real-time reverse transcription-PCR expression profiling of the complete human ATP-binding cassette transporter superfamily in various tissues. *Clin Chem,* 49(2): 230-238.

Lankas GR, Wise LD, Cartwright ME, Pippert T, Umbenhauer DR. 1998. Placental Pglycoprotein deficiency enhances susceptibility to chemically induced birth defects in mice. *Reprod Toxicol,* 12(4): 457-463.

Lawn RM, Wade DP, Garvin MR, Wang X, Schwartz K, Porter JG, Seilhamer JJ, Vaughan AM, Oram JF. 1999. The Tangier disease gene product ABC1 controls the cellular apolipoprotein-mediated lipid removal pathway. *J Clin Invest,* 104(8): R25–R31.

Leazer TM, Klaassen CD. 2003. The presence of xenobiotic transporters in rat placenta. *Drug Metab Dispos,* 31(2): 153-167.

Li Q, Tsujita M, Yokoyama S. 1997. Selective down-regulation by protein kinase C inhibitors of apolipoprotein-mediated cellular cholesterol efflux in macrophages. *Biochemistry,* 36 (40): 12045-12052.

Lindegaard ML, Wassif CA, Vaisman B, Amar M, Wasmuth EV, Shamburek R, Nielsen LB, Remaley AT, Porter FD. 2008 Characterization of placental cholesterol transport: ABCA1 is a potential target for in utero therapy of Smith-Lemli-Opitz syndrome. *Hum Mol Genet,* 17(23): 3806-3813.

Litman T, Druley TE, Stein WD, Bates SE. 2001. From MDR to MXR: new understanding of multidrug resistance systems, their properties and clinical significance. *Cell Mol Life Sci,* 58(7): 931-959.

Litman, T., Jensen U, Hansen A, Covitz KM, Zhan Z, Fetsch P, Abati A, Hansen PR, Horn T, Skovsgaard T, Bates SE. 2002. Use of peptide antibodies to probe for the mitoxantrone resistance-associated protein MXR/BCRP/ABCP/ABCG2. *Biochim Biophys Acta,* 1565(1): 6-16.

Lue H, Kleemann R, Calandra T, Roger T, Bernhagen J. Macrophage migration inhibitory factor (MIF): mechanisms of action and role in disease. *Microbes Infect*, 4(4): 449-460.

MacFarland A, Abramovich DR, Ewen SW, Pearson CK. 1994. Stage-specific distribution of P-glycoprotein in first-trimester and full-term human placenta. *Histochem J*, 26(5): 417-423.

Martì E, Bovolenta P. 2002. Sonic hedgehog in CNS development: one signal, multiple outputs. *Trends Neurosci*, 25 (2):89-96.

Mathias AA, Hitti J, Unadkat JD. 2005. P-glycoprotein and breast cancer resistance protein expression in human placentae of various gestational ages. *Am J Physiol Regul Integr Comp Physiol*, 289(4): R963-969.

Matsuo M. 2010. ATP-binding cassette proteins involved in glucose and lipid homeostasis. *Biosci Biotechnol Biochem*,74(5):899-907.

McConihay JA, Horn PS, Woollett LA. 2001. Effect of maternal hypercholesterolemia on fetal sterol metabolism in the Golden Syrian hamster. *J Lipid Res*, 42(7):1111-1119.

McNeish J, Aiello RJ, Guyot D, Turi T, Gabel C, Aldinger C, Hoppe KL, Roach ML, Royer LJ, de Wet J, Broccardo C, Chimini G, Francone OL. 2000. High density lipoprotein deficiency and foam cell accumulation in mice with targeted disruption of ATP-binding cassette transporter-1. *Proc Natl Acad Sci U S A*, 97(8):4245-4250.

McNeish J, Aiello RJ, Guyot D, Turi T, Gabel C, Aldinger C, Hoppe KL, Roach ML, Royer LJ, de Wet J, Broccardo C, Chimini G, Francone OL. 2000. High density lipoprotein deficiency and foam cell accumulation in mice with targeted disruption of ATP-binding cassette transporter-1. *Proc Natl Acad Sci U S A*, 97(8):4245-4250.

Mendez AJ, Lin G, Wade DP, Lawn RM, Oram JF. 2001. Membrane lipid domains distinct from cholesterol/sphingomyelin-rich rafts are involved in the ABCA1 mediated lipid secretory pathway. *J Biol Chem*, 276(5): 3158-3166.

Mitchell RA, Bucala R. 2000. Tumor growth-promoting properties of macrophage migration inhibitory factor (MIF). *Semin Cancer Biol*, 10(5): 359-366.

Murphy AJ, Woollard KJ, Hoang A, Mukhamedova N, Stirzaker RA, McCormick SP, Remaley AT, Sviridov D, Chin-Dusting J. 2008. High-density lipoprotein reduces the human monocyte inflammatory response. *Arterioscler Thromb.Vasc Biol*, 28 (11):2071-2077.

Nagashige M, Ushigome F, Koyabu N, Hirata K, Kawabuchi M, Hirakawa T, Satoh S, Tsukimori K, Nakano H, Uchiumi T, Kuwano M, Ohtani H, Sawada Y. 2003. Basal membrane localization of MRP1 in human placental trophoblast. *Placenta*, 24(10): 951-958.

Napoli C, D'Armiento FP, Mancini FP, Postiglione A, Witztum JL, Palumbo G, Palinski W. 1997. Fatty streak formation occurs in human fetal aortas and is greatly enhanced by maternal hypercholesterolemia. Intimal accumulation of low density lipoprotein and its oxidation precede monocyte recruitment into early atherosclerotic lesions. *J Clin Invest*, 100(11):2680-2690.

Neufeld EB, Stonik JA, Demosky SJ Jr, Knapper CL, Combs CA, Cooney A, Comly M, Dwyer N, Blanchette-Mackie J, Remaley AT, Santamarina-Fojo S, Brewer HB Jr. 2001. The ABCA1 transporter modulates late endocytic trafficking: insight from the correction of the genetic defect in Tangier disease. *J Biol Chem*, 279(15): 27584-27590.

Oram J F. 2003. HDL apolipoproteins and ABCA1: partners in the removal of excess cellular cholesterol. *Arterioscler Thromb Vasc Biol*, 23(5): 720-727.

Oram J F.2002. ATP-binding cassette transportes A1 and cholesterol trafficking.*Curr Opin Lipidol*, 13(4): 373-381.

Oram JF, Lawn RM, Garvin MR, Wade DP. 2000. ABCA1 is the cAMP-inducible apolipoprotein receptor that mediates cholesterol secretion from macrophages. *J Biol Chem*, 275(44): 34508-34511.

Oram JF, Mendez AJ, Slotte JP, Johnson TF. 1991. High density lipoprotein apolipoproteins mediate removal of sterol from intracellular pools but not from plasma membranes of cholesterol-loaded fibroblasts. *Atheroscler Thromb*, 11(2): 403-414.

Oram JF, Vaughan AM, Stocker R. 2001. ATP-binding cassette transporter A1 mediates cellular secretion of alpha-tocopherol. *J Biol Chem* 2001;276(43): 39898-39902.

Ozvegy C, Litman T, Szakács G, Nagy Z, Bates S, Váradi A, Sarkadi B. 2001. Functional characterization of the human multidrug transporter, ABCG2, expressed in insect cells. *Biochem Biophys Res Commun*, 285(1): 111-117.

Palinski W, Napoli C. 2002. The fetal origins of atherosclerosis: maternal hypercholesterolemia, and cholesterol-lowering or antioxidant treatment during pregnancy influence in utero programming and postnatal susceptibility to atherogenesis. *FASEB J*, 16(11): 1348-1360.

Pascolo L, Fernetti C, Pirulli D, Crovella S, Amoroso A, Tiribelli C. 2003. Effects of maturation on RNA transcription and protein expression of four MRP genes in human placenta and in BeWo cells. *Biochem Biophys Res Commun*, 303(1): 259-265.

Perda J, Correr S, Motta PM. 1994. The structure of the human yolk sac: a scanning and transmission electron microscopic analysis. *Arch Histol Cytol* 57(2):107–117

Porter JA, Young KE, Beachy PA. 1996. Cholesterol modification of hedgehog signaling proteins in animal development. *Science* , 274 (5285):255-259.

Rothblat GH, de la Llera-Moya M, Atger V, Kellner-Weibel G, Williams DL, Phillips MC. 1999. Cell cholesterol efflux: integration of old and new observations provides new insights. *J Lipid Res* 40(5):781-796.

Rust S, Rosier M, Funke H, Real J, Amoura Z, Piette JC, Deleuze JF, Brewer HB, Duverger N, Denèfle P, Assmann G. 1999. Tangier disease is caused by mutations in the gene encoding ATP-binding cassette transporter 1. *Nat Genet*, 22(4):352-355.

Samtani MN, Schwab M, Nathanielsz PW, Jusko WJ. 2004. Area/moment and compartmental modeling of pharmacokinetics during pregnancy: applications to maternal/fetal exposures to corticosteroids in sheep and rats. *Pharm Res*, 21(12): 2279-2292.

Santamarina-Fojo S, Remaley AT, Neufeld EB, Brewer HB Jr. 2001. Regulation and intracellular trafficking of the ABCA1 transporter. *J Lipid Res*, 42(9): 1339-1345.

Sarkadi B, Ozvegy-Laczka C, Német K, Váradi A. 2004. ABCG2 -- a transporter for all seasons. *FEBS Lett*, 2004; 567(1): 116-120.

Sato K, Sugawara J, Sato T, Mizutamari H, Suzuki T, Ito A, Mikkaichi T, Onogawa T, Tanemoto M, Unno M, Abe T, Okamura K. 2003. Expression of organic anion transporting polypeptide E (OATP-E) in human placenta. *Placenta*, 24(2-3): 144-148.

Schmid KE, Davidson WS, Myatt L,Woollett LA. 2003. Transport of cholesterol across a BeWo cell monolayer: implications for net transport of sterol from maternal to fetal circulation. *J Lipid Res*, 44(10):1909-1918.

Schmitz G, Grandl M. 2008. Lipid homeostasis in macrophages - implications for atherosclerosis. *Rev Physiol Biochem Pharmacol*, 160:93-125.

Schmitz G, Kaminski WE, Porsch-Ozcürümez M, Klucken J, Orsó E, Bodzioch M, Büchler C, Drobnik W. 1999. ATP-binding cassette transporter A1 (ABCA1) in macrophages: a dual function in inflammation and lipid metabolism? *Pathobiology*, 67(5-6):236-240.

Shi W-K, Hopkins B, Thompson S, Heath JK, LukeBM,Graham CF. 1985. Synthesis of apolipoproteins, alphafoetoprotein, albumin, and transferrin by the human foetal yolk sack and other foetal organs. *J Embryol Exp Morphol* 85:191–206.

Shi W-K, Hopkins B, Thompson S, Heath JK, LukeBM,Graham CF. 1985. Synthesis of apolipoproteins, alphafoetoprotein, albumin, and transferrin by the human foetal yolk sack and other foetal organs. *J. Embryol. Exp. Morphol.* 85:191–206

Smit JW, Huisman MT, van Tellingen O, Wiltshire HR, Schinkel AH. 1999. Absence or pharmacological blocking of placental P-glycoprotein profoundly increases fetal drug exposure. *J Clin Invest*, 104(10): 1441 -1447.

Smith JD, Waelde C, Horwitz A, Zheng P. 2002. Evaluation of the role of phosphatidylserine translocase activity in ABCA1-mediated lipid efflux.*J Biol Chem*, 277(20): 17797-17803.

Stefulj J, Panzenboeck U, Becker T, Hirschmugl B, Schweinzer C, Lang I, Marsche G, Sadjak A, Lang U, Desoye G, Wadsack C . 2009. Human endothelial cells of the placental barrier efficiently deliver cholesterol to the fetal circulation via ABCA1 and ABCG1. *Circ Res*, 104(5): 600-608.

St-Pierre MV, Hagenbuch B, Ugele B, Meier PJ, Stallmach T. 2002. Characterization of an organic anion-transporting polypeptide (OATP-B) in human placenta. *J Clin Endocrinol Metab*, 87(4): 1856-1863.

Takahashi Y, Smith J D. 1996. Cholesterol efflux to apolipoprotein AI involves endocytosis and resecreation in a calcium-dependent pathway.*Proc Natl Acad Sci USA*, 96(20): 11358-11363.

Takahashi Y, Smith J D. 1999. Cholesterol efflux to apolipoprotein AI involves endocytosis and resecreation in a calcium-dependent pathway.*Proc Natl Acad Sci USA*, 96(20): 11358-11363.

Tall AR. 2008. Cholesterol efflux pathways and other potential mechanisms involved in the athero-protective effect of high density lipoproteins. *J Intern Med*, 263(3): 256-273.

Tanabe M, Ieiri I, Nagata N, Inoue K, Ito S, Kanamori Y, Takahashi M, Kurata Y, Kigawa J, Higuchi S, Terakawa N, Otsubo K. 2001. Expression of P-glycoprotein in human placenta: relation to genetic polymorphism of the multidrug resitance (MDR)-1 gene. *J Pharmacol Exp Ther*, 297(3): 1137-1143.

Tanc C, Liu Y, Kessler PS, Vaughan AM, Oram JF. The macrophage cholesterol exporter ABCA1 functions as an anti-inflammatory receptor. *J Biol Chem*, 284: 32336-43.

Tellier E, Canault M, Poggi M, Bonardo B, Nicolay A, Alessi MC, Nalbone G, Peiretti F. 2008. HDLs activate ADAM17-dependent shedding. *J Cel Physiol*, 214 (3):687-693.

Ushigome F, Takanaga H, Matsuo H, Yanai S, Tsukimori K, Nakano H, Uchiumi T, Nakamura T, Kuwano M, Ohtani H, Sawada Y. 2000. Human placental transport of vinblastine, vincristine,digoxin and progesterone: contribution of Pglycoprotein. *Eur J Pharmacol*, 408(1): 1 -10.

Vaughan A M, Oram J F. 2003. ABCA1 redistributes membrane cholesterol independent of apolipoprotein interactions. *J Lipid Res* 2003; 44(7): 1373-1380.

Von Eckardstein A, Langer C, Engel T, Schaukal I, Cignarella A, Reinhardt J, Lorkowski S, Li Z, Zhou X, Cullen P, Assmann G. 2001. ATP binding cassette transporter ABCA1 modulates the secretion of apolipoprotein E from human monocyte-derived macrophages. *FASEB J* 2001; 15(9): 1555-1561.

Wadsack C, Hammer A, Levak-Frank S, Desoye G, Kozarsky KF, Hirschmugl B, Sattler W, Malle E. 2003. Selective cholesterol ester uptake from high density lipoprotein by human first trimester and villous trophoblast cells. *Placenta*, 24 (2-3):131-143.

Wang N, Silver DL, Costet P, Tall AR. 2000. Specific binding of ApoA-I, enhanced cholesterol efflux, and altered plasma membrane morphology in cells expressing ABC1. *J Biol Chem*, 275(42): 33053-33058.

Wang N, Silver DL, Thiele C, Tall AR. 2001. ATP-binding cassette transporter A1 (ABCA1) functions as a cholesterol efflux regulatory protein. *J Biol Chem*, 276(26): 23742-23747.

Woollett LA. 2001. The origins and roles of cholesterol and fatty acids in the fetus. *Curr Opin Lipidol*, 2001;12(3): 305-312.

Woollett LA. 2005. Maternal cholesterol in fetal development: transport of cholesterol from the maternal to the fetal circulation. *Am J Clin Nutr* 82(6):1155-1161.

Woollett LA. 2008. Where does fetal and embryonic cholesterol originate and what does it do? *Annu Rev Nutr*, 28:97-114.

Wyne KL, Woollett LA. 1998. Transport of maternal LDL and HDL to the fetal membranes and placenta of the Golden Syrian hamster is mediated by receptor-dependent and receptor-independent processes. *J Lipid Res*, 39 (3):518-530.

Yancey PG, Bortnick AE, Kellner-Weibel G, de la Llera-Moya M, Phillips MC, Rothblat GH. 2003. Importance of different pathways of cellular cholesterol efflux. *Arterioscler Thromb Vasc Biol* 23(5):712-719.

Yoshida S, Wada Y. 2005. Transfer of maternal cholesterol to embryo and fetus in pregnant mice. *J Lipid Res*, 46 (10):2168-2174.

Young AM, Allen CE, Audus KL. 2003. Efflux transporters of the human placenta. *Adv Drug Deliv Rev*, 55(1):125-132.

Yvan-Charvet L, Pagler T, Gautier EL, Avagyan S, Siry RL, Han S, Welch CL, Wang N, Randolph GJ, Snoeck HW, Tall AR. 2010. ATP-binding cassette transporters and HDL suppress hematopoietic stem cell proliferation. *Science*, 328(5986):1689-1693.

Yvan-Charvet L, Wang N, Tall AR. 2010. Role of HDL, ABCA1, and ABCG1 transporters in cholesterol efflux and immune responses. *Atherioscler Thromb Vasc Biol*, 30(2): 139-143.

Yvan-Charvet L, Welch C, Pagler TA, Ranalletta M, Lamkanfi M, Han S, Ishibashi M, Li R, Wang N, Tall AR. 2008. Increased inflammatory gene expression in ABC transporter-deficient macrophages: free cholesterol accumulation, increased signaling via toll-like receptors, and neutrophil infiltration of atherosclerotic lesions. *Circulation,* 118(18):1837–1847.

Zhou X, Engel T, Goepfert C, Erren M, Assmann G, von Eckardstein A. 2002. The ATP-binding cassette transporter A1 contributes to the secretion of interleukin 1beta from macrophages but not from monocytes. *Biochem Biophys Res Commun,* 291(3): 598-604.

Zhu X, Lee JY, Timmins JM, Brown JM, Boudyguina E, Mulya A, Gebre AK, Willingham MC, Hiltbold EM, Mishra N, Maeda N, Parks JS. 2008. Increased cellular free cholesterol in macrophage-specific Abca1 knock-out mice enhances proinflammatory response of macrophages. *J Biol Chem,* 283(34):22930-22941.

Part 6

Key Factors and Cellular Organelles in Placental Development

17

The Role of Mitochondria in Syncytiotrophoblast Cells: Bioenergetics and Steroidogenesis

Federico Martinez, Rebeca Milan, Oscar Flores-Herrera, Sofia Olvera-Sanchez, Erika Gomez-Chang and Maria Teresa Espinosa-Garcia
Universidad Nacional Autónoma de México, Departamento de Bioquímica, Facultad de Medicina, Distrito Federal, Mexico

1. Introduction

Human placenta maintains pregnancy. The mitochondria of this tissue synthesize pregnenolone (P5) from cholesterol through a transport chain formed by adrenodoxin, adrenodoxin reductase and cytochrome P450scc (CYP11A1; EC 1.14.15.6) , which breaks up the lateral chain of cholesterol. P5 is transformed into progesterone (P4) within mitochondria by the 3β-OH-steroid-dehydrogenase-Δ^{5-6}isomerase (3HSD). The particular hormone(s) or substance(s) that modulate P4 synthesis during pregnancy is currently unknown (Strauss et al., 1996; Martinez & Strauss, 1997); nevertheless, the presence of cAMP analogues stimulated P4 synthesis in trophoblastic cells, suggesting that a hormonal signal or another kind of signal may modulate the concentration of this second messenger into the cells (Ringler et al., 1989; Strauss et al., 1992). Although P4 synthesis was suggested to be the main function of the placenta, the analysis of P450scc cytochrome concentration shows that placental mitochondria have a lower content of P450scc than respiratory chain cytochromes (Table 1), even when it is compared to adrenal gland mitochondria, suggesting that placental mitochondria participate in other functions different to that from steroidogenesis.

	Human Placenta			Adrenal Glands			
Cytochrome	nmol/mg of mitochondrial protein			nmol/mg of mitochondrial protein			
$a_1 + a_3$	0.140	0.10	-	0.23	0.75		
b	0.089	0.07	-	0.17	0.32		
$c + c_1$	0.125	0.13		0.29	0.67		
P450scc	0.110	0.10	0.123	1.50	1.30	0.39	1.0
Reference	Négrié et al., 1979	Simpson & Miller, 1978	Meigs & Ryan, 1968	Cammer & Estabrook, 1967	Harding & Nelson, 1966	I. Hanukoglu & Z. Hanukoglu, 1986	Jefcoate et al., 1973

Table 1. Concentration of cytochromes in human placenta and adrenal gland mitochondria

It seems that ATP synthesis in placental mitochondria is not related to its consumption at the cytoplasm, but rather it is related to the mitochondrial metabolism and, although seemingly contradictory, this allows pregnancy to reach full-term delivery.

2. Transport

2.1 Transport of carbohydrates, lipids, and amino acids

The development of both placenta and fetus is metabolically related. The mother supplies the essential nutrients for the fetus and the placenta, and their transport is strictly controlled in the placenta by the expression and the activity of specific transporters in the plasma membrane of syncytiotrophoblast (Angiolini et al., 2006). When the development of the fetus is optimal, some transporters of nutrients and ions are downregulated in the placenta; then a decrease of cellular receptors for specific molecules is observed (Hahn et al., 1999).

The placenta uses mainly glucose for its metabolism and at the same time transports it to the fetus that requires 4-8 mg/kg/min of glucose for the oxidative phosphorylation (OXPHOS) process (Aldoreta & Hay, 1995). Two isoforms of GLUT have been identified: GLUT1 and GLUT3 (Kahn & Flier, 1990). GLUT 1 is responsible of glucose uptake from the maternal circulation and its activity is independent of insulin. Glucose itself down-regulates the placental GLUT1 providing a fetal protection mechanism when maternal glucose is high (Hahn, 1998). GLUT3 is relevant during implantation and establishment of the placenta, and thereafter GLUT3 is not required; suggesting that GLUT3 has no relevance in glucose uptake after the first trimester (Clarson et al., 1997).

Glucose placental transport is accomplished by facilitated diffusion through GLUT1 transporter, but its expression is not affected by the concentration of extracellular glucose (3.7 mM o 70 mg/dl maternal and 3.2 mM o 61 mg/dl fetal) (Ingermann, 1987). It has been reported that the placenta is in constant hypoxia, for which it has a glycolytic metabolism, where 70% of total glucose is used to produce ATP through anaerobic glycolysis (Hanguel et al., 1986).

Glycogen is synthesized by the human placenta only as a primary response to maternal hyperglycemia. Although glycogen during pregnancy has been reported (Ville, 1953), the placenta does not synthesize glycogen efficiently (Barash et al., 1991). There are data showing the presence of gluconeogenic enzymes (Matalon & Michals, 1984), and Prendergast et al. demonstrate that the placenta synthesizes glucose, and evidence of the presence of glucose-6-phosphatase has been published (Matsubara et al., 1999; Prendergast et al., 1999); however, it is unknown whether the glucose synthesis might have any physiologic relevance.

The incubation of trophoblastic cells, perfused explants or placentas, produces lactic acid as a result of anaerobic glycolysis used by the fetus (Battaglia, 1989; Piquard et al., 1990). The radioactivity of glucose labeled with ^{14}C showed the following distribution: lactate 60-69%, glycogen 1.3-4.8%, pentose pathway 5%, fatty acids 0.7-1.4% and CO_2 1.6-2.4% (Desoye & Shafrir, 1994). Similarly, in slices of human placenta from middle gestation, 73% of glucose was degraded through glycolysis, 10% through pentose pathway and the rest through lipids formation and glycogen synthesis. Although pentose pathway has been described in the placenta (Shelley, 1979), reports suggest that it does not make an important contribution to glucose metabolism (Moe et al., 1991). The placenta can also use fructose or lactate as energy sources.

Condition	Glucose consumption	Lactate production
	mmol/h/g	
95% O_2 + 5% CO_2	6.96 ± 2.50	21.23 ± 7.79
95% N_2 + 5% CO_2	12.50 ± 3.36	24.06 ± 5.24

Table 2. Glucose consumption and lactate production in human placenta (Modified from Schneider et al., 1988).

The placenta transports 50% of fatty acids to the fetus during the last trimester of pregnancy; that is the reason why β-oxidation is not a good candidate for ATP generation. In addition, placental membranes have a lipoprotein lipase which catalyzes the degradation of lipoproteins, mainly VLDL (Coleman, 1986). Fatty acids and glycerol are transported by simple diffusion and, once inside the trophoblast, they are bound to proteins and are transported to the basal stratus to diffuse to the fetus.

The following proteins have been related to the transport of lipids, the plasma membrane fatty acid binding protein (pFABPpm), fatty acid transporter protein (FATP) and the cytoplasmic fatty acid binding protein family (FABP) (Hornstra et al., 1995). pFABPpm makes up about 4% of cytosolic proteins, it is responsible for the intracellular distribution of fatty acids and to the membrane, and mainly binds essential long chain fatty acids. Also, the transport of essential fatty acids by the placenta is important, since these acids are implicated in cell-cell signaling and contribute to the development of the fetal brain, as well as cardiovascular and lung development (Wollet, 2005; Cunningham et al., 2009).

Cholesterol is the precursor of steroid hormones but it is not synthesized by the human placenta. Trophoblast cells express receptors for lipoproteins like LDL, VLDL, and class A scavenger receptors, as well as for the LDL receptor-related protein (LRP), the apolipoprotein E (apoE) receptor 2, and the scavenger receptor class B type (SR-BI). The cholesterol required for the synthesis of P4 is provided by maternal lipoproteins (Strauss et al., 1996; Palinski, 2009) (Fig.1).

Protein synthesis is essential for fetal development; the human placenta has at least three different amino acid transporters (neutral, cationic and anionic) coupled to an ionic energy dependent process. Two cationic amino acid transporter systems called y^+ (Hoeltzli & Smith, 1989) and y^+L (Fei et al., 1995) are specific for cationic amino acids and are widely expressed in both maternal and fetal sides. System "y" is Na^+-independent (Moe, 1995) and system y^+L has higher affinity for lysine and neutral amino acids. Transport of neutral amino acids involves the transporters A, ASC and L. Type A is a Na^+-dependent transporter with affinity for amino acids with short polar or linear side chains. System ASC is a Na^+-dependent transport for serine, cysteine, threonine and glutamine. The system L is a Na^+ independent transporter for large aromatic or non-polar branched side chains of amino acids (Yudilevich & Sweiry, 1985).

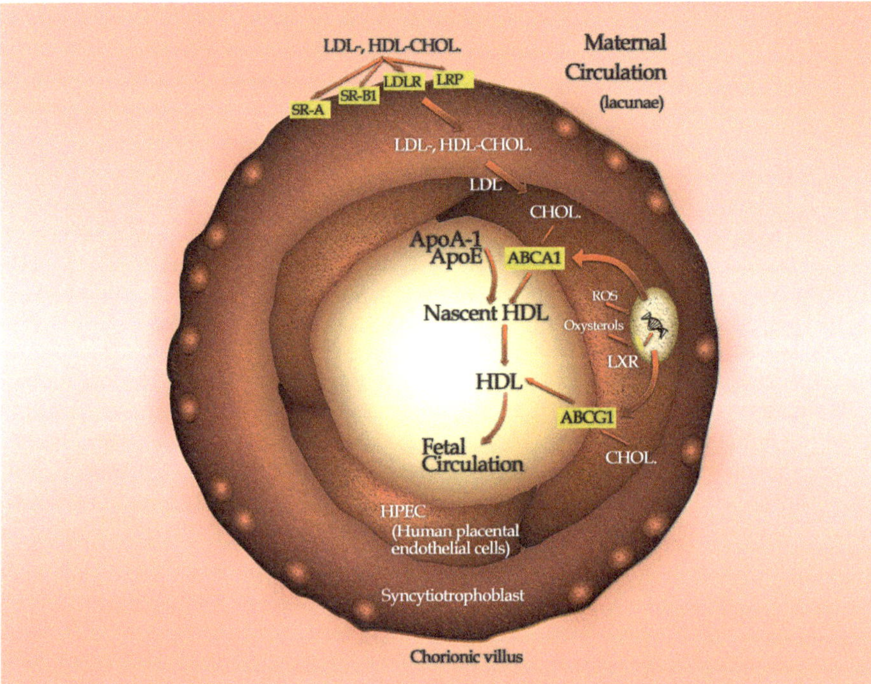

Fig. 1 Maternal-fetal cholesterol transport in the placenta (Modified from Palinski, 2009).

2.2 Transport of relevant ions

Ions are needed for fetus growth and metabolism, due to their contribution to cell homeostasis. The ions are not only related to amino acid transport, because ion transporters are necessary for other cellular functions. Na^+ is transported actively (Stulc et al., 1995). Carter has reported that 30% of the ATP produced by the placenta is used for the synthesis of proteins and steroids; while Na^+/K^+ ATPase consumes another 20-30%, making these processes the most costly and the main consumers of placental energy (Carter, 2000).

Chloride is co-transported with Na^+ or K^+; it is bidirectional and almost symmetrical and apparently associated with the maintenance of cell volume. Calcium is transported to the fetus against a concentration gradient reaching a fetal plasma concentration higher than maternal plasma concentration (Stulc, 1997).

Potassium is taken by the Na^+-K^+-ATPase and its efflux through the K^+-channel (K_{ATP}); the fetal transport of K^+ is against a concentration gradient and independent of the maternal potassium status (Stulc, 1997).

The movement of ions in the cell has relevance in the mitochondrial metabolism; the increase of K^+ in the cytoplasm in adrenal cells stimulates aldosterone synthesis (Spät & Pitter, 2004). The mechanism involves the release of Ca^{2+} from its cellular reservoirs modifying the mitochondria metabolism. Human placental mitochondria have a vectorial influx of Ca^{2+}, and changes in its concentration modifies P4 synthesis (García-Pérez et al.,

2002), although this transport can be modified by K^+. It has been observed that the increases of K^+ also modify mitochondrial steroidogenesis (Martinez, 1995). The transport of K^+ in the mitochondria has not been clarified, but it has been proposed that it could be through the mitoK_{ATP} channel described by Garlid (Garlid & Paucek, 2003).

3. Energetic metabolism

3.1 Architecture of the human placental mitochondria

The size, aspect and organization of mitochondrial membranes vary between species, tissues and physiological conditions. Using isolated mitochondria and cultured cells, Hackenbrock revealed a close coupling between ultrastructure and energetic state (Hackenbrock et al., 1971). In the energized state, when low ADP concentrations are limited for OXPHOS (the so-called respiratory state IV), mitochondria display the common, orthodox conformation: filamentous electron-dense cristae within a matrix of intermediate electron density. When high ADP concentrations accelerate OXPHOS (the respiratory state III), mitochondria adopt the condensed conformation: the matrix is condensed and electron dense, while the intermembrane space and cristae-lumen appears swollen and electron light. Reversible changes between the orthodox and condensed conformation are modulated by metabolites, by drugs that inhibit respiratory complexes or by ionophores that uncouple respiration and phosphorylation (Hackenbrock, 1968, 1971). Decades ago, several authors confirmed that stimulation of respiration induces the condensed conformation, with a characteristic electron-dense matrix in mitochondria (Malka et al., 2005; Rossignol et al., 2004). It is reasonable to assume that mitochondrial ultrastructure, morphology and dynamics are linked and thus, that mitochondrial morphology and dynamics are also modulated by OXPHOS.

Although many types of mitochondrial cristae structure have been described (Munn, 1974), from recent electron microscopic tomography studies, the differences between typical mitochondria are now evident; e.g., liver (Mannella, 1994, 1997), neuronal (Perkins, 1997, 2001a), brown adipose tissue (Perkins et al., 1998), fungus (Nicastro et al., 2000; Perkins et al., 2001b), rods and cones (Perkins, 2003), and those from steroidogenic tissues, e.g., Leydig cells (Prince, 2002). In general, cristae from typical mitochondria are lamellar while in steroidogenic cells are tubular, vesicular, or tubulovesicular (Reichert et al., 2002). It has been suggested that due to this particular morphology of the cristae, mitochondria of Leydig cells should not be able to produce ATP, since the narrow gap between lamellae would not allow the location of the F_1 subunit of ATP synthase (Prince, 2002); however, a recent publication indicates that mitochondrial membrane potential ($\Delta\psi m$), mitochondrial ATP synthesis, and mitochondrial respiration are all required to support Leydig cell steroidogenesis (Allen et al., 2006).

In our laboratory, two kinds of mitochondria were isolated from human placenta: non steroidogenic mitochondria with typical cristae from cytotrophoblast, and steroidogenic mitochondria with vesicular cristae from syncytiotrophoblast. *In situ*, large mitochondria were observed in cytotrophoblast cells, with morphology similar to the typical liver mitochondria, and containing lamellar cristae in an orthodox configuration (Fig. 2). In contrast, the syncytiotrophoblast contains smaller mitochondria with a condensed matrix and cristae composed by vesicular regions connected by narrow tubules. The larger cytotrophoblast mitochondria have a round shape, whereas syncytiotrophoblast mitochondria display an irregular shape with protuberances of the outer and inner membranes (De Los Rios Castillo et al., 2011).

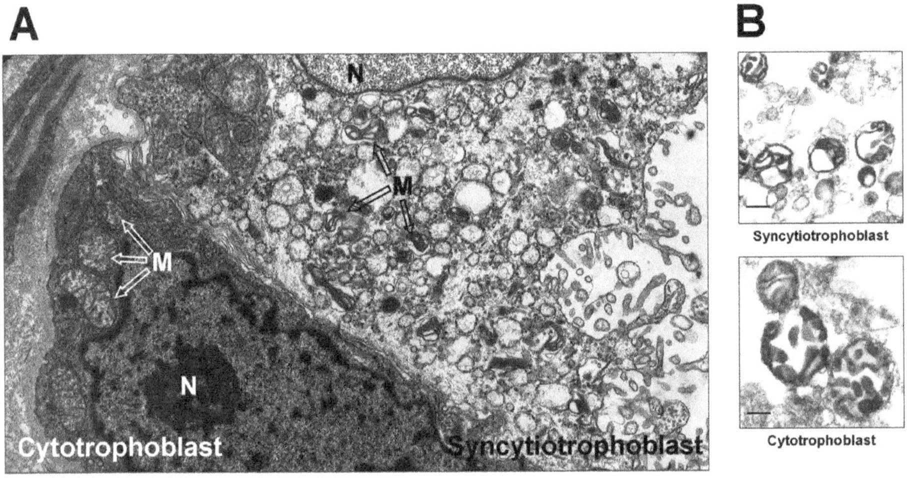

Fig. 2. Ultrastructure of human syncytiotrophoblast and cytotrophoblast cells. (A) Electron micrograph of term placenta villus showing syncytiotrophoblast and underlying cytotrophoblast. N, nucleus; M, mitochondria. 10,000 X. (B) Isolated mitochondria from human cytotrophoblast and syncytiotrophoblast. Scale bar, 200 nm (Modified from De Los Rios Castillo et al., 2011)

Isolated cytotrophoblast and syncytiotrophoblast mitochondria showed values for respiratory control higher than those previously reported for this tissue (Olivera & Meigs, 1975) and the oxygen uptake was coupled to ATP synthesis, reaching 151 ± 16 and 153 ± 13 nmol ATP/mg/min, respectively (De Los Rios Castillo et al., 2011). These observations demonstrate the presence of functional mitochondria in both cell types, retaining the ability to increase the consumption of oxygen and the synthesis of ATP upon the addition of ADP.

3.2 Energetic pathways

The metabolism of mitochondria involves two major pathways: energy production and P4 synthesis, and several evidences show that both are closely related, as suggested by the similar content of cytochromes from the electron transport chain cytochrome P450scc, suggesting the alternating activity of both pathways, which can generate ATP for cell function and for P4 synthesis to maintain pregnancy. A mechanism to regulate the functioning of both pathways could be the presence of alternative enzymes, e.g. an NADP-dependent isocitrate dehydrogenase is associated to the inner mitochondrial membrane; isocitrate, the substrate for this enzyme supports progesterone synthesis, while succinate promotes the synthesis of ATP.

It has been described that ATP-diphosphohydrolase and ADPase enzymes are tightly bound to mitochondrial membranes and their activities are involved in steroidogenesis. Particularly, the activity of ATP-diphosphohydrolase was described as supporting P4 synthesis, probably providing the energy requirement for cholesterol transport between the mitochondrial membranes, similar to the activity of mitochondrial GDPase reported in adrenal gland (Fig. 3) Additionally, these enzymes could participate in the transformation of ATP to adenosine, which can be released into the blood vessels to promote oxygenation of the placenta.

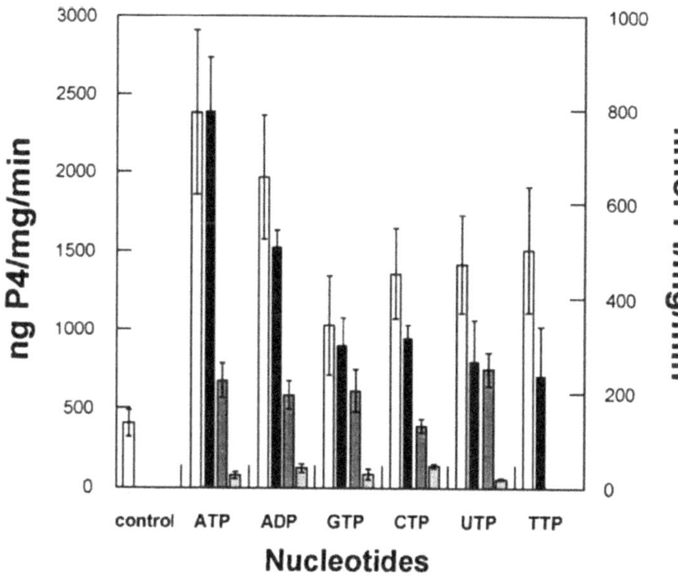

Fig. 3. Effect of several nucleotides on progesterone synthesis and their hydrolysis by human placental apyrase. Mitochondria were incubated in progesterone synthesis medium with or without 1 mM 5′p-fluorsulfonyl benzoyl adenosine (FSBA). Nucleotide hydrolysis was also performed in progesterone synthesis medium. Progesterone synthesis (□); nucleotide hydrolysis (■); progesterone synthesis + FSBA (▩); nucleotide hydrolysis + FSBA (░) (Modified from Flores-Herrera et al., 2002).

The concentration of adenine nucleotides is another way to analyze the pathways that produce energy in the form of ATP. The total amount of nucleotides at the time of expelling is 0.766 a 0.816 mmol/g wet weight, ATP 0.49, ADP 0.23, and AMP 0.12 nmol/g wet weight (Young & Schneider, 1984). In mitochondria isolated from full-term human placenta the concentrations of nucleotides are 1.24 5.78 y 1.09 nmol of ATP, ADP, and AMP/mg of protein, respectively (Martinez et al., 1987). These data suggest that in spite of the anoxia produced by labor, the placenta synthesizes mainly ATP, whereas glycogen levels do not vary significantly until 60 minutes after labor (Bloxam & Bobinski, 1984). The fact that mitochondria synthesize ATP does not imply that they supply the trophoblast with ATP for its cellular functioning in an important amount.

3.3 The relevance of nucleotide hydrolysis

With regard to their steroidogenic role, syncytiotrophoblast mitochondria synthesize P4 (35.7 ± 0.9 ng P4/mg/min) due to the presence of 3HSD in their inner membrane (Cherradi et al., 1994; Martinez et al., 1997; Brand et al., 1998). Their steroidogenic activity was ten times higher than cytotrophoblast mitochondria (3.6 ± 1.34 ng P4/mg/min). In both cases,

22(*R*)-hydroxycholesterol, a soluble substrate used to assess maximal steroidogenesis (Tuckey, 1992) increased steroidogenic activity to 92.2 ± 3.4 and 10.1 ± 3.95 ng P4/mg/h in syncytiotrophoblast and cytotrophoblast mitochondria, respectively (De Los Rios Castillo et al., 2011). Additionally we demonstrated that ATP is essential for progesterone synthesis (Flores-Herrera et al., 2002). These results agree with the specialized role of each placental cell (Martinez et al., 1997) and demonstrate that isolated mitochondria from syncytiotrophoblast are intact and retain their physiological function.

Nevertheless, human syncytiotrophoblast mitochondria have bioenergetics and steroidogenic functions, which raise an interesting question: why do they have an irregular shape with tubular, vesicular, or tubulovesicular cristae? At present, there is interest concerning proteins that govern mitochondrial ultrastructure, but few of such proteins have been identified (Pellegrini & Scorrano, 2007). It has been speculated that the dimer of F_0F_1-ATP synthase (complex V for oxidative phosphorylation of ATP) may play a major role in determining cristae formation (Paumard et al., 2002; Minauro-Sanmiguel et al., 2005; Dudkina et al., 2005; Strauss et al., 2008). Dimerization of F_0F_1-ATP synthase in the mitochondrial inner membrane has been described in yeast (Arnold et al., 1998) and bovine mitochondria (Schägger & Pfeiffer, 2000). A critical role in the stability of the mammalian dimeric complex V has been proposed for the inhibitory F_1 moiety protein (IF_1) (García et al., 2006). IF_1 is known to dimerize in solution (Gordon-Smith et al., 2001), and this dimer has been recently shown to interact with two molecules of soluble F_1 simultaneously (Cabezón et al., 2000; Dominguez-Ramirez et al., 2001). If the same interaction occurs in the membrane, it might be responsible for the dimerization of the F_0F_1-ATP synthase complex, and in mammalian cells, changes in IF_1 concentration affect the degree of F_0F_1-ATP synthase dimerization, which in turn could alter the formation of cristae (García et al., 2006). In this sense, the density of mitochondrial cristae in HeLa cells is increased by IF_1 overexpression and decreased by IF_1 suppression (Campanella et al., 2008); interestingly, IF_1 overexpression increases both the formation of dimeric F_0F_1-ATP synthase and F_0F_1-ATP synthase activity (Campanella et al., 2008).

The analysis of the electron transport chain and oxidative phosphorylation complexes from human syncytiotrophoblast and cytotrophoblast mitochondria allow us to demonstrate that the dimeric form of the F_0F_1-ATP synthase (complex V) is involved in the cristae architecture in trophoblast cells (De Los Rios Castillo et al., 2011). In this sense, we found that the dimer of mitochondrial F_0F_1-ATP synthase is scarce in syncytiotrophoblast associated to a low IF_1 concentration. Due to the fact that human placenta cells are ontogenetically related, i.e. cytotrophoblast cells differentiate into syncytiotrophoblast cells, the amounts of IF_1 found in the steroidogenic cells could be the result of cell differentiation and have a significant effect on their mitochondrial architecture (tubulovesicular cristae) and physiology (P4 synthesis). The amount of IF_1 and F_0F_1-ATP synthase dimer present in these mitochondria is probably related to its physiological functions.

But, why do syncytiotrophoblast cells have mitochondria with atypical cristae morphology? Since the human placenta does not express StAR (Tuckey, 2005) and TSPO (Maldonado-Mercado et al., 2008), two proteins involved in mitochondrial cholesterol flow, it has been suggested that the reduction in the size of syncytiotrophoblast mitochondria and the change in the structure of cristae may improve the steroidogenic activity of syncytiotrophoblast cells (Martinez et al., 1997). In this sense, the translocation of cholesterol to P450scc has been well known to be the rate-limiting step in steroidogenesis; thus, a greater surface could enhance the movement of cholesterol to the inner membrane where P450scc is located. It is tempting to speculate that the non-ortodox cristae structure in mitochondria from steroidogenic tissue allows cholesterol to flow from the outer to the inner mitochondrial membranes and improves hormone production.

3.4 Mitochondrial accessory proteins involved in progesterone synthesis

For P4 synthesis by human syncytiotrophoblast mitochondria, the cristae architecture could not be considered as the only and most important issue; we have identified a set of different proteins involved in hormone production as a heat shock protein-60 kDa (HSP60), associated to the increases of progesterone synthesis through its association with the MLN64-like protein (Olvera-Sanchez et al., 2011); an ADPase, and an ATP-diphosphohydrolase associated to mitochondrial membranes (Uribe et al., 1999; Flores-Herrera et al., 1999).

ATP-diphosphohydrolase is anchored to mitochondrial membranes whit its nucleotide-hydrolyzing activity oriented to the intermembrane space. The kinetic characterization of its activity in a detergent solubilized fraction revealed that it can use ATP, ADP, GTP, GDP, UTP, UDP, CTP, CDP, TTP and TDP in a cation (Mg^{+2}, Ca^{+2}, and Zn^{+2}) dependent fashion as substrates (Flores-Herrera et al., 1999) (Fig. 4). ATP hydrolysis by this ATP-diphosphohydrolase can stimulate oxygen uptake in intact mitochondria from syncytiotrophoblast coupling with ATP synthesis (Martinez et al., 1993). Since one main function of mitochondria is the synthesis of ATP through the F_0F_1-ATPase activity, the presence of external mitochondria ATP-diphosphohydrolase and an ADPase in the human

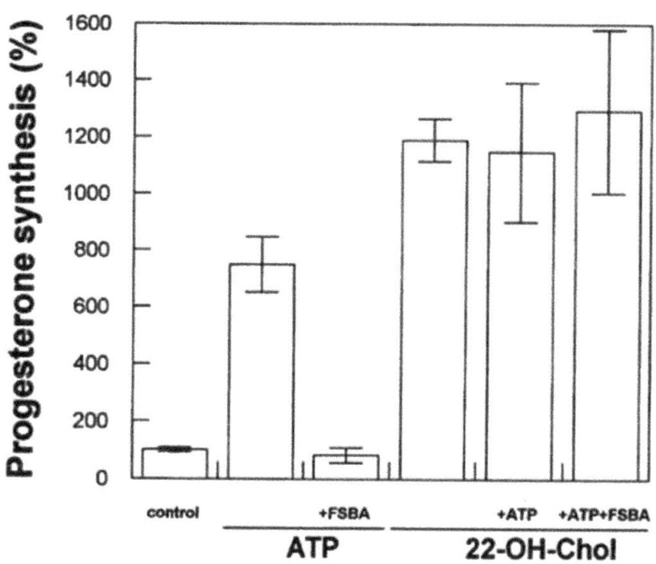

Fig. 4. Effect of 22(*R*)-hydroxycholesterol (22-OH-Chol) on progesterone synthesis. Mitochondria were incubated in progesterone synthesis medium with or without 1 mM FSBA. Where indicated, 1 mM ATP or 15 μM 22-OH-Chol was added. 100% progesterone synthesis = 142 ng progesterone/mg/min (Modified from Flores-Herrera et al., 2002).

placental mitochondria could produce a futile cycle due to the combination of the F_0F_1-ATPase and ATP-diphosphohydrolase activities, being lethal for trophoblast cells. However, the futile cycle is not observed, because the addition of ATP (or ADP) to isolated mitochondria induces oxygen consumption without uncoupling the respiration, suggesting the presence of mechanisms that regulate the activity of ATP-diphosphohydrolase in a way that trophoblast cells remain alive (Martinez et al., 1993). Indeed, ATP-diphosphohydrolase activity and its substrate specificity seem to be regulated by the proton electrochemical potential ($\Delta\mu_{H+}$), i.e. if mitochondrial inner membrane is energized, ATP-diphosphohydrolase selectively hydrolyzes ATP, while dissipation of $\Delta\mu_{H+}$ by CCCP produces a loss of substrate specificity, and is able to hydrolyze ATP and GTP equally (O. Flores-Herrera, et al., manuscript in preparation).

With respect to ATP-diphosphohydrolase role in syncytiotrophoblast mitochondria steroidogenesis, its activity in presence of ATP is involved in cholesterol transport between mitochondrial membranes (Flores-Herrera et al., 1999; Flores-Herrera et al., 2002). In addition, other nucleotide hydrolase activities have been determined in mitochondria from other steroidogenic tissues; in particular, in adrenal mitochondria GTP enhances steroidogenesis, a process modulated by a GTPase (X. Xu & T. Xu, 1989); however, no conclusion can be drawn yet in this steroidogenic tissue. However, syncytiotrophoblast mitochondria hydrolyze several nucleosides tri- and di-phosphatides increasing P4 synthesis, which is sensitive to ATP-diphosphohydrolase inhibition by FSBA, a non-hydrolysable ATP analog (Flores-Herrera et al., 2002) (Fig. 4). Finally, although the mechanisms of regulation of this enzyme have to be elucidated, we conclude that ATP-diphosphohydrolase is anchored to syncytiotrophoblast mitochondrial membranes, which nucleotide hydrolysis activity is involved in cholesterol transport between mitochondrial membranes and in oxygen uptake by mitochondrial electron transport chain (Flores-Herrera et al., 2002).

4. Signaling pathway in placental steroidogenesis

4.1 The role of mitochondria in the phosphorylation cell signaling

Progesterone synthesis by human placenta is essential for the maintenance of pregnancy. In the human being, P4 is produced in the corpus luteum cells during the secretory phase of the menstrual cycle; whereas in the early stages of pregnancy its production continues due to the stimulus of the Chorionic Gonadotropin hormone (hCG); however, between the 6th and 8th week of gestation, the corpus luteum decreases its production of P4, which is now synthesized by the trophoblastic cells of the placenta (Tuckey, 2005).

Unlike the other steroidogenic tissues, placental steroidogenesis is chronically regulated. Both regulation systems are under the control of diverse factors or hormones that activate signal transduction pathways in different forms, allowing either short-term or long-term regulation. In general, the chronic response is started within hours after the initiating stimulus and involves the activation of certain signaling pathways, among them the cAMP-dependent protein kinase (PKA) cascade is the most important.

The effect mediated by PKA/cAMP in long-term and short-term regulation of steroidogenesis is the main pathway stimulated by trophic hormones which acts through G protein-coupled receptors, which in turn activates the enzyme adenylate cyclase, which increases the content of cAMP. cAMP has pleiotropic effects such as the activation of PKA, which phosphorylates proteins and transcription factors such as the steroidogenic factor (SF-1) and the protein cAMP response element binding (CREB), the latter being the main mediator of positive changes in gene expression (Sands, 2008); for example, the activation of StAR gene (Stocco et al., 2005) or even its phosphorylation (Fig. 5).

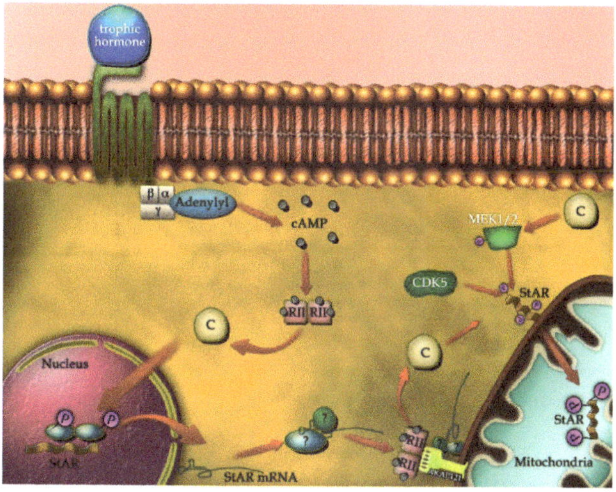

Fig. 5. The model illustrates the activation of the transduction pathway mediated by PKA/cAMP in the postranscriptional and postranslational regulation StAR protein (Modified from Manna, 2009).

Although other PKA-dependent and -independent signaling pathways have been reported, the responses generated are generally less potent than those mediated by PKA/cAMP (Manna et al., 2006).

During pregnancy, the production of P4 gradually increases with no substantial variations observed (Tuckey, 2005). It has been reported that a plasmatic decrease of P4 is associated with a higher probability of abortion (Duan et al., 2010).

The addition of 8Br-cAMP or dibutyryl-cAMP to cultured trophoblast cells stimulated the P4 synthesis by increasing the transcription and translation of P450scc and adrenodoxin. Nevertheless, independent of the factors involved modulating the intracellular concentration of cAMP, the likely participation of different hormones and the trophic factors and cytokines that could have endocrine, paracrine, autocrine or intracrine effect in the regulation of steroidogenesis through the signaling pathway mediated by PKA is still unknown; since, as it has been said, there are other pathways that can participate in the regulation of P4 synthesis (Manna et al., 2006; Stocco et al., 2005) (Fig. 6).

In trophoblast choriocarcinoma-derived cells of human placenta (BeWo) the addition of hCG increased P4 synthesis through PKA. Other factors also increased in a variable way the production of P4; nevertheless, it has been suggested that its main effect would be predominantly as a regulator and just in a few cases as a stimulant of steroidogenesis, although through the activation of cAMP-dependent pathways and PKA activation (Manna et al., 2006).

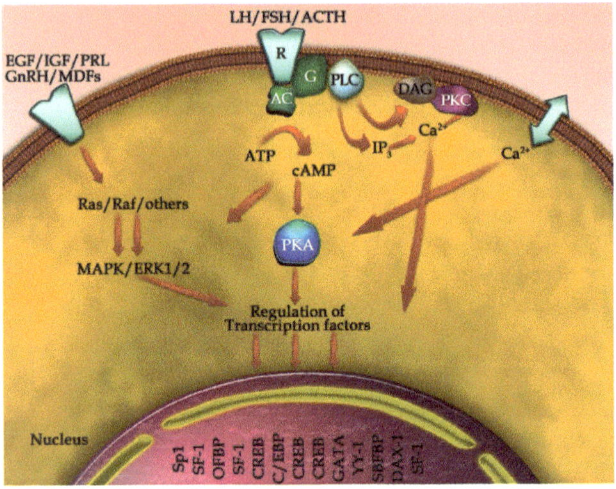

Fig. 6. Model proposed to illustrate the cAMP-dependent and -independent pathways in the regulation of StAR expression and steroidogenesis in adrenal gland and gonads (Modified from Manna, 2009).

Although the signaling pathways associated with P4 synthesis in human placenta are unknown, one of the best studied mechanism is the one mediated by PKA activation. Unlike gonads, adrenal cortex, and the corpus luteum, P4 synthesis by placental cells in the presence of cAMP soluble derivatives produce no acute response, not even in cells obtained from first-trimester placentas (Zosmer et al., 1997).

Previous data confirm that trophoblast cells have the machinery to produce cAMP, which may increase its concentration in cytoplasm through the stimulation of β_2 adrenergic receptors in full-term placentas (Kasugai et al., 1987). Interestingly, in first-trimester placentas, norepinephrine increased the content of cAMP mediated by α_1-adrenergic receptors (Shi & Zhuang, 1993). There is also evidence of the potential effect of other hormones that may stimulate placental P4 synthesis through cAMP-dependent pathways, just like it happens in the case of estrogens (Pepe & Albretch, 1999), insulin (Lavy et al., 1987), insulin-like growth factor 1 (Nestler, 1987) and epidermal growth factor (Ritvos, 1988). The results suggest the possibility of different stimuli for specific effectors according to the gestational age.

The function of PKA in cells is vital, since its activity is aimed at specific functions, which include the differential expression of regulatory and catalytic subunits in different tissues. Thus, anchor proteins (AKAP's, **A**-**k**inase **a**nchor **p**roteins) in certain cellular locations place PKA close to its substrates, making its activity more efficient (Fig. 7). For instance, in Leydig tumoral cells from mice the association of AKAP 121 with the regulatory subunit α of PKA II in mitochondria in response to cAMP was observed, which was interpreted as a powering effect of steroidogenesis on directing the synthesis and activation of StAR to the mitochondrion in response to cAMP (Dyson et al., 2008).

In a similar way, mitochondria isolated from human placenta show the interaction of PKA, AKAP-121, and PTPD1 (Gómez-Concha et al., 2011) (Fig. 8). In addition, it was seen that in the presence of radioactive ATP several proteins were phosphorylated in less than 5 min on

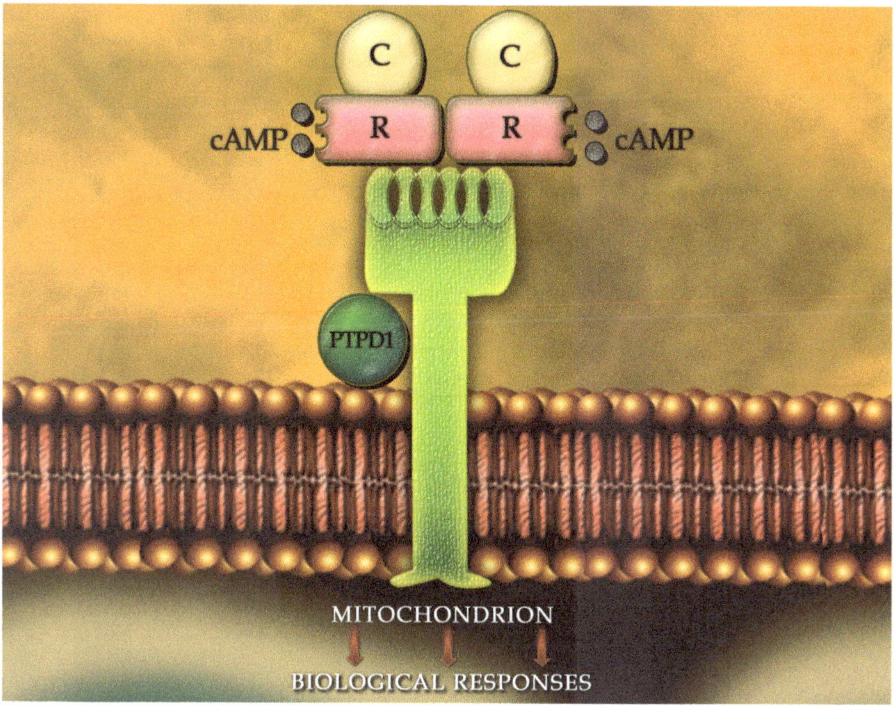

Fig. 7. A signaling complex made up by AKAP 121, which anchors PKA close to the mitochondrion, thus facilitating the phosphorylation of mitochondrial proteins (Modified from Feliciello, 2005).

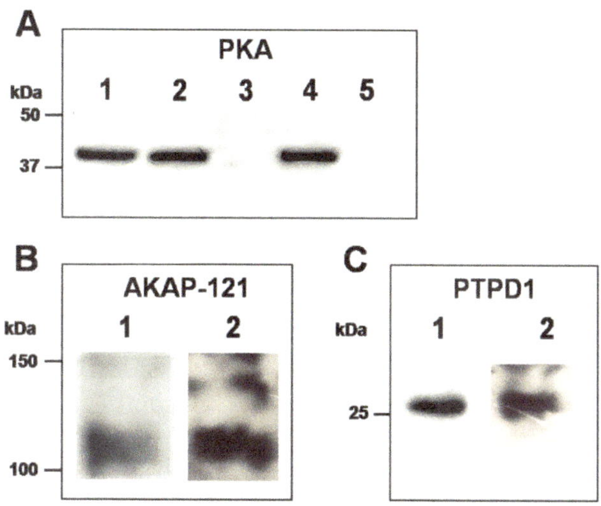

Fig. 8. Immunodetection of PKA (A), AKAP-121 (B) and PTPD1 (C) (see Material and Methods from Gómez Concha, 2011.)

serine and threonine, and to a lesser degree on tyrosine, suggesting the potential activity of kinases. Likewise, the importance of cAMP-PKA pathway in BeWo cells and in mitochondria isolated from human placenta was shown using H89, an inhibitor of PKA activity (Maldonado-Mercado et al., 2008). In mitochondria isolated from syncytiotrophoblast, steroidogenesis was inhibited 50% with 100 μM of H89, whereas in BeWo cells with concentrations of 10 and 20 μM, an inhibition of steroidogenesis of 70% and 90% was found, respectively. The addition of 22(*R*)-hydroxycholesterol to the isolated mitochondria previously inhibited with H89, reestablishes P4 synthesis, thus confirming that the activities of P450scc and 3HSD are not affected by H89.

The results show that to the maximal concentration of H89 inhibited the synthesis of P4 in 99%, but only 50% of protein phosphorylation, which suggests that there are other kinase activities in mitochondria isolated from the human placenta, suggesting the pathway mediated by PKA could be associated to another pathways that ensures the production of P4; then it is relevant to determine the kinases that participate and their associations with the steroidogenesis by the human placenta as it was proposed (Maldonado-Mercado et al., 2008; Gómez -Concha et al., 2011) (Fig. 9).

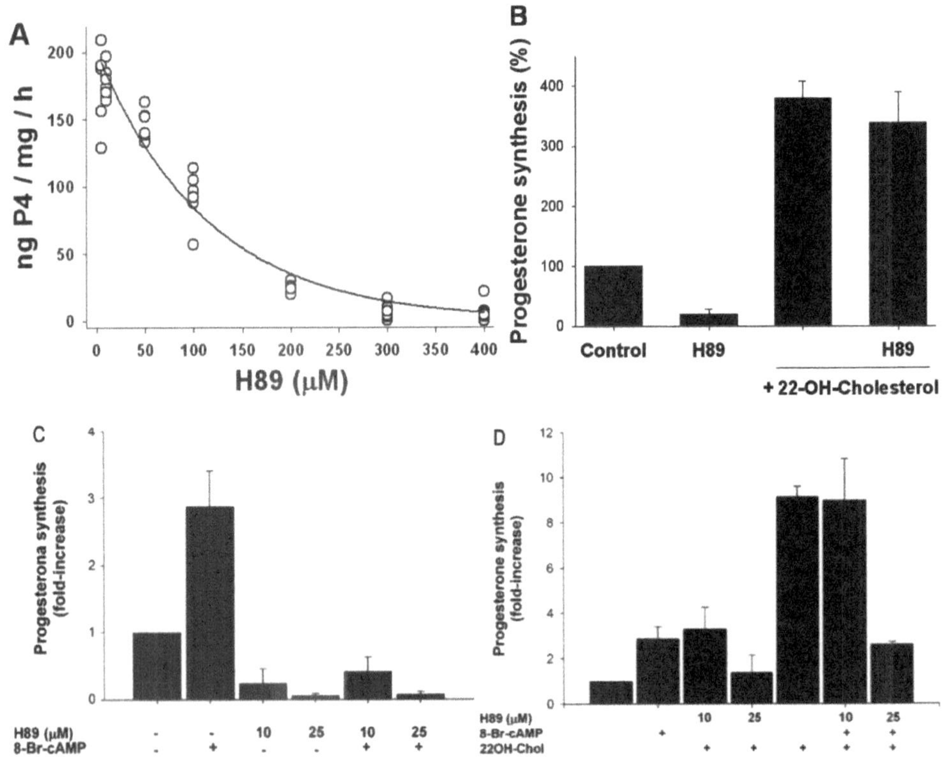

Fig. 9. Progesterone syntheses by syncytiotrophoblast mitochondria (A and B) and progesterone synthesis in BeWo cells (C and D) (see Material and Methods from Maldonado-Mercado et al., 2008, and Gómez-Concha et al., 2011). 22(*R*)-hydroxycholesterol (22-OH-Cholesterol or 22OH-Chol).

Interestingly, in cultured human placenta cells, the stimulus of an acute signaling pathway associated with steroidogenesis as the one observed in isolated mitochondria has not been described; nevertheless it has been suggested that the pathway mediated by PKA/cAMP plays an important role in the regulation of placental steroidogenesis, perhaps with the potential participation of other signal transduction pathways, as it has been observed in other tissues (Dodge-Kafka & Kapiloff, 2006). The endocrine, paracrine, autocrine, and even intracrine mechanisms that modulate this process are still to be described. No matter which one is the signaling pathway activated, the importance of the events of dynamic phosphorylation of proteins with pleiotropic effects in cellular functions as hormonal synthesis is the most relevant (Corso & Thomson, 2001; Gorostizaga et al., 2007; Thomson, 2002).

4.2 Protein phosphorylation in the control of steroidogenesis

Protein phosphorylation is one of the most studied postranslational modifications. The modification of target proteins on specific residues allows structural changes, changes in the protein-protein interaction, and favors their activation or inactivation (Chang & Karin, 2001), thus achieving the regulation of their functions (Matthews, 1995; Klumpp & Krieglstein, 2005; Puttick et al, 2008).

It has been shown that the activity of certain proteins modulated by phosphorylation/ dephosphorylation has a temporary effect in specific cellular regions such as the plasma membrane, endoplasmic reticulum, and nucleus, regulating the cellular metabolism (Trost, 2010; Bauman & Scott, 2002), a system that seems to be associated with steroidogenesis (Gómez-Concha et al., 2011), similar to StAR protein (Steroidogenic acute regulatory protein) in adrenal glands and gonads. StAR protein phosphorylation mediated by PKA stimulates the transport of cholesterol from the cytoplasm into mitochondrial membranes (Stocco, 2000; Thomson, 1998; Manna & Stocco, 2005), apparently through a multiprotein complex associated to this organelle (Thomson, 2002) (Fig.10).

It has been suggested that a tyrosine phosphatases is the key for the regulation of StAR and the transport of cholesterol, where phosphorylation/dephosphorylation of intermediary proteins is fundamental in the regulation of steroids biosynthesis (Cooke et al, 2011). Although the placenta does not synthesize StAR protein, data suggest that trophoblast cells have a phosphorylation/dephosphorylation system associated with steroidogenesis.

It has been described that the PKA activity associated with mitochondria is different from that of cytoplasm, suggesting a differential regulation according to their subcellular location, maybe related to the complex formed by PKA, AKAP 121, and PTPD1 (Feliciello et al, 2001; Gómez-Concha et al., 2011). This way, the identification of proteins phosphorylated on their serine, tyrosine, and threonine residues suggests that the metabolism of placental mitochondria has important kinase activity (Gómez-Concha et al., 2011).

In BeWo cells and in isolated mitochondria from placenta, the phosphorylated proteins of 46, 42 and 36 kDa appear to be a potential target of kinases and phosphatases system, where the H89 change the balance of phosphorylation/ dephosphorylation between proteins of 42 and 36 kDa (Maldonado-Mercado et al., 2008; Gómez-Concha et al., 2011) (Fig. 11 and 12).

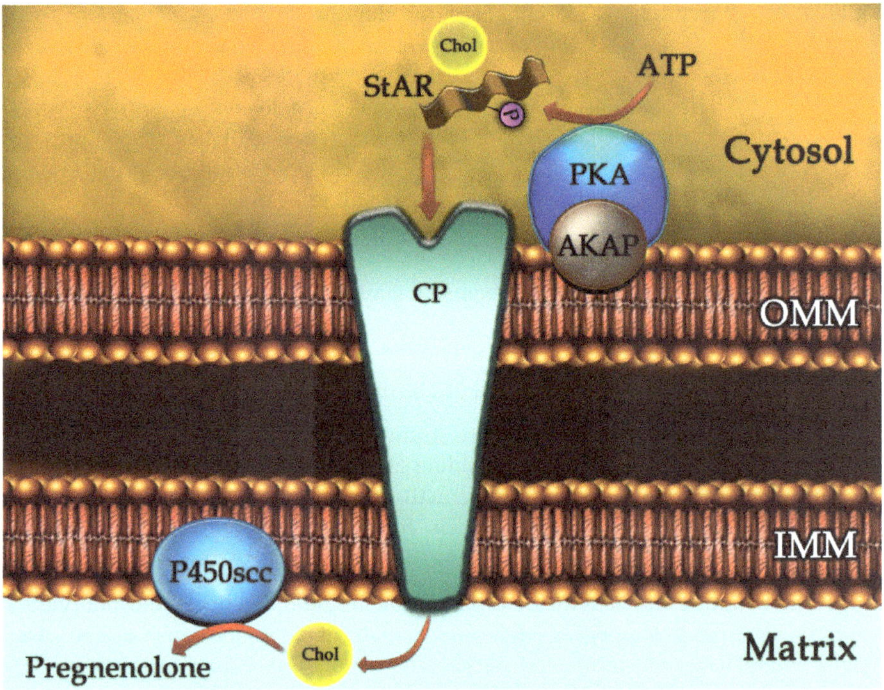

Fig. 10. Propose model for steroidogenic modulation by mitochondrial PKA (Modified from Thomson, 2002).

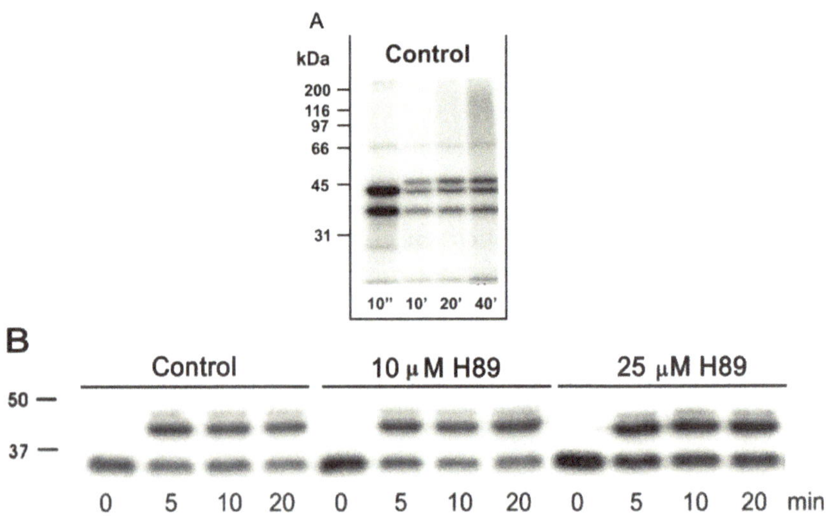

Fig. 11. Incorporation of ($\gamma^{32}P$) to syncytiotrophoblast mitochondria proteins (A) and isolated mitochondria from BeWo cells in the presence of H89 (B). (see Material and Methods from Maldonado-Mercado et al., 2008; Gómez -Concha et al., 2011)

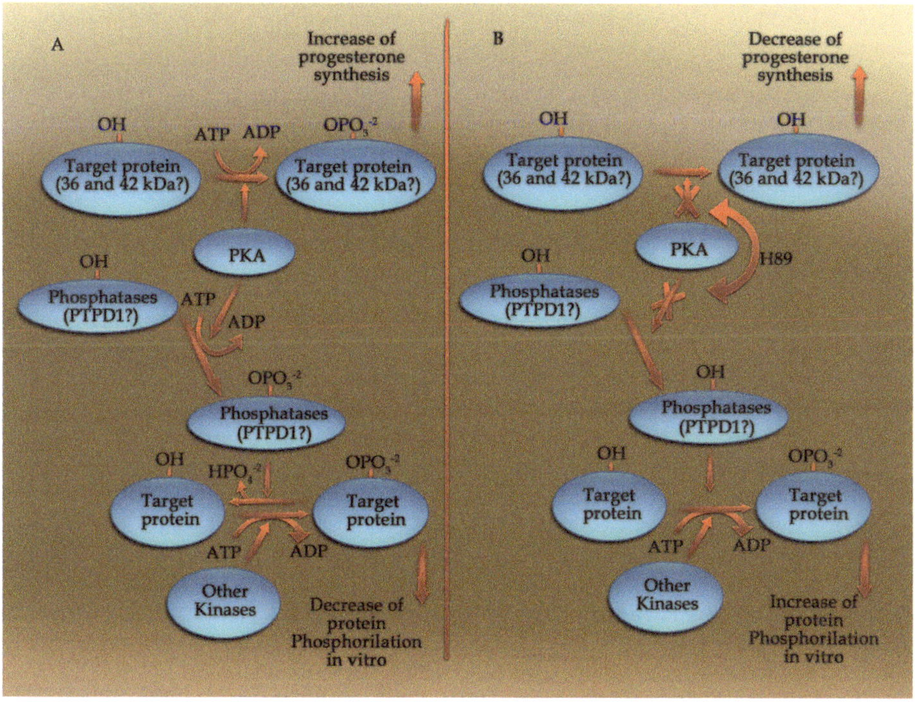

Fig. 12. Model proposed for the participation of PKA in steroidogenesis by syncytiotrophoblast mitochondria (Modified from Gómez -Concha et al., 2011).

5. Steroidogenesis

The transport of cholesterol to mitochondria by proteins is required for steroidogenesis. Deep differences between the placenta and adrenal glands have been observed, which are tightly associated to the permanent production of progesterone.

Meanwhile the cellular movement of cholesterol from cytoplasm to different organelles is accomplished by StAR, i.e. adrenal glands, gonads, liver, brain and others; human placenta does not express the StAR protein. A metastatic lymph node 64 protein (MLN64), which has similar characteristics to StAR protein to recognize cholesterol and transport it to the mitochondria, has been implicated in the movement of cholesterol in the human placenta; also, other proteins have been associated with cholesterol transport, such as the heat shock protein 60 (HSP60) (Olvera-Sanchez et al, 2011) and porine (Espinosa-Garcia et al., 2000).

In the previous sections of this chapter, several aspects of the trophoblast cells have been described. As it was observed, the human placenta possesses special characteristics basically oriented to maintain the relationship between mother and fetus in order to reach a successful delivery. The human placenta works as a mechanical barrier, being highly specific about the molecules that can cross it. In a sense, it controls by itself the mechanisms that regulate the metabolism and hormone production to assure nutrient supply by using different metabolic and signaling pathways, also modulating the mitochondrial activity through ATP-diphosphohydrolase and other enzymatic activities due to the relevant role that mitochondria play in both ATP synthesis and steroidogenesis.

As mentioned before, cholesterol is the source of steroid hormones, but the human placenta is unable to synthesize it, so the cholesterol must be obtained from mother´s lipoproteins. During pregnancy, the amount of progesterone required is high, and during the first trimester its production is responsibility of the corpus luteum, while the egg implantation in the maternal epithelium of the uterus occurs.

5.1 Electron transport chain coupled to cytochrome P450scc

Placental steroidogenesis is an essential process for reproduction. Syncytiotrophoblast cells are the P4-producing cells in the human placenta (Martinez et al., 1997). By full-term pregnancy, placenta produces about 300 mg of P4 per day (Strauss et al., 1996). The first enzymatic stage in its production is the conversion of cholesterol into P5 by P450scc type I (CYP11A1; EC 1.14.15.6), composed by approximately 530 amino acids, including the signal peptide necessary for its association to the mitochondrial inner membrane and only one heme group. P450scc receives six electrons from 3 moles of NADPH through a 54 kDa flavoprotein, ferredoxin reductase (adrenodoxin reductase), and ferredoxin (adrenodoxin) a 2Fe-2S protein with a molecular weight of 13.5 kDa. Both are found in the mitochondrial matrix. Studies of the molecular mechanism about the formation of this complex and electron transport have proposed a stoichiometry for proteins 1:1:1 or 1:2:1, and it has been suggested that adrenodoxin behaves as a mobile electron transporter from adrenodoxin reductase to P450scc (Miller, 2005), and the interaction between CYP11A and adrenodoxin reductase has been shown by molecular biology technics (Payne & Hales, 2004; Strushkevicha, 2011) (Fig. 13).

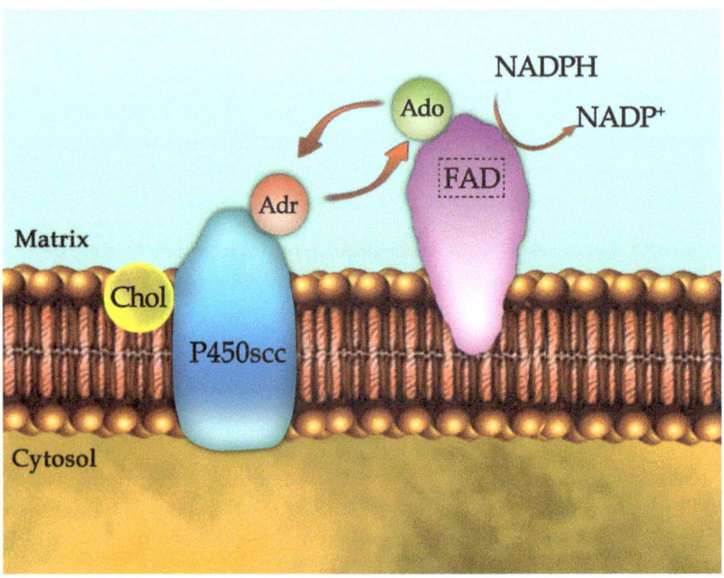

Fig. 13. Electron transport from adrenodoxin reductase to P450scc. Ado = adrenodoxin; Adr = Adrenodoxin reduced; FAD = adrenodoxin reductase (Modified from Payne and Hales, 2004).

The transformation of cholesterol into P5 requires three mono-oxygenation reactions, using molecular oxygen, involving two stereo-specific hydroxylations with the formation of 22(*R*)-hydroxycholesterol and 20(*R*),22(*R*)-dihydroxycholesterol followed by the breaking of the bond C-C between carbons 20 and 22 to release the lateral chain, yielding isocaproaldehyde and P5, which is changed into P4 through two consecutive reactions that require NAD^+ and are catalyzed by the same enzyme 3HSD type 1 (EC 5.3.3.1) with no release of intermediaries. Two isoenzymes of 3HSD are known in humans, product of different genes (Payne & Hales, 2004). In the placenta, 3HSD is found in the mitochondria, unlike other steroiodogenic tissues in which it is found in the endoplasmic reticulum. The activity of this enzyme is higher than P450scc activity; therefore, it is not a limiting step in P4 synthesis (Tuckey, 2005). On the other hand, no disease involving the loss of 3HSD activity in the placenta is known, suggesting that its absence is incompatible with pregnancy.

5.2 Systems for cholesterol transport and mitochondrial contact sites

The cholesterol that participates in P4 synthesis comes from maternal circulation as lipoprotein complexes (LDL or HDL) which bind to their receptors in the plasma membrane. LDLs are released from their endosomal receptors to make late endosomes/lysosomes and obtain free cholesterol as substrate for P450scc (Hu et al., 2010).

The transport of cholesterol from the cytoplasm into the outer mitochondrial membrane in most steroidogenic tissues is associated to many proteins; the StAR, is the first protein identified as part of a family that contains the START domain (StAR-related lipid transfer domain) of about 210 amino acids. It is synthesized as a 37 kDa protein with a signal peptide aimed to the mitochondrion to yield cholesterol to the outer mitochondrial membrane and, then is transformed into a 30 kDa intramitochondrial protein (Manna & Stocco, 2005). This protein is phosphorylated and activated in response to hormonal stimulation in steroidogenic cells (Arakane et al., 1996). The constructs lacking the 62 amino acid residues from the amino-terminal of StAR yields a truncated protein still able to participate in steroidogenesis. These results suggest that the translocation of the StAR protein to the interior of the mitochondria is not a requisite for cholesterol transport, and suggests that cholesterol may be transferred to another soluble acceptor protein or transporter in the outer mitochondrial membrane which finally allows it to reach P450scc for P4 synthesis (Bose et al., 2000; Alpy & Tomasetto, 2006). Nevertheless, the human placenta does not express StAR, and it has been proposed that the protein MLN64 (Moog-Lutz, 1997) could perform the activity of cholesterol transporter. MLN64 is a 54 kDa protein (445 amino acids), isolated from a metastatic nodule of breast cancer. MLN64 is found in late endosomes and has two functional domains, one in the amino end with four transmembrane domains and another at the carboxyl end, corresponding to the START domain, oriented towards the cytoplasm, composed by 227 amino acids with an identity of 37% of StAR sequence. The tridimensional organization of its crystals shows the formation of a hydrophobic tunnel which allows the collocation of one molecule of cholesterol. This location supports the theory of MLN64 substituting StAR in human placenta to promote the flow of cholesterol.

Full-term human placenta isolated mitochondria synthesize P4 without the addition of exogenous cholesterol (Martinez et al., 1997). It has been reported that cholesterol transport between human placenta mitochondrial membranes requires proteins, since when treated with trypsin they are unable to transport cholesterol and, therefore, synthesize P4.

Nevertheless, mitochondria treated with trypsin were able to efficiently transform 22(*R*)-hydroxycholesterol into P4, a substrate that does not need a protein membrane transport system, showing that the P450scc chain is not modified by such treatment; thus making human placenta isolated mitochondria an adequate model for the study of cholesterol transport and steroidogenesis (Espinosa-García et al., 2000).

The transport of cholesterol towards the inner mitochondrial membrane requires many proteins associated with the contact sites; these are dynamic structures formed by proteins coming from both the outer and inner membrane and work as complexes that are assembled and degraded according to specific mitochondria conditions. Hence, contact sites might represent the most efficient route for cholesterol to reach P450scc (Thomson, 2003).

It has been reported that during the isolation of mitochondrial contact sites from full-term human placenta, 3 fractions were obtained from the outer membrane and 4 from the inner membrane. The protein composition was specific for each one of them and only one fraction of the inner membrane was able to transform cholesterol into P4. In such fraction, reported as steroidogenic site, porine, creatine kinase, the translocator of adenine nucleotides, ATP-diphosphohydrolase, MLN64, and HSP90, HSP72, HSP40 and HSP27, enzymes of the P450scc chain, and $NADP^+$-dependent isocitrate dehydrogenase were identified. These results support the theory that binding sites are an efficient system for cholesterol transit in the human placenta mitochondria (Uribe et al., 2003) (Fig. 14).

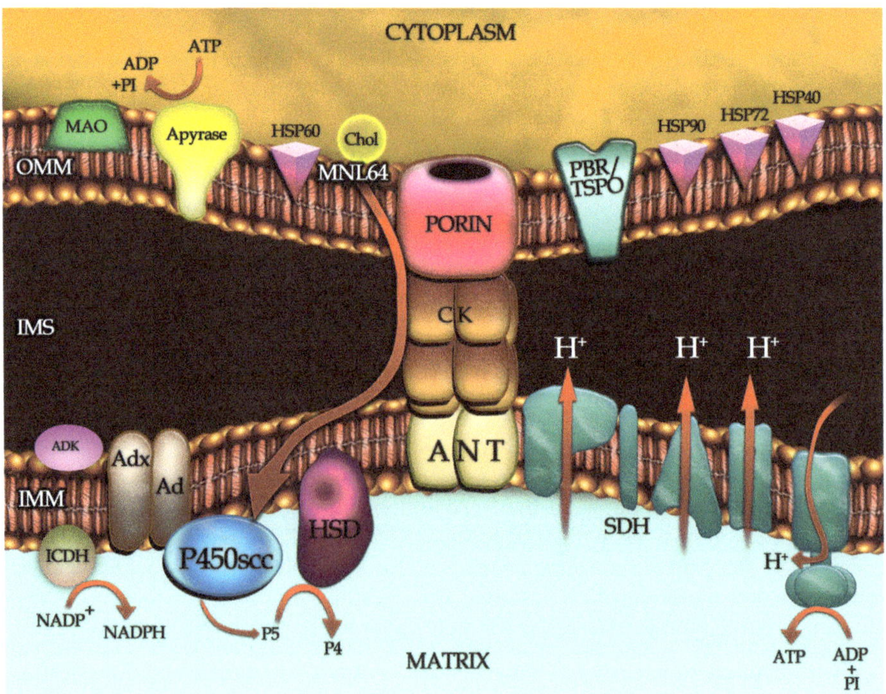

Fig. 14. Model of isolated contact sites from human placental syncytiotrophoblast mitochondria. (Modified from Uribe et al., 2003).

The use of MLN64 antibodies allowed the recognition of a 60 KDa protein identified as an HSP and another 30 kDa protein corresponding to the START domain of MLN64, in human placenta isolated mitochondria. Results suggest that both proteins participate in placental seteroidogenesis, favoring both cholesterol movement towards mitochondrial membranes and the release of P4 from mitochondria (Olvera-Sanchez et al., 2011).

5.3 Steroidogenesis regulation

P4 biosynthesis regulation in placenta seems to be at two levels. One is related to hormones and/or factors currently unknown, which initiates a signal transduction cascade involving PKA activation cAMP mediated, as explained before, and another level involving the mitochondria.

As for the mechanism at mitochondrial level, it has been proposed that the activity of P450scc might be regulated by the concentration of adrenodoxin reductase which causes a decrease of P450scc affinity for cholesterol, and makes it work just at 16% of its capacity (Tuckey & Headlam, 2002). Nevertheless, the results obtained from mitochondria isolated from the placenta in the presence of 22(*R*)-hydroxycholesterol show no limitation in their capacity to produce P4. Therefore, it is unlikely that in physiologic conditions the activity of adrenodoxin reductase is a controlling factor.

Just like other steroidogenic tissues, the limiting step in P4 production is the access of cholesterol to mitochondria. So far, no evidence of any protein limiting transport is available, surely because it would be incompatible with pregnancy. Data available suggest that placental cells have the necessary mechanisms to allow cholesterol to reach mitochondria constantly, making P4 synthesis a constitutive metabolic pathway that assures, independently of nutritional conditions, physical or related to mother's health, that the fetus reaches the full term of pregnancy. In this context, the knowledge of the endocrine, paracrine, etc., signaling pathways would allow the development of therapeutic strategies that favor the integral development of the fetus.

Nevertheless, it is important to mention that acute regulation at mitochondrial level is necessarily accompanied by a chronic modulation mediated by the control of the transcription/translation of the genes that encode for the different steroidogenic enzymes, in a tissue-specific fashion. As for the placenta, it has been observed that there are mechanisms controlling the expression of the genes of the steroidogenic enzymes in which cAMP has no prominent role.

In gonads or adrenal glands, mutations of the genes encoding for proteins STARD1, CYP11A1 or 3HSD affects steroid production, being SF-1 the main factor regulating P450scc expression (Schimmer & White, 2010). Nevertheless, SF-1 factor is not found in human placenta. It has been suggested that P450scc expression is regulated by AP-2 factors that bind to cis elements overlapped to the sequences required for the recognition of SF-1 in other steroidogenic tissues (Ben-Zimra, 2002). It has also been proposed that LBP (Long Terminal Repeat Binding Proteins) identified in the syncytiotrophoblast might assume the regulator role of SF-1, binding to the region -155 to -131 of the promoter of the genes that allow the expression of P450scc. LBP-1b would act as an activator of the expression of P450scc, whereas LBP-9 and LBP-32 would act as repressors (Henderson et al., 2008; LaVoie & King., 2009).

6. Conclusion

On the whole, the information shows that mitochondria isolated from human placenta are an appropriate model to study the mechanisms of cholesterol transport. The physiological difference between human placenta and other steroidogenic organs make the human syncytiotrophoblast a particular tissue, which maintains a functional independence while allowing the interaction between the mother and the fetus to successfully reach the full term of pregnancy in order to perpetuate the species.

7. Acknowledgements

The present work has the partial support of DGAPA, UNAM (IN202496, IN200399, IN203006, IN 217609), and CONACYT (26096M). The author thanks Dr. José Luis Pérez-García in the translation of the present chapter.

8. References

Aldoreta, P.W. & Hay, W.W. (1995). Metabolic Substrates for Fetal Energy Metabolism and Growth. *Clinics in Perinatology*, Vol.22, No.1, (March 1995), pp.15-37, ISSN 0095-5108

Allen, J.A; Shankara, T.; Janus, P.; Buck, S.; Diemer, T.; Hales, K.H. & Hales, D.B. (2006). Energized, Polarized, and Actively Respiring Mitochondria are Required for Acute Leydig Cell Steroidogenesis. *Endocrinology*, Vol.147, No.8, (August 2006), pp. 3924–3935, ISSN 0013-7227

Alpy, F. & Tomasetto, C. (2006). MLN64 and MENTHO, Two Mediators of Endosomal Cholesterol Transport. *Biochemical Society Transactions*, Vol. 34, Pt.3, (June 2006), pp. 343- 345, ISSN 0300-5127

Angiolini, E.; Fowden, A.; Coan, P.; Sandovici, I.; Smith, P.; Dean, W.; Burton, G.; Tycko, B.; Reik, W.; Sibley, C. & Contância, M. (2006). Regulation of Placental Efficiency for Nutrient Transport by Imprinted Genes. *Placenta*, Vol.27, Suppl A, (April 2006), pp. S98-102, ISSN 0143-4004

Arakane, F.; Sugawara, T.; Nishino, H.; Liu, Z.; Holt, J.A.; Pain, D.; Stocco, D.M.; Miller, W.L. & Strauss J.F. 3rd. (1996). Steroidogenic Acute Regulatory Protein (StAR) Retains Activity in the Absence of its Aitochondrial Import Sequence: Implications for the Mechanism of StAR Action. *Proceedings of the National Academy of Sciences. U.S.A.*, Vol. 93, No. 24, (November 1996), pp. 13731-13736, ISSN 0027-8424

Arnold, I.; Pfeiffer, K.; Neuport, W.; Stuart, R.A. & Schägger, H. (1998). Yeast Mitochondrial F1F0-ATP Synthase Exists as a Dimer: Identification of Three Dimer-Specific Subunits. *The EMBO Journal*, Vol.17, No.24, (December 1998), pp. 7170- 7178, ISSN 0261-4189

Barash, V.; Reskin, A.; Shafrir, E.; Waddell, I.D. & Burchell, A. (1991). Kinetic and Immunologic Evidence for the Absence of Glucose-6-phosphatase in Early Human Chorionic Villi and Term Human Placenta. *Biochimica et Biophysica Acta*, Vol.1073, No.1, (January 1991), pp. 161-167, ISSN 0304-4165

Battaglia, F.C. (1989). An Update Off and Placental Metabolism: Carbohydrate and Amino Acids. *Biology of the Neonate*, Vol.55, No.6, pp. 347-354, ISSN 0006-3126

Bauman, A.L. & Scott, J.D. (2002). Kinase- and Phosphatase-Anchoring Proteins: Harnessing the Dynamic Duo. *Nature Cell Biology,* Vol.4, No.8, (August 2002), pp. E203–E206, ISSN1465-7392

Ben-Zimra, M.; Koler, M. & Orly, J. (2002). Transcription of Cholesterol Side-Chain Cleavage Cytochrome P450 in the Placenta: Activating Protein-2 Assumes the Role of Steroidogenic Factor-1by Binding to an Overlapping Promoter Element. *Molecular Endocrinology,* Vol.16, No.8, (August 2002), pp. 1864–1880, ISSN 0888-8809

Bloxam, D.L. & Bobinski, P.M. (1984). Energy Metabolism and Glycolysis in the Human Placenta During Ischaemia and in Normal Labour. *Placenta,* Vol.5, No.5, (September-October 1984), pp. 381-394, ISSN 0143-4004

Bose, H.S.; Whittal, R.M.; Huang, M.C.; Baldwin, M.A. & Miller, W.L. (2000). N-218 MLN64, a Protein with StAR-like Steroidogenic Activity, Is Folded and Cleaved Similarly to StAR. *Biochemistry,* Vol.39, No.38, (September 2000), pp. 11722-11731, ISSN 0006-2960

Brand, C.; Cherradi, N.; Defaye, G.; Chinn, A.; Chambaz, E.M.; Feige, J.J. & Bailly, S. (1998). Transforming Growth Factor Beta1 Decreases Cholesterol Supply to Mitochondria Via Repression of Steroidogenic Acute Regulatory Protein Expression. *Journal of Biological Chemistry,* Vol.273, No.11, (March 1998), pp. 6410-6416, ISSN 0021-9258

Cabezón, E.; Arechaga, I.; Jonathan, P.; Butler, G. & Walker, J.E. (2000). Dimerization of Bovine F1-ATPase by Binding the Inhibitor Protein, IF1. *Journal of Biological Chemistry,* Vol.275, No.37, (September 2000), pp. 28353-28355, ISSN 0021-9258

Cammer, W. & Estabrook, R.W. (1967). Spectrophotometric Studies of the Pigments of Adrenal Cortex Mitochondria. *Archives of Biochemistry and Biophysics,* Vol.122, No.3, (December 1967), pp. 735-747, ISSN 0003-9861

Campanella, M.; Casswell, E.; Chong, S.; Farah, Z.; Wieckowski, M.R.; Abramov, A.; Y. Tinker, A. & Duchen, M.R. (2008). Regulation of Mitochondrial Structure and Function by the F1Fo-Atpase Inhibitor Protein, IF1. *Cell Metabolism,* Vol.8, No.1, (July 2008), pp. 13–25. ISSN 1550-4131

Carter, A.M. (2000). Placental Oxygen Consumption. Part I: in vivo Studies-a Review. *Placenta,* Vol.21, Suppl. A, (March-April 2000), pp. S31-37, ISSN 0143-4004

Chang, L. & Karin, M. (2001). Mammalian MAP Kinase Signalling Cascades. *Nature,* Vol.410, No.6824, (March 2001), pp. 37–40, ISSN0028-0836

Cherradi, N.; Defaye, G. & Chambaz, E.M. (1994). Characterization of the 3 beta-hydroxysteroid dehydrogenase Activity Associated With Bovine Adrenocortical Mitochondria. *Endocrinology,* Vol.134, No.3, (March 1994), pp. 1358-1364. ISSN 0013-7227

Clarson, L.H.; Glazier, J.D.; Sides, M.K. & Sibley, C.P. (1997). Expression of the Facilated Glucose Transporters (GLUT1 and GLUT3) by a Choriocarcionoma Cell Line (Jar) and Cytotrophoblast Cell in Culture. *Placenta,* Vol.18, No.4, (May 1997), pp. 333-339, ISSN 0143-4004

Coleman, R.A. (1986). Placental Metabolism and Transport of Lipids. *Federation Proceedings,* Vol.45, No.10, (September 1986), pp. 2519-2523, ISSN 0014-9446

Cooke, M.; Mele, P.; Maloberti, P.; Duarte, A.; Poderoso, C.; Orlando, U.; Paz, C.; Cornejo Maciel, F. & Podestá, E.J. (2011). Tyrosine Phosphatases as Key Regulators of Star Induction and Cholesterol Transport: SHP2 as a Potential Tyrosine Phosphatase

Involved in Steroid Synthesis. *Molecular and Cellular Endocrinology*, Vol.336, No.1-2, (April 2011), pp. 63-69, ISSN 0303-7207

Corso, M. & Thomson, M. (2001). Protein Phosphorylation in Mitochondria from Human Placenta. *Placenta*, Vol.22, No.5, (May 2001), pp. 432-439, ISSN 0143-4004

Cunningham, P. & McDermott, L. (2009). Long Chain PUFA Transport in Human Term Placenta. *The American Journal of Clinical Nutrition*, Vol.139, No.4, (February-April 2009), pp. 636-639, ISSN 0002-9165

De Los Rios Castillo, D.; Zarco-Zavala, M.; Olvera-Sanchez, S.; Pardo, J.P.; Juarez, O.; Martinez, F.; Mendoza-Hernandez, G.; García-Trejo J.J. & Flores-Herrera O. (2011). Atypical Cristae Morphology of Human Syncytiotrophoblast Mitochondria. Role for Complex V. *The Journal of Biological Chemistry*. Vol.286, No.27, (July 2011), pp. 23911-23919, ISSN 0021-9258

Desoye, G. & Shafrir, E. (1994). Placental Metabolisms and its Regulation in Health and Diabetes. *Molecular Aspects of Medicine*, Vol.15, No.6, pp. 505-682, ISSN 0098-2997

Dodge-Kafka, K.L. & Kapiloff, M.S. (2006). The mAKAP Signaling Complex: Integration of AMPc, Calcium, and MAP Kinase Signaling Pathways. *European Journal of Cell Biology*, Vol.85, No.7, (July 2006), pp.593-602, ISSN 0171-9335

Dominguez-Ramirez, L.; Mendoza-Hernandez, G.; Carabez-Trejo, A.; Gomez-Puyou, A. & Tuena de Gomez-Puyou, M. (2001). Equilibrium Between Monomeric and Dimeric Mitochondrial F1-inhibitor Protein Complexes. *FEBS Lett*, Vol.507, No.2, (October 2001), pp. 191- 194, ISSN 0014-5793

Duan. L.; Yan, D.; Zeng, W.; Yang, X. & Wei, Q. (2010). Effect of Progesterone Treatment Due to Threatened Abortion in Early Pregnancy for Obstetric and Perinatal Outcomes. *Early Human Development*, Vol.86, No.1, (January 2010), pp. 41-3, ISSN 0378-3782

Dudkina, N.V.; Heinemeyer, J.; Keegstra, W.; Boekema, E.J. & Braun, H.P. (2005). Structure of Dimeric ATP Synthase from Mitochondria: an Angular Association of Monomers Induces the Strong Curvature of the Inner Membrane. *FEBS Lett*, Vol.579, No.25, (October 2005), pp. 5769-5772, ISSN 0014-5793

Dyson, M.T.; Jones, J.K.; Kowalewski, M.P.; Manna, P.R.; Alonso, M.; Gottesman, M.E. & Stocco, D.M. (2008). Mitochondrial A-Kinase Anchoring Protein 121 Binds Type II Protein Kinase A and Enhances Steroidogenic Acute Regulatory Protein-Mediated Steroidogenesis in MA-10 Mouse Leydig Tumor Cells. *Biology of Reproduction*, Vol.78, No.2, (February 2008), pp. 267-77, ISSN 0006-3363

Espinosa-Garcia, M.T.; Strauss J.F. III & Martinez, F. (2000). A Trypsin-Sensitive Protein is Required for Utilization of Exogenous Cholesterol for Pregnenolone Synthesis by Placental Mitochondria. *Placenta*, Vol.21, No.7, (September 2000), pp. 654 -660, ISSN 0143-4004

Fei, Y.J.; Prasad, P.D.; Leibach, F.H. & Ganapathy, V. (1995). The Amino Acid Transport System $y^{+}L$ Induced in *Xenopus laevis* Oocytes by Human Choriocarcinoma Cell (JAR) mRNA is Functionally Related to the Heavy Chain of the 4F2 Cell Surface Antigen. *Biochemistry*, Vol.34, No.27, (July 1995), pp. 8744-8751, ISSN 0006-2960

Feliciello, A.; Gottesman, M.E. & Avvedimento, E.V. (2001). The Biological Functions of A-kinase Anchor Proteins. *Journal of Molecular Biology*, Vol.308, No.2, (April 2001), pp. 99-114, ISSN 0022-2836

Feliciello, A.; Gottesman, M.E. & Avvedimento EV. (2005). cAMP-PKA Signaling to the Mitochondria: Protein Scaffolds, mRNA and Phosphatases. *Cell Signal*, Vol.17, No.3, (March2005), pp. 279-87, ISSN 0898-6568

Flores-Herrera, O.; Uribe, A.; Pardo, J.P.; Rendón, J.L. & Martinez, F. (1999). A Novel ATP-diphosphohydrolase from Human Term Placental Mitochondria. *Placenta*, Vol.20, No.5-6, (July-August 1999), pp. 475–484, ISSN 0143-4004

Flores-Herrera, O.; Uribe, A.; García-Pérez, C.; Milán, R. & Martinez, F. (2002). 5-p-Fluorosulfonylbenzoyl Adenosine Inhibits Progesterone Synthesis in Human Placental Mitocondria. *Biochimica et Biophysica Acta, Molecular and Cell Biology of Lipids*, Vol.1585, No.1, (November 2002), pp. 11-18, ISSN 1388-1981

García, J.J.; Morales-Ríos, E.; Cortés-Hernandez, P. & Rodríguez-Zavala, J.S. (2006). The Inhibitor Protein (IF1) Promotes Dimerization of the Mitochondrial F1F0-ATP Synthase. *Biochemistry*, Vol.45, No.42, (October 2006), pp. 12695-12703, ISSN 0006-2960

García-Pérez, C.; Pardo, J.P. & Martinez, F. (2002). $Ca^{(2+)}$ Modulates Respiratory and Steroidogenic Activities of Human Term Placental Mitochondria. *Archives of Biochemistry and Biophysics*, Vol.405, No.1, (September 2002), pp. 104-111, ISSN0003-9861

Garlid, K.D. & Paucek, P. (2003). Mitochondrial Potassium Transport: the K^+ Cycle. *Biochimica et Biophys Acta, Bioenergetics*, Vol.1606, No.1-3, (September 2003), pp. 23-41, ISSN 0005-2728

Gómez-Concha, C.; Flores-Herrera, O.; Olvera-Sanchez, S.; Espinosa-Garcia, M.T. & Martinez, F. (2011). Progesterone Synthesis by Human Placental Mitochondria is Sensitive to PKA Inhibition by H89. *The International Journal of Biochemistry & Cell Biology*, Vol.43 No.9, (September 2011), pp. 1402-11, ISSN: 1357-2725

Gordon-Smith, D.J.; Carbajo, R.J.; Yang, J.; Videler, H.; Runswick, M.J.; Walker, J.E. & Neuhaus, D. (2001). Solution Structure of a C-terminal Coiled-coil Domain From Bovine IF(1): the Inhibitor Protein of F(1) ATPase. *Journal of Molecular Biology*, Vol.308, No.2, (April2001), pp. 325–339, ISNN 0022-2836

Gorostizaga A, Cornejo Maciel F, Brion L, Maloberti P, Podestá EJ, & Paz C. (2007). Tyrosine Phosphatases in Steroidogenic Cells: Regulation and Function. *Molecular and Cellular Endocrinology*, Vol.265-266, (February 2007), pp. 131-137, ISSN 0303-7207

Hahn, T.; Barth, S.; Weiss, U.; Mosgoeeller, W. & Desoye, G. (1998). Sustained Hyperglycemia In Vitro Down-Regulates the GLUT1 Glucose Transport System of Cultured Human Term Placental Trophoblast: a Mechanism to Protect Fetal Development? *Federation of American Societies for Experimental Biology*, Vol. 12, No.12, (September 1998), pp. 1221-1231, ISSN 0892-6638

Hahn, T.; Barth, S.; Graf, R.; Engelmann, M.; Beslagic, D.; Reul, J.M.; Holsboer, F.; Dohr, G. & Desoye, G. (1999). Placenta Glucose Transport Expression is Regulated by Glucorticoids. *The Journal of Clinical Endocrinology and Metabolism*, Vol. 84, No.4, (April 1999), pp. 1445-1452, ISSN 0021-972X

Hackenbrock, C.R. (1968). Ultrastructural Bases for Metabolically Linked Mechanical Activity in Mitochondria. II. Electron Transport-linked Ultrastructural Transformations in Mitochondria. *The Journal of Cell Biology*, Vol.37, (May 1968), No.2, pp. 345–69, ISSN 0021-9525

Hackenbrock, C.R.; Rehn, T.G.; Weinbach, E.C. & Lemasters, J.J. (1971). Oxidative Phosphorylation and Ultrastructural Transformation in Mitochondria in the Intact Ascites Tumor Cell. *The Journal of Cell Biology*, Vol.51, (October 1971), No. 1, pp. 123–37, ISSN 0021-9525

Hanguel, S.; Dezmaizieres, V. & Challier, J.C. (1986). Glucose Uptake, Utilization, and Transfer by The Human Placenta As Functions of Maternal Glucose Concentration. *Pediatric Research*, Vol.20, No.3, (March 1986), pp. 269-273, ISSN 0031-3998

Hanukoglu, I. & Hanukoglu, Z. (1986). Stoichiometry of Mitochondrial Cytochromes P-450, Adrenodoxin and Adrenodoxin Reductase in Adrenal Cortex and Corpus Luteum. Implications for Membrane Organization and Gene Regulation. *European Journal of Biochemistry*, Vol.157, No.1, (Mayo 1986), pp. 27-31, ISSN 0014-2956

Harding, B.W. & Nelson, D.H. (1966). Electron Carriers of the Bovine Adrenal Cortical Respiratory Chain and Hydroxylating Pathways. *The Journal of Biological Chemistry*, Vol.241, No.10 (May 1966), pp. 2212-2219, ISSN 1864-6158

Henderson,Y C.; Frederick, M.J.; Wang, M.T.; Hollier, L.M. & Clayman, G.L. (2008). LBP-1b, LBP-9, and LBP-32/MGR Detected in Syncytiotrophoblasts from First-Trimester Human Placental Tissue and Their Transcriptional Regulation. *DNA and Cell Biology*, Vol.27, No.2, (February 2008), pp. 71–79, ISSN 1044-5498

Hoeltzli, S.D. & Smith, C.H. (1989). Alanine Transport System in Isolated Basal Plasma Membrane of Human Placenta. *The American Journal of Physiology*, Vol.256, No.3-Pt1, (March 1989), pp. C630-C637, ISSN 0002-9513

Hornstra, G.; Al, M.D.; van Houwelingen, A.C. & Foreman-van D. (1995). Essential Fatty Acids in Pregnancy and Early Human Development. *European Journal of Obstetrics and Gynecology and Reproductive Biology*, Vol.61, No.1, (July 1995), pp. 57-62, ISNN 0301-2115

Hu, J.; Zhang, Z.; Shen, W.J. & Azhar, S. (2010). Review Cellular Cholesterol Delivery, Intracellular Processing and Utilization for Biosynthesis of Steroid Hormones. *Nutrition and Metabolism*, Vol.7, (June 2010), pp. 47- 72, ISSN 1743-7075

Ingermann, R.L. (1987). Control of Placental Glucose Transfer. *Placenta*, Vol.8, no.6, (November-December 1987), pp. 557-571, ISSN 0143-4004

Jefcoate, C.R.; Simpson, E.R.; Boyd, G.S.; Brownie, A.C. & Orme-Johnson, W.H. (1973). The Detection of Different States of the P-450 Cytochromes in Adrenal Mitochondria: Changes Induced by ACTH. *Annals of the New York Academy of Sciences*, Vol.212, (June 1973), pp. 243-61, ISSN 0077-8923

Kahn, B.B & Flier, J.S. (1990). Regulation of Glucose-Transporter Gene Expression in Vitro and In Vivo. *American Diabetes Association*, Vol.13, No. 6, (June 1990), pp. 548-564, ISSN 0149-5992

Kasugai M, Kato H, Iriyama H, Kato M, Ninagawa T, & Tomoda Y. (1987). The Roles of Ca2+ and Adenosine 3′, 5′-Monophosphate in the Regulation of Progesterone Production by Human Placental Tissue. *The Journal of Clinical Endocrinology & Metabolism*, Vol.65, No.1, (July 1987), pp. 122-126, ISSN0021-972X

Lavy, G.; Barnea, E.R. & Decherney, A.H. (1987). The Effect of Insulin on Oestradiol and Progesterone Release by Normal and Diabetic Placentae In Vitro. *Placenta*, Vol.8, No.4, (July-August 1987), pp. 443-8, ISSN 0143-4004

LaVoie, H.A. & King, S.R. (2009). Transcriptional Regulation of Steroidogenic Genes: STARD1, CYP11A1 and HSD3B. *Experimental Biology and Medicine*. Vol.234, No.8, (August 2009), pp. 880–907, ISSN 1535-3702

Maldonado-Mercado, G.; Espinosa-Garcia, M.T.; Gomez-Concha, C.; Monreal-Flores, J. & Martinez, F. (2008). Steroidogenesis in BeWo Cells: Role of Protein Kinase A and Benzodiazepines. *The International Journal of Biochemistry & Cell Biology*, Vol. 40, No.5, pp. 901-908, ISSN 1357-2725

Malka, F.; Guillery O.; Cifuentes-Diaz, C.; Guillou, E.; Belenguer, P.; Lombes, A. & Rojo, M. (2005). Separate Fusion of Outer and Inner Mitochondrial Membranes. *European Molecular Biology Organization reports*, Vol.6, (September 2005), No.9, pp.853–859, ISSN 1469-221X

Manna, P.R. & Stocco, D.M. (2005). Regulation of the Steroidogenic Acute Regulatory Protein Expression: Functional and Physiological Consequences. *Current Drug Targets–Immune. Endocrine & Metabolic Disorders*, Vol.5, No.1, (March 2005), pp. 93 – 108, ISSN 1568-0088

Manna, P.R.; Chandrala, S.P.; Jo, Y. & Stocco, D.M. (2006). cAMP-Independent Signaling Regulates Steroidogenesis in Mouse Leydig Cells in the Absence of StAR Phosphorylation. *Journal of Molecular Endocrinology*, Vol.37, No.1, (August 2006), pp. 81-95, ISSN 0952-5041

Manna, P.R.; Dyson, M.T. & Stocco, D.M. (2009). Regulation of the Steroidogenic Acute Regulatory Protein Gene Expression: Present and Future Perspectives. *Molecular Human Reproduction*, Vol.15, No.6, 8June 2009), pp. 321-33 ISSN 1360-9947

Mannella, C.A.; Marko, M.; Penczek, P.; Barnard, D. & Frank, J. (1994). The Internal Compartamentation of Rat-Liver Mitochondria: Tomographic Study Using the High-Voltage Transmission Electron Microscope. *Microscopy Research Technique*, Vol.27, No.4, (March 1994), pp. 278–283, ISSN 1097-0029

Mannella, C.A.; Marko, M. & Buttle, K. (1997). Reconsidering Mitochondrial Structure: New Views of an Old Organelle. *Trends in Biochemical Sciences*, Vol.22, No.2, (February 1997), pp. 37–38, ISSN 0968-0004

Martinez, F.; Chávez, E. & Echegoyen, S. (1987). Decreased Exchange of Adenine Nucleotides in Human Placental Mitochondria. *International Journal of Biochemistry*, Vol.19, No.3, pp. 275-279, ISSN 1357-2725

Martinez, F.; Espinosa-García, M.T.; Flores-Herrera, O. & Pardo, J.P. (1993). Respiratory Control Induced by ATP in Human Term Placental Mitochondria. *Placenta*, Vol.14, No.3, (May-June 1993), pp. 321-331. ISSN 0143-4004

Martinez, F.; Pardo, J.P.; Fores-Herrera. O. & Espinosa-García, M.T. (1995). The Effect of Osmolarity on Human Placental Mitochondria Function. *The International Journal of Biochemistry & Cell Biology*, Vol.27, No.8, (August 1995), pp. 795-803, ISSN 1357-2725

Martinez, F. & Strauss J.F. III (1997). Regulation of Mitochondrial Cholesterol Metabolism. In: *Subcellular Biochemistry: Cholesterol: its Functions and Metabolism in Biology and Medicine*. Bittman, R., pp. 205-234, Plenum Press, ISBN 0306454785/0-306-45478-5, N.Y., USA.

Martinez, F.; Kiriakidou, M. & Strauss J.F. III (1997). Structural and Functional Changes in Mitochondria Associated with Trophoblast Differentiation: Methods to Isolate Enriched Preparations of Syncytiotrophoblast Mitochondria. *Endocrinology*, Vol.138, No.5 (May 1997), pp. 2172–2183, ISSN 0013-7227

Matalon, R. & Michals, K. (1984). Gluconeogenic Enzymes in the Human Placenta. *Journal of Inherited Metabolic Disease*, Vol.7, No.4, (1984), pp. 179-181, ISSN 0141-8955

Matthews, H.R. (1995). Protein Kinases and Phosphatases that Act on Histidine, Lysine, or Arginine Residues in Eukaryotic Proteins: A Possible Regulator of the Mitogen-Activated Protein Kinase Cascade. *Pharmacology & Therapeutics*, Vol.67, No.3, pp. 323–350, ISSN 0163-7258

Matsubara, S.; Takizawa, T. & Sato, I. (1999). Glucose-6-Phosphatase is Present in Normal and Preeclamptic Placental Trophoblasts: Ultrastructural Enzyme-Histochemical Evidence. *Placenta*, Vol. 20, No.1, (January 1999), pp. 81-85, ISSN 0143-4004

Milan, R.; Flores-Herrera, O.; Espinosa-Garcia, M.T.; Olvera-Sanchez, S. & Martinez, F. (2010). Contribution of Potassium in Human Placental Steroidogenesis. *Placenta*, Vol.31, No.10, (August-October 2010), pp. 860-866, ISSN 0143-4004

Miller, W.L. (2005). Minireview: Regulation of Steroidogenesis by Electron Transfer. *Endocrinology*, Vol.146, No.6, (June 2005), pp.2544–2550, ISSN 0013-7227

Meigs, R.A. & Ryan, K.J. (1968). Cytochrome P-450 and Steroid Biosynthesis in the Human Placenta. *Biochimica et Biophysica Acta*, Vol.165, No.3, (October 1968), pp. 476-82, ISSN 0006-3002

Minauro-Sanmiguel, F.; Wilkens, S. & Garcia, J.J. (2005). Structure of Dimeric Mitochondrial ATP Synthase: Novel F0 Bridging Features and the Structural Basis of Mitochondrial Cristae Biogenesis. *Proceedings of the National Academy of Sciences, U.S.A.*, Vol.102, No.35, (August 2005), pp. 12356-12358, ISSN 1091-6490

Moe, A.J. (1995). Placental Amino Acid Transport. *The American Journal of Physiology*, Vol.268, No.6, Pt1, (June 1995), pp. C1321-C1331, ISSN 0002-9513

Moe, A.J.; Farmer, D.R.; Nelson, D.M. & Smith, C.H. (1991). Pentose Phosphate Pathway in Cellular Trophoblast From Full-Term Human Placentas. *The American Journal of Physiology*, Vol.261, No.6Pt1, (December 1991), PP. C1042-1047, ISSN 0363-6127

Moog-Lutz, C.; Tomasetto, C.; Régnier, C.H.; Wendling, C.; Lutz, Y.; Muller, D.M.; Chenard, B.P. & Rio, M. (1997). MLN64 Exhibits homology with the Steroidogenic Acute Regulatory Protein (StAR) and is Over-Expressed in Human Breast Carcinomas. *International Journal of Cancer*, Vol.71, No.2, (April 1997), pp. 183–191, ISSN 0020-7136

Munn, E.A. (1974). The Structure of Mitochondria, In: *The cell*, Saunders, W.B., pp. 414-419, Academic Press, ISBN 0-7216-3584-9, Germany.

Négrié, C.; Triadou, N.; Michel, O.; Bouhnik, J. & Michel, R. (1979). Oxidative Phosphorylation Reactions and Cholesterol Hydroxylation Mechanisms in Human Term Placental Mitochondria. *Journal of Steroid Biochemistry*, Vol.11, No.2, (August 1979), pp. 1135-40, ISSN 0022-4731

Nestler, J.E. (1987). Modulation of Aromatase and P450 Cholesterol Side-Chain Cleavage Enzyme Activities of Human Placental Cytotrophoblasts by Insulin and Insulin-Like Growth Factor I. *Endocrinology*, vol.121, No.5, (November 1987), pp. 1845-1852, ISSN 0013-7227

Nicastro, D.; Frangakis, A.S.; Typke, D. & Baumeister, W. (2000). Cryo-Electron Tomography of Neurospora Mitochondria. *Journal of Structural Biology*, Vol.129, No.1, (February 2000), pp. 48–56, ISSN 1047-8477

Olivera, A.A. & Meigs, R.A. (1975). Mitochondria From human Term Placenta. I. Isolation and Assay Conditions for Oxidative Phosphorylation. *Biochimica et Biophysica Acta, Bioenergetics*, Vol.376, No.3, (March 1975), pp. 426-435, ISSN 0005-2728

Olvera-Sanchez, S.; Espinosa-Garcia, M.T.; Monreal, J.; Flores-Herrera, O. & Martinez F. (2011). Mitochondrial Heat Shock Protein Participates in Placental Steroidogenesis. *Placenta,* Vol.32, No.3, (March-June 2011), pp. 222-229. ISSN 0143-4004

Palinski, W. (2009). Maternal- Fetal cholesterol transport in the placenta. Good, Bad and Target for Modulation. *Circulation Research,* Vol.104, No.5, (March 2009), pp. 569-571, ISSN 0009-7330

Paumard, P.; Vaillier, J.; Coulary, B.; Schaeffer, J.; Soubannier, V.; Mueller, D.M.; Brethes, D.; di Rago, J.P. & Velours, J. (2002). The ATP Synthase is Involved in Generating Mitochondrial Cristae Morphology. *The EMBO Journal,* Vol.21, No.3, (February 2002), pp. 221–230, ISSN 0261-4189

Payne, A.H. & Hales, D.B. (2004). Overview of Steroidogenic Enzymes in the Pathway from Cholesterol to Active Steroid Hormones. *Endocrine Reviews,* Vol.25, No.6, (December 2004), pp. 947-970, ISSN 0163-769X

Pellegrini, L. & Scorrano, L. (2007). A Cut Short to Death: Parl and Opa1 in the Regulation of Mitochondrial Morphology and Apoptosis. *Cell Death & Differentiation,* Vol.14, No.4, (July 2007), pp. 1275–1284, ISSN 1350-9047

Pepe, G.J. & Albretch, E.D. (1999). Regulation of Functional Differentiation of the Placental Villous Syncytiotrophoblast by Estrogen During Primate Pregnancy. *Steroids,* Vol.64, No.9, (September 1999), pp. 624-627 ISSN: 0039-128X

Perkins, G.A.; Renken, C.W.; Martone, M.E.; Young, S.J.; Ellisman, M. & Frey, T. (1997). Electron Tomography of Neuronal Mitochondria: Three-Dimensional Structure and Organization of Cristae and Membrane Contacts. *Journal of Structural Biology,* Vol.119, No.3, (August 1997), pp. 260-272, ISSN 1047-8477

Perkins, G.A.; Song, J.Y.; Tarsa, L.; Deerinck, T.J.; Ellisman, M.H. & Frey, T.G. (1998). Electron Tomography of Mitochondria from Brown Adipocytes Reveals Crista Junctions. *Journal of Bioenergetics and Biomembranes,* Vol.30, No.5, (October 1998), pp. 431–442, ISSN 0145-479X

Perkins, G.A; Renken, C.W.; Frey, T.G. & Ellisman, M.H. (2001a). Membrane Architecture of Mitochondria in Neurons of the Central Nervous System. *Journal of neuroscience research,* Vol.66, No.5, (December 2001), pp. 857–865, ISSN 0360-4012

Perkins, G.A.; Renken, C.W.; van der Klei, I.J.; Ellisman, M.H. & Neupert, W. (2001b). Electron Tomography of Mitochondria After the Arrest of Protein Import Associated with Tom19 Depletion. *European Journal of Cell Biology,* Vol.80, No.2, (February 2001), pp. 139–150, ISSN 0171-9335

Perkins, G.A.; Ellisman, M.H. & Fox, D.A. (2003). Three-Dimensional Analysis of Mouse Rod and Cone Mitochondrial Cristae Architecture: Bioenergetic and Functional Implications. *Molecular Vision,* Vol.9, (March 2003), pp. 60–73, ISSN 1090-0535

Piquard, F.; Schaefer, A.; Dellenbach, P. & Haberey, P. (1990). Lactate Movements in the Human Placenta In Situ. *Biology of the Neonate,* Vol.58, No.2, pp. 61-68, ISSN 0006-3126

Prendergast, C.H.; Parker, K.H.; Gray, R.; Venkatesan, S.; Bannister, P.; Castro-Soares, J.; Murphy, K.W.; Beard, R.W.; Regan, L.; Robinson, S.; Steer, P.; Halliday, D. &

Johnston, D.G. (1999). Glucose Production by the Human Placenta In Vivo. *Placenta*, Vol.20, No.7, (September 1999), pp. 591-598, ISSN 0143-4004

Prince, F.P. (2002). Lamellar and Tubular Associations of the Mitochondrial Cristae: Unique Forms of the Cristae Present in Steroid-Producing Cells. *Mitochondrion*, Vol.1, No.4, (February 2002), pp. 381–389, ISSN 1567-7249

Puttick, J.; Baker, E.N. & Delbaere, L.T. (2008). Histidine Phosphorylation in Biological Systems. *Biochimica et Biophysica Acta, Proteins and Proteomics*, Vol.1784, No.1, (January 2008), pp. 100-105, ISSN 1570-9639

Reichert, A.S. & Neupert, W. (2002). Contact Sites Between the Outer and Inner Membrane of Mitochondria-Role in Protein Transport, *Biophysica Acta Molecular Cell Research*, Vol.1592, No.1, (September 2002), pp. 41–49, ISSN 0167-4889

Ringler, G.E.; Kao, L.C.; Miller, W.L. & Strauss, J.F. III (1989). Effects of 8-Bromo-cAMP on Expression of Endocrine Functions by Cultured Human Trophoblast cells. Regulation of Specific mRNAs. *Molecular and Cellular Endocrinology*, Vol.61, No.1, (Jan 1989), pp. 13-21, ISSN 0303-7207.

Ritvos, O. (1988). Modulation of Steroidogenesis in Choriocarcinoma Cells by Cholera Toxin, Phorbol Ester, Epidermal Growth Factor and Insulin-Like Growth Factor I. *Molecular and Cellular Endocrinology*, Vol.59, No.1-2, (September 1988), pp. 125-133, ISSN 0303-7207

Rossignol, R.; Gilkerson, R.; Aggeler R.; Yamagata, K.; Remington, S.J. & Capaldi, R.A. (2004). Energy Substrate Modulates Mitochondrial Structure and Oxidative Capacity in Cancer Cells. *American Association for Cancer Research*, vol.64, (February 2004), No.3, pp. 985–893, ISSN 0008-5472

Sands, W. & Palmer, T.M. (2008). Regulating Gene Transcription in Response to Cyclic AMP Elevation. *Cellular Signaling*, Vol.20 No.3, (March 2008), pp.460-466, ISSN 0898-6568

Schimmer, B.P. & White, P.C. (2010). Steroidogenic Factor 1: Its Roles in Differentiation, Development, and Disease. *Molecular Endocrinology*, Vol.24, No.7, (July 2010), pp. 1322–1337, ISSN 0888-8809

Schneider, H.; Malek, A.; Duft, R. & Bersinger, N. (1988). Evaluation of an In Vitro Dual Perfusion System for the Study of Placental Proteins: Energy Metabolism. In: *Placenta as a model and a source*, Genbacev, O.; Klopper, A. & Beaconsfield. R., pp. 39-50, Plenum Press, ISBN 0306432382, New York, USA

Schägger, H. & Pfeiffer, K. (2000). Supercomplexes in the Respiratory Chains of Yeast and Mammalian Mitochondria. *The EMBO Journal*, Vol.19, No.8, (April 2000), pp. 1777-1783, ISSN 0261-4189

Shelley, H.J. (1979). Transfer of Carbohydrates, In: *Placental transfer*, Chamberlain, G. & Wilkinson, A.W. pp. 118-1412, Pitman Medical, ISBN 0272795313, Ithaca, New York, USA

Shi, C.Z. & Zhuang, L.Z. (1993). Stimulatory Effect of Norepinephrine on Progesterone Production by Human First Trimester Placenta Explants In Vitro. *Life Sciences*, Vol.52, No.20, pp. 1657-65, ISSN 0024-3205

Simpson, E.R. & Miller, D.A. (1978). Cholesterol Side-Chain Cleavage, Cytochrome P450, and Iron-Sulfur Protein in Human Placental Mitochondria. *Molecular and Cellular Endocrinology*, Vol.190, No.2, (October 1978), pp. 800-808, ISSN 0303-7207

Spät, A. & Pitter, J.G. (2004). The Effect of Cytoplasmic Ca2+ Signal on the Redox State of Mitochondrial Pyridine Nucleotides. *Molecular and Cellular Endocrinology*, Vol. 215, No.1-2, (February 2004), pp. 115–118, ISSN 0303-7207

Stocco, D.M. (2000). Intramitochondrial Cholesterol Transfer. *Biochimica et Biophysica Acta, Molecular and Cell Biology of Lipids*, Vol.1486, No.1, (June 2000), pp.184-197, ISSN 1388-1981

Stocco, D.M.; Wang, X.; Jo, Y. & Manna, P.R. (2005). Multiple Signaling Pathways Regulating Steroidogenesis and Steroidogenic Acute Regulatory Protein Expression: More Complicated than we Thought. *Molecular Endocrinology*, Vol.19, No.11, (November 2005), pp.2647-2659, ISSN0888-8809

Strauss, J.F. III; Kido, S.; Sayegh, R.; Sakuragi, N. & Gafvels, M.E. (1992). The cAMP Signalling System and Human Trophoblast Function. *Placenta*, Vol.13, No.5, (September-October 1992), pp. 389-403, ISSN 0143-4004

Strauss, J.F. III; Martinez, F. & Kiriakidou, M. (1996). Placental Steroid Hormone Synthesis: Unique Features and Unanswered Questions. *Biology of Reproduction*, Vol.54, No.2, (February 1996), pp. 303-311, ISSN 0006-3363

Strauss, M.; Hofhaus, G.; Schröder, R.R. & Kühlbrandt, W. (2008). Dimer Ribbons of ATP Synthase Shape the Inner Mitochondrial Membrane. *The EMBO Journal*, Vol.27, No.7, (April 2008), pp. 1154-1160, ISSN 0261-4189

Strushkevicha, N.; MacKenziea, F.; Cherkesovab, T.; Grabovecb, I.; Usanovb, S. & Parka, H.W. (2011). Structural Basis for Pregnenolone Biosynthesis by the Mitochondrial Monooxygenase System. *Proceedings of the National Academy of Sciences, USA*. Vol.108, No.25, (June 2011), pp. 10139–10143 ISSN 0027-8424

Stulc, J.; Stulcová, B. & Sibley, C.P. (1995). Mechanisms of the Fetomaternal Transfer of Na^+ Across the Dually Perfused Placentaof the Rat. *Placenta*, Vol.16, No.2, (March 1995), pp. 127-135, ISSN 0143-4004

Stulc, J. (1997). Placental Transfer of Inorganic Ions and Water. *Physiological Reviews*, Vol.77, No.3, (July 1997), pp. 805-836, ISNN 0031-9333

Thomson, M. (2002). Evidence of Undiscovered Cell Regulatory Mechanisms: Phosphoproteins and Protein Kinases in Mitochondria. *Cellular and Molecular Life Sciences*, Vol.59, No.2, (February 2002), pp. 213-219, ISSN: 1420-682X

Trost, M.; Bridon, G.; Desjardins, M. & Thibault, P. (2010). Subcellular Phosphoproteomics, In: *Mass Spectrometry Reviews*, Vol.29, No.6, (November-December 2010), pp. 962–990 ISNN 1098-2787

Tuckey, R.C. (1992). Cholesterol Side-Chain Cleavage by Mitochondria from the Human Placenta. Studies Using Hydroxycholesterols as Substrates. *Journal of Steroid Biochemistry and Molecular Biology*, Vol.42, No.8, (September 1992), pp. 883-890, ISSN 0960-0760

Tuckey, R.C. & Headlam, M.J. (2002). Placental Cytochrome P450scc (CYP11A1): Comparison of Catalytic Properties Between Conditions of Limiting and Saturating Adrenodoxin Reductase. *The Journal of Steroid Biochemistry and Molecular Biology*, Vol.81, No.2, (June 2002), pp. 153–158, ISSN 0960-0760

Tuckey, R. C. (2005). Progesterone Synthesis by the Human Placenta, *Placenta*, Vol.26, No.4, (April 2005), pp. 273-281. ISSN 0143-4004

Uribe, A.; Flores-Herrera, O.; Rendón, J.L.; Espinosa-García, M.T. & Martinez, F. (1999). Presence of Two Enzymes, Different from the F_1F_0-ATPase, Hydrolyzing

Nucleotides in Human Term Placental Mitochondria. *The International Journal of Biochemistry & Cell Biology*, Vol.31, No.2, (February 1999), pp. 319-330. 1357-2725

Uribe, A.; Strauss J.F. III & Martinez, F. (2003). Contact Sites from Human Placental Mitochondria. Characterization and Role in Progesterone Synthesis. *Archives of Biochemistry and Biophysics*, Vol.413, No.2, (May 2003), pp. 172-181, ISSN 0003-9861

Ville, C.A. (1953). The Metabolism of Human Placenta In Vitro. *The Journal of Biological Chemistry*, Vol.205, No.1, (November 1953), pp. 113-123, ISSN 0021-9258

Wollet, L. (2005). Maternal Cholesterol in Fetal Development: Transport of Cholesterol from Maternal to the Fetal Circulation. *The American journal of clinical nutrition*, Vol.82, No.6, (December 2005), pp. 1155-1161, ISSN 0002-9165

Xu, X.; Xu, T.; Robertson, D.G & Lamberth, J.D. (1989). GTP Stimulates Pregnenolone Generation in Isolated Rat Adrenal Mitochondria. *Journal of Molecular Biology*, Vol.264, No.30, (October 1989), pp. 17674–17680, ISSN 0022-2836

Young, M.P. & Schneider, H. (1984). Metabolic Integrity of the Isolated Perfused Lobule of Human Placenta. *Placenta*, Vol.5, No.2, (March-April 1984), pp. 95-104. ISSN 0143-4004

Yudilevich D.L. & Sweiry J.H. (1985). Transport of Amino Acids in the Placenta. *Biochemica et Biophys Acta*, Vol.822, No.2, (September 1985), pp. 169-201, ISSN 0006-3002

Zosmer, A.; Elder, M.G. & Sullivan, M.F. (1997). Second Messenger and the Control of Progesterone Production from First Trimester Trophoblast. *The Journal of Steroid Biochemistry and Molecular Biology*, Vol.62, No.2-3, (June 1997), pp. 201-205, ISSN 0960-0760

18

Role of Nuclear Receptors Peroxisome Proliferator-Activated Receptors (PPARs) and Liver X Receptors (LXRs) in the Human Placental Pathophysiology

Geoffroy Marceau, Loïc Blanchon, Jean-Marc Lobaccaro and Vincent Sapin
Université d'Auvergne,
France

1. Introduction

The placenta is a transitory structure indispensable for the proper development of the embryo and fetus during mammalian gestation. Like other members of the nuclear receptor family, the peroxisome proliferator-activated receptors (PPARs) and the liver X receptors (LXRs) are known to be involved in the physiological and pathological events occurring during the placentation. This placental involvement has been recently confirmed focusing on the early stages of placental development (implantation and invasion....), mouse knockout phenotypes and cyto/syncytio-trophoblastic physiology. In this review, we describe the involvement of PPARs and LXRs in placenta and in the amniotic membrane during gestation (e.g., fat transport and metabolism...), in pathological process (e.g., chorioamnionitis, preeclampsia...), metabolic disorders (e.g., diabetes) and parturition.

2. The peroxisome proliferator-activated receptors (PPARs)

Discovered in 1990, PPARs are known for their biological role in inducing the proliferation of peroxisomes in rodents (Issemann & Green, 1990). They are transcription factors belonging to the ligand-activated nuclear hormone receptor superfamily (Michalik et al., 2002) and have been identified in different species such as the xenopus, mouse, rat, and humans.

2.1 Nomenclature and structure of PPARs

In all these species, PPARs present three isotypes encoded by distinct single-copy genes: PPARα (NR1C1), PPARβ/δ (also called NUC1 or NR1C2), and PPARγ (NR1C3), located on chromosomes 22, 6, 3 in humans. The PPARγ gene alternative promoters give rise to three different isoforms named γ1, γ2, and γ3 which differ at their 5_ends (Fajas et al., 1997). PPAR α, β, $\gamma 1/\gamma 3$, γ2 translation produces proteins of 468, 441, 475, and 505 amino acids, respectively, with a molecular weight of 49 to 56 kDa (Fournier et al., 2007). By performing multiple PPAR nucleotide/protein alignments in different species, a strong interspecies identity (human, mouse, rat, bovine, ≈84%) has been established, illustrating a strong evolutionary conservation among species by derivation from a common ancestor (Table 1).

Like several other members of the nuclear receptor superfamily, PPARs possess the typical structure organized in six domains named A to F (Figure 1) (Escher et al., 2000). Domain C (DBD: DNA binding domain) contains two zinc fingers and allows promoter target genes interaction and dimerization with its preferential nuclear receptor: retinoid X receptor (RXR). The PPAR/RXR heterodimer binds to the target gene promoter response element named peroxisome proliferator response element (PPRE) which is made up of two half site AGGTCA separated by one or two nucleotides (also called DR1 or DR2 for direct repeat 1 or 2). Domain E/F allows ligand binding and contains a ligand-dependent transactivation function called AF2 (activating function 2). It is also involved in dimerization and interaction with cofactors.

		cDNA homology (%)			Protein homology (%)		
		Mouse	Rat	Bovine	Mouse	Rat	Bovine
Human relative identity percent	PPARα	44	64	72	92	92	94
	PPARβ	60	69	75	92	91	95
	PPARγ1	79	84	78	98	97	97
	PPARγ2	86	86	88	96	95	95

Table 1. Percentage of nucleotide and amino acid identity between human and mouse, rat and bovine PPAR sequences respectively. No PPARγ3 alignment was carried out owing to lack of data on different species. The different sequences came from Ensembl and were aligned with Genomatix software (Borel et al., 2008).

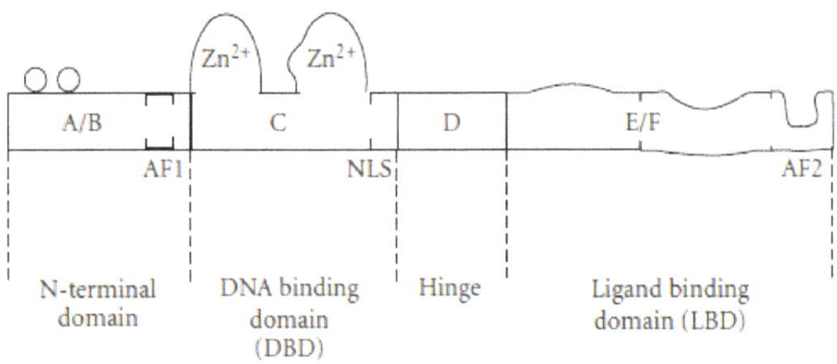

Fig. 1. Schematic representation of typical nuclear receptor structure. AF1: activating function 1 (ligand-independent function), AF2: activating function 2 (ligand-dependent function), NLS: nuclear signal localization (Borel et al., 2008).

2.2 PPAR ligands

As with the other nuclear receptors, the binding of the ligand is a key step in the control of PPAR transcriptional activity. In the absence of a ligand, corepressors and histone deacetylases (HDAC) bind to PPARs and inhibit the transcription of target genes. PPAR ligands have the ability to dissociate the corepressor complexes from the PPAR/RXR heterodimer, allowing the binding of the coactivators in order to initiate and activate transcription. There are two kinds of ligands for the PPARs: natural and synthetic. Among the natural ligands the monounsaturated fatty acids (FA) (e.g., oleic acid) and the polyunsaturated fatty acids (PUFA) (e.g., linoleic acid, linolenic acid and arachidonic acid) are described as ligands for PPARα, PPARβ and PPARγ. They act with concentrations consistent with those found in human serum (Desvergne & Wahli, 1999). The different PUFA metabolites: 8(S)- and 15-hydroxyeicosatetraenoic acid (8(S)- and 15-HETE), leukotriene B4 (LTB4), 9- and 13- hydroxyoctadedienoic acid (9-HODE and 13-HODE) and 15-deoxy-Δ12,14-prostaglandin J2 (PGJ2) are potent selective activators of PPAR*a* and PPAR*γ*.

More recently, it has been demonstrated that P450 eicosanoids are potent PPAR*a* and PPAR*γ* ligands (Ng et al., 2007). These ligands induce PPAR binding to PPRE and can modify the expression of PPARα responsive genes like apoA-I or apoA-II in the same way than synthetic ligands. Thus the finely regulated conversion of PUFAs to eicosanoids through either the lipoxygenase, cyclooxygenase, or cytochrome P450 monooxygenase pathways may provide a mechanism for the differential regulation of PPAR*a* and PPAR*γ* and their respective target genes. PPAR*β* can be activated by different types of eicosanoids including prostaglandinA1 (PGA1) and prostaglandin D2 (PGD2). Many synthetic ligands exist and have been used in PPAR work. These ligands include prostaglandin 12 analogs, pirinixic acid (Wy-14643) for PPAR*a*, hypolipidemic and hypoglycemic agents (nonthiazolidinedione) for PPAR*β*, and thiazolidinediones (e.g., rosiglitasone, troglitazone) for PPAR*γ* (Michalik et al., 2002).

2.3 Placental PPAR expression patterns

The three PPAR isoforms are been shown to be expressed in the villous trophoblastic cells and syncytiotrophoblasts of the human term placenta (Fournier et al., 2007). Furthermore, the three PPARs are present in total placenta, amnion, chorion, and in amnion-derived WISH epithelial cell line at the mRNA and protein levels. But the expression of PPAR*a* and PPAR*γ* seems to be weaker than that observed for PPARβ/δ. In addition, PPAR*γ* is more express in chorion than in amnion (Borel et al., 2008).

2.4 Implications of PPARs in placenta and fetal membranes

2.4.1 Placental and amniotic presence of PPARs ligands

The lipids of human amnion and chorion are enriched in the essential fatty acid arachidonic acid, which is the precursor of all the prostaglandins of the 2 series (Schwarz et al., 1975). Sixty-six percent of the arachidonic acid of the human fetal membranes are available in the glycerophospholipids of these tissues and can easily be converted into PGD2 (Okita et al., 1982). The placenta produces considerable amounts of PGD2 (Mitchell et al., 1982). The enzymes necessary to convert PGD2 into prostaglandin J2 (PGJ2) are present and co expressed with PPAR*γ* in placenta. 15 Deoxy-Δ12,14-PGJ2 (15dPGJ2) and its precursor PGD2 are present in amniotic fluid at concentrations that do not exceed 3 nM (Helliwell et al., 2006). However, this amniotic fluid concentration cannot be an exact representation of the physiological placental reality for PPARs ligands because the nuclear concentration is not measured. The maternal blood may also be a source of PPAR ligands for the human placenta and the fetal membranes. It has been established that a heatstable compound (not a protein, but rather a prostanoid or a fatty acid) is detected in maternal blood serum and is able to activate the PPAR*γ* (Waite et al., 2000). The presence of classical and new PPARs ligands (e.g., P450 eicosanoids, PUFA metabolites) in placenta and fetal membranes suggests that they could activate PPAR, induce PPAR binding to PPREs and modify the expression of PPAR target genes.

2.4.2 Fundamental implications of PPARs during early placentation

As a determining result, the knockout of the PPARγ in mice (Barak et al., 1999) yielded the first findings indicating the importance of this factor in early embryonic and perinatal development. These results are concomitant with those obtained by the generation of RXRα or β null mice (PPARγ partner in the functional heterodimer), also showing an embryonic lethality explained by the lack of generation of a functional labyrinthine zone (Sapin et al., 2001; Parrast et al., 2009). Furthermore, complementary studies conducted by the inactivation of PPARγ coactivators or coregulators, such as peroxisome proliferators activator receptor-binding protein (PBP) and peroxisome proliferator-activated receptor-interacting protein (PRIP), also lead to severe placental dysfunction, such as inadequate vascularisation of the structure (Antonson et al., 2003; Zhu et al., 2000; Zhu et al., 2003). Furthermore, the inactivation of PPARβ/δ led to the formation of abnormal gaps and a thinner but fully differentiated vascular structure in the placentodecidual interface (Barak et al., 2002). These results establish the no redundant roles of PPARγ and PPARβ/δ in early mouse placental development. Recent analysis of PPARγ null mice also demonstrated that PPARγ plays a pivotal role in controlling placental vascular proliferation and contributes to its termination in late pregnancy [Nadra et al., 2010]. In human, PPARβ/δ plays a central role at various stages of pregnancy like implantation, decidualization, and placentation (Wang et al., 2007). By contrast, the inactivation of PPARα has no effect on placental formation or on the developing fetus and by the way theirs possible roles during pregnancy had to be clarified (Michalik et al., 2002). In humans, the studies are almost exclusively focused on the PPARγ roles during early placentation. It has been clearly established that all three PPARs can stimulate or inhibit the differentiation and/or proliferation of the villous cytotrophoblasts into syncytiotrophoblasts and the synthesis of chorionic gonadotrophic hormone and may hamper extravillous trophoblastic cell invasion (Fournier et al., 2007). It's also clearly established that hCG gene expression is differentially regulated in the villous and extra-villous trophoblast lineages during their in vitro differentiation and modulated in an opposite way by PPARγ (Handschuh et al., 2009).

2.4.3 Roles of PPARs in the uptake and transport of trophoblastic lipids

As one of the first functions described for PPARγ in other tissues, trophoblastic lipid uptake and accumulation are also regulated in part by this factor (Schaiff et al., 2007). The PPARγ ligands seem to increase the uptake and accumulation of the fatty acids in human placenta (Schaiff et al., 2005). This regulation is associated with an enhanced expression of adipophilin (fat droplet-associated protein) and fatty acid transport proteins (1 and 4) in human trophoblasts (Schaiff et al., 2005; Bildirici et al., 2003; Duttaroy, 2004). These results were confirmed by the *in vivo* activation of PPARγ by its agonist rosiglitazone in mice, which also leads to the enhancement of the previous described genes plus two new ones involved in the lipid transport: S3-12 (plasma associated protein) and myocardial lipid droplet protein/MLDP (Schaiff et al., 2007). Taken together, these results confirm the results obtained on PPARγ-null mutants: the absence of the lipid droplets normally present around the fetal vessels in the wild-type placenta (Barak et al., 1999).

2.4.4 PPARs in placental inflammatory response and in the parturition signaling

At this stage of our knowledge of PPARs, the most interesting results have been obtained with the study of their involvement in the inflammation process, which may be linked to labor at term and also to the premature rupture of fetal membranes (Figure 2). Term labor is associated with an increase in proinflammatory proteins and cytokines such as IL1β, IL6, IL8, IL10, and TNF-a. This increase in proinflammatory proteins and cytokines induces uterine contractions. PPARγ ligands have been demonstrated to inhibit the secretion of IL6, IL8, and TNF-a in amnion and chorion (Lappas et al., 2006), highlighting the role of PPARs in the regulation of the inflammatory response in human gestational tissues and cells (Kniss, 1999; Lappas et al., 2002; Ackerman et al., 2005; Berry et al., 2005). The parathyroid hormone-related protein (presenting a cytokine-like action) is involved in many processes during normal and pathological pregnancies, and is decreased by PPARγ stimulation (Lappas & Rice, 2004), which also blocks proinflammatory cytokine release by adiponectin and leptin (Lappas et al., 2005). The production of prostaglandins by the endometrium, the myometrium, and the fetal membranes induces the contraction of the myometrium during labor. This generation of uterotonic prostaglandins correlates with the increased prostaglandin-endoperoxide synthase type 2/cyclooxygenase type 2 (COX-2) activity and the increased secretory phospholipase A2-IIA (sPLA2) mRNA, proteins and activities. By inhibiting the production of the COX-2 and sPLA2 in fetal membranes, PPARγ promotes the quiescence of the uterus during gestation (Ackerman et al., 2005). The PPARγ level of expression remains stable throughout gestation, except for the period just before labor, when its expression in fetal membranes declines. This reduction is coincidental with a

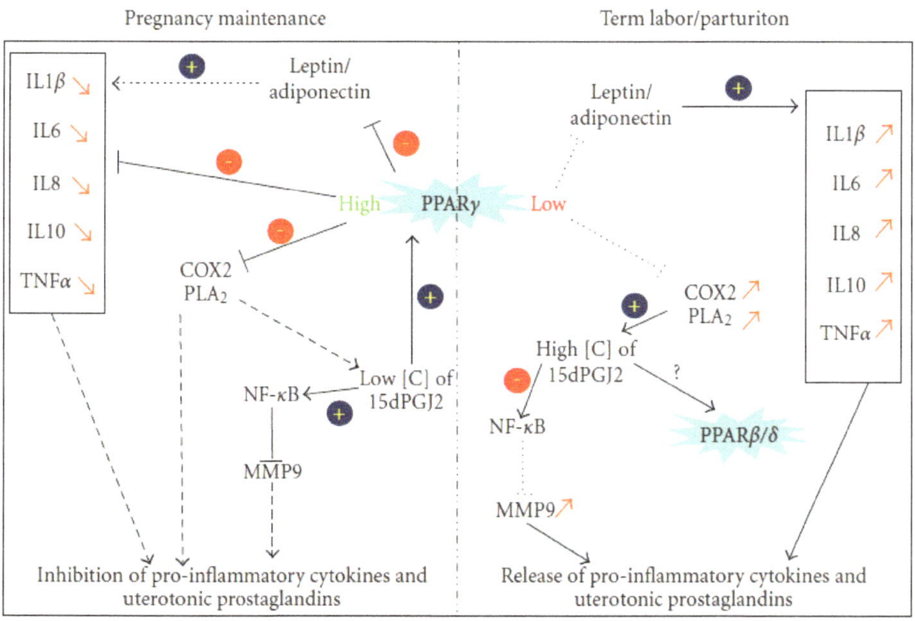

Fig. 2. Schematic representation of PPARγ implication in pregnancy maintenance and labor. IL1β: Interleukin 1β; IL6: Interleukin 6; IL8: Interleukin 8; IL10: Interleukin 10, TNFa: Tumor Necrosis Factor a; COX2: Cyclo-oxygenase type 2; PLA2: Phospholipase A2; NF-κB: Nuclear Factor-Kappa B; MMP9: Matrix Metalloproteinase 9; 15dPGJ2: 15-Deoxy-Δ12, 14 prostaglandin J2 (Borel et al., 2008).

relative increase in COX-2 expression (Dunn-Albanese et al., 2004). The PPAR action seems to be concentration-dependent. A small amount of 15dPGJ2 (<0.1 μM) acts through the PPARγ signaling pathway, where at high concentration (1 μM) its actions are most probably mediated through other pathways: PPARβ/δ and/or an inhibition of NF-κB independent of PPARs (Berry et al., 2005). Furthermore, 15dPGJ2 and troglitazone were also demonstrated to have some anti-inflammatory or apoptosis-induction specific effects by PPARγ-independent pathways (Lappas et al., 2006).

2.4.5 PPARs in placental and amniotic membranes pathologies

In contrast to the different roles described for PPARs during human placentation, only a few studies on PPARs and placental pathologies have been conducted. PPARs may be involved in the pathophysiology of gestational diabetes mellitus, intrauterine growth restriction and preeclampsia (Holdsworth-Carson et al., 2010). In choriocarcinoma and hydatiform moles, a downregulation of the PPARγ expression is observed but this real influence needs to be elucidated (Capparuccia et al., 2002). The potential involvement of PPARγ on preeclampsia is suggested by the fact that this pathology is associated with an increased peroxidation in trophoblasts (Roberts et al., 1999; Ware Branche et al., 1994). An overproduction of 15-HETE has also been noted, suggesting a deregulation of PPARγ (Johnson et al., 1998). This can cause a strong transactivation of PPARγ during early pregnancy, resulting in a reduction of extravillous trophoblastic invasion, one cellular explanation often cited in the physiopathology of preeclampsia (Schild et al., 2002; Fournier et al., 2002; Fournier et al., 2008a). It is also established that deletion of PPARγ, PPARβ/δ, and some of their coactivators (PBP, PRIP, and RAP250) induce abnormal placental phenotypes (abruption, reduction of fetomaternal exchanges, and alterations of trophoblastic differentiation) in null mutants (Barak et al., 1999; Antonson et al., 2003; Zhu et al., 2000; Barak et al., 2002; Kuang et al., 2002; Nadra et al., 2006). Chromosomal and/or genetic alterations (point mutation or deletion) may occur for these genes, inducing human placental alterations. The placental 11β hydroxysteroid dehydrogenase type 2 is a target gene of PPARs (Julan et al., 2005). This enzyme plays a key role in fetal development by controlling fetal exposure to maternal glucocorticoids. An abnormal regulation by PPARs may result in an absence of fetal protection. In the rat placental HRP-1 established cell line, the phthalate and derivatives transactivate PPARs (α and γ) induced an increase in uptake rates of fetal essential fatty acid and the transport of arachidonic and docosahexaenoic acid (Xu et al., 2005). If such a mechanism can be induced by the phthalates during human placentation, this may strongly affect the fetal essential fatty acid content during growth.

Gestational diabetes is linked to impaired lipids metabolism (Capobianco et al., 2003) and the increase of PPARγ observe in human trophoblastic cells culture might be involved in the impairment of placental development induced by high glucose conditions (Suwaki et al., 2007). Decreased 15dPGJ2 in blood of diabetic mothers is also linked to a decrease in placental PPARγ expression. The inhibition of PPARγ results in an induction of a placental proinflammatory environment associated with an increase in nitrogen monoxide production and release, which can impair fetoplacental development (Jawerbaum et al., 2004; Jawerbaum & González, 2006; Jawerbaum & Capobianco , 2011). The PPAR regulation of inflammation may be very important in another obstetrical pathology of the amniotic membranes: the chorioamnionitis. This pathology, usually due to an ascendant colonization of pathogenic microorganisms from the vagina to the uterus, is closely associated with preterm labor and premature rupture of membranes (chorion and amnion). These ruptures of membranes seem to arise from deregulated proinflammatory factor synthesis. It has already been reported in this pathology that IL1β, IL6, IL8, TNF-α, and prostaglandinE(2) show inadequate concentrations in placental membrane and in amniotic fluid (Willi et al., 2002; Zaga et al., 2004; Jacobsson et al., 2005; Zaga-Clavellina et al., 2006). As PPARs may be involved in the occurrence and control of this inflammatory response, further studies are needed to assess their importance in this process and to find new possible therapeutic strategies to prevent this damaging pathology.

More generally, the use of natural and synthetic PPAR ligands looks to be a promising way in preventing placental pathologies such as endometriosis, preeclampsia or diabetes (Giaginis et al., 2008). An interesting study also demonstrates that the reduction of LPS induction of cytokines is reduced by PPARγ ligands in fetal membranes. Nevertheless, the few studies already conducted were done practically only on animal (rodent) models and looks to have positive effects on the pathologies (Toth et al., 2007). Till now, the major problem using, for example, TZD (thiazolidinediones) linking to the PPARγ pathways still the numerous adverse effects of this kind of treatment (e.g., weight gain, anemia, leukopenia, etc.). Perhaps, at the level of clinician actual knowledge, PPARγ and its ligands could be used in a first time, only as good early marker candidates for the diagnosis of pregnancy pathologies like, for example, preeclampsia.

3. The liver x receptor (LXRs)

First discovered and defined as orphan receptors, liver X receptors (LXRs) were subsequently identified as the nuclear receptor target of the cholesterol metabolites, oxysterols (Apfel et al., 1994; Janowski et al., 1996). LXR pathway regulates lipid metabolism and inflammation via both the induction and repression of target genes (Calkin & Tontonoz, 2010) and have been identified in different species such as the vase tunicate, xenopus, zebrafish, mouse, rat, and humans.

3.1 Nomenclature and structure of LXRs

LXRα (NR1H3) and LXRβ (NR1H2) belong to a subclass of the nuclear receptor superfamily, that form obligatory heterodimers with retinoid X receptor (RXR), the receptor of 9-cis retinoic acid. In humans LXRα and LXRβ are encoded by two distinct genes located on chromosomes 11 and 19, respectively. LXR were initially isolated from a human liver cDNA library as orphan receptors. Later, oxysterols, which are oxidized derivatives of cholesterol, were identified as their natural ligands and the first physiological functions were associated with cholesterol homeostasis. By performing multiple LXR nucleotide/protein alignments of LXRs in different species, a strong interspecies identity (human, mouse, rat, bovine, $\approx$87%) has been established, illustrating a strong evolutionary conservation among species by derivation from a common ancestor (Table 2).

Similar to other nuclear receptors, both LXR isoforms comprise four distinct domains: 1) an amino-terminal activation domain (AF-1), recruiting ligand-independent co-activators (domain A/B), 2) a DNA-binding domain containing two zinc fingers (domain C), 3) a hinge domain, binding co-repressors in absence of ligand (domain D) and 4) a multi-functional carboxy-terminal domain, required for dimerization, containing a hydrophobic ligand binding site and a transactivation domain (AF-2) recruiting co-activators (domain E/F) (Figure 1). Interestingly, even though both DNA and ligand-binding pockets share 80% identity, human and mouse LXR*β* are shorter than LXR*a* in their N-terminal domain (12 and 11 amino acids, respectively) and longer in the hinge region (23 and 18 amino acids, respectively). This fact could account for the lack of redundancy *in vivo*, even though both LXR isoforms bind similar DNA sequences and ligands *in vitro* (Viennois et al., 2011). LXR *a*, *β*, translation produces proteins of 447, 461 amino acids, respectively, with a molecular weight of 55 kDa for both (Michael et al., 2005). LXR*a* exists in three variants originating from alternative promoter usage and mRNA splicing: LXR*a*1, LXR*a*2, and LXR*a*3 (Chen et al., 2005).

		cDNA homology (%)			Protein homology (%)		
		Mouse	Rat	Bovine	Mouse	Rat	Bovine
Human relative identity percent	LXRα	88	89	91	91	92	92
	LXRβ	87	87	87	81	81	78

Table 2. Percentage of nucleotide and amino acid identity between the human, mouse, rat, and bovine LXR sequences. No LXR *a*1, *a*2 and *a*3 alignment was carried out owing to lack of data on different species. The different sequences came from Ensembl and were aligned with Genomatix software.

3.2 LXR ligands

As with PPARs, there are two kinds of ligands for the LXRs: natural and synthetic. The physiological LXR agonist ligands are oxysterols, oxidized metabolites of cholesterol. In mammals, there are two sources of plasmatic oxysterols, *in vivo* production by enzymatic or chemical pathways, and exogenous nutritional supply (Viennois et al., 2011). Natural activating oxysterols include 22(R) hydroxycholesterol in steroidogenic tissues, 24(S)-hydroxycholesterol in brain and plasma, 24(S),25-epoxycholesterol mainly found in the liver and 27-hydroxycholesterol in macrophages. These oxysterols have been reported to activate both LXR*a* and LXR*β* (Janowski et al., 1996). Likewise, desmosterol, a cholesterol precursor produced from zymosterol, could also activate LXR (Yang et al., 2006). Molecules derived from the bile acid pathway in particular natural 6α-hydroxylated bile acids have been proposed as putative ligands inducing transcriptional activity of LXR*a* (Song et al., 2000). Some ligands naturally present in the serum may also have an antagonistic effect on LXR as 7-ketocholesterol (Song et al., 2001).

Many pharmaceutical companies have screened potential LXR ligands. Among them T0901317 (Schultz et al., 2000) and GW3965 (Collins et al., 2002), two nonsteroidal synthetic LXR agonists, are commonly used in experimental studies. T0901317, in contrast with GW3965, is not completely selective for LXR (Viennois et al., 2011).

3.3 LXR expression patterns

LXR*α* was initially described as being highly expressed in a restricted subset of tissues known to play an important role in lipid metabolism such as liver, small intestine, kidney, spleen and adipose tissue whereas LXR*β* was found to be ubiquitously expressed (Viennois et al., 2011).

In the human placenta, both LXRα and LXRβ have been identified as early as the 6th week of gestation and can also be detected during gestation (Marceau et al., 2005). Indeed, mRNA expression is lowest in the first and second trimester of pregnancy (25 and 24% of term for LXRα, 33 and 16% for LXRβ, respectively). Expression levels in preterm and term placentae are similar to each other, but significantly higher than in the first two trimesters of gestation. The obligate heterodimeric partner of the LXRs, RXR, was found to be constitutively expressed throughout gestation (Plösch et al., 2010). Furthermore, both LXRs have been demonstrated to be expressed in choriocarcinoma trophoblast cell lines, e.g., JAR and BeWo (Weedon-Fekjaer et al., 2005).

3.4 Implications of LXRs in placenta and fetal membranes

3.4.1 Placental and amniotic presence of LXRs ligands

Placenta is an organ in which oxysterols are detected at a high concentration range (Schroepfer, 2000). Moreover, oxysterols such as 25-hydroxycholesterol (25-OHC) and 7-ketocholesterol (7-ketoC) circulate at low concentrations in normal conditions, but increase in maternal plasma as pregnancy advances (Aye et al., 2011). At low concentrations (2.5 μM) the oxysterol 22 (R)-OHC was shown to prevent first trimester extravillous cytotrophoblast invasion through the liver X receptor (LXR) which recognizes oxysterols as endogenous ligands (Pavan et al., 2004; Fournier et al., 2008b). Furthermore, the 7-ketocholesterol inhibit extravillous cytotrophoblast invasion. The role of LXR ligands in the placenta was confirmed using the LXR agonist T0901317, demonstrating the role of this nuclear receptor and its ligands in modulating the human trophoblast invasion (Pavan et al., 2004).

3.4.2 Fundamental implications of LXRs during early placentation

Little is known about the function of LXR during the placentation. A potential function of LXR in the placenta may be the regulation of cholesterol transport from the maternal to the fetal circulation. Indeed, cholesterol may be transported from the mother to the fetus to supplement the fetal cholesterol pool (Bełtowski & Semczuk, 2010). Conceptus implantation involves invasion of the uterine epithelium and the underlying stroma by extraembryonic trophoblast cells that undergo a complex process of proliferation, migration and differentiation. A specific feature of human placentation is the high degree of trophoblast invasion, greater than in other mammals. T0901317 has been shown to inhibit the invasiveness of cultured cytotrophoblast cells *in vitro* (Pavan et al., 2004). In addition, LXR mediates the inhibitory effect of oxidized LDL on trophoblast invasiveness.

3.4.3 Roles of LXRs in the uptake and transport of trophoblastic lipids

Compared with the liver, placenta secretes 50-200 times more fatty acid (Coleman & Haynes, 1987), indicating the importance of fatty acid as a mode of delivery of lipids to the fetus (Duttaroy, 2000). Noted that a new target gene, the long -chain acyl-coA synthetase 3 (ACSL3) was recently identified to illustrate the role of LXR as a regulator in fatty acid metabolism (Weedson-Fekjaer et al., 2010a). LXR has been demonstrated to be expressed in the placenta and in trophoblast-like cell lines, e.g., JAR and BeWo (Peet et al., 1998; Weedon-Fekjaer, 2005; Pavan et al., 2004). The increased fatty acid secretion by BeWo cells mediated by LXRs indicates its importance in placental lipid transport. Moreover, LXR activation in trophoblasts would lead to increased expression of its target genes, e.g., ATP-binding cassette transporter A1 (ABCA1) and ATP-binding cassette transporter G1 (ABCG1). Based on the localization of the ABCG1 and ABCA1 proteins to the basolateral (fetal) side of the trophoblast, one could assume that LXR activation would increase cholesterol flux from the maternal to the fetal circulation. Depending on the lipidation status of acceptor particles in the fetal circulation, both ABCG1- or ABCA1-dependent pathways seem to be possible, or even a combination of both. Therefore, LXR activation may be considered as a stimulus for increased transport of maternal cholesterol via the placenta to the fetal circulation (Plösch et al.,2007). Added to the fact that ABCA1 and ABCG1 are present on the syncytiotropholast (the maternal facing placental membrane), these results identify the inducible placental cholesterol transport by LXR as a preventive mechanism of placental accumulation of cytotoxic oxysterols (Aye et al., 2010).

3.4.4 LXRs in trophoblast invasion

Human implantation involves invasion of the uterine wall by trophoblastic cells and remodeling of uterine arteries by extravillous cytotrophoblasts (Henry-Berger et al., 2008). Several lines of evidence support the involvement of the LXR pathway in trophoblast biology. Firstly, trophoblast invasion is accompanied by an increased degradation of extracellular matrix proteins by members of the matrix metalloproteinases (MMPs) family (Caniggia et al.,1997), and expression of matrix metalloprotease-9 (MMP9) is regulated in macrophages by a mechanism dependent on LXR activation (Castrillo et al., 2003); secondly, T0901317 and oxidized LDLs (oxLDL), rich in oxysterols, significantly reduce trophoblast invasion via a mechanism involving LXRβ (Pavan et al., 2004; Fournier et al., 2008; Bełtowski & Semczuk, 2010). Recently Aye et al have shown that oxysterols inhibit syncytialisation and differentiation of term placental trophoblasts by activating LXRs. Excessive oxysterol exposure during pregnancy as a result of increased oxidative stress may, therefore, compromise placental formation and regeneration via inhibition of syncytialisation, thereby contributing to placental pathologies (Aye et al., 2011).

3.4.5 LXRs in placental pathologies

The pregnancy disease preeclampsia, a multisystemic disorder affecting about 5-10% of pregnancies towards the end of the second trimester of gestation, is still one of the leading causes of pregnancy-related maternal and fetal morbidity and mortality (Sibai et al., 2005; Myatt, 2002). Among its complications, intrauterine growth restriction and premature birth are of clinical relevance. Maternal predisposing factors such as diabetes, hypertension and obesity contribute to the consequences of this condition. Strong evidence supports that preeclampsia is generated by shallow invasion of the extravillous trophoblast into the decidua and an incomplete remodeling of the maternal uterine spiral arteries (Myatt, 2002). LXRβ mediates the inhibitory effect of oxidized LDL on trophoblast invasiveness, thus LXR agonists might interfere with the implantation process (Fournier et al., 2008). Moreover, inefficient trophoblast invasion may lead to subsequent impairment of placental perfusion, which is a main pathogenetic factor in preeclampsia. Furthermore, LXR agonists reduce the synthesis and secretion of hCG from trophoblast cells, which is mandatory for maintaining pregnancy in the first trimester (Weedon-Fekjaer et al., 2005). An increase in LXR and ABCA1 transporter levels point to an important role of ligands such as the oxysterols, which may be increased in preeclampsia (Plösch et al., 2010). A positive correlation between placental LXRβ mRNA expression and placental free fatty acids was found in preeclampsia (Weedon-Fekjaer et al., 2010b).

Recently, T0901317 has been shown to increase the expression of endoglin, part of the transforming growth factor-β receptor complex. Endoglin is highly expressed in syncytiotrophoblast and inhibits trophoblast invasion (Henry-Berger et al., 2008). The human endoglin gene promoter contains six putative LXRE sequences and at least one of them binds the LXR/RXR heterodimer to stimulate transcription in response to 22(R)-hydroxycholesterol, T0901317 or synthetic RXR agonists (Henry-Berger et al., 2008). Interestingly, circulating endoglin level is increased in preeclampsia and may contribute to endothelial dysfunction associated with this disorder (Legry et al., 2008). Apart from stimulating endoglin, LXR agonists may reduce trophoblast invasiveness by down-regulating MMP9, as has been demonstrated in macrophages (Castrillo et al., 2003). The demonstration that LXRα together with ABCA1 can be regulated by hypoxia is another argument of the LXR involvement in preeclampsia, where the oxygen tension is described as abnormal (Plösch et al., 2010).

4. Conclusion

Since the discovery of the PPARs, there has been a marked increase in available data on their involvement in mammalian development. Concerning the placenta, all PPARs, but particularly PPARγ, are essential for multiple physiological functions of the trophoblastic and amniotic parts, leading to major involvement of PPARs in the pathophysiology of gestational diseases. However, special care must be taken when this particular PPAR signalling cascade is involved, because part of the regulation may involve PPAR ligand signalling but may be transduced by independent nuclear receptor pathways. This last point introduces a new level of complexity in PPAR biology. It does not close preclusion of the eventual use of PPARs for therapeutic treatment during pregnancy, but future medical applications seem still to be a long way off. We can reasonably expect to see some obstetrical use of PPARs in diagnosis (detection of PPARs mutations in intrauterine growth retardation, predisposition of preeclampsia) and therapeutics (tocolysis or treatment of chorioamniotis).

About LXR, a few recent publications show its involvement in obstetric pathologies such as preeclampsia, where he would reduce the invasiveness of extravillous trophoblast. Besides, the potential therapeutic application of LXR agonists may include increasing uterine contractility, (especially in conditions expected to increase cholesterol content in uterine myocytes, such as obesity, hypercholesterolemia or gestational diabetes mellitus) and stimulation of transplacental cholesterol transport for the prenatal treatment of inborn errors of cholesterol synthesis.

5. Acknowledgment

Thank to Loïc Blanchon for help in drafting the section on PPAR.

Thank to Valerie Borel for participation in the drafting the section on PPAR.

Thank to Jean-Marc Lobaccaro for reviewing the section on LXR.

Thank to Vincent Sapin for proofreading and corrections throughout the chapter.

6. References

Ackerman, W. E.; Zhang, X. L.; Rovin, B. H. & Kniss, D. A. (2005). Modulation of cytokine-induced cyclooxygenase 2 expression by PPARG ligands through NFκB signal disruption in human WISH and amnion cells. *Biology of reproduction*, Vol. 73, No. 3, pp. 527–535.

Antonson, P.; Schuster, G. U.; Wang, L.; Rozell, B.; Holter, E. ; Flodby, P. ; Treuter, E. ; Holmgren, L. & Gustafsson, J.A. (2003). Inactivation of the nuclear receptor coactivator RAP250 in mice results in placental vascular dysfunction. *Molecular and Cellular Biology*, Vol. 23, No. 4, pp. 1260–1268.

Apfel, R.; Benbrook, D.; Lernhardt, E.; Ortiz, M.A.; Salbert, G. & Pfahl, M. (1994). A novel orphan receptor specific for a subset of thyroid hormone-responsive elements and its interaction with the retinoid/thyroid hormone receptor subfamily. *Molecular and cellular biology*, Vol. 14, No. 10, pp. 7025-7035.

Aye, I.L.; Waddell, B.J.; Mark, P.J. & Keelan, J.A. (2010). Placental ABCA1 and ABCG1 transporters efflux cholesterol and protect trophoblasts from oxysterol induced toxicity. *Biochim Biophys Acta*, Vol.1801, No9, pp.1013-1024.

Aye, I.L.; Waddell, B.J.; Mark, P.J. & Keelan, J.A. (2011). Oxysterols inhibit differentiation and fusion of term primary trophoblasts by activating liver X receptors. *Placenta*, Vol. 32, No. 2, pp 183-191.

Barak, Y.; Nelson, M. C.; Ong, E. S.; Jones Y.Z.; Ruiz-Lozano, P.; Chien, K.R.; Koder, A. & Evans R.M. (1999). PPAR γ is required for placental, cardiac, and adipose tissue development. *Molecular Cell*, Vol. 4, No. 4, pp. 585–595.

Barak, Y.; Liao, D. ; He, W.; Ong, E.S.; Nelson, M.C.; Olefsky, J.M.; Boland, R. & Evans, R.M. (2002). Effects of peroxisome proliferator-activated receptor δ on placentation, adiposity, and colorectal cancer. *Proceedings of the National Academy of Sciences of the United States of America*, Vol. 99, No. 1, pp. 303–308.

Bełtowski, J. & Semczuk, A. (2010). Liver X receptor (LXR) and the reproductive system--a potential novel target for therapeutic intervention. *Pharmacological Reports*, Vol. 62, No. 1, pp 15-27.

Berry, E. B.; Keelan, J. A.; Helliwell, R. J.; Gilmour, R. S. & Mitchell, M. D. (2005). Nanomolar and micromolar effects of 15- deoxy- Δ12,14-prostaglandin J2 on amnion-derived wish epithelial cells: differential roles of peroxisome proliferator activated receptors γ and δ and nuclear factor *Kb*. *Molecular Pharmacology*, Vol. 68, No. 1, pp. 169–178.

Bildirici, I.; Roh, C.-R. ; Schaiff, W. T.; Lewkowski, B. M.; Nelson, D. M. & Sadovsky, Y. (2003). The lipid droplet-associated protein adipophilin is expressed in human trophoblasts and is regulated by peroxisomal proliferator-activated receptor-γ/Retinoid X Receptor. *Journal of Clinical Endocrinology and Metabolism*, Vol. 88, No. 12, pp. 6056–6062.

Borel, V. ; Gallot, D. ; Marceau, G.; Sapin, V. & Blanchon, L. (2008). Placental implications of peroxisome proliferator-activated receptors in gestation and parturition. *PPAR research*, pp. 758762.

Calkin, A.C. & Tontonoz, P. (2010). Liver x receptor signaling pathways and atherosclerosis. *Arteriosclerosis, thrombosis, and vascular biology*, Vol. 30, No. 8, pp1513-1518.

Caniggia, I.; Taylor, C.V.; Ritchie, J.W.; Lye, S.J. & Letarte M. (1997). Endoglin regulates trophoblast differentiation along the invasive pathway in human placental villous explants. *Endocrinology*, Vol. 138, No. 11, pp 4977–4988.

Capobianco, E.; Jawerbaum, A.; White, V.; Pustovrh, C.; Sinner, D. & Gonzalez, E. T. (2003). Elevated levels of endothelin-1 and prostaglandin E2 and their effect on nitric oxide generation in placental tissue from neonatal streptozotocin-induced diabetic rats. *Prostaglandins Leukotrienes and Essential Fatty Acids*, Vol. 68, No. 3, pp. 225–231.

Capparuccia, L.; Marzioni, D.; Giordano, A.; Fazioli, F. ; De Nictolis, M. ; Busso, N. ; Todros, T. & Castellucci, M. (2002). PPARγ expression in normal human placenta, hydatidiform mole and choriocarcinoma. *Molecular Human Reproduction*, Vol. 8, No. 6, pp. 574–579.

Castrillo, A.; Joseph, S.B.; Marathe, C.; Mangelsdorf, D.J. & Tontonoz P. (2003). Liver X receptor-dependent repression of matrix metalloproteinase-9 expression in macrophages. *The Journal of Biological Chemistry*, Vol. 278, No. 12, pp 10443–10449.

Chen, M.; Beaven, S. & Tontonoz P. Identification and characterization of two alternatively spliced transcript variants of human liver X receptor alpha. *Journal of lipid research*, Vol. 46, No. 12, pp 2570-2579.

Coleman, R.A. & Haynes, E.B. (1987). Synthesis and release of fatty-acids by human trophoblast cells in culture. *Journal of Lipid Research*, Vol. 28, No. 11, pp 1335-1341.

Collins, J.L.; Fivush, A.M.; Watson, M.A.; Galardi, C.M.; Lewis, M.C.; Moore, L.B.; Parks, D.J.; Wilson, J.G.; Tippin, T.K.; Binz, J.G.; Plunket, K.D.; Morgan, D.G.; Beaudet, E.J.; Whitney, K.D.; Kliewer, S.A. & Willson, T.M. Identification of a nonsteroidal liver X receptor agonist through parallel array synthesis of tertiary amines. *Journal of medicinal chemistry*, Vol. 9, No. 45 pp 1963-1966.

Desvergne, B. & Wahli W. (1999). Peroxisome proliferator activated receptors: nuclear control of metabolism. *Endocrine Reviews*, Vol. 20, No. 5, pp. 649–688.

Dunn-Albanese, L. R.; Ackerman, W. E.; Xie, Y.; Iams, J. D. & Kniss, D. A. (2004). Reciprocal expression of peroxisome proliferator-activated receptor-γ and cyclooxygenase-2 in human term parturition. *American Journal of Obstetrics and Gynecology*, Vol. 190, No. 3, pp. 809–816.

DuttaRoy, A.K. (2000). Transport mechanisms for long-chain polyunsaturated fatty acids in the human placenta. *The American Journal of Clinical Nutrition*, Vol. 71, No. 1 suppl, pp 315S-322S.

Duttaroy, A. K. (2004). Fetal growth and development: roles of fatty acid transport proteins and nuclear transcription factors in human placenta. *Indian Journal of Experimental Biology*, Vol. 42, No. 8, pp. 747–757.

Escher, P. & Wahli W. (2000). Peroxisome proliferator-activated receptors: insight into multiple cellular functions. *Mutation Research*, Vol. 448, No. 2, pp. 121–138.

Escher, P.; Braissant, O.; Basu-Modak, S.; Michalik, L.; Wahli, W. & Desvergne, B. (2001).Rat PPARs: quantitative analysis in adult rat tissues and regulation in fasting and refeeding. *Endocrinology*, Vol. 142, No. 10, pp. 4195–4202.

Fajas, L.; Auboeuf, D.; E. Raspe, Schoonjans, K.; Lefebvre, A.M.; Saladin, R.; Najib, J.; Laville, M.; Fruchart, J.C.; Deeb, S.; Vidal-Puig, A.; Flier, J.; Briggs, M.R.; Staels, B.; Vidal, H. & Auwerx, J. (1997). The organization, promoter analysis, and expression of the human PPARγ gene. *The Journal of Biological Chemistry*, Vol. 272, No. 30, pp. 18779–18789.

Fournier, T.; Pavan, L.; Tarrade, A.; Schoonjans, K. ; Auwerx, J.; Rochette-Egly, C. & Evain-Brion D. (2002). The role of PPAR- γ/RXR-a heterodimers in the regulation of human trophoblast invasion. *Annals of the New York Academy of Sciences*, vol. 973, pp. 26–30.

Fournier, T.; Tsatsaris, V.; Handschuh, K. & Evain-Brion D. (2007). PPARs and the placenta. *Placenta*, Vol. 28, No. 2-3, pp. 65–76.

Fournier, T. ; Thérond, P. ; Handschuh, K. ; Tsatsaris, V. & Evain-Brion, D. (2008a). PPARgamma and early human placental development. *Current medicinal Chemistry*, Vol. 15, No. 28, pp 3011-3024.

Fournier, T.; Handschuh, K.; Tsatsaris, V.; Guibourdenche, J. & Evain-Brion D. (2008b). Role of nuclear receptors and their ligands in human trophoblast invasion. *Journal of Reproductive Immunology*, Vol. 77, No. 2, pp 161-170.

Giaginis, C.; Spanopoulou, E. & Theocharis, S. (2008). PPAR-gamma signaling pathway in placental development and function: a potential therapeutic target in the treatment of gestational diseases. *Expert opinion on therapeutic targets*, Vol. 12, No. 8, pp 1049-1063.

Handschuh, F.; Guibourdenche, J.; Cocquebert, M.; Tsatsaris, V.; Vidaud, M.; Evain-Brion , D.; Fournier, T. (2009) Expression and regulation by PPARgamma of hCG alpha- and beta-subunits : comparison between villous and invasive extravillous trophoblastic cells. *Placenta*, Vol. 30, No.12, pp. 1016-1022.

Helliwell, R. J.; Keelan, J. A.; Marvin, K. W.; Adams, L.; Chang, M.C.; Anand, A.; Sato, T.A.; O'Carroll, S.; Chaiworapongsa, T.; Romero, R.J. & Mitchell M.D. (2006). Gestational age-dependent up-regulation of prostaglandin D synthase (PGDS) and production of PGDS-derived anti-inflammatory prostaglandins in human placenta. *Journal of Clinical Endocrinology &Metabolism*, Vol. 91, No. 2, pp. 597–606.

Henry-Berger, J.; Mouzat, K.; Baron, S.; Bernabeu, C.; Marceau, G.; Saru, J.P.; Sapin, V.; Lobaccaro, J.M. & Caira, F. (2008). Endoglin (CD105) expression is regulated by the liver X receptor alpha (NR1H3) in human trophoblast cell line JAR. *Biology of Reproduction*, Vol. 78, No. 6, pp 968-975.

Holdsworth-Carson, S.J.; Lim, R.; Mitton, A.; Whitehead, C.; Rice, G.E.; Permezel, M. & Lappas M. (2010). Peroxisome proliferator-activated receptors are altered in pathologies of the human placenta: gestational diabetes mellitus, intrauterine growth restriction and preeclampsia. *Placenta*, Vol. 31, No. 3, pp 222-229.

Issemann, I. & Green S. (1990). Activation of a member of the steroid hormone receptor superfamily by peroxisome proliferators. *Nature*, Vol. 347, No. 6294, pp. 645–650.

Jacobsson, B.; Mattsby-Baltzer, I. & Hagberg, H. (2005). Interleukin-6 and interleukin-8 in cervical and amniotic fluid: relationship to microbial invasion of the chorioamniotic membranes. *Journal of Obstetrics and Gynaecology*, Vol. 112, No. 6, pp. 719–724.

Janowski, B.A.; Willy, P.J.; Devi, T.R.; Falck, J.R. & Mangelsdorf, D.J. (1996). An oxysterol signalling pathway mediated by the nuclear receptor LXR alpha. *Nature*, Vol. 383, No. 6602, pp 728–731.

Jawerbaum, A.; Capobianco, E.; Pustovrh, C.; White, V.; Baier, M.; Salzberg, S.; Pesaresi, M. & Gonzalez, E. (2004). Influence of peroxisome proliferator-activated receptor γ activation by its endogenous ligand 15-deoxy Δ12,14 prostaglandin J2 on nitric oxide production in term placental tissues from diabetic women. *Molecular Human Reproduction*, Vol. 10, No. 9, pp. 671–676.

Jawerbaum, A. & González, E. (2006). Diabetic pregnancies: the challenge of developing in a pro-inflammatory environment. *Current Medicinal Chemistry*, Vol. 13, No. 18, pp. 2127–2138.

Jawerbaum, A. & Capobianco, E. (2011). Review: Effects of PPAR activation in the placenta and the fetus: implications in maternal diabetes. *Placenta*, Vol. 32, Suppl No. 2, pp 212-217.

Julan, L.; Guan, H.; Van Beek, J. P. & Yang, K. (2005). Peroxisome proliferator-activated receptor δ suppresses 11β- hydroxysteroid dehydrogenase type 2 gene expression in human placental trophoblast cells. *Endocrinology*, Vol. 146, No. 3, pp. 1482–1490.

Johnson, R. D.; Polakoski, K. L.; Huang, X.; Sadovsky, Y. & Nelson, D. M. (1998). The release of 15-hydroxyeicosatetraenoic acid by human placental trophoblast is increased in preeclampsia. *American Journal of Obstetrics and Gynecology*, Vol. 178, No. 1 part 1, pp. 54–58.

Kniss, D. A. (1999). Cyclooxygenases in reproductive medicine and biology. *Journal of the Society for Gynecologic Investigation*, Vol. 6, No. 6, pp. 285–292.

Kuang, S.-Q.; Liao, L.; Zhang, H.; Pereira, F.A.; Yuan, Y.; DeMayo, F.J.; Ko, L. & Xu, J. (2002). Deletion of the cancer-amplified coactivator AIB3 results in defective placentation and embryonic lethality. *Journal of Biological Chemistry*, Vol. 277, No. 47, pp. 45356–45360.

Lappas, M.; Permezel, M.; Georgiou, H. M. & Rice, G. E. (2002). Regulation of proinflammatory cytokines in human gestational tissues by peroxisome proliferator-activated receptor- γ: effect of 15-deoxy-Δ12,14-PGJ2 and troglitazone. *Journal of Clinical Endocrinology &Metabolism*, Vol. 87, No. 10, pp. 4667- 4672.

Lappas, M. & Rice, G. E. (2004). Phospholipase A2 isozymes in pregnancy and parturition. *Prostaglandins Leukotrienes and Essential Fatty Acids*, Vol. 70, No. 2, pp. 87–100.

Lappas, M.; Permezel, M. & Rice, G. E. (2005). Leptin and adiponectin stimulate the release of proinflammatory cytokines and prostaglandins from human placenta and maternal adipose tissue via nuclear factor-κB, peroxisomal proliferator-activated receptor-γ and extracellularly regulated kinase ½. *Endocrinology*, Vol. 146, No. 8, pp. 3334–3342.

Lappas, M.; Yee, K.; Permezel, M. & Rice, G. E. (2006). Lipopolysaccharide and TNF-*a* activate the nuclear factor kappa B pathway in the human placental JEG-3 cells. *Placenta*, Vol. 27, No. 6-7, pp. 568–575.

Legry, V.; Cottel, D.; Ferrières, J.; Chinetti, G.; Deroide, T.; Staels, B.; Amouyel, P. & Meirhaeghe, A. (2008). Association between liver X receptor _ gene polymorphisms and risk of metabolic syndrome in French populations. *International Journal of Obesity*, Vol. 32, No. 3, pp 421–428.

Marceau, G.; Volle, D.H.; Gallot, D.; Mangelsdorf, D.J.; Sapin, V. & Lobaccaro, J.M. (2005). Placental expression of the nuclear receptors for oxysterols LXRalpha and LXRbeta during mouse and human development. *The Anatomical Record. Part A, Discoveries in Molecular Cellular and Evolutionary Biology*, Vol. 283, No. 1, pp 175-181.

Michael, L.F.; Schkeryantz, J.M. & Burris T.P. (2005). The pharmacology of LXR. *Mini reviews in medicinal chemistry*, Vol. 5, No. 8, pp729-740.

Michalik, L.; Desvergne, B.; Dreyer, C.; Gavillet, M.; Laurini, R. N. & W.Wahli. (2002) PPAR expression and function during vertebrate development. *International Journal of Developmental Biology*, Vol. 46, No. 1, pp. 105–114.

Mitchell, M. D.; Kraemer, D. L. & Strickland, D. M. (1982). The human placenta: a major source of prostaglandin D_2. *Prostaglandins Leukotrienes and Medicine*, Vol. 8, No. 4, pp. 383–387.

Myatt L. (2002). Role of placenta in preeclampsia. *Endocrine*, Vol; 19, No. 1, pp 103-111.Nadra, K.; Anghel, S. I.; Joye, E.; Tan, N.S. ; Basu-Modak, S. ; Trono, D. ; Wahli, W. & Desvergne B. (2006). Differentiation of trophoblast giant cells and their metabolic functions are dependent on peroxisome proliferator-activated receptor *β/δ*. *Molecular and Cellular Biology*, Vol. 26, No. 8, pp. 3266–3281.

Nadra, K.; Quignodon, L.; Sardella, C.; Joye, E. ; Mucciolo, A. ; Chrast, R. ; Desvergne, B. (2010) PPARgamma in placental angiogenesis. *Endocrinology*, Vol.15, No.10, pp. 4969-4981.

Ng, V. Y.; Huang, Y.; Reddy, L. M.; Falck, J. R.; Lin, E. T. & Kroetz, D. L. (2007). CytochromeP450 eicosanoids are activators of peroxisome proliferator-activated receptor *a*.. *Drug Metabolism and Disposition*, Vol. 35, No. 7, pp. 1126–1134.

Okita, J. R.; MacDonald, P. C. & Johnston, J. M. (1982). Mobilization of arachidonic acid from specific glycerophospholipids of human fetal membranes during early labor. *Journal of Biological Chemistry*, Vol. 257, No. 23, pp. 14029–14034.

Parast, MM.; Yu, H.; Ciric, A.; Salata, MW.; Davis, V.; Milstone DS. (2009) PPARgamma regulates trophoblast proliferation and promotes labyrinthine trilineage differentiation. *PLoS One*, Vol. 4, No. 11: e8055.

Pavan, L.; Hermouet, A.; Tsatsaris, V.; Thérond, P.; Sawamura, T. ; Evain-Brion, D. & Fournier, T. (2004). Lipids from oxidized low-density lipoprotein modulate human trophoblast invasion: involvement of nuclear liver X receptors. *Endocrinology*, Vol. 145, No. 10, pp 4583-4591.

Peet, D.J. Janowski, B.A. & Mangelsdorf, D.J. (1998). The LXRs: a new class of oxysterol receptors. *Current Opinion in Genetics and Development*, Vol. 8, No. 5, pp 571-575.

Plösch, T.; van Straten, E.M. & Kuipers, F. (2007). Cholesterol transport by the placenta: placental liver X receptor activity as a modulator of fetal cholesterol metabolism? *Placenta*, Vol. 28, No. 7, pp 604-610.

Plösch, T.; Gellhaus, A.; van Straten, E.M.; Wolf, N.; Huijkman, N.C.; Schmidt, M.; Dunk, C.E.; Kuipers, F. & Winterhager, E. (2010). The liver X receptor (LXR) and its target gene ABCA1 are regulated upon low oxygen in human trophoblast cells: a reason for alterations in preeclampsia? *Placenta*, Vol. 31, No. 10, pp 910-918.

Roberts, J.M.; Taylor, R. N.; Musci, T. J.; Rodgers, G. M.; Hubel, C. A. & McLaughlin, M. K. (1989). Preeclampsia: an endothelial cell disorder. *American Journal of Obstetrics and Gynecology*, Vol. 161, No. 5, pp. 1200–1204.

Sapin, V.; Blanchon, L.; Serre, A. F.; Lemery, D.; Dastugue, B. & Ward, S. J. (2001). Use of transgenic mice model for understanding the placentation: towards clinical applications in human obstetrical pathologies? *Transgenic Research*, Vol. 10, No. 5, pp. 377–398.

Sibai, B. ; Dekker, G. & Kupferminc, M. (2005). Pre-eclampsia. *Lancet*, Vol. 365, pp785-799.

Schaiff, W. T.; Bildirici, I.; Cheong, M.; Chern, P. L.; Nelson, D. M. & Sadovsky, Y. (2005). Peroxisome proliferator-activated receptor-γ and retinoid X receptor signaling regulate fatty acid uptake by primary human placental trophoblasts. *Journal of Clinical Endocrinology and Metabolism*, Vol. 90, No. 7, pp. 4267–4275.

Schaiff, W. T.; Knapp Jr., F. F.; Barak, Y.; Biron-Shental, T.; Nelson, D. M. & Sadovsky, Y. (2007). Ligand-activated PPARγ alters placental morphology and placental fatty acid uptake in mice. *Endocrinology*, Vol. 148, No. 8, pp. 3625–3634.

Schild, R. L.; Schaiff, W. T.; Carlson, M. G.; Cronbach, E. J.; Nelson, D.M. & Sadovsky, Y. (2002). The activity of PPAR γ in primary human trophoblasts is enhanced by oxidized lipids. *Journal of Clinical Endocrinology and Metabolism*, Vol. 87, No. 3, pp. 1105–1110.

Schroepfer, G.J. (2000). Oxysterols: modulators of cholesterol metabolism and other processes. *Physiological Reviews*, Vol. 80, No. 1, pp 361–554.

Schultz, J.R.; Tu, H.; Luk, A.; Repa, J.J.; Medina, J.C.; Li, L.; Schwendner, S.; Wang, S.; Thoolen, M.; Mangelsdorf, D.J.; Lustig, K.D. & Shan B. (2000). Role of LXRs in control of lipogenesis. *Genes and development*, Vol. 14, No. 22, pp 2831-2838.

Schwarz, B. E.; Schultz, F. M.; Macdonald, P. C. & Johnston J. M. (1975). Initiation of human parturition. III. fetal membrane content of prostaglandin E2 and F2*a* precursor. *Obstetrics and Gynecology*, Vol. 46, No. 5, pp. 564–568.

Song, C.; Hiipakka, R.A. & Liao S. (2000). Selective activation of liver X receptor alpha by 6alpha-hydroxy bile acids and analogs. *Steroids*, Vol. 65, No. 8, pp 423-427.

Song, C.; Hiipakka, R.A. & Liao, S. (2001). Auto-oxidized cholesterol sulfates are antagonistic ligands of liver X receptors: implications for the development and treatment of atherosclerosis. *Steroids*, Vol. 66, No. 6, pp 473-479.

Suwaki, N.; Masuyama, H.; Masumoto, A.; Takamoto, N. & Hiramatsu, Y. (2007).Expression and potential role of peroxisome proliferator-activated receptor gamma in the placenta of diabetic pregnancy. *Placenta*, Vol. 28, No. 4, pp 315-323.

Toth, B.; Hornung, D.; Scholz, C.; Djalali, S.; Friese, K. & Jeschke, U. (2007). Peroxisome proliferator-activated receptors: new players in the field of reproduction. *American Journal of Reproductive Immunology*, Vol. 58, No. 3, pp. 289–310.

Viennois, E.; Pommier, A.J.; Mouzat, K.; Oumeddour, A.; El Hajjaji, F.Z.; Dufour, J.; Caira, F.; Volle, D.H.; Baron, S. & Lobaccaro, J.M. (2011). Targeting liver X receptors in human health: deadlock or promising trail? *Expet opinion on therapeutics targets*, Vol. 15, No. 2, pp 219-232.

Waite, L. L.; Person, E. C.; Zhou, Y.; Lim, K. H.; Scanlan, T. S. & Taylor, R. N. (2000). Placental peroxisome proliferator-activated receptor-γ is up-regulated by pregnancy serum. *Journal of Clinical Endocrinology &Metabolism*, Vol. 85, No. 10, pp. 3808– 3814.

Wang, H.; Xie, H.; Sun, X.; Tranguch, S.; Zhang, H.; Jia, X.; Wang, D.; Das, SK.; Desvergne, B.; Wahli, W.; DuBois, R.N. & Dey, S.K. (2007). Stage-specific integration of maternal and embryonic peroxisome proliferator-activated receptor delta signaling is critical to pregnancy success. *The Journal of Biological Chemistry*, Vol. 282, No. 52, pp 3770-37782.

Ware Branch, D.; Mitchell, M. D.; Miller, E.; Palinski, W. & Witztum, J. L. (1994). Pre-eclampsia and serum antibodies to oxidized low-density lipoprotein. *Lancet*, Vol. 343, No. 8898, pp. 645– 646.

Weedon-Fekjaer, M.S. Duttaroy, A.K. & Nebb, H.I. (2005). Liver X receptors mediate inhibition of hCG secretion in a human placental trophoblast cell line. *Placenta*, Vol. 26, No. 10, pp 721-728.

Weedon -Fekjaer, M.S.; Johnsen, G.M.; Anthonisen, E.H.; Sugulle, M.; Nebb, H.I.; Duttaroy, A.K.; Staff, A.C. (2010a) Expression of liver X receptors in pregnancies complicated by preeclampsia. *Placenta*, Vol. 31, No.9, pp. 818-824.

Weedon-Fekjaer, M.S.; Dalen, K.T., Solaas, K.; Staff, A.C.; Duttaroy, A.K.; Nebb, H.I. (2010b) Activation of LXR increases acyl-CoA synthetase activity through direct regulation of ACSL3 in human placental trophoblast cells. J Lip Res, Vol. 51, No.7, pp.1886-1896.

Willi, M. J.; Winkler, M.; Fischer, D.-C.; Reineke, T.; Maul, H. & Rath, W. (2002).Chorioamnionitis: elevated interleukin-6 and interleukin-8 concentrations in the lower uterine segment. *Journal of PerinatalMedicine*, Vol. 30, No. 4, pp. 292–296.

Xu, Y.; Cook, T. J. & Knipp, G. T. (2005). Effects of di-(2-ethylhexyl)-phthalate (DEHP) and its metabolites on fatty acid homeostasis regulating proteins in rat placental HRP-1 trophoblast cells. *Toxicological Sciences*, Vol. 84, No. 2, pp. 287–300.

Yang, C.; McDonald, J.G.; Patel, A;. Zhang, Y.; Umetani, M.; Xu, F.; Westover, E.J.; Covey, D.F.; Mangelsdorf, D.J.; Cohen, J.C. & Hobbs, H.H. (2006). Sterol intermediates from cholesterol biosynthetic pathway as liver X receptor ligands. *The journal of biological chemistry*, Vol. 281, No. 38, pp 27816-27826.

Zaga, V.; Estrada-Gutierrez, G. ; Beltran-Montoya, J. ; Maida-Claros, R.; Lopez-Vancell, R. & Vadillo-Ortega, F. (2004). "Secretions of interleukin-1β and tumor necrosis factor a by whole fetal membranes depend on initial interactions of amnion or choriodecidua with lipopolysaccharides or group B streptococci. *Biology of Reproduction*, Vol. 71, No. 4, pp. 1296–1302.

Zaga-Clavellina, V.; Lopez, G. G.; Estrada-Gutierrez, G.; Martinez-Flores, A. ; Maida-Claros, R.; Beltran-Montoya, J. & Vadillo-Ortega F. (2006). Incubation of human chorioamniotic membranes with Candida albicans induces differential synthesis and secretion of interleukin-1β, interleukin-6, prostaglandin E2, and 92 kDa type IV collagenase. *Mycoses*, vol. 49, no. 1, pp. 6–13.

Zhu, Y.; Qi, C.; Jia, Y.; Nye, J. S.; Rao, M. S. & Reddy, J.K. (2000). Deletion of PBP/PARBP, the gene for nuclear receptor coactivator peroxisome proliferator-activated receptor-binding protein, results in embryonic lethality. *Journal of Biological Chemistry*, Vol. 275, No. 20, pp. 14779–14782.

Zhu, Y.J.; Crawford, S. E.; Stellmach, V.; Dwivedi, R.S.; Rao, M.S.; Gonzalez, F.J.; Qi, C. & Reddy, J.K. (2003). Coactivator PRIP, the peroxisome proliferator-activated receptor interacting protein, is a modulator of placental, cardiac, hepatic, and embryonic development. *Journal of Biological Chemistry*, Vol. 278, No. 3, pp. 1986–1990.

19

Genomic Imprinting in Human Placenta

Luca Lambertini[1,2], Men-Jean Lee[3], Carmen J. Marsit[4] and Jia Chen[1,5,6]
[1]*Department of Preventive Medicine, Mount Sinai School of Medicine, New York,*
[2]*Department of Obstetrics, Gynecology and Reproductive Science, Mount Sinai School of Medicine, New York,*
[3]*Department of Obstetrics and Gynecology, Indiana University-Purdue University, Indianapolis,*
[4]*Department of Pharmacology and Toxicology, Dartmouth Medical School, Hanover,*
[5]*Department of Pediatrics, Mount Sinai School of Medicine, New York,*
[6]*Department of Oncological Sciences, Mount Sinai School of Medicine, New York,*
USA

1. Introduction

The placenta is a unique organ that supports and drives embryonic development by providing an environment for the growth of the fetus, coordinating the different phases of embryogenesis, and serving as an interface for maternal-fetal interactions. The placenta is a very dynamic organ, where a continuum of phenotypic and morphological changes takes place over the course of gestation. Such plasticity is achieved due to a unique epigenetic profile that allows for: 1) a rapid growth to timely accommodate the embryo; 2) a marked invasiveness that allows implantation and invasion of fetal cells into the maternal endometrium; and 3) a specific metabolic activity that spans from growth in a hypoxic environment, accession to the maternal blood supply, remodeling of endothelial cell functions, to evasion of the immune system, allocation of nutrient resources, disposal of fetal waste products, and production of pregnancy-associated hormones (Hu & Cross, 2010).

Consistently, since the early 1980s, the placenta has been proven to possess an unusual epigenetic profile with the lowest level of genomic DNA methylation of all organs across different species (Ehrlich *et al.*, 1982; Gama-Sosa *et al.*, 1983). Under the assumption that DNA methylation leads to gene silencing, this hypomethylated profile has been attributed to the need for the placenta to sustain implantation with promotion of rapid and highly coordinated fetoplacental growth and maturation. Somewhat supportive of this hypothesis is the discovery that the placenta shares common epigenetic features with tumor tissues which display fast growth and invasive morphologic characteristics as well (Guilleret *et al.*, 2009; Harada, 1978; Perry *et al.*, 2010).

1.1 Placenta epigenetics and genomic imprinting

The intricate network of epigenetic mechanisms that act on the genome modifying its expression to determine the phenotype is, as of yet, only poorly understood. DNA methylation, histone modification and long non-protein-coding RNAs (lncRNAs) activity are the best known of such mechanisms. While studies that explored each of these phenomena individually, either in a genome-wide or targeted fashion, struggled to determine the full extent of their importance (Lambertini *et al.*, 2011), the integrated investigation of their interplay, in the framework of specific molecular pathways linked to phenotypical outcomes, is gaining momentum (Q. Li *et al.*, 2011; Qureshi & Mehler, 2011).

Genomic imprinting is probably the best example of how multiple epigenetic mechanisms act on the phenotype. It has in fact been shown that DNA methylation, histone modification and lncRNAs, coordinately act in regulating the monoallelic expression of a small subset of genes (~1%) in the human genome accordingly to their parent-of-origin. As for all other epigenetic mechanisms, imprinting shows tissue-specificity, i.e. genes that are imprinted in the placenta are biallelically expressed in other tissues (T.H. Vu *et al.*, 2010). The loss of genomic imprinting (LOI) during the early stages of embryogenesis, can lead to placental and fetal growth restriction and influence the fetal development into adulthood (Sasaky & Ishino, 2006; Tycko, 2006; American Journal of Medical Genetics, 2010).

Accordingly, experiments on mice showed that induced pluripotent stem cells (iPCs) and embryonic stem (ES) cells have indistinguishable global mRNA profiles; however iPCs fail to support the development of all-iPCs animals contrary to ES cells. A closer investigation of the iPCs and ES mRNA profiles however revealed a reproducible expression difference for only 2 transcripts, the lncRNA *Meg3* and the small nucleolar RNA *Rian*, two imprinted genes belonging to the *Dlk1-Dio3* imprinted domain. Additionally, the expression profiles of other imprinted gene sets were found to vary from clone to clone further supporting the critical role played by imprinted genes in development (Stadtfeld *et al.*, 2010).

In another mouse model, bi-maternal embryos obtained from immature primordial oocytes, with no established epigenetic imprinting marks, and fully developed oocytes with complete sex-specific imprinting signals, were not viable. Placentas of these embryos showed both severe growth restriction and abnormal histology. The engineered deletion in primordial oocytes of two relatively small regions encompassing the two imprinted gene clusters *Igf2-H19* and *Dlk1-Dio3*, alone rescued the phenotype. The placenta was then found to develop normally and the associated conceptuses grew normally into adulthood. Interestingly, embryos from one normal and one primordial oocyte, alternatively carrying only one of the imprinting deletions, resulted in phenotypes affecting placental growth and fetal development as well as size and general health status of the progeny (Kawahara *et al.*, 2009).

These findings support the fundamental role that imprinted genes play in development while contemporaneously highlighting the need, for embryogenesis to proceed regularly, of the contribution of genotypes carrying different epigenetic marks (i.e. paternal and maternal), as shown in the early 1980s from studies in mice (McGrath & Solter, 1984). This condition has been addressed by the "parental conflict theory" which proposes that the parent-of-origin specific epigenetic marks of genomic imprinting evolved in animals to properly allow for the distribution of maternal resources to each developing embryo (Haig

& Graham, 1991; Moore & Haig, 1991). Under this theory a tug-of-war takes place between the paternally expressed genes that promote fetal growth to generate a stronger offspring, and the maternally expressed genes that have the opposite effect in order to preserve maternal energies (McGrath & Solter, 1984). In line with this theory are the findings that paternal uniparental disomy (UPD) (paternalization) of the imprinted region of chromosome 11, which carries several imprinted gene clusters, results in the Beckwith-Wiedemann syndrome characterized by a birthweight 50% above normal, accompanied by other overgrowth symptoms. On the other hand, maternal UPD (maternalization) of this same region leads to Silver-Russell syndrome characterized by perinatal and postnatal growth deficiency (Barlow *et al.*, 1991).

There are also evolutionary findings that support the parental conflict theory. Humans in fact show a diminished degree of conservation of the genomic imprinting, particularly for maternally expressed genes (Hutter *et al.*, 2010), compared to lower species. This is consistent with the observation that singleton pregnancies are much more common in humans therefore reducing the need of conservation of maternal energy (Isles, 2009; Monk *et al.*, 2006).

Analysis of the LOI in normal placenta provides additional clues on possible relaxation of the imprinting status in humans. Normal placenta samples in fact returned appreciable LOI values (>3%) for genes like *IGF2*, *MEST*, *PEG3*, *SLC22A18* and *TP73* in a pilot study run by measuring LOI in a highly quantitative allele-specific real-time PCR (RT-PCR) on 22 placental RNA samples across 14 imprinted genes (Diplas *et al.*, 2009a; Lambertini *et al.*, 2008; Lambertini *et al.*, 2009). It has however to be noticed that 3 out of the 5 genes identified were paternally expressed (or maternally imprinted) and 2 maternally expressed (or paternally imprinted) which speaks more directly for a generalized LOI of imprinted genes independently from their parent-of-origin.

1.2 Genomic imprinting characteristics

The mechanism by which DNA methylation, histone modification and lncRNAs operate in silencing genes accordingly to their parent-of-origin is becoming more and more clear as evidence accumulates, even though several points still remain obscure.

Imprinted genes often reside in clusters spread across all human genome and are expected to represent only around 1% of the expressed genes or ~200 genes; of these at present only ~90 have been experimentally proven. Imprinted genes, both when alone or clustered, are invariably regulated by imprinting control regions (ICRs) that determine the silent/active status of one of the alleles. ICRs are short DNA sequences with limited shared features that show allele-specific methylation at consensus CpG dinucleotides involved in the binding with regulatory proteins. Functional CpG dinucleotides invariably appear as 50% methylated. Such attributes were discovered in a total of 8 imprinted clusters both in mice and humans overlooking the allele-specific expression of a total of nearly 30 genes (Lewis & Reik, 2006). ICR-like features have been shown for 5 other regions which have at present been linked to a single imprinted gene. The remaining imprinted genes returned mostly parent-of-origin specific methylation of the promoter region. ICRs can ultimately be located several kilobase pairs (kbp) away from a specific imprinted gene, in non-coding genomic areas or in the promoter or gene body of other imprinted genes (Lewis & Reik, 2006).

DNA methylation was for several years thought to be the only epigenetic mechanism regulating imprinting, recently however experiments on histone modification showed that ICRs carry characteristic features of allele-specific methylation of histone H3, acetylation of histones H3 and H4 and ubiquitination of histone H2 over specific lysine aminoacidic residues. These epigenetic signals have been linked with the stabilization of the active/silenced status of each allele (Gieni & Hendzel, 2009; Yang & Kuroda, 2007).

One question has however always been left unanswered, how can an ICR regulate the silencing of one allele of a gene located up to 100 kbp away? The answer to this question was tentatively provided by the discovery of lncRNAs. These molecules, which are not translated into proteins, are actively transcribed, have lengths often above 1,000 bp and carry consensus sequences for the binding of regulatory proteins complexes that can also bind ICRs (Bernstein & Allis, 2005). Accordingly, lncRNAs are ideal candidates for determining spatial and temporal specificity as transcription regulators by interacting with their promoters in a temporally regulated fashion (Mohammad *et al.*, 2009; Yazgan & Krebs, 2007). From the mechanistic point of view it has been proposed that lncRNAs act by directly recruiting chromatin modifying proteins that would participate in the formation of DNA loops intended to activate/silence genes and even select between promoters with different strength (Lefevre *et al.*, 2008).

Interestingly only 1.5% of our entire genome encodes mRNAs that are translated into proteins while 60-80% of the genome is transcribed into non-protein-coding RNAs (Lee, 2009). Also while the number of nucleotides encoding protein sequences is relatively constant, the number of nucleotides for non-protein-coding sequences increases over a wide range of eukaryotic complexity, suggesting that increased complexity itself may be explained by an increase in *cis*-acting regulatory elements driving *trans*-acting lncRNAs (Taft *et al.*, 2007). It has now been proposed that lncRNAs act on silencing specific alleles much the same way that the *XIST* lncRNA acts on silencing one of the X chromosome copies in females. In this model, DNA methylation and histone modification marks would act as readout signals for lncRNA-protein complexes (Heard *et al.*, 2004). Accordingly, each of the identified imprinted clusters expresses at least one lncRNA (Bartolomei, 2009).

An indirect confirmation of this model comes from the discovery that LOI is a cell-specific phenomenon. It has been in fact shown in cell lines that the administration of 5-aza-2'-deoxycytidine (AZA) induces complete bi-allelic expression in individual clones (Diplas et al., 2009b). This finding is thus consistent with a total erasure of the DNA methylation readout code therefore leading to a complete binding inhibition of the protein complexes that would otherwise drive the allele silencing.

2. Imprinted genes and development

Epigenetic imprinting signals are timely reset during the zygote pre-implantation and early implantation phases. It has been hypothesized that at this stage the embryo undergoes to a basic programming in order to develop according to the environmental conditions it would face after birth (Santos & Dean, 2004).

During pre-implantation the zygote is subjected to a genome-wide wave of de-methylation intended to reset this epigenetic signal brought about by the parents. Re-methylation of genomic regions takes place accordingly to the new fetal programming. ICRs and ICR-like elements on paternal and maternal alleles are however protected from such changes and maintain their parent-of-origin original configuration (Figure 1) (Perera & Herbstman, 2011). The hypothesis behind this phenomenon is that, at fertilization, paternal and maternal haploid genomes still carry their own epigenetic effector protein complexes that act by differentially binding to chromosomal regions to generate sex-specific tridimensional organization of the genome. This theory finds a further explanation while looking at the first genome-wide de-methylation wave of non-imprinted regions; paternal and maternal genomes are in fact stripped at this stage of their DNA methylation signals at a different rate with the paternal genotype becoming quickly unmethylated after fertilization while the maternal de-methylation proceeds slowly (Reik *et al.*, 2001). Following the resetting of the DNA methylation profiles in a cell type specific fashion, the histone code is reset to further

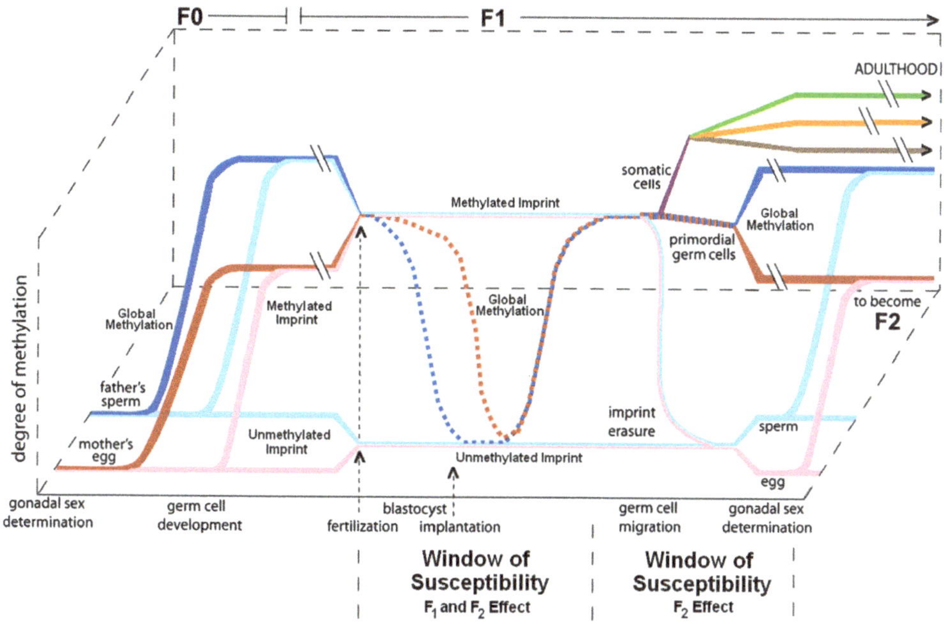

Fig. 1. Fetal imprinting reprogramming of DNA methylation marks during the early zygote developmental phases. F_0 sperm and egg carry global (red and blue lines) and imprinting-specific methylation signals (pink and light blue). After fertilization global methylation is reprogrammed at the blastocyst stadium. Imprinting signals are however maintained unaltered to generate an embryo with distinct parental contributions. Imprinting reprogramming takes place only in the primordial germ cells later in development to generate gametes carrying imprinting marks according to the sex of the developing embryo. Perturbations of the imprinting profiles at the blastocyst stage can directly affect the embryo and also the gametes (F_1 and F_2 windows) Perturbations happening later affect specifically imprinting reprogramming of gametes (F_2 window). Somatic cells separately develop from the embryo carrying the parental imprinting signals and the newly reprogrammed global methylation setting (purple line). They later rearrange their methylation status coherently with the adult tissue they will originate (green, orange and brown lines). [Adapted from (Perera & Herbstman, 2011)].

stabilize the DNA methylation profile providing the embryo with the articulated network of epigenetic signaling carrying the essential parent-of-origin specific setup of the genome (Santos & Dean, 2004).

Later in fetal development a subset of embryonal cells are selected to become primordial germ cells (PGCs). In order to guarantee the generation of mature haploid germ cells with imprinting marks consistent with the sex of the developing embryo, PGCs undergo to a second DNA de/re-methylation programming and histone coding this time specifically targeted to imprinted domains (Reik *et al.*, 2001).

Embryonic DNA methylation and histone modification signals placed in the early zygote during these developmental stages together constitute the "code" for lncRNAs to later "read" to drive, similarly to the X inactivation process, the gene silencing/activation in a plastic and adaptable system during subsequent developmental phases. This same system would also determine the tissue specificity of imprinting as shown in the liver where the *IGF2-H19* ICR is still paternally methylated but *IGF2* is biallelically expressed (T.H. Vu *et al.*, 2010).

This highly coordinated system of epigenetic reprogramming creates windows of vulnerability during the early phases of the fetal development that extends into the later phases, as well as exerting a trans-generational effect when perturbing the correct PGCs programming. Such perturbations, depending from the time of occurrence, can in fact extend their effect across at least the second generation (Figure 1) and possibly even beyond. In this framework, it has been hypothesized that several fetal outcomes can be associated with perturbations of the embryo epigenetic reprogramming at different times across the windows of susceptibility (Table 1).

Between these episodes, the prenatal and periconceptional exposure to insufficient maternal caloric intake has been found to leave lasting signals on the methylation profile of several imprinted genes like *INS*, *IGF2*, *GNASAS* and *MEG3* up to 60 years after the triggering event. This environmental phenomenon has also been reported to act in a sex-specific way with a strict dependence from the exposure timing. Exposures happening late in the pregnancy in fact do not leave persistent changes on the methylation profiles (Tobi *et al.*, 2009). Epidemiologic investigations on exposed subjects concomitantly revealed high rates of behavioral disorders and obesity (Lumey, 1998; Roseboom *et al.*, 2006; Susser *et al.*, 1998), as confirmed by other investigations in populations with similar exposures (Song *et al.*, 2009).

The key role of imprinted genes in placental and fetal development is further shown when investigating the other genes with which they network by using informatics tools such as Ingenuity Pathway Analysis (IPA) (Ingenuity® Systems - www.ingenuity.com). Imprinted gene pathway analyses in fact link these genes to three main areas: 1) cell proliferation, assembly, organization, cycling and death; 2) metabolism of lipids and other small intracellular signaling molecules that bind proteins and nucleic acids to regulate their activity and/or function; and 3) development and function of nervous system, respiratory system and other organs. At the same time these genes are listed in the pathways leading to developmental, neurological, psychological, skeletal, muscular, genetic, cardiovascular, gastrointestinal, hepatic and connective tissue disorders together with cancer in agreement with the common epigenetic setting of placental and tumor tissues (Table 2).

Event	Reference
1. Phocomelia from prenatal exposure to thalidomide as antiemetic in early pregnancy	(McBride, 1961) (Taussig, 1962)
2. Cerebral palsy, mental retardation, and convulsions from prenatal exposure to methyl mercury from contaminated fish	(Ordonez *et al.*, 1966) (Pierce *et al.*, 1972) (Bakir *et al.*, 1973) (Harada, 1978)
3. Reduced birth weight and increased incidence of preterm birth from prenatal exposure to maternal smoking	(Underwood *et al.*, 1967) (Meyer *et al.*, 1976)
4. The fetal alcohol syndrome	(Lemoine *et al.*, 1968) (Ulleland, 1972) (Jones & Smith, 1973)
5. Diminished intelligence and shortening of attention span from prenatal exposure to lead	(Landrigan *et al.*, 1975)
6. Clear cell adenocarcinoma of the vagina in young women from prenatal exposure to the synthetic estrogen diethylstilbestrol administered in pregnancy to prevent premature labor	(Herbst *et al.*, 1981)
7. Neural tube defect from prenatal exposure to folic acid deficiency	(Molloy *et al.*, 1985)
8. Low birth weight from prenatal treatment with multiple courses of antenatal glucocorticoids	(Doyle *et al.*, 1989) (Thorp *et al.*, 2002)
9. Behavioral disorders and obesity from prenatal and periconceptional exposure to insufficient maternal caloric intake	(Susser *et al.*, 1996) (Lumey, 1998) (Roseboom *et al.*, 2006)
10. Reduced head circumference at birth from prenatal exposure to organophosphate insecticides	(Perera *et al.*, 2003) (Eskenazi *et al.*, 2004)
11. Shorter anogenital distance and poorer semen quality in males from prenatal exposure to phthalates	(Swan *et al.*, 2005) (Mendiola *et al.*, 2011)
12. Reduced intelligence from prenatal exposure to polychlorinated biphenyls (PCBs)	(Engel *et al.*, 2007) (Wolff *et al.*, 2007)
13. Reduced intelligence and slowed mentation from prenatal exposures to arsenic and manganese in drinking water	(Khan *et al.*, 2011) (Parvez *et al.*, 2011)

Table 1. Neonatal outcomes associated with perturbations of the embryo epigenetic reprogramming at different times across the windows of susceptibility.

Imprinted Genes by Network(2)	Networks	
	Functional Areas	Associated Disease
1. *CCNE1, CDKN1C, CYR61, DLK1, E2F7, GDNF, GRB10, H19, HOXD10, IGF2, KCNQ1, MAPK12, NGFB, NNAT, PCNA, SNURF, TP73, WT1*	Cellular Growth Proliferation	Developmental Disorders Genetic Disorders
2. *BMPR2, DLGAP2, GRIA1, HOXA11, HTR2A, INS, MAGI2, NEDD9, PEG3, PPP1R9A, SHANK2, SNRPN, UBE3A*	Nervous System Dev & Funct	Cancer Skeletal & Muscular Disorders Reproductive System Diseases
3. *CD44, DIRAS3, DLX5, EPS15, IL1B, ILK, NDN, NLRP2, TFPI2*	Cellular Development Cell Cycle	Cardiovascular Diseases
4. *ATP10A, CCDC86, CDKAL1, SGCE, SLC22A3, SLC22A18AS*	Small Molecule Biochemistry	Gastrointestinal Diseases Hepatic System Diseases
5. *CTAG2, CTNND2, L3MBTL, MEST, OSBPL5, PLAGL1, TCEB3C*	Gene Expression	Cancer Connective Tissue Disorders
6. *COPG2, CPA4, DHCR24, PEG10, ZNF331*	Cell Cycle Cellular Development	Cancer
7. *CTNNA3, KCNQ1OT1, PHLDA2*	Organ Development Respiratory System Dev & Funct Cell Assembly & Organization	-
8. *GFI1, GNAS, LASS4, LMO1*	Lipid Metabolism Small Molecule Biochemistry Cell Death	-
9. *GABRA5, GABRB3, GABRG3*	-	Neurological Diseases Developmental Disorders Psychological Disorders
10. *KCNK9*	Cell Death	Neurological Diseases
11. *MEG3*	Connective Tissue Dev & Funct	Behavioral Syndromes
12. *SDHD*	-	Cancer Endocrine System Disorders Genetic Disorders
13. *SLC22A18*	-	Cancer Developmental Disorders

(1): it includes only those genes for which a gene network of reference could be found by imputing all imprinted genes experimentally proven.
(2): networks include biallelically expressed genes not listed here for ease of reading.

Table 2. Function and Disease Association of IPA networks including imprinted genes(1)

It is not surprising that studies in animal models pointed out the importance of imprinted genes in the placental and fetal development and phenotype determination (Bressan *et al.*, 2009). Around 70% of the known imprinted genes are in fact expressed in placenta (Diplas *et al.*, 2009a). A first classification of the role that imprinted genes play in development has been recently carried out in mice that divided them into genes express exclusively in the placenta and genes expressed in both placenta and embryo. The first group is made out of genes that regulate the exchange of resources between mother and fetus and are often found imprinted only in the placenta. The second group has instead been further subdivided into: 1) genes that program the metabolism in the early postnatal period to determine growth and metabolic phenotype that greatly affect the survival of the offspring; and 2) genes that participate in the development of metabolic organs such as the pituitary and pancreas, energy processing and storage organs like liver and fat, the hypothalamus and the placenta. Imprinted genes of this subgroup have been linked to growth retardation, and brain, bone, muscle and liver disorders (Charalambous *et al.*, 2007).

Characteristic expression profiles of imprinted genes have also been described for the placenta and endocrine tissues across species with an associated specific pattern of transcription factor binding sites suggestive of the critical role they play in these tissues (Steinhoff *et al.*, 2009).

Additionally it has been shown that the expression of imprinted genes in placenta is tightly regulated compared to other genes (Diplas *et al.*, 2009a). Low transcriptional noise has been reported for genes that substantially affect the phenotype (Elowitz *et al.*, 2002; Ozbudak *et al.*, 2002), lead to lethality (Blake *et al.*, 2003; Fraser *et al.*, 2004), show haploinsufficiency (Batada & Hurst, 2007). Given their role and their functionally haploid status, imprinted genes have been proposed to belong to this group (Zaitoun *et al.*, 2010).

3. Imprinted genes dysregulation in fetoplacental development

Intra-uterine growth restriction (IUGR) and preeclampsia (PE) are by far the most common pregnancy outcomes and alone they account for about a third of all preterm births (Little, 2009). Both IUGR and PE are considered placentation disorders that arise from shallow trophoblast invasion with characteristic tissue morphology that leads to uteroplacental insufficiency. At the same time a vast body of literature has linked poor placentation with numerous chronic and developmental disorders in children (Barker, 1997; Godfrey & Barker, 2000; Heijmans *et al.*, 2007) spanning from asthma (Federal Interagency Forum on Child and Family Statistics, 2011; US Environmental Protection Agency [US EPA], 2010;) and obesity (Centers for Disease Control [CDC], 2011) to neurodevelopmental syndromes (Boyle *et al.*, 1994; CDC, 2009), learning disabilities (Pastor & Reuben, 2008), birth defects (Paulozzi *et al.*, 1997; L.T. Vu *et al.*, 2008) to even cancer (National Institutes of Health/National Cancer Institute [NIH/NCI], 2011).

Together these diseases all fall in the category of those that would greatly benefit from the availability of early diagnostic tools to give healthcare providers an opportunity for intervention/prevention to impact the quality of life of the affected subjects and to substantially contain the public health expenditure. The development of such epigenetic tools into biomarkers for prenatal diagnosis during pregnancy would also extend their clinical utility.

Analyses of the epigenetic profiles associated with IUGR and PE have revealed a substantial correlation with perturbations of the genomic imprinting settings particularly for growth restriction. These findings are not surprising in light of the role of imprinted genes in regulating placental and fetal development. However links are still lacking that unequivocally connect LOI to chronic and developmental syndromes.

3.1 Pregnancy outcomes

The first approach developed to investigate the correlation between LOI and IUGR was simply based on the analysis of the ICRs methylation status in placentas from uncomplicated fetuses and placentas from IUGR fetuses at term. Studies have focused on the first identified and extensively characterized *IGF2-H19* ICR, also known as IC1 or ICR1, because of the experimentally proven opposite effects of IGF2 paternalization and maternalization on the embryonic growth. The *IGF2-H19* ICR displays typical silencing features on the paternal allele including DNA methylation and histone inactivation signals absent on the maternal allele, which result in *IGF2* expression from the paternal allele and *H19* from the maternal (Lewis & Reik, 2006). Such studies however failed to provide a clear answer, while in fact some investigations found a correlation with loss of methylation at the IGF2-H19 ICR and IUGR (Bourque et al., 2010) others showed no differences (Tabano et al., 2010).

At the same time it has been shown that IUGR induces contained dysregulation of a small subset of imprinted genes (Diplas et al., 2009a). Between them there is *PHLDA2*, a gene that showed a very consisted but contained upregulation in IUGR. This conclusion, while in line with previous studies (McMinn et al., 2006), has also been recently proven in studies on mice where animals were engineerized to double the *Phlda2* dosage. Mice placentas showed a dramatic reduction of the junctional zone and perturbations of the glycogen metabolism that led to the restriction of the embryonic growth (Tunster et al., 2010). Such findings are consistent with the putative role attributed to *PHLDA2* as a pleckstrin-homology protein involved in intracellular signaling via the binding of lipids within biological membranes. There is however no evidence that correlates the expression upregulation of *PHLDA2* with methylation changes of the *PHLDA2* ICR (KvDMR). The same has been shown for other dysregulated imprinted genes in IUGR (Diplas et al., 2009a ; Guo et al., 2008).

Recently a new approach has been developed that determines LOI by highly quantitative allele-specific RT-PCR using non-functional single nucleotide polymorphisms (SNPs) at the RNA level (Lambertini et al., 2008). By measuring the RNA relative amounts produced by each allele, the effect of all known epigenetic signals is taken into account. The analysis of these values in normal and IUGR placentas produced two main conclusions: 1) LOI is a common phenomenon in human placenta affecting different genes at different extents even in morphologically normal tissues; and 2) LOI differentially affects imprinted genes with some of them showing widespread appreciable values unrelated to the tissue morphology (e.g. *IGF2, MEST, PEG3, SLC22A18, TP73*), some others that are invariably imprinted with again no morphological correlation (e.g. *CD44, EPS15, MEG3, PEG10, PHLDA2*), and some other genes that show consistent LOI values only in IUGR placentas (e.g. *DLK1, H19, PLAGL1, SNRPN*).

Quantitative LOI data however showed no correlation with gene expression which, challenges the dogma that LOI leads to the reactivation of a silent allele and results in increased expression of the affected gene(s). These findings are however in line with new studies that instead tie genomic imprinting to the tridimensional chromosome organization into physically organized expression networks. In this model lncRNAs, while still tethered to the genome during their transcription, would act by recruiting DNA binding proteins into complexes that interact with ICRs generating anchoring points for structural proteins that would pull genomic regions together into transcriptional hotspots (Court *et al.*, 2011; Horike *et al.*, 2005). The disruption of this genomic architecture would lead to uncoordinated activation/silencing of imprinted genes (Minard *et al.*, 2009; Zlatanova & Caiafa, 2009). In this framework, still to be clarified is the differential role played by the parental origins.

PE and IUGR share common pathological features even though they develop into distinct outcomes with also different clinical progression. It is therefore expected that the two outcomes also share common LOI profiles. While logical however this conclusion cannot be drawn as of yet. Few data in fact exist on the correlation of genomic imprinting with PE. A study on mice in fact proved that dysregulation in pregnant females of the expression of the paternally imprinted/maternally expressed *Cdkn1c* imprinted gene, a potent inhibitor of several cyclin/cyclin dependent kinase complexes, leads to PE-like symptoms including hypertension, proteinuria, thrombocytopenia, decreased anti-thrombin III activity, and increased endothelin levels in late pregnancy. However no data exist that reported LOI of *CDKN1C* in human preeclampsia (Kanayama *et al.*, 2002). More recently instead correlations have been found between LOI of *H19* and PE in humans (L. Yu *et al.*, 2009).

Association of perturbations of genomic imprinting with other outcomes has mostly been hypothesized about preterm birth given the substantial contribution of the female line (Boyd *et al.*, 2009; Little, 2009).

3.2 Fetal neurodevelopment

There is a growing recognition of the importance of the intrauterine period of development on health and disease throughout life, including mental health. Particularly, research is focused on the placenta which serves as the master regulator of the intrauterine environment and plays a functional role in shaping fetal development including neurodevelopment. These effects are modulated by simultaneous production of many pregnancy related hormones, proteins and growth factors thereby fulfilling a critical role in proper intrauterine development. Specifically, the placenta has been shown to produce an array of neuropeptide hormones that are analogous to those produced by the hypothalamus and pituitary of the brain, including GnRH, TRH, GHRH, CRH, and oxytocin (Liu, 2009). Rapid advancements in discovery of integrated regulation of neuropeptide homeostasis within and outside the brain as well as placenta (Petraglia *et al.*, 1991; Yen, 1991, 1994) has led to the formulation of a new concept that the placenta acts as the "third brain" that links the developed (maternal) and developing (fetal) brains (Yen, 1994). In turn, alterations to this critical neurodevelopmental function may be a major contributor to the pathophysiology of intrauterine insults including illicit drug exposures (Lester & Padbury, 2009).

Although alterations to the development of the hypothalamic-pituitary-adrenal (HPA) axis are likely critical mediators of appropriate infant neurodevelopment, it is also clear that additional genes and pathways may be affected by the maternal environment (Fink *et al.*, 2010), and specifically that alterations to imprinted genes can play a crucial role in neurodevelopment. A high proportion of identified imprinted genes are expressed in the central nervous system. Maternally expressed imprinted genes are thought to favor the development of larger brains (Davies *et al.*, 2005). Children with Beckwith-Wiedemann syndrome, which results in part from inappropriate imprinting of specific imprinted gene clusters, demonstrate greater than expected proportions of abnormal scores on emotional and behavioral scales (Kent *et al.*, 2008). These observation were also confirmed in animal models, wherein female mice engineered to be null for the paternally expressed imprinted *Peg3* gene, exhibit a reduced number of oxytocin-producing neurons in the hypothalamus, linking imprinted gene expression to neurodevelopment (L. Li *et al.*, 1999). Recent work has also demonstrated that alterations in imprinted gene expression in the placenta are associated with infant neurodevelopmental outcome as reflected in prospectively validated neurobehavioral measures, and that specifically imprinted genes such as *MEG3*, *HOXA11*, and *HOXD10*, which are involved in nervous system, skeletal, and muscular development may be mediating these effects (Marsit *et al.*, 2011). Additional research is needed to better dissect the roles of individual imprinted genes on infant neurodevelopment and to link these alterations to later life mental health and disease.

3.3 Obesity

As expected by the role that imprinted genes play in the development of metabolic organs that we previously outlined, obesity has been linked to imprinted genes dysregulations both in experimental animals and in epidemiologic investigations.

Knockout mouse models of heterozygous disruption of the imprinted gene *Gnas*, encoding the heterotrimeric G protein alpha-subunit that coordinates the stimulation of the adenylyl cyclase, returned obese mice following the inactivation of the maternal allele and slim mice when the paternal allele was disrupted. Interestingly homozygous knockout mice were not viable (L. Yu *et al.*, 2009; S. Yu *et al.*, 2000). These data were later confirmed in humans (Plagge *et al.*, 2008) and support the link between obesity and imprinted genes dysregulation that was already describe in the mid 1970s while analyzing a population of young men conceived during a famine episode in the Netherlands (Ravelli *et al.*, 1976). This same population was later shown to carry an altered DNA methylation profile in the *IGF2-H19* region (Heijmans *et al.*, 2007; Tobi *et al.*, 2009). In agreement with these are the numerous studies that linked metabolic alteration and overgrowth with disturbances of the imprinting profile (Barlow *et al.*, 1991; Bressan *et al.*, 2009).

4. The proposed role of genomic imprinting in fetoplacental development

Placental and fetal developments are accomplished across the relative short period of time of the pregnancy, therefore requiring a highly coordinated regulation of the genome to support the different phases of this process. The correct development can thus be achieved only by the activation of plastic and adaptable systems that are able to timely rearrange the functioning genes based on changes in the environment and the developmental program. Genomic imprinting is emerging as the best candidate for such role. It has been in fact shown that imprinted genes have a different level of imprinting in placenta during pregnancy. First trimester placentas return widespread higher LOI values compared to term placentas (Pozharny *et al.*, 2010; L. Yu *et al.*, 2009).

Specifically genes like *CD44* and *EPS15* show a drastic LOI reduction from the first to third trimester of pregnancy (Pozharny *et al.*, 2010). These data are particular interesting if we consider that *CD44* is translated into a protein that participates in cell-cell interactions, adhesion and migration, and it has been tied to tumor metastasis promotion. Given the very fast growing and invasive nature of the placenta in the first trimester, *CD44* would therefore be critical for supporting this phase. *EPS15* instead encodes a peptide involved in receptor-mediated endocytosis of the epidermal growth factor; this gene has been linked to acute myelogenous leukemia. *EPS15* would thus represent a key player in the process of establishing the appropriate maternal blood supply in the placenta to assist the fetal growth. The analysis of these findings supports the hypothesis that the "gain of imprinting" of imprinted genes during the different stages of fetoplacental development would add an additional layer of control on their activity. It has been proposed that this phenomenon is driven by the timely activation of effectors lncRNAs (Kacem & Feil, 2009), of which imprinted genes are substantially provided, that act by silencing one gene copy accordingly to the parent-of-origin, similarly to other known lncRNAs as *XIST* and *HOTAIR* (Gupta *et al.*, 2010; Lee, 2009). It is however not known why this process silence one specific allele and take place without altering the resulting expression profile of these genes.

Similar findings were recently reported in cultured human PGCs. In this model imprinting of some genes appeared very early after fertilization, while other genes showed complete imprinting only starting at 5 to 11 weeks after fertilization (Crane *et al.*, 2009), again demonstrating the plasticity of this epigenetically driven phenomenon.

The common opinion that is gaining support is that genomic imprinting bimodally acts by adding layers of controls on the genome to regulate its activity according to environmental signals. This theory is supported by experiments on animals that showed that both in early developmental phases and in adult life, environmental signals trigger the activation of pathways that modify the complex epigenetic signaling controlling gene expression (Reik *et al.*, 2001; Santos & Dean, 2004). These studies provide critical information on the effect of the gene-environment interplay on the physiology of organisms (Zhang & Meaney, 2010). An example of this condition in humans is represented by the data indicating that common environmental changes (such as dietary changes) may result in statistically significant epigenetic variations on DNA methylation of imprinted loci (Tobi *et al.*, 2009).

In the bimodal imprinting model, DNA methylation and histone modification signals are placed on the genome very early in development when the zygote reprogramming takes place. They represent the first event leading to imprinting. Perturbations of this phase would most probably lead to the more severe effects on growth and development because it deprives the genome of the critical anchors for the imprinting machinery to recognize the areas to act upon. This hypothesis is confirmed, both at the genetic and epigenetic level, by studies on severe neurodevelopmental syndromes such as Prader-Willi and Angelman which have been correlated to inappropriate imprinting at the chromosome location 15q11 (Driscoll *et al.*, 1992; Hamabe *et al.*, 1991; Williams *et al.*, 1990). Additionally, immediately after implantation, PGCs are selected to be programmed accordingly to the sex of the developing embryo; at this stage the improper placement of epigenetic signals acquires its transgenerational meaning. PGCs programming in fact is supposed to work by applying the epigenetic "code" of the allele consistent with the fetal sex, to the other allele. If "code" perturbations have been generated during the zygote reprogramming, they are therefore passed into PGCs. Accordingly, it has recently been shown that, during pregnancy, maternal exposure to phthalates, a family of chemicals with known potential for the perturbation of the epigenetic profile, specifically target the correct male fetal development. Male babies from exposed mothers show reduced anogenital distance and, later in life, low sperm count (Mendiola *et al.*, 2011).

lncRNAs represent instead the second level of imprinting. lncRNAs act by assembling protein complexes that have several functions spanning from the regulation of the activity of enhancers (Mohammad *et al.*, 2009), assembly of transcription complexes (Royo & Cavaille, 2008) to generation of transcriptional hotspots (Yang & Kuroda, 2007). The timely expression of these molecules is critical for the proper activation/silencing of gene sets. Later in life, lncRNAs would also restore biallelic expression of genes accordingly to the tissue, possibly also leading to a loss of methylation of unused and unprotected ICRs (Gieni & Hendzel, 2009). Perturbations of this second regulation layer would give way to other, possibly less severe and reversible, syndromes.

LOI has been implicated in the etiology of growth restriction syndromes and both conditions have been independently associated with chronic and developmental disorders that greatly impact the health of children - Barker Hypothesis (Barker, 1997) - with the potential of limiting their quality of life into adulthood, often resulting in reduced life expectancy. Chronic disorders in young adults also entail a great deal of expenditure due to the necessary life-long treatments (Landrigan & Goldman, 2011; Trasande, 2011; Trasande & Liu, 2011). The study of perturbations in genomic imprinting can shed light into the mechanisms leading to these disorders. The complete characterization of LOI also bears the promise of developing its highly quantitative measurement into new groundbreaking biomarkers that could have a major impact on public health by allowing early diagnosis of several pathologies correlated with placentation disorders, as well as on biomedical, behavioral and clinical research (Maccani & Marsit, 2009). The completion of the analysis of the imprinting in placenta at different developmental stages is critical to achieve this goal (Pozharny *et al.*, 2010).

After this, the next logical step is to develop a method that allows monitoring the imprinting status during pregnancy. New technological tools are now available to carry out quantitative RT-PCR experiments on single DNA/RNA molecules therefore opening the way to the challenge of measuring LOI in cells isolated from the amniocentesis fluid or from chorionic villi sampling (CVS). These advancements could be an opportunity to predict those pregnancies at risk of developing obstertrical disorders such as PE or IUGR and even fetuses at risk for future diagnosis of developmental diseases back to the first trimester of pregnancy.

5. Acknowledgments

This work was supported by the Venture Capital Research Funding Program of the Mount Sinai Children's Environmental Health Center and Mount Sinai Child Health and Development Institute.

6. References

American Journal of Medical Genetics (2010). Special Issue: Imprinted Genes and Human Disease, Am J Med Genet C Semin Med Genet 154C(3).

Bakir F, Damluji SF, Amin-Zaki L, Murtadha M, Khalidi A, al-Rawi NY, Tikriti S, Dahahir HI, Clarkson TW, *et al.* (1973). Methylmercury poisoning in Iraq. Science 181 (96): 230-41.

Barker DJ (1997). Maternal nutrition, fetal nutrition, and disease in later life. Nutrition 13 (9): 807-13.

Barlow DP, Stoger R, Herrmann BG, Saito K & Schweifer N (1991). The mouse insulin-like growth factor type-2 receptor is imprinted and closely linked to the Tme locus. Nature 349 (6304): 84-7.

Bartolomei MS (2009). Genomic imprinting: employing and avoiding epigenetic processes. Genes Dev 23 (18): 2124-33.

Batada NN & Hurst LD (2007). Evolution of chromosome organization driven by selection for reduced gene expression noise. Nat Genet 39 (8): 945-9.

Bernstein E & Allis CD (2005). RNA meets chromatin. Genes Dev 19 (14): 1635-55.

Blake WJ, Kaern M, Cantor CR & Collins JJ (2003). Noise in eukaryotic gene expression. Nature 422 (6932): 633-7.

Bourque DK, Avila L, Penaherrera M, von Dadelszen P & Robinson WP (2010). Decreased placental methylation at the H19/IGF2 imprinting control region is associated with normotensive intrauterine growth restriction but not preeclampsia. Placenta 31 (3): 197-202.

Boyd HA, Poulsen G, Wohlfahrt J, Murray JC, Feenstra B & Melbye M (2009). Maternal contributions to preterm delivery. Am J Epidemiol 170 (11): 1358-64.

Boyle CA, Decoufle P & Yeargin-Allsopp M (1994). Prevalence and health impact of developmental disabilities in US children. Pediatrics 93 (3): 399-403.

Bressan FF, De Bem TH, Perecin F, Lopes FL, Ambrosio CE, Meirelles FV & Miglino MA (2009). Unearthing the roles of imprinted genes in the placenta. Placenta 30 (10): 823-34.

Centers for Disease Control and Prevention (CDC) (2009). Prevalence of autism spectrum disorders - Autism and Developmental Disabilities Monitoring Network, United States, 2006. MMWR Surveill Summ 58 (10): 1-20.

Centers for Disease Control and Prevention (CDC) (2011). Overweight and obesity: US obesity trends. Trends by state 1985–2009. Atlanta (GA): CDC; 2011 Mar 3. Available at: http://www.cdc.gov/obesity/data/trends.html

Charalambous M, da Rocha ST & Ferguson-Smith AC (2007). Genomic imprinting, growth control and the allocation of nutritional resources: consequences for postnatal life. Curr Opin Endocrinol Diabetes Obes 14 (1): 3-12.

Court F, Baniol M, Hagege H, Petit JS, Lelay-Taha MN, Carbonell F, Weber M, Cathala G & Forne T (2011). Long-range chromatin interactions at the mouse Igf2/H19 locus reveal a novel paternally expressed long non-coding RNA. Nucleic Acids Res: [Epub ahead of print].

Crane JL, Shamblott MJ, Axelman J, Hsu S, Levine MA & Germain-Lee EL (2009). Imprinting Status of Galpha(s), NESP55, and XLalphas in cell cultures derived from human embryonic germ cells: GNAS imprinting in human embryonic germ cells. Clin Transl Sci 2 (5): 355-60.

Davies W, Isles AR & Wilkinson LS (2005). Imprinted gene expression in the brain. Neurosci Biobehav Rev 29 (3): 421-30.

Diplas AI, Lambertini L, Lee MJ, Sperling R, Lee YL, Wetmur J & Chen J (2009a). Differential expression of imprinted genes in normal and IUGR human placentas. Epigenetics 4 (4): 235-40.

Diplas AI, Hu J, Lee MJ, Ma YY, Lee YL, Lambertini L, Chen J & Wetmur JG (2009b). Demonstration of all-or-none loss of imprinting in mRNA expression in single cells. Nucleic Acids Res 37 (21): 7039-46.

Doyle LW, Kitchen WH, Ford GW, Rickards AL & Kelly EA (1989). Antenatal steroid therapy and 5-year outcome of extremely low birth weight infants. Obstet Gynecol 73 (5 Pt 1): 743-6.

Driscoll DJ, Waters MF, Williams CA, Zori RT, Glenn CC, Avidano KM & Nicholls RD (1992). A DNA methylation imprint, determined by the sex of the parent, distinguishes the Angelman and Prader-Willi syndromes. Genomics 13 (4): 917-24.

Ehrlich M, Gama-Sosa MA, Huang LH, Midgett RM, Kuo KC, McCune RA & Gehrke C (1982). Amount and distribution of 5-methylcytosine in human DNA from different types of tissues of cells. Nucleic Acids Res 10 (8): 2709-21.

Elowitz MB, Levine AJ, Siggia ED & Swain PS (2002). Stochastic gene expression in a single cell. Science 297 (5584): 1183-6.

Engel SM, Berkowitz GS, Barr DB, Teitelbaum SL, Siskind J, Meisel SJ, Wetmur JG & Wolff MS (2007). Prenatal organophosphate metabolite and organochlorine levels and performance on the Brazelton Neonatal Behavioral Assessment Scale in a multiethnic pregnancy cohort. Am J Epidemiol 165 (12): 1397-404.

Environmental Protection Agency (EPA) (2010). America's children and the environment (ACE), measure D1: percentage of children with asthma. Washington (DC):EPA; 2010 Nov 19. Available at: http://www.epa.gov/economics/children/child_illness/d1-graph.html.

Eskenazi B, Harley K, Bradman A, Weltzien E, Jewell NA, Barr DB, Furlong CE & Holland NT (2004). Association of in utero organophosphate pesticide exposure and fetal growth and length of gestation in an agricultural population. Environ Health Perspect 112 (10): 1116-24.

Federal Interagency Forum on Child and Family Statistics (2011). America's children in brief: key national indicators of well-being, 2010. Merrifield (VA): The Forum. Available at: http://www.childstats.gov/americaschildren/health.asp

Fink NS, Urech C, Berger CT, Hoesli I, Holzgreve W, Bitzer J & Alder J (2010). Maternal laboratory stress influences fetal neurobehavior: Cortisol does not provide all answers. Journal of Maternal-Fetal & Neonatal Medicine 23 (6): 488-500.

Fraser HB, Hirsh AE, Giaever G, Kumm J & Eisen MB (2004). Noise minimization in eukaryotic gene expression. PLoS Biol 2 (6): e137.

Gama-Sosa MA, Midgett RM, Slagel VA, Githens S, Kuo KC, Gehrke CW & Ehrlich M (1983). Tissue-specific differences in DNA methylation in various mammals. Biochim Biophys Acta 740 (2): 212-9.

Gieni RS & Hendzel MJ (2009). Polycomb group protein gene silencing, non-coding RNA, stem cells, and cancer. Biochem Cell Biol 87 (5): 711-46.

Godfrey KM & Barker DJ (2000). Fetal nutrition and adult disease. Am J Clin Nutr 71 (5 Suppl): 1344S-52S.

Guilleret I, Osterheld MC, Braunschweig R, Gastineau V, Taillens S & Benhattar J (2009). Imprinting of tumor-suppressor genes in human placenta. Epigenetics 4 (1): 62-8.

Guo L, Choufani S, Ferreira J, Smith A, Chitayat D, Shuman C, Uxa R, Keating S, Kingdom J, *et al.* (2008). Altered gene expression and methylation of the human chromosome 11 imprinted region in small for gestational age (SGA) placentae. Dev Biol 320 (1): 79-91.

Gupta RA, Shah N, Wang KC, Kim J, Horlings HM, Wong DJ, Tsai MC, Hung T, Argani P, *et al.* (2010). Long non-coding RNA HOTAIR reprograms chromatin state to promote cancer metastasis. Nature 464 (7291): 1071-6.

Haig D & Graham C (1991). Genomic imprinting and the strange case of the insulin-like growth factor II receptor. Cell 64 (6): 1045-6.

Hamabe J, Kuroki Y, Imaizumi K, Sugimoto T, Fukushima Y, Yamaguchi A, Izumikawa Y & Niikawa N (1991). DNA deletion and its parental origin in Angelman syndrome patients. Am J Med Genet 41 (1): 64-8.

Harada M (1978). Congenital Minamata disease: intrauterine methylmercury poisoning. Teratology 18 (2): 285-8.

Heard E, Chaumeil J, Masui O & Okamoto I (2004). Mammalian X-chromosome inactivation: an epigenetics paradigm. Cold Spring Harb Symp Quant Biol 69: 89-102.

Heijmans BT, Kremer D, Tobi EW, Boomsma DI & Slagboom PE (2007). Heritable rather than age-related environmental and stochastic factors dominate variation in DNA methylation of the human IGF2/H19 locus. Hum Mol Genet 16 (5): 547-54.

Herbst AL, Hubby MM, Azizi F & Makii MM (1981). Reproductive and gynecologic surgical experience in diethylstilbestrol-exposed daughters. Am J Obstet Gynecol 141 (8): 1019-28.

Horike S, Cai S, Miyano M, Cheng JF & Kohwi-Shigematsu T (2005). Loss of silent-chromatin looping and impaired imprinting of DLX5 in Rett syndrome. Nat Genet 37 (1): 31-40.

Hu D & Cross JC (2010). Development and function of trophoblast giant cells in the rodent placenta. Int J Dev Biol 54 (2-3): 341-54.

Hutter B, Bieg M, Helms V & Paulsen M (2010). Divergence of imprinted genes during mammalian evolution. BMC Evol Biol 10 (1): 116.

Isles AR (2009). Evolution of genomic imprinting in humans: does bipedalism have a role? Trends Genet 25 (11): 495-500.

Jones KL & Smith DW (1973). Recognition of the fetal alcohol syndrome in early infancy. Lancet 302 (7836): 999-1001.

Kacem S & Feil R (2009). Chromatin mechanisms in genomic imprinting. Mamm Genome 20 (9-10): 544-56.

Kanayama N, Takahashi K, Matsuura T, Sugimura M, Kobayashi T, Moniwa N, Tomita M & Nakayama K (2002). Deficiency in p57Kip2 expression induces preeclampsia-like symptoms in mice. Mol Hum Reprod 8 (12): 1129-35.

Kawahara M, Morita S, Takahashi N & Kono T (2009). Defining contributions of paternally methylated imprinted genes at the Igf2-H19 and Dlk1-Gtl2 domains to mouse placentation by transcriptomic analysis. J Biol Chem 284 (26): 17751-65.

Kent L, Bowdin S, Kirby GA, Cooper WN & Maher ER (2008). Beckwith Weidemann syndrome: a behavioral phenotype-genotype study. Am J Med Genet B Neuropsychiatr Genet 147B (7): 1295-7.

Khan K, Factor-Litvak P, Wasserman GA, Liu X, Ahmed E, Parvez F, Slavkovich V, Levy D, Mey J, *et al.* (2011). Manganese Exposure from Drinking Water and Children's

Classroom Behavior in Bangladesh. Environ Health Perspect: [Epub ahead of print].

Lambertini L, Diplas AI, Lee MJ, Sperling R, Chen J & Wetmur J (2008). A sensitive functional assay reveals frequent loss of genomic imprinting in human placenta. Epigenetics 3 (5): 261-9.

Lambertini L, Diplas AI, Wetmur J, Lee MJ & Chen J (2009). Evaluation of genomic imprinting employing the analysis of Loss Of Imprinting (LOI) at the RNA level: preliminary results. Eur J Oncol 14 (3): 161-9.

Lambertini L, Lee TL, Chan WY, Lee MJ, Diplas AI, Wetmur JG & Chen J (2011). Differential methylation of imprinted genes in growth-restricted placentas. Reprod Sci: [Epub ahead of print].

Landrigan PJ, Whitworth RH, Baloh RW, Staehling NW, Barthel WF & Rosenblum BF (1975). Neuropsychological dysfunction in children with chronic low-level lead absorption. Lancet 1 (7909): 708-12.

Landrigan PJ & Goldman LR (2011). Children's vulnerability to toxic chemicals: a challenge and opportunity to strengthen health and environmental policy. Health Aff (Millwood) 30 (5): 842-50.

Lee JT (2009). Lessons from X-chromosome inactivation: long ncRNA as guides and tethers to the epigenome. Genes Dev 23 (16): 1831-42.

Lefevre P, Witham J, Lacroix CE, Cockerill PN & Bonifer C (2008). The LPS-induced transcriptional upregulation of the chicken lysozyme locus involves CTCF eviction and noncoding RNA transcription. Mol Cell 32 (1): 129-39.

Lemoine P, Harousseau H, Borteyru JP & Menuet JC (1968). Les enfants des parents alcooliques: Anomalies observées. A propos de 127 cas. Ouest Medical 21: 476-82.

Lester BM & Padbury JF (2009). Third pathophysiology of prenatal cocaine exposure. Dev Neurosci 31 (1-2): 23-35.

Lewis A & Reik W (2006). How imprinting centres work. Cytogenet Genome Res 113 (1-4): 81-9.

Li L, Keverne EB, Aparicio SA, Ishino F, Barton SC & Surani MA (1999). Regulation of maternal behavior and offspring growth by paternally expressed Peg3. Science 284 (5412): 330-3.

Li Q, O'Malley ME, Bartlett DL & Guo ZS (2011). Homeobox gene Rhox5 is regulated by epigenetic mechanisms in cancer and stem cells and promotes cancer growth. Mol Cancer 10: 63.

Little J (2009). Invited commentary: maternal effects in preterm birth--effects of maternal genotype, mitochondrial DNA, imprinting, or environment? Am J Epidemiol 170 (11): 1382-5.

Liu JH (2009). Endocrinology of Pregnancy. In: Maternal-Fetal Medicine, Principles and Practice. 6th Edition. Resnik C ed., 111-24, Saunders Elsevier. Philadelphia (PA), USA.

Lumey LH (1998). Reproductive outcomes in women prenatally exposed to undernutrition: a review of findings from the Dutch famine birth cohort. Proc Nutr Soc 57 (1): 129-35.

Maccani MA & Marsit CJ (2009). Epigenetics in the placenta. Am J Reprod Immunol 62 (2): 78-89.

Marsit CJ, Lambertini L, Maccani M, Koestler D, Houseman EA, Gagne L, Padbury JF, Lester BM & Chen J (2011). Imprinted Gene Expression in the Placenta is Associated with Infant Neurobehavioral Outcomes. J Pediatr; e-pub ahead of print.

McBride WG (1961). Thalidomide and Congenital Abnormalities. Lancet 2: 1358.

McGrath J & Solter D (1984). Completion of mouse embryogenesis requires both the maternal and paternal genomes. Cell 37 (1): 179-83.

McMinn J, Wei M, Schupf N, Cusmai J, Johnson EB, Smith AC, Weksberg R, Thaker HM & Tycko B (2006). Unbalanced placental expression of imprinted genes in human intrauterine growth restriction. Placenta 27 (6-7): 540-9.

Mendiola J, Stahlhut RW, Jorgensen N, Liu F & Swan SH (2011). Shorter anogenital distance predicts poorer semen quality in young men in Rochester, new york. Environ Health Perspect 119 (7): 958-63.

Meyer MB, Jonas BS & Tonascia JA (1976). Perinatal events associated with maternal smoking during pregnancy. Am J Epidemiol 103 (5): 464-76.

Minard ME, Jain AK & Barton MC (2009). Analysis of epigenetic alterations to chromatin during development. Genesis 47 (8): 559-72.

Mohammad F, Mondal T & Kanduri C (2009). Epigenetics of imprinted long noncoding RNAs. Epigenetics 4 (5): 277-86.

Molloy AM, Kirke P, Hillary I, Weir DG & Scott JM (1985). Maternal serum folate and vitamin B12 concentrations in pregnancies associated with neural tube defects. Arch Dis Child 60 (7): 660-5.

Monk D, Arnaud P, Apostolidou S, Hills FA, Kelsey G, Stanier P, Feil R & Moore GE (2006). Limited evolutionary conservation of imprinting in the human placenta. Proc Natl Acad Sci U S A 103 (17): 6623-8.

Moore T & Haig D (1991). Genomic imprinting in mammalian development: a parental tug-of-war. Trends Genet 7 (2): 45-9.

National Institutes of Health /National Cancer Institute (NIH/NCI) (2011). Surveillance epidemiology and end results (Homepage). Rockville (MD). Available at: http://seer.cancer.gov

Ordonez JV, Carrillo JA, Miranda M & Gale JL (1966). [Epidemiologic study of a disease believed to be encephalitis in the region of the highlands of Guatemala]. Bol Oficina Sanit Panam 60 (6): 510-9.

Ozbudak EM, Thattai M, Kurtser I, Grossman AD & van Oudenaarden A (2002). Regulation of noise in the expression of a single gene. Nat Genet 31 (1): 69-73.

Parvez F, Wasserman GA, Factor-Litvak P, Liu X, Slavkovich V, Siddique AB, Sultana R, Islam T, Levy D, *et al.* (2011). Arsenic Exposure and Motor Function among Children in Bangladesh. Environ Health Perspect: [Epub ahead of print].

Pastor PN & Reuben CA (2008). Diagnosed attention deficit hyperactivity disorder and learning disability: United States, 2004-2006. Vital Health Stat 10 (237): 1-14.

Paulozzi LJ, Erickson JD & Jackson RJ (1997). Hypospadias trends in two US surveillance systems. Pediatrics 100 (5): 831-4.

Perera FP, Rauh V, Tsai WY, Kinney P, Camann D, Barr D, Bernert T, Garfinkel R, Tu YH, *et al.* (2003). Effects of transplacental exposure to environmental pollutants on birth outcomes in a multiethnic population. Environ Health Perspect 111 (2): 201-5.

Perera FP & Herbstman J (2011). Prenatal Environmental Exposures, Epigenetics, and Disease. Reprod Toxicol 31 (3): 363-73.

Perry JK, Lins RJ, Lobie PE & Mitchell MD (2010). Regulation of invasive growth: similar epigenetic mechanisms underpin tumour progression and implantation in human pregnancy. Clin Sci (Lond) 118 (7): 451-7.

Petraglia F, Coukos G, Volpe A, Genazzani AR & Vale W (1991). Involvement of placental neurohormones in human parturition. Ann N Y Acad Sci 622: 331-40.

Pierce PE, Thompson JF, Likosky WH, Nickey LN, Barthel WF & Hinman AR (1972). Alkyl mercury poisoning in humans. Report of an outbreak. JAMA 220 (11): 1439-42.

Plagge A, Kelsey G & Germain-Lee EL (2008). Physiological functions of the imprinted Gnas locus and its protein variants Galpha(s) and XLalpha(s) in human and mouse. J Endocrinol 196 (2): 193-214.

Pozharny Y, Lambertini L, Ma Y, Ferrara L, Litton CG, Diplas A, Jacobs AR, Chen J, Stone JL, *et al.* (2010). Genomic loss of imprinting in first-trimester human placenta. Am J Obstet Gynecol 202 (4): 391 e1-8.

Qureshi IA & Mehler MF (2011). Advances in Epigenetics and Epigenomics for Neurodegenerative Diseases. Curr Neurol Neurosci Rep: [Epub ahead of print].

Ravelli GP, Stein ZA & Susser MW (1976). Obesity in young men after famine exposure in utero and early infancy. N Engl J Med 295 (7): 349-53.

Reik W, Dean W & Walter J (2001). Epigenetic reprogramming in mammalian development. Science 293 (5532): 1089-93.

Roseboom T, de Rooij S & Painter R (2006). The Dutch famine and its long-term consequences for adult health. Early Hum Dev 82 (8): 485-91.

Royo H & Cavaille J (2008). Non-coding RNAs in imprinted gene clusters. Biol Cell 100 (3): 149-66.

Santos F & Dean W (2004). Epigenetic reprogramming during early development in mammals. Reproduction 127 (6): 643-51.

Sasaky H & Ishino I, Eds. (2006). Genomic Imprinting, Cytogenet Genome Res 113 (Complete Issue).

Song S, Wang W & Hu P (2009). Famine, death, and madness: schizophrenia in early adulthood after prenatal exposure to the Chinese Great Leap Forward Famine. Soc Sci Med 68 (7): 1315-21.

Stadtfeld M, Apostolou E, Akutsu H, Fukuda A, Follett P, Natesan S, Kono T, Shioda T & Hochedlinger K (2010). Aberrant silencing of imprinted genes on chromosome 12qF1 in mouse induced pluripotent stem cells. Nature 465 (7295): 175-81.

Steinhoff C, Paulsen M, Kielbasa S, Walter J & Vingron M (2009). Expression profile and transcription factor binding site exploration of imprinted genes in human and mouse. BMC Genomics 10: 144.

Susser E, Neugebauer R, Hoek HW, Brown AS, Lin S, Labovitz D & Gorman JM (1996). Schizophrenia after prenatal famine. Further evidence. Arch Gen Psychiatry 53 (1): 25-31.

Susser E, Hoek HW & Brown A (1998). Neurodevelopmental disorders after prenatal famine: The story of the Dutch Famine Study. Am J Epidemiol 147 (3): 213-6.

Swan SH, Main KM, Liu F, Stewart SL, Kruse RL, Calafat AM, Mao CS, Redmon JB, Ternand CL, *et al.* (2005). Decrease in anogenital distance among male infants with prenatal phthalate exposure. Environ Health Perspect 113 (8): 1056-61.

Tabano S, Colapietro P, Cetin I, Grati FR, Zanutto S, Mando C, Antonazzo P, Pileri P, Rossella F, *et al.* (2010). Epigenetic modulation of the IGF2/H19 imprinted domain

in human embryonic and extra-embryonic compartments and its possible role in fetal growth restriction. Epigenetics 5 (4): 313-24.
Taft RJ, Pheasant M & Mattick JS (2007). The relationship between non-protein-coding DNA and eukaryotic complexity. Bioessays 29 (3): 288-99.
Taussig HB (1962). A study of the German outbreak of phocomelia. The thalidomide syndrome. JAMA 180: 1106-14.
Thorp JA, Jones PG, Knox E & Clark RH (2002). Does antenatal corticosteroid therapy affect birth weight and head circumference? Obstet Gynecol 99 (1): 101-8.
Tobi EW, Lumey LH, Talens RP, Kremer D, Putter H, Stein AD, Slagboom PE & Heijmans BT (2009). DNA methylation differences after exposure to prenatal famine are common and timing- and sex-specific. Hum Mol Genet 18 (21): 4046-53.
Trasande L (2011). Quantifying the economic consequences of childhood obesity and potential benefits of interventions. Expert Rev Pharmacoecon Outcomes Res 11 (1): 47-50.
Trasande L & Liu Y (2011). Reducing the staggering costs of environmental disease in children, estimated at $76.6 billion in 2008. Health Aff (Millwood) 30 (5): 863-70.
Tunster SJ, Tycko B & John RM (2010). The imprinted Phlda2 gene regulates extraembryonic energy stores. Mol Cell Biol 30 (1): 295-306.
Tycko B (2006). Imprinted genes in placental growth and obstetric disorders. Cytogenet Genome Res 113 (1-4): 271-8.
Ulleland CN (1972). The offspring of alcoholic mothers. Ann N Y Acad Sci 197: 167-9.
Underwood PB, Kesler KF, O'Lane JM & Callagan DA (1967). Parental smoking empirically related to pregnancy outcome. Obstet Gynecol 29 (1): 1-8.
Vu LT, Nobuhara KK, Laurent C & Shaw GM (2008). Increasing prevalence of gastroschisis: population-based study in California. J Pediatr 152 (6): 807-11.
Vu TH, Nguyen AH & Hoffman AR (2010). Loss of IGF2 imprinting is associated with abrogation of long-range intrachromosomal interactions in human cancer cells. Hum Mol Genet 19 (5): 901-19.
Williams CA, Zori RT, Stone JW, Gray BA, Cantu ES & Ostrer H (1990). Maternal origin of 15q11-13 deletions in Angelman syndrome suggests a role for genomic imprinting. Am J Med Genet 35 (3): 350-3.
Wolff MS, Engel S, Berkowitz G, Teitelbaum S, Siskind J, Barr DB & Wetmur J (2007). Prenatal pesticide and PCB exposures and birth outcomes. Pediatr Res 61 (2): 243-50.
Yang PK & Kuroda MI (2007). Noncoding RNAs and intranuclear positioning in monoallelic gene expression. Cell 128 (4): 777-86.
Yazgan O & Krebs JE (2007). Noncoding but nonexpendable: transcriptional regulation by large noncoding RNA in eukaryotes. Biochem Cell Biol 85 (4): 484-96.
Yen SS (1991). Endocrine-metabolic adaptions in pregnancy. In: Reproductive Endocrinology. 3rd Edition. Yen SS and Jaffe RB eds, 963-70, WB Saunders. Philadelphia (PA), USA.
Yen SS (1994). The placenta as the third brain. J Reprod Med 39 (4): 277-80.
Yu L, Chen M, Zhao D, Yi P, Lu L, Han J, Zheng X, Zhou Y & Li L (2009). The H19 gene imprinting in normal pregnancy and pre-eclampsia. Placenta 30 (5): 443-7.
Yu S, Gavrilova O, Chen H, Lee R, Liu J, Pacak K, Parlow AF, Quon MJ, Reitman ML, *et al.* (2000). Paternal versus maternal transmission of a stimulatory G-protein alpha

subunit knockout produces opposite effects on energy metabolism. J Clin Invest 105 (5): 615-23.
Zaitoun I, Downs KM, Rosa GJ & Khatib H (2010). Upregulation of imprinted genes in mice: an insight into the intensity of gene expression and the evolution of genomic imprinting. Epigenetics 5 (2): 149-58.
Zhang TY & Meaney MJ (2010). Epigenetics and the environmental regulation of the genome and its function. Annu Rev Psychol 61: 439-66, C1-3.
Zlatanova J & Caiafa P (2009). CCCTC-binding factor: to loop or to bridge. Cell Mol Life Sci 66 (10): 1647-60.

Permissions

The contributors of this book come from diverse backgrounds, making this book a truly international effort. This book will bring forth new frontiers with its revolutionizing research information and detailed analysis of the nascent developments around the world.

We would like to thank Jing Zheng, Ph.D., for lending his expertise to make the book truly unique. He has played a crucial role in the development of this book. Without his invaluable contribution this book wouldn't have been possible. He has made vital efforts to compile up to date information on the varied aspects of this subject to make this book a valuable addition to the collection of many professionals and students.

This book was conceptualized with the vision of imparting up-to-date information and advanced data in this field. To ensure the same, a matchless editorial board was set up. Every individual on the board went through rigorous rounds of assessment to prove their worth. After which they invested a large part of their time researching and compiling the most relevant data for our readers. Conferences and sessions were held from time to time between the editorial board and the contributing authors to present the data in the most comprehensible form. The editorial team has worked tirelessly to provide valuable and valid information to help people across the globe.

Every chapter published in this book has been scrutinized by our experts. Their significance has been extensively debated. The topics covered herein carry significant findings which will fuel the growth of the discipline. They may even be implemented as practical applications or may be referred to as a beginning point for another development. Chapters in this book were first published by InTech; hereby published with permission under the Creative Commons Attribution License or equivalent.

The editorial board has been involved in producing this book since its inception. They have spent rigorous hours researching and exploring the diverse topics which have resulted in the successful publishing of this book. They have passed on their knowledge of decades through this book. To expedite this challenging task, the publisher supported the team at every step. A small team of assistant editors was also appointed to further simplify the editing procedure and attain best results for the readers.

Our editorial team has been hand-picked from every corner of the world. Their multi-ethnicity adds dynamic inputs to the discussions which result in innovative outcomes. These outcomes are then further discussed with the researchers and contributors who give their valuable feedback and opinion regarding the same. The feedback is then collaborated with the researches and they are edited in a comprehensive manner to aid the understanding of the subject.

Apart from the editorial board, the designing team has also invested a significant amount of their time in understanding the subject and creating the most relevant covers. They scrutinized every image to scout for the most suitable representation of the subject and create an appropriate cover for the book.

The publishing team has been involved in this book since its early stages. They were actively engaged in every process, be it collecting the data, connecting with the contributors or procuring relevant information. The team has been an ardent support to the editorial, designing and production team. Their endless efforts to recruit the best for this project, has resulted in the accomplishment of this book. They are a veteran in the field of academics and their pool of knowledge is as vast as their experience in printing. Their expertise and guidance has proved useful at every step. Their uncompromising quality standards have made this book an exceptional effort. Their encouragement from time to time has been an inspiration for everyone.

The publisher and the editorial board hope that this book will prove to be a valuable piece of knowledge for researchers, students, practitioners and scholars across the globe.

List of Contributors

Monika Zadrożna, Barbara Nowak, Maria Żołnierek, Lucyna Zamorska and Józef Niweliński
Department of Pharmacobiology, Medical College, Jagiellonian University, Poland

Murray D. Mitchell and Gregory E. Rice
University of Queensland Centre for Clinical Research, Herston, Queensland, Australia

Piyali Datta Chakraborty
Albert David Ltd, Kolkata, India

Debasish Bhattacharyya
Division of Structural Biology and Bioinformatics, CSIR- Indian Institute of Chemical Biology, Kolkata, India

Celena Heazlewood and Matthew Cook
Mater Medical Research Institute, Level 3, Aubigny Place, Raymond Terrace, South Brisbane, Australia
University of Queensland, School of Medicine, Brisbane, Australia

Nina Ilic
Mater Adult Hospital, South Brisbane, Australia

Kerry Atkinson
Mater Medical Research Institute, Level 3, Aubigny Place, Raymond Terrace, South Brisbane, Australia
Mater Adult Hospital, South Brisbane, Australia
University of Queensland, School of Medicine, Brisbane, Australia

Gladis Magnarelli and Natalia Guiñazú
IDEPA-CONICET, Universidad Nacional del Comahue, Argentina

Ricardo E. Fretes
Placenta and Chagas Laboratory, Cell Biology, Histology and Embryology Department, Medicine Faculty, Universidad Nacional Córdoba, Cordoba, Argentina
IICSHUM and Cathedra of Histology, Embryology and Genetic, Health Department, Universidad Nacional La Rioja, La Rioja, Argentina

Cintia Diaz-Luján, Maria Fernanda Triquell and Luciana Mezzano
Placenta and Chagas Laboratory, Cell Biology, Histology and Embryology Department, Medicine Faculty, Universidad Nacional Córdoba, Cordoba, Argentina

Qian Zhou and Kai Wang
Clinical and Translational Research Center, Shanghai First Maternity and Infant Hospital, Tongji University School of Medicine, Shanghai, P.R. China

Qi-zhi He
Department of Pathology, Shanghai First Maternity and Infant Hospital, Tongji University School of Medicine, Shanghai, P.R. China

Jing Zheng
Department of Obstetrics and Gynecology, Perinatal Research Laboratories, University of Wisconsin, Madison, WI, USA

Ke-hong Hao
Department of Obstetrics, Shanghai First Maternity and Infant Hospital, Tongji University School of Medicine, Shanghai, P.R. China

Juan Duaso, Christian Castillo and Ulrike Kemmerling
Institute for Biomedical Sciences, Faculty of Medicine, University of Chile, Chile

Andrzej Plewka
Department of Proteomics, Medical University of Silesia in Sosnowiec, Poland

Grażyna Nowaczyk
Department of Physiology, School of Health Care, Medical University of Silesia, Katowice, Poland

Danuta Plewka
Department of Histology, Medical University of Silesia in Katowice, Poland

Lucia Mincheva-Nilsson and Vladimir Baranov
Umeå University, Medical Faculty, Department of Clinical Microbiology Division of Clinical Immunology, Umeå, Sweden

Aled H. Bryant and Catherine A. Thornton
Institute of Life Science, Swansea University, UK

Jorge M. Tolosa
Mothers and Babies Research Centre, University of Newcastle, New Lambton Heights, NSW, Australia
Faculty of Medical Sciences, University of Santiago of Chile, Santiago, Chile

Vicki L. Clifton
Robinson Institute, Lyell McEwin Hospital, Elizabeth Vale, SA, Australia

John E. Schjenken, Jonathan W. Paul and Roger Smith
Mothers and Babies Research Centre, University of Newcastle, New Lambton Heights, NSW, Australia

P. Hoffmann, S. Brouillet, M. Benharouga, J.J. Feige and N. Alfaidy
University Joseph Fourier, INSERM U1036, CEA - Grenoble, France

Marie Jirkovská
Charles University in Prague, First Faculty of Medicine, Czech Republic

Kerry Richard, Huika Li, Kelly A. Landers, Jatin Patel and Robin H. Mortimer
Royal Brisbane and Women's Hospital and The University of Queensland, Australia

Jayonta Bhattacharjee
Department of Physiology, University of Siena, Siena, Italy
Samuel Lunenfeld Research Institute, Mount Sinai Hospital, Toronto, Canada

Isabella Caniggia
Samuel Lunenfeld Research Institute, Mount Sinai Hospital, Toronto, Canada

Francesca Ietta, Roberta Romagnoli, Nicoletta Bechi and Luana Paulesu
Department of Physiology, University of Siena, Siena, Italy

Federico Martinez, Rebeca Milan, Oscar Flores-Herrera, Sofia Olvera-Sanchez, Erika Gomez-Chang and Maria Teresa Espinosa-Garcia
Universidad Nacional Autónoma de México, Departamento de Bioquímica, Facultad de Medicina, Distrito Federal, Mexico

Geoffroy Marceau, Loïc Blanchon, Jean-Marc Lobaccaro and Vincent Sapin
Université d'Auvergne, France

Jia Chen
Department of Preventive Medicine, Mount Sinai School of Medicine, New York, USA
Department of Pediatrics, Mount Sinai School of Medicine, New York, USA
Department of Oncological Sciences, Mount Sinai School of Medicine, New York, USA

Men-Jean Lee
Department of Obstetrics and Gynecology Indiana University-Purdue University, Indianapolis, USA

Carmen J. Marsit
Department of Pharmacology and Toxicology, Dartmouth Medical School, Hanover, USA

Luca Lambertini
Department of Preventive Medicine, Mount Sinai School of Medicine, New York, USA
Department of Obstetrics, Gynecology and Reproductive Science, Mount Sinai School of Medicine, New York, USA